Toxicological Testing Handbook

Toxicological Testing Handbook

Principles, Applications, and Data Interpretation

Second Edition

edited by

David Jacobson-Kram
U.S. Food and Drug Administration
Silver Spring, Maryland, U.S.A.

Kit A. Keller
Toxicology Consultant
Washington, D.C., U.S.A.

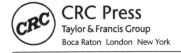

CRC Press
Taylor & Francis Group
Boca Raton London New York

CRC Press is an imprint of the
Taylor & Francis Group, an **informa** business

CRC Press
Taylor & Francis Group
6000 Broken Sound Parkway NW, Suite 300
Boca Raton, FL 33487-2742

First issued in paperback 2019

© 2006 by Taylor & Francis Group, LLC
CRC Press is an imprint of Taylor & Francis Group, an Informa business

No claim to original U.S. Government works

ISBN-13: 978-0-8247-3858-8 (hbk)
ISBN-13: 978-0-367-39060-0 (pbk)
Library of Congress Card Number 2006040380

Library of Congress Cataloging-in-Publication Data

Toxicological testing handbook : principles, applications, and data interpretation / edited by David
  Jacobson-Kram, Kit A. Keller.--2nd ed.
      p. ; cm.
  Rev. ed. of: Toxicology testing handbook : principles, applications, and data interpretation /
edited by David Jacobson-Kram, Kit A. Keller. c2001.
  Includes bibliographical references and index.
  ISBN-13: 978-0-8493-3858-8 (alk. paper)
  ISBN-10: 0-8493-3858-1 (alk. paper)
  1. Toxicity testing--Handbooks, manuals, etc. 2. Health risk assessment--Handbooks, manuals,
etc. I. Jacobson-Kram, David, 1949- II. Keller, Kit A. III. Toxicology testing handbook.
  [DNLM: 1. Toxicity Tests--Handbooks. QV 607 T7542 2006]

RA1199.T695 2006
615.9'07--dc22   2006040380

Visit the Taylor & Francis Web site at
http://www.taylorandfrancis.com

and the CRC Press Web site at
http://www.crcpress.com

Preface

This updated and expanded second edition provides practical guidance to people responsible for developing toxicology data, evaluating results from toxicology studies, and performing risk assessments. It will be particularly useful to those using outside laboratories to perform studies for regulatory submission. Individuals charged with developing a safety profile on a new material may be nontoxicologists, inexperienced entry-level toxicologists, or toxicologists with expertise in a particular subdiscipline but lacking experience in other areas. Individuals with responsibility for assuring the safety of new products and materials are found in an array of businesses, including the pharmaceutical industry; biotechnology companies; medical device manufacturers; formulators of cosmetics and personal care products; herbal, food, and supplement companies; and the chemical, pesticide, and petroleum industries.

This text serves as a guide for proper study design to help ensure regulatory acceptance. It addresses such issues as species selection, dose level and dosing regimen, animal number, routes of exposure, and proper statistical evaluation. Chapters focused on particular subdisciplines examine the purpose of the study, choice of species and the conditions under which the animals are maintained, experimental design, route of exposure, the duration of the study, choice of vehicles, and endpoints evaluated. This second edition updates each chapter, with particular efforts made to add more help in data interpretation and hazard assessment.

New chapters have been added to reflect changing regulatory requirements. These include chapters on safety pharmacology, juvenile studies, health safety assessment of pharmaceuticals, and heath assessment strategies in the food and cosmetic industry. We have also included a separate and expanded chapter on carcinogenicity studies and the "good laboratory practices" chapter contains new information on how to evaluate the quality of a contract research organization prior to study placement.

The current business environment is dominated by downsized workforces, consolidated corporate functions, and lean start-ups. Often companies have a single individual responsible for all regulatory compliance issues. If that person has a background in toxicology at all, it is often general and cursory. This text can help lessen the dependence on outside consultants to design product safety studies and facilitate regulatory approval. It can serve as a principal textbook for courses in regulatory affairs and quality assurance and complements other texts in basic and advanced toxicology courses. Since similarities and differences in regulatory requirements in the United States, Europe, and Japan are an important topic in each chapter, it could serve as a resource to individuals responsible for registering products in overseas markets.

David Jacobson-Kram
Kit A. Keller

Contents

Contents vii

Contributors

Christopher Banks   CTBR Bio-Research, Inc., Senneville, Quebec, Canada

Jane J. Clarke   Genetic Toxicology Department, BioReliance, Invitrogen Bioservices, Rockville, Maryland, U.S.A.

Raymond M. David   Health and Environment Laboratories, Eastman Kodak Company, Rochester, New York, U.S.A.

Kerry L. Dearfield   Office of the Science Advisor, U.S. Environmental Protection Agency, Washington, D.C., U.S.A.

Amy L. Ellis   Office of New Drugs, Center for Drug Evaluation and Research, U.S. Food and Drug Administration, Silver Spring, Maryland, U.S.A.

J. Caroline English   Health and Environment Laboratories, Eastman Kodak Company, Rochester, New York, U.S.A.

Patricia Escobar   Genetic Toxicology Department, BioReliance, Invitrogen Bioservices, Rockville, Maryland, U.S.A.

William H. Farland   Office of Research and Development, U.S. Environmental Protection Agency, Washington, D.C., U.S.A.

Linda J. Frederick   Hospira, Inc., Lake Forest, Illinois, U.S.A.

Dori R. Germolec   National Institutes of Environmental Health Sciences, National Toxicology Program, National Institutes of Health, Research Triangle Park, North Carolina, U.S.A.

Ramadevi Gudi   Genetic Toxicology Department, BioReliance, Invitrogen Bioservices, Rockville, Maryland, U.S.A.

Kenneth L. Hastings   Office of New Drugs, Center for Drug Evaluation and Research, U.S. Food and Drug Administration, Silver Spring, Maryland, U.S.A.

Kok Wah Hew   Non-clinical Safety and Efficacy, Takeda Global Research and Development, Lincolnshire, Illinois, U.S.A.

Robert V. House   Science and Technical Operations, DynPort Vaccine Company LLC, Frederick, Maryland, U.S.A.

Abigail C. Jacobs   Center for Drug Evaluation and Research/Food and Drug Administration, Silver Spring, Maryland, U.S.A.

David Jacobson-Kram   Office of New Drugs, U.S. Food and Drug Administration, Silver Spring, Maryland, U.S.A.

Kit A. Keller   Toxicology Consultant, Washington, D.C., U.S.A.

Ljubica S. Krsmanovic   Genetic Toxicology Department, BioReliance, Invitrogen Bioservices, Rockville, Maryland, U.S.A.

Lynda L. Lanning   Otsuka Maryland Research Institute, Rockville, Maryland, U.S.A.

Robert W. Luebke   Immunotoxicology Branch, U.S. Environmental Protection Agency, Research Triangle Park, North Carolina, U.S.A.

Kamala Pant   Genetic Toxicology Department, BioReliance, Invitrogen Bioservices, Rockville, Maryland, U.S.A.

Donald L. Putman   Genetic Toxicology Department, BioReliance, Invitrogen Bioservices, Rockville, Maryland, U.S.A.

Kathleen C. Raffaele   Health Effects Division, Office of Pesticide Programs, U.S. Environmental Protection Agency, Washington, D.C., U.S.A.

Elmer J. Rauckman   Toxicology and Regulatory Affairs, Freeburg, Illinois, U.S.A.

William S. Redfern   Safety Pharmacology Department, Safety Assessment U.K., AstraZeneca R&D Alderley Park, Macclesfield, Cheshire, U.K.

Gary J. Rosenthal   Drug Development, RxKinetix, Inc., Boulder, Colorado, U.S.A.

Richard H. C. San   Genetic Toxicology Department, BioReliance, Invitrogen Bioservices, Rockville, Maryland, U.S.A.

Andrew I. Soiefer   North Jersey Toxicology Associates LLC, Randolph, New Jersey, U.S.A.

Linnea Steiger   Innovative Science Solutions, Morristown, New Jersey, U.S.A.

Valentine O. Wagner III   Genetic Toxicology Department, BioReliance, Invitrogen Bioservices, Rockville, Maryland, U.S.A.

Ian D. Wakefield   Nonclinical Development, UCB Celltech, Slough, U.K.

Walter P. Weisenburger   Advanced Neuro Health LLC, Kalispell, Montana, U.S.A.

Steven M. Weisman   Innovative Science Solutions, Morristown, New Jersey, U.S.A.

William P. Wood   Office of Research and Development, U.S. Environmental Protection Agency, Washington, D.C., U.S.A.

1

Regulatory Toxicology Testing: Laboratories and Good Laboratory Practices

Linda J. Frederick
Hospira, Inc., Lake Forest, Illinois, U.S.A.

INTRODUCTION

Your study report is only as good as the supporting data. If you do not exercise due diligence in qualifying a Contract Research Organization (CRO) before placing your study, you might face business and regulatory risks later. It is important to ensure that systems are in place at the CRO that guarantee the integrity of your data and regulatory compliance of the study with Good Laboratory Practice (GLP) Regulations (1). The study report is the product of your scientific efforts and labor. If the report is not accurate, complete, and substantiated by the raw data, the conduct of a nonclinical study is of no real value to the sponsor or the U.S. Food and Drug Administration (FDA). Often the health and safety of the general public may well depend upon the results of a single toxicology safety study.

STUDY MONITOR/SPONSOR REPRESENTATIVE AND THE AUDIT

Your role as the Study Monitor or Sponsor Representative, hereafter referred to as simply "Study Monitor," is to initiate and support the study conduct, approve study documentation, and assist the Study Director with scientific decisions impacting the study design. Although you are not formally charged with the responsibility of interpreting the GLP regulations, current industry standards would require that you have a basic understanding of them. A Quality Assurance (QA) professional has the background, training, and experience to determine the regulatory compliance of a CRO and should be enlisted to assist you with the preplacement inspection. Because the QA representative focuses primarily on the compliance of the facility, it is strongly recommended that you, the scientific expert, participate in the technical review of the CRO. This team approach assures that a comprehensive review is performed from both the scientific and regulatory perspectives. A second set of eyes and ears is a distinct benefit when covering so much material in a condensed timeframe.

An audit report should contain all findings from the inspection and a rating status for the CRO. Follow-up and action plan acceptance for the audit is the responsibility of the QA professional with input from the Study Monitor. The need for a reinspection should be based upon the number and severity of audit observations and the responses from the CRO. This decision should be made by the Study Monitor and the QA representative after audit documentation and correspondences have been reviewed and discussed.

To be an effective sponsor Study Monitor you need to be aware of the history, scope, and subparts of the GLP regulations. The following review of the regulations is not all-inclusive but is intended to provide a high-level overview of key information to aid you in your role as a Study Monitor.

BACKGROUND OF THE GOOD LABORATORY PRACTICES

The GLPs were developed in response to FDA concerns about the quality of drug and chemical safety testing. Prior to the GLPs the agency periodically conducted "for cause" inspections that resulted in findings of incomplete reporting of results, lack of documentation, improper data corrections, missing data, studies of questionable purpose/design, and unqualified personnel. In 1975 the FDA "for cause" compliance program revealed deeply disturbing findings that included falsification of laboratory work, replacement of animals that died on test with no supporting documentation, fabrication of test results, and exclusion of unfavorable results. The U.S. Senate Health Subcommittee became deeply involved. The chairman, Senator Ted Kennedy, relentlessly sought facts about drug and chemical testing in the U.S.A. As a direct result of his efforts, the FDA established the GLP regulations. In addition to the GLPs, which became effective in June 1979, the agency initiated another surveillance program of industry and academia, developed a compliance program, trained GLP inspectors, and identified facilities involved in nonclinical testing. Continued FDA monitoring revealed that experiments were deficient, technical personnel were not trained, management review was not adequate, protocols lacked sufficient detail, personnel qualifications were inadequate, procedures were disregarded, study sponsors were not involved, and reports were not verified or reviewed.

There are important lessons to be learned from the surveillance program. History has taught us the following:

- People make mistakes
- People can be disorganized and in a hurry
- Complex work requires a documented plan
- Every team needs a leader
- Personnel training is essential for consistency and reproducibility of results
- There is no deliverable if record keeping is not adequate
- All work requires a secondary reviewer for accuracy
- Records and specimens must be securely stored and inventoried
- Only a small percentage of people intentionally commit fraud.

To summarize, the majority of laboratory mistakes are due to simple human error and not malicious intent. Implementing the GLP regulations can help to avoid common problems and guarantee consistent, efficient operations. The GLPs are designed to combine good scientific practices with regulatory compliance to assure studies are well planned, properly conducted, and accurately reported. The GLP regulations will aid you in the overall management of studies and allow you to adequately demonstrate safety while increasing efficiency and productivity.

The scope of the GLP regulations prescribes practices for conducting nonclinical laboratory studies that support applications for research or marketing permits for products regulated by the FDA. These products include food and color additives, animal food additives, human and animal drugs, medical devices for human use, biological products, and electronic products.

The GLPs are comprised of subparts A through K, which detail general provisions, organization and personnel, facilities, equipment, testing facilities operation, test and control articles, protocol records and reports, and disqualification of testing facilities. Although all 144 provisions in the regulations are equally important to assess, there are several key sections that should be focused upon during the preplacement inspection. Limited time and resources are a reality when conducting these audits, but with the proper understanding of the critical areas that need to be assessed a thorough audit can be performed with maximum efficiency.

CONDUCTING THE PREPLACEMENT AUDIT

Facility Organization and Personnel

The facility organization and personnel are critical to the successful conduct of your study and its compliance. The GLPs do not prescribe personnel qualifications or academic standards but do require that all individuals engaged in the supervision or conduct of a study have education, training, and experience to enable them to perform their assigned functions. The best way to determine the adequacy of the personnel is to review summaries of training, experience, and job descriptions that must be present as stated in the regulations. Request these documents for specific individuals that you select from the organizational chart, that you interview during the facility tour, or that are assigned to work on your study.

Review records for Management and Study Directors, as well as technical and scientific personnel. Look for revision dates on curricula vitae that should be updated at periodic intervals. The FDA expects that all employees will receive annual GLP training and quite often will ask for a copy of the training material. Include a review of employee GLP training records and the qualifications of the instructor providing the training. Employee files should not contain salary, performance, or human resource information. If this type of confidential information is made available to you during an audit, you should seriously question the professionalism of the CRO. Another important record to request is the GLP job descriptions. This document should contain concise, general statements of the job duties associated with each job title. You should not be supplied with human resource position criteria or a help wanted advertisement. As you review employee records, be sure to note work experience and number of years with the current employer. Increased numbers of new employees may be evidence of organization management issues and will not guarantee well-trained, seasoned employees to work on your studies. Consistency and completeness of training records are easy to review and a good indicator as to the level of detail for all facility documentation. If these records are not current, incomplete, or have improper error corrections, they set the tone for the remainder of the inspection.

Organization and personnel are broken down into the following four categories:

- Testing facility management
- Study director
- Quality assurance unit (QAU)
- Scientific and technical personnel.

Testing facility management plays the most important role in the development and maintenance of a successful compliance program. They are tasked with the designation and replacement of Study Directors, establishment of a QAU and must guarantee that deviations from the regulations, as reported by the QAU, are communicated to the Study Director and corrective actions are taken. Management has the responsibility for scientific operations encompassing the study control, conduct, reporting, and quality. This includes personnel, resources, facilities, equipment, materials, and methodologies. The challenge Management faces is to implement a compliant system that guarantees the quality and integrity of studies and data.

The Study Director has the overall responsibility for the technical conduct of the study, i.e., interpretation, analysis, documentation, and reporting of results. The Study Director represents the single point of study control. It is essential that the Study Monitor establish good communications with the Study Director to keep apprised of study status and any protocol changes. Should serious concerns surface regarding study compliance, the Study Monitor needs to alert the sponsor QAU for follow-up action. The Study Director is pivotal to the success or failure of the study. Your periodic monitoring of study activities via contact with the Study Director demonstrates your commitment to the study and guarantees his/her continuous study involvement.

The QAU assures Management that the facilities, equipment, personnel, methods, practices, records, and controls conform to the regulations. The QA professional performs internal audits as well as CRO/vendor audits at periodic intervals to ensure a continued state of compliance. To maintain objectivity, the QAU must be entirely separate from and independent of the personnel engaged in the direction and conduct of the study. In a small CRO it is acceptable for QA personnel to be involved in study conduct as long as different QAU personnel perform the inspection functions for that study. This allows for maximum utilization of resources through cross-training and careful assignment of study role responsibilities. It is important for all study participants to understand why the QAU exists and what its functions are.

When the GLPs were introduced, QA was a part of every industry except for the laboratory sciences. The FDA intended that an on-site QAU would be their "man in the plant" and serve as a means to ensure constant compliance in between their routine surveillance inspections. To further assure the effectiveness of the QAU, the FDA clearly stated in their compliance program manual that the agency would not be allowed access to actual audit observations but may request proof those inspections were performed, documented, and followed up upon by the QAU. Armed with the knowledge that the FDA is not privy to specific audit findings, except by subpoena, the QAU has no fear of retaliation for the number, type, or severity of observations it cites. The QAU is allowed to effectively perform the duties of inspecting each study at intervals adequate to assure study integrity.

The QAU also maintains copies of all protocols, provides status reports to Management and the Study Director, maintains a master schedule of all GLP studies being conducted, reviews final study reports, maintains inspection records, reports any problems found to Management and the Study Director immediately, and prepares and signs a QA statement for every final study report.

The QAU is a valuable resource and team member whose sole purpose is to assure compliance with the GLP regulations. Through diligent QAU auditing activities Management can expect accurate reporting and data integrity.

Study personnel are the backbone of the nonclinical study. Toxicologists, pathologists, statisticians, veterinarians, chemists, histologists, laboratory technicians, formulation scientists, and supervisors are just a few of the individuals involved in the conduct and support of the study. The GLP regulations say very little about the responsibilities of study and support personnel other than there shall be a sufficient number for timely and proper conduct of a study and proper sanitation, health, and safety requirements should be followed to avoid contamination of test systems and test and control articles.

Facilities and Equipment

Facilities and equipment are best evaluated by first performing a walk-through tour that enables the QA professional to jot down specific model numbers, asset tags, and physically inspect their condition. After the tour, documentation should be requested for key pieces of equipment and facility support operations. The tour is also instrumental in determining what Standard Operating Procedures (SOPs) should be reviewed. In general, the testing facility shall be of suitable size and construction to allow for proper study conduct. The design shall allow for a degree of separation that will prevent any function or activity from having an adverse effect on the study. The animal care areas shall have separation of species or test systems, isolation of individual projects, quarantine of animals, and proper collection and disposal of waste. Storage of feed and bedding shall be separated from areas housing test systems and protected against infestation or contamination. Similarly, facilities for handling test and control articles need to prevent contamination or mix-ups. This equates to separate areas for receipt, storage, and mixing. Lastly, laboratory and archive spaces should also be provided.

When assessing facilities, attention should be paid to the condition of the ceilings, floors, and walls. Notice if areas are cluttered. Observe the amount of facility traffic and the level of activity. Are the temperature and humidity being monitored and controlled? Is there a back-up power source in case of an interruption of service? What is the water source, and how is it treated and tested? Do you see standing water or debris on the floors? Are there signs of pests or insects? Do you notice any odors? What security monitoring systems are in place? Is there separation of clean and dirty equipment, and is it appropriately labeled? Are feed and bedding rotated with the oldest lots being used first? Are supplies stored directly on the floor or on pallets? Is there proper labeling and identification of equipment, supplies, and test systems? Is there limited access to the archive? Are personnel in proper attire? Are equipment and instrumentation in a calibration program? What type of fire suppression system is used? Look into the animal rooms. Are there racks of animals or are most of the rooms empty? A facility that has few or no studies in process is cause for concern and further investigation. These are the types of issues the QA professional will address and include in the audit report.

The concerns surrounding equipment stem from the earlier agency inspections that revealed inadequate balance maintenance and calibration, no documentation of failures, use of unsuitable equipment, equipment located in unclean areas, and balance accuracy checks not performed at point of use. So as you tour the facility, identify equipment used in the generation, measurement, or assessment of data and equipment used for facility environmental control. Make sure it is of appropriate design and adequate capacity to function according to the study protocol. Equipment must be suitably located for operation, inspection, cleaning, and maintenance. To demonstrate sufficient design and function, equipment needs to be qualified and validated. This principle also applies to computerized equipment and systems.

Volumes have been written on the computer validation process and electronic records/electronic signatures (2), so for the purposes of performing a GLP compliance inspection we will just review the basics. Validation involves a validation plan that details the process and test protocols. Validation occurs in a controlled test environment by qualified personnel following appropriate SOPs and using good documentation practices.

A report is issued with evidence of plan execution and results that are reviewed and signed by appropriate personnel. QA is always a part of this process.

In 2003 the FDA issued draft and final guidances on how the agency would interpret 21 CFR Part 11 during its reevaluation of the regulation. FDA will narrowly interpret the scope of Part 11 and exercise enforcement discretion regarding certain Part 11 requirements. By definition, the scope of Part 11 applies to records required by predicate rules that are kept electronically in lieu of paper records or that are relied upon for regulated activities, including submissions to the agency. Enforcement discretion affects the following areas:

- Audit trail requirements
- Validation requirements
- Copying of electronic records
- Electronic record retention
- Legacy system data.

It will not be applied to the establishment of controls for closed and open systems or to the requirements for electronic signatures.

Sponsors and CROs should focus efforts on documenting risk assessments based upon the system's impact on the quality of the product, patient safety, and integrity of the records generated. The primary force guiding your validation decisions and the mandatory records to be maintained should be the appropriate predicate rule(s).

During the course of the CRO inspection the QA professional should identify at least one computer validation package for review. This audit will be cursory but nonetheless can adequately determine whether SOPs and the validation plan were followed and proper documentation of error resolution of test protocols occurred.

Equipment maintenance and calibration records also need to be assessed. The regulations require that all equipment be adequately inspected, cleaned, maintained, tested, calibrated, and/or standardized. They further state that SOPs shall detail those methods, materials, and schedules and discuss remedial action to be taken for failure or malfunction. It is necessary to designate the person responsible for each of the above-mentioned operations in these SOPs. According to FDA standards, if it is not documented it never happened, therefore written records of all equipment activities must be generated. These records need to capture the date of operation, whether the maintenance was routine or nonroutine, the nature of the defect, how, and when the defect was discovered, and the remedial action taken.

Refer to the model numbers and asset tag information collected during the facility tour, and request specific equipment records for review. These records should be used in combination with the appropriate equipment SOPs to confirm compliance with the regulations and the CRO's policies.

Standard Operating Procedures

All CROs must have SOPs in writing that detail the study methods and are approved by Management. SOPs are intended to insure the quality and integrity of the data generated. If there are any changes to SOPs, those changes need to be authorized in writing by Management. To be effective, SOPs need to be accurate, current, and immediately available in each laboratory area. The ultimate success of SOPs relies upon trained users who properly execute, and follow them. For reconstruction purposes a historical file of SOPs and all revisions shall be maintained by the CRO. SOPs are the framework for the organization and require an in-depth review during the preplacement inspection.

Request an SOP index and copies of SOPs critical to your study conduct and support. Review the SOPs for sufficient detail that will allow users to accurately perform the functions described. They should not be so specific that executing them would be cumbersome and prohibitive. Good SOPs are clear and concise. The effective date on an SOP should allow enough time for training of personnel to be completed once all management approvals have been obtained. They should not contain vague wording, such as "may" or "should." Checking compliance with SOPs is a straightforward process. For example, if an equipment SOP states that calibration occurs semiannually and routine maintenance is performed every twelve months, then this documentation should be captured in the equipment log. If facility pest control is performed quarterly, then the documentation can be checked to confirm that this time period complies with the frequency stated in the SOP.

The SOP review should continue in this manner until you gain a level of confidence with compliance to SOPs and facility documentation practices. SOPs should be updated as needed, but certainly an annual review should be performed by facility management to assure current SOPs are still applicable. Whether SOPs are revised or not, documentation should be present that a Management review has been performed. The most common SOP observations listed on a FDA form FD483 (an agency form used to list objectionable conditions observed during the conduct of the inspection that is presented to a representative of the company at the conclusion of the inspection) are that SOPs did not exist, were not followed, were inadequate, or were not official, e.g., lacked Management approval. SOPs are the single most important facility document. They tell the entire story of the CRO's operations, processes, and commitment to data integrity and compliance. Having the SOPs to review is analogous to having the answers to a test; to not utilize that information and spot-check documentation against them would be a gross injustice to the audit process.

Study Protocol and Amendments

The study protocol answers the why, what, and when of study conduct. A protocol supplies the plan for orderly progression of events, a framework for designing data collection tools, and a document telling all study participants what to do. The GLPs require an approved written protocol that indicates the objectives and methods for the conduct of the study. The protocol is a living document and, as such, is subject to change. All changes and revisions need to be documented in a protocol amendment, along with the reason and accompanied by the dated signature of the Study Director. Amendments are proactive revisions to the protocol and are always preferable to issuing deviations, which occur after the fact. Deviations should truly be reserved for those unplanned departures from the study protocol.

An example of a protocol deviation would be if clinical chemistry and hematology parameters are scheduled for all animals during week one of the study, but on the way to the lab one test tube rack of samples is dropped and several of the collection tubes shatter and cannot be analyzed. This was an accident that has resulted in noncompliance with the protocol. It could not have been planned for in advance and is therefore documented as a protocol deviation. The FDA realizes that protocol deviations can and will occur and has accepted departures from the study design with proper documentation approved by Management.

An amendment to the protocol is a planned revision and should be issued in advance of the actual change taking place. An example of a protocol amendment would be a decision to add extra animals on test to be used for pharmacokinetic evaluations. This is a conscious decision to revise the protocol. Proper approvals and documentation can be in place prior to the animals being placed on test.

The biggest problem seen with study conduct is the lack of timely and approved documentation for protocol amendments and deviations. I cannot emphasize enough the need for the sponsor Study Monitor to keep in contact with the Study Director. You need to be an active participant in decisions regarding the study design and authorize any changes in writing.

Study communications are necessary for reconstruction and to demonstrate Management's awareness. Telephone conversations and electronic correspondences are not sufficient stand-alone documentation. A conversation needs to be captured to a permanent storage medium and must be signed and dated to be considered official. Similarly, e-mails or faxes must be signed and dated and filed with other study supporting documentation in the archives at the testing facility. Remember the FDA mentality: if it is not documented, it didn't happen. Adequate study documentation is the key to a successful submission to the agency.

Study Report

The study final report is the deliverable to the FDA. It is the final product of all study labor. Without an accurate and complete report, all time and effort in conducting a nonclinical study is useless to the study sponsor and the agency. The GLPs supply a detailed list of report content requirements, which should be confirmed as adequately addressed in the final report. Do not leave the review of the final report to the Study Director and QAU at the CRO; it is the sponsor's responsibility to verify the conclusions made in the report. Invest the time as the Study Monitor to assess the report and engage the help of the sponsor QAU for yet another independent review. The final report should be compared to the protocol and any amendments or deviations to ensure it reflects the study conduct.

For reports being issued from a CRO you are using for the first time, I would encourage the sponsor QAU to arrange to visit the facility to check the raw data against the final report results. Because there is no prior history with this CRO, the extra effort on the part of the sponsor representatives to confirm that raw data exists, is compliant with the regulations, and substantiates the conclusions stated in the final report is well worth the investment of time.

Study raw data, protocols, amendments, and final reports cannot be assessed during a preplacement audit as these records are only generated once the sponsor signs a contract and initiates the study with the CRO. During the preplacement inspection you can request SOPs discussing content of protocols, final reports, and how raw data are recorded, but at best you are dealing with templates that only give you a glimpse as to how your specific study will be handled. A preplacement audit is a good start to assuring compliance, but without follow-up inspections and periodic monitoring of study conduct, there is no assurance of a quality product being delivered. The best way to illustrate this point is to take you on a journey of GLP noncompliance based on actual study events I have encountered during my years of auditing.

CASE STUDY OF NONCOMPLIANCE

Background

Big Pharmaceutical Company (BPC) has developed a drug with distinct therapeutic advantages compared to those currently on the market. BPC management and marketing personnel estimated potential sales in the billions of dollars. Even though other pharmaceutical companies had similar products in development, it was well worth BPC's time and efforts to enter the race to market with their blockbuster drug.

The FDA requested BPC to perform a special study to determine the drug's potential to produce certain physiological changes that could affect the cardiovascular system. BPC's toxicology team hurriedly searched for a CRO with the scientific expertise to conduct the cutting-edge drug safety study.

The BPC team identified three CROs with the capabilities to conduct the study. One of the sites was a laboratory associated with a prominent university and directed by a world-renowned physiologist who had served on a grass roots committee that had established the guidelines for the type of tests to be conducted. This physiologist and two other colleagues started a nonprofit organization involved in basic research and development activities, which had been in operation for three years. The BPC team decided to pursue negotiations with University Affiliated Laboratory (UAL) and requested that the BPC QA professional perform a GLP preplacement audit.

The QA representative met with the BPC team to determine the services being requested of UAL and to identify the sponsor point-of-contact for the project. BPC Management appointed a Study Monitor who was a doctorate level scientist with project management experience and a background in Good Manufacturing Practices and Good Clinical Practices. The Study Monitor had no formal training or experience with the GLP regulations.

The University Affiliated Laboratory Audit

The preplacement inspection of UAL was conducted using the auditing techniques described earlier in this chapter. The sponsor QAU reviewed personnel and training records, CVs, job descriptions, and organizational charts. UAL SOPs and records for the QAU functions were examined. Purged copies of the master schedule, study inspection reports to Management, and QA statements were in compliance with the GLPs. Checklists for protocol and report audits were also acceptable.

A facility tour was conducted with emphasis on the following:

- building diagrams
- pest control program
- water analysis results
- back-up power source
- air filtration, HVAC systems, frequency of air changes/hour
- temperature, humidity, and light cycle records
- security and alarm systems
- feed and bedding storage and monitoring
- veterinary care
- cage wash area—monitoring of water temperature and validated cleaning methods
- test and control article receipt, storage, tracking, and handling
- proper labeling of reagents, chemicals, and solutions
- equipment calibration, standardization, cleaning, and maintenance
- validation packages
- SOP availability and adequacy
- archive security, fire protection, and indexing systems

- data retention times
- review of previous agency inspections, warning letters, FD483s, etc.

The Study Monitor from BPC did a separate inspection that focused solely on the scientific and technical aspects of the study. Emphasis was placed on test methods, study design and scientific qualifications of the UAL Study Director.

Based upon the initial GLP inspection and the reputation of the facility, BPC selected UAL as the contract laboratory to perform the special FDA requested study.

Study Design

The BPC Study Monitor and the Study Director from UAL developed the study protocol and sent it to both QAUs for simultaneous inspections. The sponsor QAU noticed areas of noncompliance with the GLPs, which included no information regarding test article characterization or concentration analysis of formulations and insufficient discussion of test systems. The protocol was finalized incorporating the suggested wording from the BPC QAU and signed by UAL Management, Study Director, and the BPC Study Monitor. Copies were provided to both QAUs for retention in their protocol files.

The study design placed the animals in the one-month treatment group on test first. Animals for the three- and six-month arms of the study would be placed on test at 30-day intervals thereafter.

The study methods included the use of telemetry devices that would be surgically implanted into the abdominal cavity of each adult test animal one week prior to the first day of treatment. The physiological data would be transmitted to a computerized data capture system. Daily observations of animal health, weekly body weights and detailed physical examinations were also to be performed throughout the study period.

Study Conduct

The BPC Study Monitor decided to order the animals for the one-month study. When the animals arrived at the UAL facility the Study Director noticed they had not been neutered. Apparently the Study Monitor was not aware that all animals on telemetry studies are routinely neutered to reduce aggressive behavior. The Study Director had ordered neutered animals for the three- and six-month treatment groups already. Realizing the dilemma, the Study Monitor and the Study Director decided to neuter the animals for the one-month study at the same time they were anesthetized for implantation of the telemetry devices.

More than 30 percent of the animals in the one-month treatment groups died; 3 died prior to drug treatment, and 10 additional animals died within the first week of dosing for the study. The Study Monitor and Study Director decided to allocate 13 animals assigned to the three- and six-month treatment arms to the one-month group as replacements. The Study Director then ordered additional animals for the three- and six-month treatment groups. As the study progressed, other changes to the protocol were made in response to the data being generated from the study. Additional dose groups were added on and start and termination dates were extended. These protocol changes were not properly documented as amendments, and the sponsor QAU was not informed of the changes to the initial study design.

During a professional QA society meeting, the sponsor QAU and the QAU from UAL had an opportunity to discuss the status of this study. The QAU from the contract laboratory told the sponsor QAU about the study deaths and the reasons behind them.

The extensive modifications to the study protocol were also mentioned. The sponsor QAU requested the UAL QAU to immediately furnish all protocol amendments and any study correspondences. Upon returning home from the meeting, faxed copies of the requested documents were available for the BPC QAU to review. The sponsor QAU contacted the UAL QAU to ask that all future amendments or study issues be properly documented, approved, and provided to the sponsor. The contract laboratory QAU promised to do this should any future changes occur.

The study proceeded according to the revised protocol, and no other contact occurred between the sponsor and contract QAUs.

Audit of the University Affiliated Laboratory Study Report

After the necropsy of the study animals and completion of all the pathology and histology analyses, a final draft report was prepared by the Study Director and sent to the BPC Study Monitor for review and approval. The Study Monitor asked a BPC toxicologist to serve as a second scientific reviewer on the draft report. The toxicologist contacted the sponsor QAU after becoming frustrated with the rather atypical style and format of the report. The BPC QAU agreed to perform a review of the draft report for compliance with the GLPs and the study protocol.

The sponsor QAU contacted the Study Director at UAL to arrange a date for the raw data to final draft report audit. The Study Director indicated the facility staff were quite busy for the next several weeks with lecture and professional meeting engagements and would be unavailable to host a QA auditor at their facility. The Study Director committed to sending verified copies of all the study raw data to the BPC QAU so the report audit could proceed in a timely manner. This is not a standard industry practice, and the sponsor QAU decided to speak with the UAL QAU regarding this oddity. In attempting to contact the QAU at the contract laboratory, the sponsor QAU was informed that this person had been involved in a serious motorcycle accident three months prior, sustained life-threatening injuries, and had not returned to work. UAL had hired a part-time QA consultant to assume the QA duties of performing study inspections, the final report audit, and issuing the QA statement as required by the GLP regulations.

With no one available to host an audit at the contract site, the final report audit was performed at BPC using verified copies of the study raw data. After two days the review of the final report was stopped due to the large number of inaccuracies and formatting errors. To continue the review would be impractical in the opinion of the sponsor QAU. The BPC team was called together to discuss a course of action, and the following errors found in the draft report:

- The report format was difficult to correlate with the raw data, and some numerical values had no units or table headers
- The protocol discussed extensive procedural details not addressed in the report, e.g., animal receipt, prestudy activities, test article administration, tissue preparation, and histology examinations
- The methods section contained broad descriptions of study methods and procedures while many of the critical details were interspersed throughout the results section
- Animal fate and physiological data tables were inaccurate, poorly formatted, and lacked critical study information
- The number of animals on test and found dead or moribund could not be verified from the information presented in the report

- Test article identification, test/control article lot numbers, dose level, sex, and disposition were missing for several animals
- Physiology data could not be located for several animals
- Extraneous values were recorded without explanation for the test article
- Data were not recorded in a timely manner, e.g., entries were made as long as one year after the study ended and by persons not directly involved in the conduct of the study
- Improper error corrections were made to the raw data
- Records were deficient and not filed to allow for expedient retrieval
- Multiple records of test article administration existed for the same day.

BPC Management took decisive action by establishing an audit team that would travel to the UAL facility and attempt to reconstruct the study from the original records and raw data. There was a critical need to determine the integrity of the study and whether the final report conclusions could be reconstructed and substantiated.

University Affiliated Laboratory Data Audit Findings

The BPC audit team arrived at UAL and requested all the study raw data and supporting documentation for immediate review. After several days of examining the study records and interviewing study personnel, the audit revealed many study-related practices and procedures that were not in compliance with the GLP regulations. Major deficiencies were noted in the following areas:

- Personnel, Study Director, and the QAU were not experienced in conducting studies for submission to regulatory agencies, documentation was incomplete, and there were not sufficient staff to support the study
- Test and control article receipt, storage, distribution, accountability, and handling were not documented
- Records of study conduct activities, observations, and measurements were inadequate or nonexistent, e.g., no animal histories, health assessments, husbandry tasks, surgical procedures, randomization to test groups, specimen processing, tissue collection at necropsy, or microscopic examinations
- Reporting of nonclinical laboratory study results did not include all of the circumstances affecting the quality and integrity of the study, did not describe the study methods, or reflect the raw data.

CONCLUSION

This nonclinical laboratory study as conducted and reported by the CRO was not adequate for submission to the FDA or any other regulatory agency in support of a drug application. This study would have to be repeated at another facility, which would further delay the development of this drug by at least one year and add more than $1 million dollars to the cost.

The take home message here is loud and clear: a preplacement inspection alone, no matter how thorough, is not sufficient to ensure GLP regulatory compliance. It is the first of many critical interfaces between the sponsor representatives and the contract research laboratory. Continuous monitoring by the Study Monitor and the QAU, combined with periodic site audits, are essential to guaranteeing regulatory compliance of the study. It is necessary for the sponsor QAU to perform in-process study inspections and review the study raw data, particularly if there is no prior history with the CRO. Equally important is involvement of the sponsor Study Monitor in study conduct coupled with a working knowledge of the GLP regulations and a strong partnership with their QAU.

Disasters of this magnitude were first noted by the FDA during the 1970s, and the GLPs were implemented in the hopes of eliminating these types of tragedies from reoccurring. Some 25 years later we can attest to the importance of those regulations, as evidenced by what can still happen today if they are not properly followed and understood by those persons involved in the conduct of nonclinical laboratory studies.

REFERENCES

1. Food and Drug Administration. Good Laboratory Practice for Nonclinical Laboratory Studies, 21 CFR Part 58. FDA; Rockville, MD, 1987.
2. Food and Drug Administration. Electronic Records; Electronic Signatures, 21 CFR Part 11. FDA; Rockville, MD, 1997.

2

Laboratory Animals and In Vitro Test Systems Used in Regulatory Toxicology

Kit A. Keller

Toxicology Consultant, Washington, D.C., U.S.A.

INTRODUCTION

The increasingly international nature of the pharmaceutical and chemical industry has resulted in many common regulatory goals in the major national regulatory agencies and development of multinational organizations, such as the Organization for Economic Co-operation and Development (OECD) and the International Conference on Harmonization (ICH), to reduce inconsistencies in regulatory burdens and reduce the number of animals used unnecessarily in regulatory testing.

Basic scientific research in the field of toxicology includes investigations utilizing a wide range of animal species, from fruit fly to fish to sheep. Over the years, in regulatory toxicology, a smaller number of "purpose bred" species (rat, mouse, guinea pig, rabbit, dog, and monkey) have become the generally accepted test models to investigate and extrapolate for human risk assessment (Table 1). Initially, species selection had more to do with availability, cost, and ease of use. As the years progressed and knowledge accumulated, selection factors—such as comparative metabolism and pharmacokinetics, available historical control databases, and other species specific factors—also began to play roles in species selection. A number of in vitro test systems have also developed into acceptable assays in regulatory toxicology.

This section is intended to give the reader a brief overview of the commonly used laboratory animals and some recommended guidelines for their care and use under current regulations, as well as a review of the various in vitro test systems currently used in regulatory toxicology.

USE OF ANIMALS IN TOXICOLOGY TESTING

Regulations

The use of animals in research is generally regulated to some extent in Europe, Japan, and the United States, as well as in other countries around the world. In the United States the primary statutory rules on the use and care of animals is contained in the Federal Animal

Table 1   Animal Species Commonly Utilized in Regulatory Toxicology Studies

Study type	Primary species	Common alternative species
Dermal and eye irritation	Rabbit	
Immunotoxicology/ sensitization	Mouse, guinea pig	Rat
Acute toxicity	Rat, mouse	
Multidose toxicity	Rodent (rat), nonrodent (dog)	Mouse, monkey
Carcinogenicity	Rat, mouse	
In vivo mutagenicity	Mouse	Rat
Development and reproduction	Rat, rabbit	Mouse, hamster, monkey
Neurotoxicology	Rat	Mouse

Welfare Act, administered by the U.S. Department of Agriculture (1). In general, this law mandates a basic standard for the care of animals used in research. It stresses adequate institutional oversight and veterinary care, including the appropriate use of anesthestics, analgesics, and tranquilizers to reduce pain and distress. A *Guide for the Care and Use of Laboratory Animals* is published by the Department of Health and Human Services (NIH Pub. No. 74–23), and a copy can be obtain on NIH's Web site (2). Other useful guidelines have also been published (3–6).

The Society of Toxicology has issued a guideline on the use of animals in toxicology testing on their Web site (7). A brief review of these principles are outlined in Table 2.

Humane Treatment of Animals

Toxicology studies can involve injury, disease, and mortality in the test species. When animals are subjected to unrelieved pain and stress, international guidelines mandate that discomfort must be limited (1,3,6). However, regulations also mandate that treatment to alleviate such distress is allowed only if it does not interfere with the study (8,9). Thus approaches to toxicity testing are evolving that entail defining criteria that would signal the early end of a test procedure or cessation of test material administration while still attaining study objectives (10–13). For example, pain and/or morbidity endpoints that

Table 2   Outline of the Society of Toxicology Guiding Principles in the Use of Animals in Toxicology

Must comply with all applicable animal welfare laws.

Protocols involving the use of animals are to be reviewed and approved by an institutional animal care and use committee before study initiation.

Care and handling of all animals must be directed by trained and experienced individuals.

Veterinary care is to be provided in a timely manner as needed.

If a surgical technique is required, appropriate aseptic technique, anesthesia, and postoperative analgesia should be provided.

Euthanasia should be conducted according to the most current guidelines of the American Veterinary Medical Association or similar bodies in different countries.

When scientifically appropriate, alternative in vitro models should be used.

If animal use is necessary, the numbers used should be kept to the minimum required to achieve scientifically valid results.

would lead to early euthanasia include such observations as impaired ambulation (which prevents the animal from reaching food or water), excessive weight loss/extreme emaciation, lack of physical or mental alertness, labored breathing, and prostration. Guidelines on safe volumes of test material administration and blood sampling volumes have also been published (14,15).

COMMON SPECIES IN REGULATORY TOXICOLOGY

There is no such thing as the perfect animal species for testing potential human toxins. No single species is predictive for man in all possible circumstances. Each species has its pros and cons, and no one species matches human physiology, organ function and morphology, or reaction to exogenous chemicals consistently (Table 3). For example, human skin is more resistant to dermal absorption of compounds than most animal models because of a thickened stratum corneum. (The pig is considered the closest model.) In addition to morphological differences, biochemical pathways also vary. For example, in rat, mouse, rabbit, guinea pig, ferret, and dog, the major plasma lipoprotein classes are the high-density lipoproteins (HDL). In contrast, the major classes in primates, including humans, are low-density lipoproteins (LDL). How exogenous chemicals are handled in the body can also vary markedly in each species. For example, rats, and dogs are considered relatively efficient biliary excreters in comparison to the guinea pig and monkey. Thus, extrapolation of toxicology findings from animals to humans in risk assessment requires expertise and a thorough knowledge of each species and the field of toxicology (16–20).

Most of the common laboratory animals used in biomedical research are purpose bred, by vendors who supply "disease-free" animals. Mice, rats, guinea pigs, other rodents, and rabbits should be specific-pathogen free (SPF). In addition, rats, and mice should also be virus-antibody-free (VAF). This is important because this ensures the general health and quality of the animals and limits factors that could complicate or interfere with the results of a study. It is also important that large animals, such as the beagle (dog) and monkey, are also supplied by reputable vendors. This is especially true of primates, which can harbor a number of pathogens that are harmful to humans. Maintaining such standards in a laboratory facility prevents a constant influx of viruses, bacteria, and parasitic organisms that could threaten the health of the entire facility's animal population and study viability. Many laboratories order additional animals for selected studies to serve as a nontreated sentinel population that are evaluated at scheduled intervals for possible viral infection.

Animals should always be examined for signs of disease when they first arrive, preferably by a veterinarian, prior to accepting any animals from an outside vendor. The animals are always allowed an acclimation period and kept separate from other animals when arriving at a facility. This period can range from a few days to many weeks, depending on the species and type of study for which they are to be utilized. The only exception to this can be circumstances when time-mated (pregnant) animals are being used in a reproduction or developmental toxicity study.

Generally more animals than needed for a study are ordered, which allows for prestudy selection of the most suitable animals for the study. Criteria for selection into the study for rodents, guinea pigs, and rabbits are usually based on acceptable body weight range (i.e., ± 2 standard deviation from the mean), normal food consumption, and acceptable health examination. When used in acute testing the condition of the eyes and skin are also considered. For large animals, one or two pre-test measurements of clinical chemistry, hematology, electrocardiographic, and

Table 3 Comparative Biological and Physiological Values in Experimental Animals and Man

	Mouse	Rat	Guinea pig	Rabbit	Dog	Monkey	Human
Average life span (years)	1.5–2	2–2.75	4.5–6	5–13	12–22	18–29	70–73
Age at puberty	35 days	50 days	62 days	7 months	7 months	2.5 years	13.5 years
Body weight (kg)	0.02–0.03	0.15–0.35	0.45–1.2	3–6	12–31	2–4	54–94
Surface area (m^2)	0.006	0.025	NA	NA	0.4	0.24	1.6
Daily food consumption (g/day)	3–6	10–20	23–34	7–186	300–500	40–300	2000
Daily water consumption (mL/day)	3.2–6.9	24–31	60–75	80–138	100–400	350–1000	2000
Energy metabolism (cal/kg/day)	NA	120–140	NA	47	34–39	49	23–26
Body temperature (°C)	36.5	37.3	37.9	38.8	38.9	38.8	36.9
Whole blood volume (mL/kg b wt)	74.5	58.0	74.0	69.4	92.6	75.0	77.8
Daily urine volume (mL)	1–2	11–15	NA	5–70	14–24	17.5–20	110–1450
Heart rate (beats/min)	330–780	250–400	150–400	123–325	60–130	165–240	41–108
Stroke volume (mL/beat)	NA	1.3–2.0	NA	1.3–3.8	14–22	8.8	62.8
Arterial blood pressure (mmHg)	113/81	116/90	77/50	110/80	148/100	159/127	120/80
Respiratory rate (breaths/min)	160–171	85–117	90	53	20	50	10–16
Inhalation rate (m^3/day)	0.052	0.29	0.40	2	4.3	5.4	20

Typical mean values or ranges collected from numerous published and unpublished sources; values may vary by age and strain within species (for comparison of reproductive parameters see Chapter 11).

ophthalmologic parameters are also factored into the decision. All animals must be "randomized" into the study treatment groups to eliminate bias.

All animals rooms and caging must be cleaned on a regular basis. For good laboratory practices (GLP) regulatory studies there is a required species specific range of allowable room temperature and humidity that must be maintained and documented. In addition, all animal rooms require a minimum number of air changes within each room, most often 12 to 15 changes each hour.

General Considerations

Rodents

Mice and rats are relatively low in cost for both purchasing and housing. In addition, they are readily available in healthy condition and are considered time efficient and relatively docile in handling and dosing with consistent results in toxicology testing. Their many years of use and their genetic stability have ensured that extensive background data is available (21,22). Both inbred and outbred strains may be used, but the former breeding system offers less genetic variation (23,24). Examples of rodent strains that are commonly used in toxicology experimentation are presented in Table 4. Rodents have a short gestation period, high fertility rate, and large litters, making them particularly economical to produce large numbers for research, as well as very useful in studying potential reproductive or developmental toxicity. Their short life spans also make them useful in chronic and lifetime studies (i.e., carcinogenicity). On the less favorable side, rats and mice have a relatively fast metabolic rate, can be stress sensitive, lack a gallbladder, have no emetic reflex, are able to produce ascorbic acid internally, and have CYP2C as their primary P450 metabolizing enzymes (compared to CYP3A in humans). Rats are also obligate nasal breathers and do not generally make a good model for humans with regard to inhalation studies. Their size can be an advantage or disadvantage, depending on what endpoint one is considering. Mice are particularly favored when test material is in short supply as they generally require much less material for a comparable study than any other commonly used species (Table 5). However, if one is trying to optimize the volume and number of blood samples for a study, rodents, particularly mice, will have some limitations. Rodents have also been found to be unsuitable test models for specific types of chemicals. For example, they are unsuitable for testing dopamine agonists for potential reproductive toxicity due to their dependence on prolactin in early pregnancy. In general, the monkey and guinea pig are better models than rodents for investigations into the potential toxic effects on gonadotropic and ovarian function.

The rat is the most commonly used species for all types of toxicology studies, including acute, multidose, developmental, reproduction, carcinogenicity, and neurotoxicity studies (Table 1). The mouse is mostly used for acute toxicity, in vivo mutagenicity, and carcinogenicity studies, although it can be used as an alternative to the rat when applicable. There are numerous publications on historical control data for rats and mice, including growth and development patterns and spontaneous disease (20,25–33). Additional background data may also be obtained from suppliers.

Guinea Pig

The guinea pig, although relatively docile and easy to handle, is generally not as well studied as other laboratory species in toxicology, and thus historical control data as well as pharmacokinetic data are often lacking. In addition, they can be very susceptible to disturbance of the alimentary tract by orally administered test materials, intravenous administration can be very difficult, and historically, guinea pigs have been found to

Table 4   Rodent Strains Frequently Used in Toxicology Studies

Strains	Description
Rat	
Sprague-Dawley (SD)	An outbred albino strain, frequently used with a very large background data base but prone to obesity and mammary neoplasms. Propensity for geriatric renal disease may limit the utility of the SD rat for studying nephrotoxic compounds.
Wistar	An outbred albino strain. Good survival for two-year bioassays, but prone to mammary and pituitary neoplasms.
Fischer 344	An inbred albino strain, small and often used, but prone to leukemia and testicular and pituitary neoplasms.
Mouse	
CD-1	An outbred albino strain, most frequently used in safety studies but prone to liver neoplasms and amyloidosis.
C3H	An inbred agouti strain. Commonly used in government laboratories, but prone to liver neoplasms.
C57BL	An inbred black strain.
BALB/c	An inbred albino strain prone to testicular atrophy.

provide a poor comparison to human metabolism of many compounds (34,35). More recently, in view of their hypersensitivity, guinea pigs have been suggested as a second species when testing biopharmaceutical products that consist of proteins or peptides.

Currently the guinea pig is used almost exclusively for acute sensitization/immuno-toxicity studies (Table 1). In recent years, there has been a push to replace this standard guinea pig assay with the newer lymph node assay in rodents (see Chapter 13 for more specifics on immuntoxicity testing methods). They have also historically been used in special cases for reproduction studies because they are similar to man and other primates in that the placenta takes over the hormonal control of pregnancy very early in gestation and thus is not dependent on active corpora lutea as are rodents and rabbits (36). However, their long gestation period (65–72 days) has generally limited their use in developmental toxicity studies.

Rabbit

Rabbits are generally docile but not as easy to handle as rodents due to their larger size and easily injured back and limbs. Rabbits are more expensive than rodents and require larger caging. The primary strains of rabbits used in regulatory toxicology are the New Zealand

Table 5   Hypothetical Test Material Requirements

Mouse	Rat	Monkey (cyno)	Dog (beagle)
Assumptions			
30 grams b wt	250 grams b wt	2.5 kg b wt.	9 kg b wt.
10/sex/group	10/sex/group	4/sex/group	4/sex/group
4 groups	4 groups	4 groups	4 groups
25, 250, and	25, 250, and	25, 250, and	25, 250, and
500 mg/kg/d	500 mg/kg/d	500 mg/kg/d	500 mg/kg/d
28 days treatment	28 days treatment	28 days treatment	28 days treatment
+20%	+20%	+20%	+20%
Test material required			
~62 grams	~520 grams	~2080 grams	~7500 grams

White or the Dutch Belted rabbit. Although "clean" rabbit suppliers are generally available, historically pasteurellosis and coccidiosis have been problems (manifested as nasal discharge, diarrhea, and congested lungs, as well as pitted kidneys and brain lesions). In addition, rabbits are very susceptible to disturbances of the gastrointestinal (GI) tract, especially when testing antibacterial agents. Clinical signs and body weight changes in rabbits can be erratic and difficult to interpret.

Rabbits are used exclusively in eye and dermal irritation studies and in developmental toxicity studies and thus often lack other available toxicity or pharmacokinetic data unless specifically generated in range-finding studies (Table 1). Although their use is somewhat limited, some background and historical control data are available in the literature (37–41).

Dog

There are more than 300 varieties of the domestic dog (*Canis familiaris*), but the beagle has become the most commonly used in nonclinical safety assessments. Though significantly more expensive than rodent species, toxicology studies with beagle dogs offer an economical large, and often required second, nonrodent animal species that is docile and easy to work with (42). The beagle is generally consistent in its genetic profile, and extensive background data are available. For inhalation studies, dogs are not an obligate nasal breather, like the rat, and therefore more closely resemble humans. In addition, aerosol deposition in alveolar region of the dog lung is closer to humans (43). Dog studies generally utilize much smaller group sizes than small animal studies and thus are less powerful statistically. In shorter studies, the usual young age of dogs can complicate interpretation of histopathology findings in the reproductive organs as sexual maturity in dogs usually dose not occur until at least 9 months of age.

Dogs are used almost exclusively for general toxicology studies ranging in duration from 2 weeks to 1 year (Table 1). They can be highly sensitive to a number of chemical classes, including cardiovascular active compounds and nonsteroidal anti-inflammatory agents. Laboratory beagles show a high spontaneous incidence of polyarteritis which can cause problems of interpretation of whether or not such a lesion, if found, represents a potential human hazard or is clinically not relevant. In general, dogs tend to have slower drug clearance than rat, more closely resembling humans (44). However, as with every species, there are marked exceptions (e.g., dissimilar pharmacokinetics with organic acids). Dogs cannot acetylate primary arylamino groups, which can also result in large differences in pharmacokinetics than humans. For example, dogs demonstrate better tolerance to the renal effects of sulphonamides than that seen in humans, due to their lack of acetylation ability.

Primates

Several taxonomic groups of primates are used in research (45). The most commonly used primate species in toxicology studies are cynomolgus monkeys, macaque monkey, rhesus monkeys, baboons, and marmosets. There can be marked physiological and pathological differences between the various taxa. For example, marmosets (a New World monkey) are glucocortcoid resistant and have higher circulating levels of steroids compared to Old World monkeys, such as the macaque. The cynomolgus monkey is usually the first choice unless the test compound can be more relevantly tested in another species. Baboons and rhesus monkeys are more difficult to obtain in numbers required for preclinical toxicity testing and generally require larger amounts of test material. There is an increasing trend in the United Kingdom to use the common marmoset (*Callithrix jacchus*). Although offering a smaller model, marmosets are less hardy, and experience is required in their specialized husbandry requirements (46,47). In all cases, primates are expensive animals to purchase and house, and only relatively recently have organized breeding programs been instituted. Wild-caught animals have always had the potential problem that the interpretation of any toxic effects could be complicated by the presence of parasites, preexisting disease, precapture lesions, and the absence of genetic consistency.

Similar to the dog, the primate would be used almost exclusively for general toxicology studies ranging in duration from 2 weeks to 1 year (Table 1). Due to the expense and risk of primate studies, such studies are initiated rather than dog studies only when there is a definite need due to such factors as poor pharmacokinetics in the dog, known overt sensitivity or toxicity to certain classes of compounds in dogs, or known antigenicity issues, as often seen with biopharmaceuticals. It should be noted that pharmacokinetics in non-human primates can differ from humans as much as with other species, and preliminary studies should be conducted before proceeding with large primate studies. Other alternatives do exist, such as the minipig or the ferret, but their use is uncommon.

Housing and Husbandry

The section below outlines current regulatory requirements for laboratory animal housing and husbandry. However, it should be noted that there is a strong effort being made for a future guideline that recommends use of solid-bottom caging and social housing in rodents and rabbits and enlarge caging and social housing for dogs and primates for better animal health and environmental enrichment (48).

Rodents

Single housing of rodents is routine in North America. Gang housing (5 rats per cage or 4 mice per cage) is the norm in Europe. Both husbandry systems have their positive and negative aspects. Gang housing of rodents does not allow individual food consumption values. Moribund animals have to be isolated, which introduces variability or, if left group housed, may result in the loss of tissue samples by cannibalism. For male mice, especially, there is the problem of fighting during the first weeks of a study. However, the housing of more than one animal per cage does contribute to animal survival (predominantly on chronic or carcinogenicity studies) and reduces the obesity evident in older rodents, particularly rats. Studies on restricting food consumption (diet "optimization") of individually housed rodents have shown similar benefits in body weight gain, morbidity, and survival. Some form of food restriction is now generally recommended on chronic and carcinogenicity studies, as well as the preceding range-finding studies. To date, no single restricted diet regime has been identified. This can present problems for interpretation of data in relation to historical controls. It should be noted that much of the background (historical control) data collected on rodent studies are specific to the type of husbandry used and, in these respects, are not interchangeable.

Caging for rodents is usually solid or mesh stainless steel. Mesh flooring allow urine and feces to fall through onto a collection tray/mat beneath the cage. This tray/mat must be changed regularly. The cages themselves and entire animal room should be on a regular cleaning schedule as well. The minimum space recommendations for single rodent caging are dependent on size/weight and range from a floor area per animal of 39 to 97 cm^2 for mice to 110 to 452 cm^2 for rats. A compromise, when designing caging, is usually made between allowing easy access and examination of the animals and the prevention of escape or injury. The cages can be suspended from permanent wall mountings or in movable racks/batteries that allow flexibility for room cleaning and periodic repositioning of the animals around the housing room to minimize environmental influences on the experimental results. Top-of-the-line caging systems are totally enclosed with full rack ventilation. In reproduction studies that require litter rearing, a larger solid floor cage with bedding for "nesting" material is required.

Rodents are extremely hardy and capable of survival in an extremely wide range of temperatures and humidity, but within the toxicology laboratory, a controlled environment is essential to eliminate variables. Mice and rats should be maintained at temperatures of 18–26° C (64–79° F) and relative humidity of 30–70%. Room illumination is usually controlled to 12 hours of light and 12 hours of darkness.

Water is supplied ad libitum by either an automatic watering system or individually filled water bottles. The daily water intake ranges from 3–7 ml in mice and 20–30 ml in rats. Feeders supplying either certified diet in the form of pellets or powdered meal, ad libitum or controlled amounts, are either attached to the caging or are free standing. Daily food requirements range from 3–6 grams in mice to 10–20 grams in rats.

Guinea Pig

Guinea pigs grow to just more than 1 kg in weight and have husbandry requirements that are similar to those of rats, though the diet should be supplemented with vitamin C, and solid floored cages with bedding that offer at least 700 cm^2 floor area and a height of 17.78 cm should be provided. Food and water should be provided ad libitum similar to rodents. Average daily requirements are 12–15 ml/100 grams of water and 20–30 grams of food. Like primates, guinea pigs require a continuous supply of vitamin C (ascorbic acid) in the diet.

Rabbit

Rabbits are also caged in stainless steel cages made of mesh or bars that are close enough together to prevent injury to the animals. The cages are usually on racks and stacked 3–4 high. Depending on the strain of rabbit, body weights of sexually mature adults range from 3.0 to 6.0 kg. Minimal recommended floor area per rabbit, depending on size and weight of the animal, ranges from 0.14 to 0.45 m^2. Rabbit generally prefer a bit cooler environment than rodents, with the room temperature kept within a range of 16–22° C (61–72° F) relative humidity should be 30–70%, and a 12-hour light and dark cycle should be maintained. Rabbits can be maintained on certified dry rabbit chow pellets but generally do better in laboratory settings when their food consumption is controlled to a set daily amount rather than allowing ad libitum feeding (49). Average daily requirements are 80–100 ml/kg of water and 75–100 grams of food.

Dog

Most dog cages are stainless steel with a floor area of at least 0.75 m^2 and a height of 82 cm for dogs up to 15 kg. These cages are usually attached to the wall or mounted in racks in tiers of two. Dogs are usually housed individually, but the exercise requirements of the animals must be considered. Communal areas, usually large joined pens, are essential to allow exercise, and social interaction. Male and female should never be exercised together and mixing of dogs from different dose groups is usually avoided. The temperature of the dog room should be kept within a range of 18–29° C (64–84° F), relative humidity should be 30–70%, and a 12-hour light and dark cycle should be maintained.

Dogs are supplied with water on an ad libitum basis (average daily intake ranges from 100–400 ml) but receive a daily measured ration of diet. For an average-weight dog on toxicity studies (8–12 kg), 400 g of certified pelleted food is usually provided, and a one hour feeding period is sufficient after training. A commercially available certified dried feed provides a satisfactory diet, but during the acclimation period or if an animal is in poor condition, this should be supplemented by moistening the pelleted food with water or supplementation with commercially available nutritional supplements or available moist canned diet. Quantitative measurement of food and water consumption is not normally attempted due to the active nature of the species. A more qualitative assessment of food consumption (i.e., all, ¾, ½, ¼ or none) is usually sufficient. Any diet modification or supplementation should be documented.

Primates

Primate caging is similar to that used to house dogs, with some additions. Primates have complex social behavior and are prone to developing abnormal behavior patterns (e.g., stereotyping or self-mutilation) if not cared for properly. When singly housed for toxicology studies, some form of environmental enrichment must be provided in the form of interactive toys and regular entertainment, such as videos. The cages used to house primates should have a screened area to allow animals to break contact with facial displays of other aggressive animals. Primates can be dangerous when handled without adequate training. A perch and a system to move the animal to the front of the cage to allow removal for examinations or study related procedures without injury to the animal or handler can be a useful addition. The recommended minimum floor area for primates is dependent on the size/weight of the monkey and ranges from 0.15 to 0.74 m^2 per animal.

The temperature in the husbandry area of nonhuman primates is usually maintained at 18–29° C (64–84° F), the humidity at 30–70% with a 12-hour light and dark cycle. Water is provided ad libitum, and a fixed amount of diet is given each day as well as a fruit supplement. Similar to dogs, quantitative measurement of food and water consumption is not normally attempted, due to their active nature and fruit supplementation. A more qualitative assessment of food consumption (i.e., all, ¾, ½, ¼ or none) is usually sufficient. Average daily requirements are 350–1000 ml of water and 40–100 grams of food. Like guinea pigs, primates require a continuous supply of vitamin C (ascorbic acid) in the diet.

Animal Identification

Identification of animals ensures the continuity of records and interpretation throughout the study. In the past, it was considered adequate to rely on the cage labeling and only discriminate between animals when gang housed. Today, each animal should be individually identified, and, if possible, the specific study identification should also be indicated. Methods of identification should be permanent (this does not include "permanent" ink). Table 6 outlines historic and current methods for identification of the common laboratory species. The use of microchip transponders implanted subcutaneously has greatly enhanced the efficiency and accuracy of animal identification in many animal facilities. Invasive methods, such as toe clipping and ear punching, are no longer used at the majority of facilities due to the pain and stress associated with such methods. Tattooing is also losing favor for many species where it requires constant shaving of the area. In some cases, animals arrive with a supplier's identification, which is often different from what is used in the actual study identification.

Routes of Administration

Laboratory animals can be administered test material by a wide variety of routes. Oral administration can be by gavage with a tube or specialized gavage needle, capsule, or diet.

Test materials can be injected as an intravenous (iv), intraperitoneal (ip), intramuscular (im), subcutaneous (sc), or intradermal (id) syringe injection. Using the lung as the route of exposure can entail such test systems as whole body chambers, nose-only exposures, aerosol canisters, or intratracheal instillations. Other miscellaneous routes, such as sublinqual, rectal, intravaginal, and topical, are also used in specialized situations. Prior to the commencement of dosing by any route, the animals should be familiarized or habituated to any restraint procedures that may be necessary.

Usually the material being tested is administered in a vehicle, such as water, saline, methylcellulose, or corn oil. There are published recommendations for maximum dosing volumes for oral gavage and injection routes for a variety of laboratory animals (Table 7) (14,15). When volume limits are a problem, systemic exposure can often be increased by increasing the frequency of administration. Common abbreviations include q.d. (once per day), b.i.d. (twice per day), q.i.d. (three times per day) and q.o.d. (every other day).

In general, for studies using an injection as the route of administration, the rate should be adjusted to avoid pain and local tissue damage, the temperature of the dosing solution/suspension should be close to the body temperature of the animal, and alternative injection sites should be used sequentially. Ideally, fluids for parenteral administration should be isotonic, however, nonisotonic fluids can be dosed by the intraperitoneal or intravenous route. A test article with any degree of irritancy is likely to produce local reactions at the dose site and in some cases ultimately prevent dosing in the area or by that particular route. An alternative method of administering irritant solutions or for repeated dose infusion studies is to use implanted catheters. Preliminary studies, such as a vein irritation test, muscle irritation test, in vitro hemolysis, or paw lick test, can anticipate problems. For oral studies, pathology of the GI tract from early range-finding studies will usually identify problems.

For studies on environmental chemicals or food additives, the test material is usually mixed into diet or drinking water. Such exposures are commonly expressed in terms of concentration (parts per million or ppm) or in terms of the actual test material received by the animal (mg/kg/day; milligram per kilogram body weight per day) based on the amount of diet or water consumed. In order to ensure consistent dosing in growing animals, the investigator is required to predict both increases in body weight and expected food consumption, based on historical control records, in order to prepare the next weeks admixtures.

Biological Sampling

Analysis of urine and blood samples from rodents is an integral part of a toxicology study. Obtaining urine samples using metabolism caging is a straightforward, noninvasive technique that requires the animals to be transferred to special cages in which urine is separated from feces and collected over a specified time period. Due to the low volumes,

Table 6 Animal Identification Methods

Species	Methods
Mouse	Toe clip (fetus/neonate), ear punch, tattoo, implant
Rat	Toe clip (fetus/neonate), ear punch, tattoo, ear tag, implant
Guinea pig	Ear punch, ear tag, tattoo, implant
Rabbit	Ear tag, tattoo, implant
Dog	Tattoo, collar, implant
Primate	Tattoo, collar, implant

Table 7 Recommended Maximum Dosing Volumes (mL/kg)

Species	Oral gavage	iv	ip	im	sc	id
Mouse	20	10	20	0.05[a]	20	0.5
Rat	20	5	10	0.1[a]	5	0.5
Guinea pig	20	5	10	0.1[a]	5	0.5
Rabbit	10	2	4	0.25	1	0.5
Dog	10	2.5	1	0.25	1	0.5
Primate	10–15	2–2.5	–	0.5	2	0.5

[a] Represents recommended total mL volume not mL/kg.

samples from mice may be pooled. Very "clean" urine samples may also be obtained at necropsy using a syringe if the bladder contains urine. In the larger animals, urine may be collected in live animals or at necropsy using a catheter.

Blood samples can be obtained by a wide variety of techniques and sites from live animals and at necropsy (Table 8). These procedures all require technical expertise to avoid harm to the animals and obtain adequate samples. Guidelines on humane sampling methods and sample volumes have been published (14,15). Anesthetics should be used in many cases to avoid unnecessary pain and stress. The selection of the most appropriate analgesic or anesthetic is dependent upon the procedure. Commonly used products include ketamine, promazines, carbon dioxide/oxygen, sodium pentobarbital, halothane, isoflurane, and sevoflurane (50). The volume of blood samples taken at any one time should not be harmful to the animal, and adequate recovery time for red blood cell regeneration needs to be factored into any protocol. Multiple sampling from the larger animal species is generally not a problem or confounding factor in data interpretation. However, for smaller species, separate satellite groups are usually added to the study specifically for blood sample collections either for PK and/or clinical pathology procedures.

Euthanasia

Euthanasia is the "act of killing animals by methods that induce rapid unconsciousness and death without pain or distress." In the United States, the selected euthanasia method is usually consistent with published recommendations (51), unless justified for scientific or medical reasons. The specific method will depend upon the species involved and the objectives of the study. Both inhalants and noninhalant chemicals, such as barbiturates, fluorinated anesthetics, and carbon dioxide/oxygen, are generally preferable to more historical physical techniques, such as cervical dislocation or decapitation.

IN VITRO TEST SYSTEMS IN REGULATORY TOXICOLOGY TESTING

A wide variety of in vitro methods are used as screening studies and in mechanistic investigations. However, few of these methods have generally been accepted in regulatory toxicology for purposes of hazard and risk assessment. The earliest accepted in vitro test systems were those for mutagenicity testing. In more recent years, the development of various additional in vitro methods are being pursued for both reasons of animal welfare and improvement of the science and predictability to human risk assessment (52,53). Validation of a new test, which usually involves multiple test sites and positive and negative controls, assures the reproducibility and relevance of the test system. The various regulatory agencies have systems in place to review the progress of such method

Table 8 Blood Sample Collection Techniques in Laboratory Animals

Technique/site	Species	Volume obtainable	Terminal procedure	Comments
Retro-orbital plexus	Rat, mouse	0.35 mL (mouse); 0.35–3.0 mL (rat)	No	Moderate volumes; relatively "dirty" samples Possible injury to eye Anesthesia should be used
Cardiac puncture	Rat, mouse	1 mL (mouse); 0.7–5 mL (rat)	Yes	Large volumes Anesthesia should be used
Lateral tail vein	Rat	0.35–2 mL	No	Heating tail aids in sampling but increases collection time Less trauma to animal Repeated collections
Jugular	Rat, rabbit	1–2 mL (rat); 0.35–5 mL (rabbit)	No	Quick method Repeated collections
Posterior vena cava	Rat, mouse, rabbit, dog, primate	1 mL (mouse); 0.7–3 mL (rat); 50–75 mL (rabbit); >75 mL (large animals)	Yes	Quick method Anesthesia should be used
Marginal ear vein	Rabbit	0.35–3 mL	No	Quick method
Vein—saphenous, cephalic, femoral	Dog, primate	1.5–5 mL	No	Quick method Repeated collections Repeated collections

developments and their validation (54,55). In general, regulators have accepted validated alternatives to whole animal studies if the new method allows classification of chemical hazards and risks similar to the way current animal tests allow them to do. Below is a brief review of some of the test systems currently accepted by at least one of the regulatory agencies.

Cellular Test Systems

A wide variety of cells are currently used for in vitro tests for regulatory toxicity testing, mostly for mutagenicity testing (see Chapter 8). This includes various bacterial strains of *S. typhimurium* and *E. coli*, as well as such human and mammalian cell lines as the mouse lymphoma L5178Y cells, human lymphobalstoid TK6 cells, Chinese hamster ovary cells, V79 cells, and AS52 cells.

The first cellular assay, other than for mutagenicity, to be accepted [by the European Commission (EC) in 2000] was an in vitro photoxicity assay that uses the mouse fibroblast cell line (3T3) with neutral red uptake (NRU) as the endpoint for cytotoxicity (56–60).

To ensure that the cells are well characterized and traceable, it is recommended that cultures be obtained from a recognized vendor. Most labs retain both a frozen permanent stock and working stocks. Each lot of cells is tested for contamination (e.g., mycoplasma) prior to use. Master "plates" are prepared by inoculating onto appropriate medium and incubation of the plates at 37° for 24 to 48 hours. Bacterial plates can be stored at 4° until needed. Master plates are usually usable for up to 5–6 weeks or for a given number of "passages."

The population of viable cells in the plate should be monitored carefully because undergrowth and overgrowth of the cultures can cause loss of assay sensitivity. Environmental factors that can alter the test results, such as pH and osmolality, must also be closely monitored. Assays using these cells generally involve repeat studies as well as positive and negative concurrent controls.

Tissue Test Systems

Historically, the only tissue widely used in regulatory testing in vitro was whole blood, usually from rabbits or humans, utilized in assessing hemolytic potential prior to intravenous injection studies or for cytogenetics studies.

More recently, two in vitro tests for skin corrosivity have been validated and accepted by the European Commission for regulatory purposes in 2000 (61–64). The first utilizes reconstructed human skin (EPISKIN™ or EpiDerm™). The second EC-approved test utilizes excised rat skin and transcutaneous electrical resistance (TER).

The Draize eye test in rabbits has historically been one of the most widely criticized toxicology studies on humane grounds. Thus, much effort has been made to find alternative in vitro methodologies to replace the use of this rabbit test. Two in vitro test systems utilizing excised animal tissues, the bovine corneal opacity and permeability test (BCOP) and the isolated rabbit eye test (IRE), developed as replacement for the Draize eye irritation test in rabbits have now gained regulatory "tolerance" in Europe for classification of eye irritancy potential (52,65,66). Another nonmammalian assay, the hen's egg test-chorioallantoic membrane (HET-CAM) has also gained general EC acceptance (67).

The dissection, handling, and use of excised tissues are highly dependent on the test system. Care must be taken to retain the viability and sensitivity of the system, and, as with cellular test systems, concurrent positive and negative controls should be utilized to ensure the integrity of the test.

REFERENCES

1. United States Department of Agriculture (USDA). Animal Welfare. Final Rules. CFR 54 Parts 1, 2, and 3, 1998.
2. http://www.nih.gov.
3. National Research Council (NRC). Guide for the Care and Use of Laboratory Animals. 7th ed. Washington DC: National Academy Press, 1996.
4. Principles for Biomedical Research Involving Animals, Council for International Organizations of Medical Sciences, International Guiding, Geneva, 1985.
5. Interdisciplinary Principles and Guidelines for the Use of Animals in Research, Testing, and Education, Adhoc Animal Research Committee, New York Academy of Science, 1988.
6. Public Health Service (PHS). Public health service policy on humane care and use of laboratory animals. Department of Health and Human Services, Washington DC, 1996.
7. www.toxicology.org.
8. Environmental Protection Agency. Federal Insecticide, Fungicide, and Rodenticide Act (FIFRA). Good Laboratory Practice Standards. Final Rule. 40 CFR Part 160, Washington DC: Government Printing Office, 1998.
9. Food and Drug Administration. Good Laboratory Practice for Non-Clinical Laboratory Studies, 21 CFR 58, Washington DC, Government Printing Office, 1999.
10. Canadian Council on Animal Care. CCAC guidelines on choosing an appropriate endpoint in experiments using animals for research, teaching, and testing. Ottawa: CCAC, 1998.
11. Organization for Economic Co-operation and Development. Guidance Document on the Recognition, Assessment, and Use of Clinical Signs as Humane Endpoints for Experimental Animals Used in Safety Evaluation. Paris: OECD ENV/JM/MONO(2000)7, 2000.
12. Hendriksen CFM, Morton DB. Humane Endpoints in Animal Experiments for Biomedical Research. Proceedings on the International Conference, November 22–25, 1998, Zeist, The Netherlands. London: Royal Society of Medicine Press, 1999.
13. Stokes WS. Humane endpoints for laboratory animals used in regulatory testing. Inst Lab Anim Res J 2002; 43:S31.
14. Hull RM. Guideline limit volumes for dosing animals in the preclinical stage of safety evaluation. Hum Exp Toxicol 1995; 14:305.
15. Diehl K-H, Hull R, Morton D, et al. A good practice guide to the administration of substances and removal of blood, including routes and volumes. J Appl Toxicol 2001; 21:15.
16. Gad SC, Chengelis CP. Animal Models in Toxicology. NY: Marcel Dekker, 1992.
17. Zbinden G. The concept of multispecies testing in industrial toxicology. Regul Toxicol Pharmacol 1993; 17:85.
18. Calabrese EJ. Suitability of animal models for predictive toxicology: theoretical and practical considerations. Drug Metab Rev 1984; 15:505.
19. Davidson IWF, Parker JC, Beliles RP. Biological basis for extrapolation across mammalian species. Regul Toxicol Pharmacol 1986; 6:211.
20. Oser BL. The rat as a model for human toxicological evaluation. J Toxicol Environ Health 1981; 8:521.
21. Baker HJ, Lindsey JR, Weisbroth SH. The laboratory rat. Biology and Disease. NY: Academic Press, 1979;1.
22. Foster HL, Small JD, Fox JG. The Mouse in Biomedical Research. NY: Academic Press, 1982;2.
23. Festing M. Use of genetically heterogeneous rats and mice in toxicological research: a personal perspective. Toxicol Appl Pharmacol 1990; 102:197.
24. Tucker MJ. Variations in disease in inbred and outbred strains of rodents. J Exp Anim Sci 1993; 35:244.
25. Attia MA. Neoplastic and non-neoplastic lesions in the mammary gland, endocrine, and genital organs in aging male and female Sprague-Dawley rats. Arch Toxicol 1996; 70:461.
26. Lillie LE, Temple NJ, Florence LZ. Reference values for young normal Sprague-Dawley rats: weight gain, hematology and clinical chemistry. Hum Exp Toxicol 1996; 15:612.

27. Haseman JK, Bourbina J, Eustis SL. Effect of individual housing and other experimental design factors on tumor incidence in B6C3F1 mice. Fund Appl Toxicol 1994; 23:44.

28. Lang PL, White WJ. Growth, development and survival of the Crl:CD(SD)BR stock and CDF(F344)/CrlBR strain. In: Mohr U, Dungworth DL, Capen CC, eds. In: Pathology of the Aging Rat. Washington DC: ILSI Press, 1994; 2:587.

29. McMartin DN, Sahota PS, Gunson DE, Hsu HH, Spaet RH. Neoplasms and related proliferative lesions in control Sprague-Dawley rats from carcinogenicity studies. Historical data and diagnostic considerations. Toxicol Pathol 1992; 20:212.

30. Chandra M, Frith CH. Spontaneous neoplasms in aged CD-1 mice. Toxicol Lett 1992; 61:67.

31. Maita K, Hirano M, Harada T, et al. Mortality, major cause of morbidity, and spontaneous tumors in CD-1 mice. Toxicol Pathol 1988; 16:340.

32. Turnbull GJ, Lee PN, Roe FJC. Relationship of body-weight gain to longevity and to risk of development of nepthropathy and neoplasia in Sprague-Dawley rats. Food Chem Toxicol 1985; 23:355.

33. Aoyama H, Kikuta M, Shirasaka N, et al. Histoical control data on reproductive abilities and incidence of spontaneous fetal malformations in Wistar Hannover GALAS rats. Congenit Anom Kyoto 2002; 42:194.

34. Wagner JE, Manning PJ. The Biology of the Guinea Pig. NY: Academic Press, 1976.

35. Smith RL, Caldwell J. Drug metabolism in non-human primates. In: Parke DZ, Smith RL, eds. Drug Metabolism From Microb to Man. London: Taylor and Francis, Ltd., 1977:331.

36. Phoenix CH. Guinea pigs. In: Hafez ESE, ed. Reproduction and breeding techniques for laboratory animals. NY: Academic Press, 1970:244.

37. Weisbroth SH, Flatt RE, Kraus AL. The Biology of the Laboratory Rabbit. NY: Academic Press, 1974.

38. Gibson JP. Use of rabbit in teratogenicity studies. Toxicol Appl Pharmacol 1966; 9:398.

39. Kameyama Y, Tanimura T, Yasuda M. Spontaneous malformations in laboratory animals—photographic atlas and reference data. Rabbit Congenit Anom 1980; 20:64.

40. Bortolotti A, Castelli D, Bonati M. Hematology and serum chemistry values of adult, pregnant, and newborn New Zealand rabbits. Lab Anim Sci 1989; 39:437.

41. Spence S. The Dutch-Belted rabbit: an alternative breed for developmental toxicity testing. Birth Defects Res B Dev Reprod Toxicol 2003; 68:439.

42. Parkinson C, Grasso P. The use of the dog in toxicity tests on pharmaceutical compounds. Hum Exp Toxicol 1993; 12:99.

43. Schlesinger RB. Comparative deposition of inhaled aerosols in experimental animals and humans: a review. J Toxicol Environ Health 1985; 15:197.

44. Tibbitts J. Issues related to the use of canines in toxicologic pathology—Issues with pharmacokinetics and metabolism. Toxicol Pathol 2003; 31:17.

45. Lowentine LJ. A primer of primate pathology: lesions and nonlesions. Toxicol Pathol 2003; 31:92.

46. Bennett BT, Abee CR, Henrickson R. Nonhuman Primates in Biomedical Research. NY: Academic Press, 1995.

47. Smith D, Trennery P, Farningham D, Klapwijk J. The selection of marmoset monkeys (Callithrix jacchus) in pharmaceutical toxicology. Lab Anim 2001; 35:117.

48. Guittin P, Decelle T. Future improvements and implementation of animal care practices within the animal testing regulatory environment. ILAR J 2002; 43:S80.

49. Clark RL, Antonello JM, Wenger JD, Deyerle-Brooks K, Duchai DM. Selection of food allotment for New Zealand White rabbits in developmental toxicity studies. Fund Appl Toxicol 1991; 17:584.

50. Kohn DF, Wixson SK, White WJ, Benson GJ. Anesthesia and Analgesia in Laboratory Animals. NY: Academic Press, 1997.

51. American Veterinary Medical Association. Report of the AVMA panel on euthanasia. J Am Vet Med Assoc 2000; 218:675.

52. Liebsch M, Spielmann H. Currently available in vitro methods used in the regulatory toxicology. Toxicol Lett 2002; 127:127.

53. Eisenbrand G, Pool-Zobel B, Baker V, et al. Methods of in vitro toxicology. Food Chem Toxicol 2002; 40:193.

54. Interagency Coordinating Committee on the Validation of Alternative Methods (ICCVAM). Validation and regulatory acceptance of toxicological test methods: A report of the ad hoc interagency coordinating committee on the validation of alternative methods (NIH publication no. 97-3981). Research Triangle Park: NIEHS. 1997. [http://iccvam.niehs.nih.gov/docs/ guidelines/validate.pdf].

55. OECD. Final Report of the OEDC Workshop on Harmonization of Validation and Acceptance Criteria for Alternative Toxicological Methods. OECD Publication Office, Paris, France, 1996.

56. European Commission. Test guideline B-41 phototoxicity—in vitro 3T3 NRU phototoxicity test of Annex V of the EU Directive 86/906/EEC for classification and labeling of hazardous chemicals. Off J Eur Comm 2000; L136:98.

57. Spielmann H, Balls M, Brand M, et al. EC/COLIPA Project on in vitro phototoxicity testing: first results obtained with the Balb/c 3T3 cell phototoxicity assay. Toxicol In Vitro 1994; 8:793.

58. Spielmann H, Lovell WW, Holzle E, et al. In vitro phototoxicity testing. The report and recommendations of ECVAM Workshop. Altern Lab Anim 1994; 22:314.

59. Spielmann H, Balls M, Dupuis J, et al. The international EU/COLIPA in vitro phototoxicity validation study: results of Phase II (blind trial). Part I: the 3T3 NRU phototoxicity test. Toxicol In Vitro 1998; 12:305.

60. Spielmann H, Balls M, Dupuis J, et al. Study on the UV filter chemicals from Annex VII of European Union Directive 76/768/EEC, in the in vitro 3T3 NRU phototoxicity test. Altern Lab Anim 1998; 26:679.

61. European Commission. Test guideline B-40 skin corrosivity-in vitro method of Annex V of the EU Directive 86/906/EEC for classification and labeling of hazardous chemicals. Off J Eur Comm 2002; L136:85.

62. ESAC-ECVAM Scientific Advisory Committee. Statement on the scientific validity of the rat skin transcutaneous resistance (TER) test and the EpiSkin™ test in vitro tests for skin corrosivity. Altern Lab Anim 1998; 26:275.

63. ESAC-ECVAM Scientific Advisory Committee. Statement on the application of the EpiDerm™ human skin model for skin corrosivity testing. Altern Lab Anim 2000; 28:365.

64. Fentem JH, Archer GEB, Balls M, et al. The ECVAM interbational validation study on in vitro test for skin corrosivity 2. Results and evaluation by the Management Team. Toxicol Vitro 1998; 12:483.

65. Spielmann H, Liebsch M, Kalweit S, et al. Results of a validation study in Germany on two in vitro alternatives to the Draize eye irritation test, the HET-CAM test and the 3T3 NRU cytotoxicity test. Altern Lab Anim 1996; 24:741.

66. Cooper KJ, Earl LK, Harbell J, Raabe H. Prediction of ocular irritancy of prototype shampoo formulations by the isolated rabbit eye (IRE) test and bovine corneal opacity and permeability (BCOP) assay. Toxicol Vitro 2001; 15:95.

67. Djabari Z, Bauza E, Dal C, Farra C, Domloge N. The HET-CAM test combined with histological studies for better evaluation of active ingredient innocuity. Int J Tissue React 2002; 24:117.

3
Safety Pharmacology

William S. Redfern
Safety Pharmacology Department, Safety Assessment U.K., AstraZeneca R&D Alderley Park, Macclesfield, Cheshire, U.K.

Ian D. Wakefield
Nonclinical Development, UCB Celltech, Slough, U.K.

BACKGROUND AND BASIC PRINCIPLES

Definition and Purpose

The International Conference on Harmonization of Technical Requirements for Registration of Pharmaceuticals for Human Use (ICH) has issued a set of international regulatory requirements and guidelines for safety pharmacology studies (ICHS7A; see Appendix A) (1). The ICHS7A regulatory guidance document provides the following definition of safety pharmacology:

> Those studies that investigate the potential undesirable pharmacodynamic effects of a substance on physiological functions in relation to exposure in the therapeutic range and above.

The document also lists the principal aims of safety pharmacology as being:

1. To identify undesirable pharmacodynamic properties of a substance that may have relevance to its human safety
2. To evaluate adverse pharmacodynamic and/or pathophysiological effects of a substance observed in toxicology and/or clinical studies
3. To investigate the mechanism of the adverse pharmacodynamic effects observed and/or suspected.

The aim of this chapter is to expand on these definitions and act as a starting point for the safety pharmacology evaluation of new active substances. Where possible we have guided the reader to reviews of specific topics and methodologies within the sphere of safety pharmacology. It is intended primarily as an entry-level guide for newcomers to this discipline, including toxicologists, and scientists in small pharmaceutical companies who have responsibility for outsourcing this work.

Historical Background

The first appearance of the term "safety pharmacology" in the published literature dates back to 1980 (2). The term was certainly in common usage in the 1980s within the pharmaceutical industry to describe nonclinical pharmacological evaluation of substances for regulatory submissions. Back then it was part of a wider "general pharmacology" assessment, which addressed actions of a compound beyond the therapeutically intended effects. Nowadays, the term "general pharmacology" is not widely used, and the ICHS7A guidelines distinguish between primary pharmacodynamics ("studies on the mode of action and/or effects of a substance in relation to its desired therapeutic target"), secondary pharmacodynamics ("studies on the mode of action and/or effects of a substance not related to its desired therapeutic target"), and safety pharmacology (definition as above).

Until relatively recently, the only detailed guidelines indicating the requirements from drug regulatory authorities for safety pharmacology studies were from the Japanese Ministry of Health & Welfare (MHW) (3). These delineated the "general pharmacology" studies into two lists: a "core" list (List A) and a list of follow-up studies (List B), from which studies would be selected on the basis of findings identified during the "List A" assessment, from the specific pharmacology of the new compound, and from the target population. Possibly the most important wording in these guidelines was "the use of novel technologies and methodologies in accordance with scientific progress should be applied actively," but this was generally overlooked by pharmaceutical companies, which tended to stick with study designs that the regulatory authorities had previously found acceptable (4). Nevertheless, several opinion leaders in the field continued to champion the strategic importance of safety pharmacology during the 1990s (5–10), and their efforts ultimately led to the ICHS7A guidance document.

A major catalyst for the renaissance in safety pharmacology was the release in 1996 of a draft "Points to Consider" document on QT prolongation by the European Medicines Agency's Committee for Proprietary Medicinal Products (CPMP), issued in final form the following year (11). This initiative had been prompted by growing concern of sudden death caused by drug-induced torsade de pointes, a potentially lethal cardiac tachyarrhythmia. One of the more controversial aspects of this document was the recommendation to incorporate screening of all noncardiac drugs for effects on cardiac action potential in vitro. The expertise to undertake this did not exist in good laboratory practices (GLP)-compliant safety pharmacology laboratories at that time.

The positive impact of the CPMP's document was that it bolstered safety pharmacology as a rigorous scientific discipline. It is, however, important also to maintain an appropriate level of vigilance towards each of the non-QT aspects of safety pharmacology, and hopefully this is reflected in this chapter.

Underlying Purpose of Safety Pharmacology Evaluations

Clearly, the ICHS7A guidelines have more than just "box-ticking" in mind when they outline the requirements for safety pharmacology. The primary purpose of safety pharmacology is "to predict and protect." In particular, the investigations are undertaken to protect Phase I clinical trials volunteers, as reflected by the requirement of ICHS7A to conclude requires safety pharmacology investigations prior to first time in humans. From the perspective of a pharmaceutical company, the safety pharmacology evaluations can achieve much more than this, but it is important first and foremost to achieve this aim.

Before assessing whether this aim has been achieved thus far, we have to define what types of clinical adverse effects could be predicted from nonclinical safety pharmacology tests. Adverse drug reactions (ADRs) in humans fall into 5 types (Table 1). Of these, acute safety pharmacology studies can only reasonably be expected to predict Type A adverse effects (i.e., dose-dependent ones). However, this still means that ~75% of clinical

Table 1 Classification of Adverse Drug Reactions in Humans

Type A	Dose-dependent; predictable from primary, secondary, and safety pharmacology	Main cause of ADRs ($\sim 75\%$), rarely lethal
Type B	Idiosyncratic response, not predictable, not dose-related	Responsible for $\sim 25\%$ of ADRs, but majority of lethal ones
Type C	Long-term adaptive changes, predictable from repeat-dose toxicity studies	Commonly occurs with some classes of drug
Type D	Delayed effects, e.g., carcinogenicity, teratogenicity	Low incidence
Type E	Rebound effects following discontinuation of therapy	Commonly occurs with some classes of drug

Abbreviation: ADRs, adverse drug reactions.
Source: From Refs. 4, 12, 13.

adverse effects are potentially predictable on the basis of preclinical safety pharmacology studies.

According to the published literature, there have only been four deaths of volunteers in clinical pharmacology studies over the last 40 years (4). Two of these were due to an undeclared existing therapy, resulting in a fatal interaction with the test drug, whereas the third was due to a delayed, neoplastic effect. More importantly, only two of these were Phase I clinical evaluations of a new candidate drug by pharmaceutical companies. Adequate safety pharmacology testing has only made a small contribution to this good safety record; the design of the Phase I trials, with ascending dose regimens, the presence of a physician, and the availability of resuscitation equipment, are probably more important in preventing lethality. Nonetheless, the main message here is that we should not be complacent. The data on "moderately severe" (and even "potentially life-threatening") adverse events leave room for improvement (4), a point re-emphasised by the catastrophic outcome in the phase I trial of TGN1412 in 2006 (14).

Looking beyond the immediate regulatory aims of safety pharmacology evaluations, throughout clinical development it is generally acknowledged that of the new chemical entities (NCEs), excluding anti-infectives, that fail prior to marketing, about 16% do so because of ADRs during clinical trials (15). After the surviving drugs make it onto the market, they are by no means free of ADRs. It has been estimated that ADRs may be the 4th leading cause of death in the U.S.A., behind heart disease, cancer, and stroke (13). Although this claim remains controversial, a similar incidence has also been reported in the United Kingdom (16).

Finally, we can look at the drugs that have been withdrawn from sale in various markets due to serious ADRs. The most topical examples of these are agents associated with torsades de pointes: nine such products have been withdrawn from various markets in the last decade (17). In terms of all drug withdrawals over a 40-year period (1960–99), those reasons for withdrawal that could conceivably have been predicted by safety pharmacology evaluations were cardiovascular (8.7%), renal (4.1%), neurological (4.1%), psychiatric (3.7%), and abuse (3.7%), giving a total of 25% (18). Thus, in principle, better safety pharmacology could reduce product withdrawals by up to 25% by removing compounds with potential safety issues preclinically.

Therefore, in reality, the aims of nonclinical safety pharmacology evaluations are threefold: to protect Phase I clinical trials volunteers from acute adverse effects of drugs;

to protect patients (including patients during clinical trials and postlicensing); and to minimise the risks of product failure. This last aim is not restricted merely to preventing withdrawal from sale: regulatory authorities may not approve new products (or permit extensions into new indications) if the safety profile is inferior to treatments already available. Even if they do, the labeling will reflect safety issues and may affect physician prescribing, and patient compliance is affected by adverse effects, even if they are not serious safety concerns. In summary, there are both tangible and intangible benefits of conducting high quality safety pharmacology assessments: prediction of up to 75% of clinical adverse effects, reduction of project failure during clinical development by up to 16%, reduction of product withdrawals by up to 25%, and improved product success through better patient compliance. There is therefore plenty of scope for improvement in the quality and predictive power of safety pharmacology evaluations, and even achieving a small fraction of these potential benefits could make a large difference to reducing pipeline attrition and improving product success.

Distinctions Between Safety Pharmacology and Toxicology

Although some toxicologists view safety pharmacology as a branch of toxicology, this can be countered by other definitions (19) that include toxicology as a branch of pharmacology! Rather than getting bogged-down in philosophical and semantic arguments, it is more worthwhile to describe the differences in aims and emphasis between the two disciplines. In broad, general terms, safety pharmacology evaluates biological *responses* to drugs, whereas toxicology assesses toxic *effects* of drugs and chemicals. Clearly there is overlap between the two disciplines, with some pharmacological responses leading to histopathological outcomes, but the emphasis between the two disciplines is subtly different (Table 2). The two disciplines are clearly complementary in preclinical risk assessment.

Safety pharmacologists have to plan for expected, potential, and unexpected effects. Therefore all compounds need to pass through a set of tests for "the unexpected," whereas

Table 2 Principal Differences Between Safety Pharmacology and General Toxicology Studies

	Safety pharmacology	General toxicology
GLP	Yes	Yes
Adverse effect type predicted	Type A	Types C–D (mainly)
Primary endpoints	Functional responses/effects	Gross clinical signs; ECG/blood pressure (dog); histopathology
Dosing regimen	Single dose (usually)	Repeat-dose (mainly)
Key exposure parameter	C_{max}	AUC
Dose-effect relationship	Can be linear or bell-shaped	Rarely bell-shaped
Knowledge of chemical structure	Usually of limited interest	Important
Sex of animals	Usually males	Males and females
Basis for risk assessment	Margins	NOAEL
Study design	Continuous innovation (fast-moving field)	Long-established techniques

Abbreviations: AUC, area under curve; C_{max}, maximum plasma concentration achieved; ECG, electrocardiogram; GLP, good laboratory practices; NOAEL, no observed adverse effect level.

additional tests should be applied where there is additional cause for concern. A penchant for "pattern recognition" is also a valuable asset to the safety pharmacologist, as sometimes the available data do not always appear to make sense.

"Need-to-Know" vs. "Nice-to-Have"

With limited, finite resources, this is an important question for safety pharmacologists. "Will the outcome of this study impact on the course of the project?" This cold logic is very seductive but makes some hidden assumptions, the main one being that we can find good products using a minimalist approach, and also misses the point. What safety pharmacology is really about is information-gathering, profiling, and getting to know our compound so as to minimize surprises later on. If an adverse effect exists, then the harder we look for it, the more likely we are to find it. If in doubt, it is better to do a well-designed study using appropriate, validated techniques, than to do nothing at all. Conversely, it is better to do nothing at all than to run the compound through an ill-conceived, mediocre study or apply an unproven technique. Therefore, the initial cost of doing "good science" pays off in the long run, even if the outcome of this particular study in isolation cannot be viewed as pivotal to the course of a project. The best starting point is to ask "What evaluations would we undertake on this compound if we had unlimited resources?," then trim it down, rather than ask "What is the minimum we need to do to satisfy the regulators?" One person's "Nice-to-know" may be a regulator's "Need-to-know!"

Selection of Methodology and Species

The following points are worth considering (4):

1. It is preferable to use the same species for in vivo tests as those used in Drug Metabolism & Pharmacokinetics (DMPK) and toxicology—generally rat and dog
2. The methods should be well-established (i.e., not a test invented internally that has not been subject to external evaluation)
3. The methods should be in common use in research and not in major decline
4. The methods should be validated in-house with at least one reference substance with known effects in humans
5. They should give reliable, reproducible results every time
6. The level of technical difficulty should be compatible with routine use.

Generally speaking, techniques traditionally used in safety pharmacology have been adapted from those applied to "discovery pharmacology," and it is therefore important for safety pharmacologists to maintain awareness of new techniques. However, safety pharmacologists also have to adopt techniques that have traditionally been the domain of neurotoxicologists and physiologists (20). It is up to each safety pharmacology department to select tests that are suited to them; adoption of a tiered, sequential approach also reduces the reliance on any one test for any particular aspect of organ function (4).

Predictive Value of Safety Pharmacology Data

Fundamental to what we are trying to achieve lies the question: *"Do safety pharmacology tests predict side effects in humans"?* The honest answer is that it is difficult to acquire hard evidence either way. If a candidate drug has an unfavorable outcome in a preclinical test, there may be limited information in the public domain, as the result may have precluded clinical development. If there has been no effect in a preclinical test, and likewise no effect in the corresponding variable in humans, these negative data may have been deemed not to be of publishable interest. What are then left are the high-profile examples of side effects in humans that were apparently not detected preclinically. Obviously, this tends to bias our perspective.

For "safety assessment" in general, even as far back as the 1960s, it was estimated on a survey of 234 drugs that toxicities detected in the rat predicted 18% of toxic effects in humans, whereas in dog this increased to 24%, with 23% of human toxic effects undetected in either species (21). The situation has improved since then with the most recent assessment indicating that studies in rodents predicted 43%, whereas studies in non-rodents predicted 63% of ADRs (22). Apart from one publication, which revealed some incongruous correlations in amongst more plausible ones (23), there has been no systematic attempt to investigate predictive power across a range of safety pharmacology endpoints. This has, however, been investigated systematically for nonclinical cardiac electrophysiology data where, for example, the margin between C_{max} (unbound) and hERG IC_{50} was found to be a good predictor of torsadogenic risk (24–26). The only other information we have available are overall measures of success or failure of development compounds and specific case histories. Clearly this is an area requiring a collaborative effort within the pharmaceutical industry. For now, we have to make intelligent judgment based on knowledge of the literature, experience with different models, and acceptability by regulatory authorities.

There are various reasons why preclinical safety pharmacology tests may not always predict human adverse effects (4):

1. Anatomical/physiological species differences (e.g., rats do not vomit)
2. Species differences in the presence, functionality, or role of the molecular target mediating the adverse effect
3. Differences in drug metabolism and pharmacokinetics between test species and humans
4. Sensitivity of the test system—observations of a qualitative nature should be followed up with specific, quantitative assessment
5. Poor optimization of test conditions—the "baseline" level has to be set correctly to detect drug-induced changes
6. Insufficiently powered studies
7. Inappropriate timing of functional measurements in relation to T_{max}
8. Delayed effects—safety pharmacology studies generally involve a single administration with monitoring for up to 24 hours postdose
9. Difficulty of detection in animals—e.g., adverse effects such as headache, disorientation, and hallucinations.

Depending on the nature of the safety pharmacology test, it may not be possible to predict with accuracy at what plasma concentration an adverse effect will appear in man, but it should at least be possible to provide a reasonable estimate. Given that safety pharmacology studies will test at multiples of therapeutic doses, even if the test system is less sensitive than humans, it should at least flag-up an effect at a high dose level.

Optimization of Methodology, Test Conditions, and Study Design

The key to obtaining good data is to involve experienced staff in the study design and execution. Often, the techniques that appear to be the "simplest" are the ones that require the most experience to obtain good data. Test conditions should be optimized and validated before use with NCEs. Validation with a reference substance may be relatively straightforward in the case of a single-variable test (e.g., rotarod), but for methods that measure multiple functions (e.g., cardiovascular telemetry), the laboratory must demonstrate that it can detect changes in each of the variables in both directions. Some of this may have to be retrospective following an effect with a candidate drug, but this runs the risk of false negatives that go undetected in an "insensitive" or even "flawed" technique.

One question that often arises is whether to use fed or fasted animals for safety pharmacology studies. Although fasting may intuitively be expected to facilitate absorption of orally administered compounds, this may not necessarily be the case. Also, fasting may increase the anxiety level in animals, which may impact on the outcome of the study. It may also affect turnover of central neurotransmitters and thereby influence behavioral responses to drugs (27). It is sometimes prudent to adjust feeding times in certain studies (e.g., to avoid effects on telemetry recordings; limit emesis in dogs), but otherwise, unless specifically required for certain gastrointestinal assessments or because of well-characterized effects of food on absorption of a particular compound, it is generally preferable to leave animals with *ad lib* access to food.

Statistical Power

For any given technique we could use group sizes most commonly used in the published literature and calculate the magnitude of change in the variable under study that this will enable us to detect. Alternatively, we can decide on the magnitude of the effect that we consider to be "biologically significant" or "cause for concern" and then estimate the sample sizes required to detect it. This latter option is not as straightforward as the first (4). Setting of thresholds for "biological significance" or "cause for concern" tend to be fairly arbitrary and are sometimes unrealistic in terms of sensitivity of the assay. For example, in a survey of the pharmaceutical industry for changes in QT, a change of $> 10\%$ was the most popular threshold of "biological significance," yet the studies were not generally of sufficient power to detect this (28). It may therefore be simpler after all to adopt group sizes in accordance with the published literature and to estimate the sensitivity of the technique using power analysis based on validation data.

Good Laboratory Practice

ICHS7A concedes that "[d]ue to the unique design of, and practical considerations for, some safety pharmacology studies, it may not be feasible to conduct these in compliance with good laboratory practice." In principle, it is possible to conduct the studies themselves to GLP; the problems arise with data acquisition software. Many state-of-the-art software packages are designed with academic research and discovery pharmacology in mind. The demand for GLP-compliant systems may not be sufficiently large to develop this feature. The deficiencies usually arise in electronic signatures, data integrity, and audit trails. Safety pharmacology laboratories are sometimes faced with the choice between a superb, non-GLP compliant package, an inferior, user-unfriendly but GLP-compliant product, or manual data handling. Because safety pharmacology techniques are quite diverse, this can be a significant problem.

ICHS7A further advises that "[t]he safety pharmacology core battery should ordinarily be conducted in compliance with GLP. Follow-up and supplemental studies should be conducted in compliance with GLP to the greatest extent feasible." This is quite achievable by safety pharmacology laboratories. The demand is usually sufficient for GLP-compliant software for the major core battery techniques (because all pharmaceutical companies are obliged to run their candidate drugs through them prior to human exposure), whereas the ICHS7A guidance document accepts the difficulty of achieving GLP compliance for less-frequently-applied follow-up and supplemental studies, which sometimes have to be outsourced to academic groups in the case of specialized techniques. Quality assurance units (or consultancy services) can advise on how to raise the standards of such noncompliant studies as high as possible, thus approaching GLP compliance "to the greatest extent feasible." Generally speaking, noncompliant studies conducted in a GLP-compliant facility (where there are GLP systems in place, the staff are used to working to GLP, and where non-GLP studies are conducted to the same standard as GLP-compliant studies) are far less of a problem than noncompliant, niche-market contract research laboratories and academic research laboratories.

ICHS7A Guidance Document—An Overview

It is not possible to summarize a regulatory guidance document such as ICHS7A, and the document itself should be read carefully. However, this section is merely intended to provide an overview to this document as an introduction to it. In summary, the guidance document recommends that appropriate safety pharmacology *core battery* studies are conducted to address potential adverse effects on the three vital organ functions: central nervous system, cardiovascular, and respiratory. *Follow-up studies* should be conducted to investigate functional adverse effects in more depth when there is cause for concern, including those identified in the core battery studies, toxicology studies, clinical investigations, and literature reports. Follow-up studies conducted in response to preclinical findings should be conducted prior to first administration to humans. In some instances, the core battery should be supplemented with additional studies on organ system functions not addressed by the core battery or repeat-dose toxicity studies, where there is cause for concern. Such *supplementary studies* should be considered if concerns arise from the pharmacological or chemical class of the test substance, from previous in vitro or in vivo studies, or from literature reports. Such organ systems include the renal/urinary system, autonomic nervous system, gastrointestinal system, skeletal muscle, immune, and endocrine systems; dependency/abuse potential would also come into this category. Sometimes these would be conducted as stand-alone studies (e.g., gastric emptying); in other instances they may involve additional measurements incorporated into the core battery studies (e.g., measurements of blood glucose if hypoglycaemia is anticipated). The subsequent sections of this chapter address each organ function separately, including core battery, supplemental, and follow-up studies.

The impact of the ICHS7A guidance document on safety pharmacology has been discussed elsewhere (29). Other regulatory guidance documents that impact on safety pharmacology are provided in a recent review (30); since its publication in 2004, further guidance documents relevant to safety pharmacology have been released (Appendix A).

ASSESSMENT OF MAJOR ORGAN FUNCTIONS

Cardiovascular System

Except for a limited number of drugs that are delivered directly to their target organ (e.g., inhaled drugs for respiratory disorders; certain drugs for gastrointestinal disorders administered orally or rectally; topically applied drugs for dermatological or ocular treatments), the overriding majority of drugs will require entry to the cardiovascular system to access their site of action. It is therefore not surprising that cardiovascular adverse effects are fairly commonplace and, given the importance of the cardiovascular system in maintaining both immediate and long-term homeostasis, potentially dangerous. The cardiovascular system is very dynamic, because it is both under the control of cardio-vascular and other reflexes and influenced by higher brain regions. It is therefore able to react rapidly to the demands of the organism, whether they be emotional (e.g., anxiety, excitement) or preparing for or responding to specific demands, e.g., postural changes, sleep-wakefulness cycle, exercise, defense ('fight-flight'), digestion, and so on. This is achieved by altering heart rate, force of cardiac contraction, blood pressure, and blood flows to different regional vascular beds. Reflexes diminish with age, and so the cardiovascular system in elderly patients may respond differently to drugs than that of a young, healthy volunteer. For example, if a neuroprotective agent targeted at stroke also causes vasodilatation, the ensuing hypotension may be minimal in animals and in young volunteers, whereas in elderly stroke patients this could be more substantial, which would mitigate against the primary neuroprotective effect by impacting on cerebral perfusion (31). Both the myocardium and vascular system respond differently to drugs in disease states (e.g., myocardial ischaemia, heart failure, diabetes), which should also be borne in mind.

Therefore there is more to evaluating safety pharmacology effects on the cardiovascular system than snapshot measurements of blood pressure, heart rate, and ECG in repeat-dose toxicity studies, and any cardiovascular recordings are susceptible to recording conditions. In safety pharmacology studies, different elements of cardiovascular function can be addressed in different tests, using a variety of species. Nonetheless, it is more efficient to restrict the species to the two used in toxicology studies (principally rat and dog) where possible.

It is also important to consider the method of administration, particularly when test compounds are administered intravenously. Highly viscous vehicles may physically restrict blood flow through the pulmonary circulation, leading to an increase in pulmonary arterial pressure, reduced pulmonary blood flow leading to impaired gaseous exchange, and all the consequences of this (respiratory stimulation, tachycardia, and increased arterial blood pressure). A large volume administered very quickly can cause a volume-loading effect and hemodilution, leading to tachycardia and respiratory stimulation. A high dose of any substance administered too quickly will result in virtually the concentration in the syringe travelling round as a bolus, which could be in the millimolar range. This could have any manner of effects on the cardiovascular system, either directly, by activating reflex afferents, or by effects on cardiovascular control regions of the CNS, particularly those outside the blood-brain barrier.

An area of intense concern both to regulatory authorities and the pharmaceutical industry is that of drug-induced torsade de pointes (17). A full consideration of this issue is outside the scope of this chapter, but numerous reviews explore the issues involved and offer strategies for the pharmaceutical industry (25,32–38). Some of the key issues involved are illustrated in Figure 1. The surface ECG represents the net sum of the electrical activity in all the individual myocytes. Delayed ventricular repolarisation leads to prolongation of the action potential duration (APD), which is reflected as prolongation of the QT interval of the ECG. This can promote the conditions for the occurrence of early after-depolarizations in individual myocytes, which may spread further as ectopic beats, and lead to the ventricular tachyarrhythmia torsade de pointes, where the QRS complexes rotate around an imaginary isoelectric line (37). This can lead to ventricular fibrillation and sudden death (36,37). Several ion channels play a role in ventricular repolarization, but of these, the rapid component of the delayed rectifier (I_{Kr}), which carries an outward potassium current, has been implicated for the vast majority of drugs that have caused

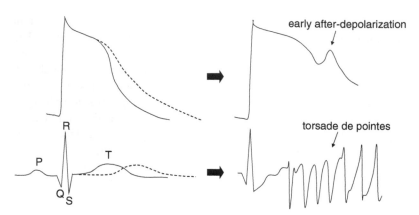

Figure 1 Relationship between increase in cardiac action potential duration, QT prolongation and torsade de pointes. Upper left panel: action potential of an individual cardiac ventricular cell (schematic), showing drug-induced prolongation of action potential duration (dotted line). Upper right panel: development of early after-depolarization during prolonged repolarization phase. Lower left panel: surface electrocardiogram (schematic), showing summation of effects of an action potential-prolonging drug on QT interval (dotted line). P-wave: atrial depolarization; QRS complex: ventricular depolarization; T-wave: ventricular repolarization. Lower right panel: degeneration into torsade de pointes, triggered by early after-depolarizations.

torsade de pointes in humans (24). This current is carried by the channel encoded by the human ether-à-go-go-related gene (hERG) (39,40).

Cardiovascular Pre–Core Battery "Screening" Techniques ("Frontloading")

Some projects carry a known cardiovascular risk and may require non-GLP evaluation of several compounds to enable selection of one or more with the lowest cardiovascular liability. The key factors at this stage influencing the choice of techniques are the number of compounds required to be tested (i.e., throughput), the quantity of material available, and the 3 Rs (replacement, refinement and reduction, with respect to the use of live animals in research).

hERG Channel Interactions.   This can be assessed using conventional whole-cell voltage clamp electrophysiology (the gold standard), automated electrophysiology, rubidium efflux, fluorescence assays, or radioligand binding, and their relative merits have been discussed elsewhere (41–44). The IC_{50} data generated are useful for selecting compounds with the lowest "QT liability." Although chemists work with hERG potency (i.e., IC_{50} values) to "design-out" hERG activity, the most important parameter to consider is the margin between the hERG IC_{50} and the predicted therapeutic free C_{max} in humans (24). hERG potency per se does not correlate well with QT prolongation, whereas "hERG margins" are a fairly good predictor of torsadogenic risk (24,25). Based on a survey of 100 marketed drugs, a margin of >30-fold between hERG IC_{50} and therapeutic free C_{max} in humans appears to confer a minimal risk of torsade de pointes (26). However, hERG margins alone are not sufficient for preclinical assessment of proarrhythmic risk; this requires evaluation of effects on hERG, QT interval in vivo, and possibly evaluation of effects on action potential characteristics in vitro. For those compounds with "low" margins in the above tests, further evaluation in a proarrhythmia model may also be required. Nonetheless, early hERG data are useful to drug discovery projects. Even if the ₒins are based on potency at either the primary molecular target or in a cell-based assay, they can help influence decision-making at an early stage. It is also possible to attempt to reduce potency at hERG at the molecular design stage, using in silico predictive modeling, although at present this is only capable of providing relatively crude estimates of hERG potency (45).

In Vivo "Screening" Methods. If a project carries a high cardiovascular liability, frontloading in vivo studies may be justified. Because of limited compound supply, these will almost certainly not involve the use of large animals, such as the dog. The two main options are the use of anesthetized animals or conscious animals implanted with telemetry transducers. The rat is suitable for measuring ECG, blood pressure, and heart rate, and it is relatively straightforward to take blood samples for bioanalysis from a tail vein. Blood pressure recordings are stable for at least 6 months in telemetered rats (46). However, ventricular repolarisation is relatively brief in the rat due to the minimal influence of the hERG K^+ current, and so this species is unsuitable for predicting "QT liability" (28). This does not preclude its usefulness for assessing effects on blood pressure, heart rate, and PR interval.

For meaningful QT measurements, the guinea pig is preferable to the rat. This species is less robust than the rat for cardiovascular recordings, and the absence of a tail implies that blood samples would have to be taken by an indwelling intravenous catheter. Nonetheless, this species is very useful for ECG recordings by telemetry (47) and for recording cardiac monophasic action potential (MAP) (48), and the blood sampling problem could be circumvented by using satellite groups.

Cardiovascular Core Battery Techniques

Here, the choices are between species (generally dog, minipig, or cynomolgus monkey) and technique (telemetry or anesthetized). The majority of safety pharmacology laboratories use beagle dogs for these evaluations (28), but minipigs are equally valid (49,50). From a 3Rs perspective, cynomolgus monkeys (and the use of primates generally) should be reserved for evaluating compounds where the primary molecular target is not present (or not functional) in the dog or minipig, for example, most biotechnology products and some conventional NCEs, or where there is dose-limiting, species-specific toxicity in the dog.

Telemetry enables 24-hour recordings of blood pressure, heart rate, core temperature, and lead II ECG from undisturbed animals in their home cage/pen. Other measurements (e.g., left ventricular pressure) are also possible, although telemetry transducers have technical limitations on the number of recordings made from a single animal. However, dog telemetry would generally be the default method for the cardiovascular core battery (28).

Anesthetized animals would be used instead of telemetry when more subtle cardiovascular effects are suspected, when prolonged emesis is likely, when untoward CNS effects are expected, or when the risks to the telemetered animals are considered too great. Anesthetized animals do have some benefits over telemetered ones: the baselines are steadier, assisting detection of small effects; more variables can be measured simultaneously (including multilead ECGs, left ventricular function, cardiac MAP, pulmonary arterial pressure, regional blood flows, respiratory function, and even renal function), and the heart can be paced if required. The disadvantages are the effects of anaesthetics, the relatively short recording period, and the requirement to use intravenous or intraduodenal routes of administration (although predosing orally is possible). Different anaesthetics have effects on cardiac ion channels, QT interval, heart rate, and blood pressure to varying extents (28).

For both conscious and anesthetised animals, a key technical issue is correction of QT interval for changes in heart rate (28,38). QT interval increases as the RR interval increases; this change is not instantaneous, so any correction should use data for RR interval or heart rate averaged over several cardiac cycles (51), particularly in view of the pronounced sinus arrhythmia in the dog. Some correction factors are better than others: Bazett's correction is unsuitable for use in dogs, whereas several others are far more appropriate (51–55). Computerized data acquisition from telemetered animals (and to a lesser extent, from anesthetized animals) enables relationships between QT and RR (or heart rate) to be plotted for individual dogs over a reasonable range of heart rates (28,56,57). This is a superior approach to the use of correction factors, although because no automated ECG software is as yet 100% reliable, more work is involved in manual checking. Nonetheless, this approach enables detection of drug-induced changes in QT interval outside the range caused by autonomic influences (57). It has even been taken one step further to assess increased beat-to-beat variability, suggested to be predictive of torsadogenic activity (58,59).

Cardiovascular Follow-Up and Supplemental Studies: "QT" Issues

Cardiac Action Potential Characteristics In Vitro (and In Vivo). Suitable preparations include Purkinje fibre (dog, sheep, rabbit, pig), papillary muscle (guinea pig, rabbit, ferret), and myocytes (any of the aforementioned species). The relative merits of each preparation are outlined elsewhere (37,60). Whereas the choice of preparation for assessing ventricular repolarisation was a source of debate ever since its inclusion in the 1997 CPMP document, the advent of the hERG assay enables safety pharmacology laboratories to use their own particular favorite action potential preparation. A consensus is unlikely, and in subsequent ICHS7B drafts, culminating in the final version, the action potential assay has been downgraded in importance compared to its preeminence in the 1997 CPMP document (61,62).

Some safety pharmacology departments include these techniques routinely or on a case-by-case basis as part of their core battery (28), although the final version of ICHS7B no longer requires this (61). It is, however, a great leap in complexity from studying effects on a single ion channel (i.e., hERG) to measuring effects on QT interval in vivo. If the hERG margin is very large (e.g., > 100-fold) and there are no effects observed on QT interval, it is probably not worthwhile investigating effects on action potential characteristics. On the other hand, such preparations will detect effects on other ion channels and will pick up changes other than just increases in repolarisation time (63–65). Particular advantages of in vitro cardiac action potential preparations over in vivo QT assessments include the ability to manipulate the experimental conditions, including assessment of rate-dependence (i.e., reverse-use dependence, by varying the rate of stimulation), use of high drug concentrations, and alterations in extracellular K^+ concentration (63,66). Derived parameters include resting membrane potential (in mV), maximum rate of depolarization (V_{max}), and APD, which is measured at different stages of repolarization, where the subscript notation indicates the percentage completeness of the repolarization (e.g., APD_{50}, APD_{90}). Some highly torsadogenic drugs (e.g., cisapride and dofetilide) will also produce early after-depolarizations in in vitro preparations at low pacing frequencies (63,65). In these assays it is important to check whether the test compound is adhering to the glass or plastic surfaces of the perfusion system or whether there are issues of solubility and stability, by comparing concentrations before and after perfusion to establish the actual tissue exposure (66). Ventricular repolarisation can also be assessed by measuring MAPs in anaesthetised guinea-pigs, a technique that bridges the gap between in vitro and in vivo (48).

Proarrhythmia Models. Delayed ventricular repolarisation per se is not life-threatening: it is merely a risk factor for torsade de pointes. Where margins between effects on hERG current, APD, or QT interval are considered low enough to give cause for concern, it is prudent to test the compound in a proarrhythmia model (24,67,68). Such models may either be in vitro or in vivo (67). In vitro models include the rabbit-isolated Langendorff heart preparation, (67,69) and the canine ventricular wedge preparation (67,70). In vivo models include the methoxamine-infused rabbit (67,71,72) and the chronic AV node-blocked dog (67,72,74). A key feature of the mechanisms underlying torsade de pointes (TdP) is that different cell types within the myocardium have different repolarization times, different contributions from the various ionic currents to their action potentials, and therefore different susceptibilities to individual hERG-blocking drugs (70). This differential effect of hERG blockers within the myocardium leads to increased dispersion of repolarization. It has been suggested that increased dispersion of repolarization across the left ventricular wall (i.e., transmural dispersion), rather than QT prolongation per se, is responsible for TdP (70). Consequently, in the presence of a hERG blocker it is possible for ectopic current flow to reenter areas that have repolarized in a circuit (70). This is only possible to study in whole hearts and ventricular wedge preparations, not in homogeneous cell preparations, such as Purkinje fibres. In the Hondeghem rabbit Langendorff model, in addition to overt arrhythmic events (such as early after-depolarizations and extrasystoles) the three cardinal indicators of proarrhythmia are reverse-use dependence (i.e., a greater prolongation of APD at lower pacing frequencies), triangulation of the action potential (where there is a greater prolongation of APD_{90} relative to earlier parts of the repolarization), and temporal instability (increased beat-to-beat variability of APD) (67,69,75).

The value of proarrhythmia models to safety pharmacology was highlighted recently in the case of the putative antianginal drug ranolazine. This drug has a relatively low margin between its IC_{50} at hERG and the therapeutic free C_{max} in humans and caused modest QT prolongation in clinical trials (76). Not surprisingly, the FDA was concerned about torsadogenic risk (77). The manufacturers opted to assess proarrhythmia in a range of models and were able to argue (successfully) that it was not proarrhythmic; if anything, it showed some antiarrhythmic properties (78–81). This also illustrates the additional safety pharmacology "baggage" accrued by a compound with a small "hERG margin," in terms of the nonclinical follow-up work that is required to establish cardiac safety. In the case of ranolazine, this was established; other candidate drugs may not be as fortunate.

Cardiovascular Follow-Up and Supplemental Studies: "Non-QT" Issues

Isolated Atria. Frequently, compounds are found to cause changes in heart rate in the core battery test (e.g., telemetered dog). The next step is to determine whether this was caused by a direct effect on the cardiac pacemaker (sinoatrial node), an effect on sympathetic, or vagal influences on the pacemaker (i.e., blocking muscarinic or β-adrenoceptors, interfering with neurotransmitter release or re-uptake, ganglionic blockade, etc.), interference with cardiovascular reflexes, or a centrally mediated effect. A reasonable starting point is to test the effects of the compound in vitro in isolated atria from guinea pig or rat, examining both direct effects and modulation of responses to adrenergic and cholinergic agonists. An alternative is to do equivalent investigations using whole-cell voltage clamp techniques to determine effects on pacemaker currents in mammalian atrial cells (82,83).

Pithed Rat.   Traditionally, the definitive pharmacological technique for assessing direct effects on the cardiovascular system was the pithed rat (84). After physical destruction of the central nervous system, the animal is maintained on a ventilator [adjusted by monitoring for arterial blood gases & pH; (85)], normotensive blood pressure may be maintained by stimulating the thoracicolumbar sympathetic vasomotor outflow, and body core temperature maintained by a heating blanket. This technique eliminates any influences of cardiovascular reflexes, the central nervous system, or of anaesthesia, and enables direct effects on the cardiovascular system to be assessed. Although once commonly used in the pharmaceutical industry (86,87), it would be very unusual to find this technique in use in safety pharmacology laboratories nowadays. Even in academic laboratories, if publications reflect the amount of research using this technique, its use has been dwindling since its heyday in the 1980s. That is not to say that the model has been superseded; we merely point this out to indicate that contract laboratories offering this technique nowadays are few and far between.

Hemodynamics.   Although the monitoring of cardiovascular effects by telemetry can provide valuable information on changes to arterial blood pressure and heart rate, it does not allow evaluation of hemodynamics or cardiac performance. Blood pressure can be a relatively insensitive measure of hemodynamic changes because there are extensive inherent buffering mechanisms to maintain homeostasis. Blood pressure is a composite variable, reflecting cardiac output and the total sum of peripheral vascular resistances, and as such, marked changes can occur in regional hemodynamics and subsequent organ/tissue blood perfusion with potentially no change in blood pressure. For example, increased blood flow in one vascular bed may be compensated for by a reduction in flow to other vascular beds with no net change in blood pressure. Similarly small reductions in cardiac output may be balanced by local and/or autonomic-derived mediators increasing vascular resistance to maintain normotension, and vice versa. Reductions in regional blood flows and tissue perfusion may have potential for adverse effects in the clinic, which could range from relatively minor (e.g., headache) to more profound events, such as decreased renal clearance and inadequate tissue perfusion to maintain normal physiological function, tissue metabolism, and/or detoxification mechanisms.

A number of methods are available to directly monitor changes in blood flow and to derive vascular conductance. These include electromagnetic, ultrasonic Doppler-based, transit-time ultrasound techniques and laser-based flow transducers placed on or around selected vessels to monitor blood flow (88–91). Typically, such flow probes may be used in anaesthetised animals, and the availability of miniature flow probes can enable blood flows to be studied in smaller species, such as the rat. Flow probes designed for longer-term use can allow repeated dose effects to be studied in chronically instrumented larger species, which when combined with telemetric blood pressure sensors and surface ECG leads provides a more comprehensive cardiovascular appraisal. Miniaturised pulsed Doppler flow probes have been implanted successfully in rats for measurement of blood flow in up to three vascular beds, together with arterial blood pressure and heart rate, in conscious, freely moving rats (92,93). Other methods using injected radioactive, fluorescent, or dye-coupled microspheres may be used to study regional blood flow and organ perfusion (90,94). A combination of perivascular probes with terminal microsphere administration can be used for investigative purposes when altered tissue perfusion is suspected as being contributory to adverse toxicological findings in organs.

More commonly, these are used in anaesthetised preparations and, when combined with methods for evaluating cardiac output and/or left ventricular function, provide a comprehensive evaluation of the responses to test agents. The aforementioned limitations of using anaesthetised preparations restricts the evaluations that can be achieved, particularly with regard to monitoring prolonged or delayed responses, and the influences of the anaesthetic agents(s) used. However, telemetry techniques exist in dogs for continuous recording of left ventricular pressure (95).

Cardiovascular Reflexes. The main cardiovascular reflexes are the baroreceptor reflex, which serves to restore blood pressure to within a normotensive range following excursions in either direction due to whatever cause; chemoreceptor reflexes, which alter autonomic and respiratory outflows due to changes in arterial blood gases and pH; and atrial reflexes, which monitor and maintain blood volume. Each of these reflexes can be affected by certain drugs acting either at the baroreceptors and chemoreceptors themselves (located at strategic locations within the circulation) or at synapses within the CNS.

The simplest method of testing the baroreceptor reflex in conscious animals is by intravenous infusion of pressor and depressor agents, such as phenylephrine and sodium nitroprusside, and to measure reflex changes in heart rate (96). Some drugs (e.g., clonidine) increase the slope (and therefore the gain) of the baroreceptor-heart rate reflex. This approach is also helpful (if not definitive) in deciding whether a drug-induced change in heart rate is of the magnitude to be expected for any given change in blood pressure. For example, if in telemetered dogs a test compound increased mean arterial blood pressure from 105 to 117 mmHg and lowered heart rate from 76 to 66 beats/min, a plot of heart rate versus blood pressure (achieved by infusing phenylephrine and/or nitroprusside) in the same dogs would indicate whether the observed change in heart rate was outside the predicted range for the associated change in blood pressure. Changes in heart rate in the opposite direction to effects on blood pressure are often explained away as being due to baroreceptor reflex changes, but this is rarely checked.

Heart Rate Variability. The advent of 24-hour monitoring of heart rate (either from an ECG signal recorded noninvasively or from a blood pressure signal obtained via a surgically implanted telemetry device) has enabled spectral power analysis of heart rate variability in both rats (97) and dogs (98). Changes in power spectra reflect changes in autonomic tone, which can be influenced by test compounds.

Nervous System

Unwanted side effects on the nervous system are commonly seen both in clinical trials of new drugs and during therapeutic use of marketed products. They have accounted for 10% of all drugs withdrawn from sale during the period 1960–99 (18). To put this in perspective, drugs withdrawn due to torsade de pointes during this period accounted for 7.5% of the total (18). The central nervous system has extremely diverse functions, ranging from the control of vegetative functions (including via the autonomic nervous system) to higher cognitive functions, such as learning, memory, and problem-solving. To address each of these functions, to the same degree of precision as that achieved in the cardiovascular core battery (where the telemetered dog is used, for example) would require an unrealistic number of tests and animals. Instead, safety pharmacology effects on the nervous system, including the central nervous system (CNS) in the core battery has to rely on a multi-observational assessment, involving a battery of tests and observations conducted on the same individual animals, covering a broad range of neurological and behavioral functions.

As mentioned under the section on the cardiovascular system, the target population is also important when assessing potential CNS adverse effects. Juvenile and geriatric patient groups may be more susceptible to impairment of cognitive processes. These considerations may influence the scale of the preclinical safety pharmacology investigations into potential CNS adverse effects. Some drugs may have the potential

Table 3 Approaches to Studying Adverse Effects of Drugs on the Nervous System

Methodology	Examples
Behavioral/neuro-logical	Functional Observational Battery/Irwin Test; locomotor activity; motor coordination; nociception; auditory function; visual function; proconvulsive tests; cognitive tests; operant tests; abuse liability, etc.
Neurophysiological recordings	EEG; ERG; EMG; BAER; nerve conduction velocity
Neuroimaging	PET; SPECT
Neurochemical	In vivo microdialysis
Neurohistopathology	(Refer to chapters elsewhere in this book)
Neuronal cultures	(Refer to chapters elsewhere in this book)
In vitro electro-physiology	Cell lines; hippocampal slices; retinal preparations; etc.

Abbreviations: BAER, brainstem auditory-evoked response; EEG, electroencephalography; EMG, electro-myography; ERG, electroretinogram; PET, positron emission tomography; SPECT, single photon emission computed tomography.

for abuse and may even cause physical dependence. Although the main classes of drugs with abuse and/or dependence liability are well known, the possibility exists that new pharmacological classes could fall into this category. The main factor mitigating against CNS adverse effects is the blood-brain barrier. Compounds that have poor access to the brain are unlikely to produce CNS adverse effects, although of course they may still have actions on the peripheral nervous system.

There are several approaches to studying adverse effects of drugs on the nervous system (Table 3). Traditionally, safety pharmacology has mainly relied on the "behavioral/neurological" testing approach, but other techniques could be applied. For all behavioral tests it is important to habituate the animals to handling, by handling daily from arrival in the animal unit until the study ends.

CNS Core Battery Studies

The two tests most commonly used are the Irwin test, originally developed for mice (99), and the Functional Observational Battery (FOB), developed for rats (100,101). Although there is a great deal of overlap in the functions they address, the two tests approach the assessments slightly differently. The Irwin test was designed to evaluate entire cages of mice rapidly, whereas the FOB is far more systematic and interactive, teasing-out hidden effects in individual rats, one animal at a time. Both methods are mentioned as being suitable for the CNS core battery in the ICHS7A guidance document (1). The Irwin test has a higher throughput compared to the FOB, which also facilitates use of multiple time points to establish the duration of any observed effects. Selection between the two tests is a trade-off between effectiveness and efficiency (Table 4); some laboratories use an Irwin test in mice as an early screen, particularly when CNS-active drugs are being evaluated, with rat Irwin test or FOB to GLP subsequently on nominated candidate drugs.

The Irwin Test. This was originally developed to detect psychoactive compounds rather than as a safety pharmacology test. Mice or rats are tested at intervals post-dose using a checklist of observations (99,102,103), including mortality, sedation, excitation, stereotypes, aggressiveness, reaction to touch, pain sensitivity, muscle relaxation, loss of

Table 4 Comparison of FOB Versus Irwin Test

	FOB	Irwin test
Species originally developed for	Rat	Mouse (subsequently adapted for rats)
Original purpose	First-tier neurotoxicity evaluation (non-pharmaceuticals)	Discovery screening for psychoactive compounds
Speed	Slow; one rat at a time	Fast; one cage at a time
Time points post-dose	Usually 1 to 3	Usually >3
Main application	In-depth assessment of both CNS and non-CNS targeted compounds; for the latter, this may be the only CNS functional evaluation performed	Rapid screening of multiple CNS-targeted compounds, to aid compound selection

Abbreviations: CNS, central nervous system; FOB, functional observational battery.

righting reflex, changes in gait and respiration, catalepsy, ptosis, corneal reflex, pupil diameter, and rectal temperature.

Functional Observational Battery. The FOB was originally developed for neurotoxicity testing in the chemical/agrochemical industries (100,101). It has been adapted successfully for use in safety pharmacology applications (104,105). The FOB is a systematic evaluation of nervous system function in the rat, comprising more than 30 parameters covering autonomic, neuromuscular, sensorimotor and behavioral domains (100,106–110). The sequence of the observations begins with those causing least disturbance to the animal, with gradual progression to more interactive assessments. Thus, the FOB assessment begins with home cage observations; the rat is then removed to assess ease of removal, handling reactivity, body tone, and the presence of autonomic signs. The animal is then placed in the center of an open field arena, and observed for 3 minutes. Rats will tend to move to the relative safety of the walls and then explore the arena, both by locomotion and rearing. This also enables observations of gait abnormalities or any unusual behavior, as well as the presence of excessive urination or loose feces. The rat is then transferred to a small containment area (e.g., open-topped plastic box or cage) for reflex testing. This includes simple tests of visual function, auditory function, touch sensitivity, nociception, and righting reflex. Respiratory function is assessed by observation of rate, depth, regularity, and any noise. Grip strength (forelimbs and hindlimbs, or forelimbs only) is quantified using a grip strength meter. Hindlimb foot splay (a simple measure of motor coordination) is tested by dropping the rat from a height of 30 cm onto a pad of paper, after painting the hindpaw insteps with ink or olive oil. Rectal temperature is measured, and finally the rat is left in a darkened room for at least 2 minutes, before testing the pupil response to light from a pencil-light. The entire assessment takes approximately 12–15 minutes per rat, therefore they have to be dosed at 15 minute intervals to accommodate this protocol.

As with the Irwin test, none of the individual tests within the FOB are definitive for the variable being measured, in that they are relatively crude and the conditions are suboptimal (see below under follow-up tests). Nonetheless, the FOB is extremely useful for hazard identification, and any flags that cause concern can be addressed in specific, optimized, follow-up studies. Some potential adverse effects on the nervous system are not addressed in the FOB, including cognitive functions, sexual function, and special senses (other than fairly crudely). Where such effects are anticipated from the pharmacology profile of the compound, specific tests may have to be considered as supplementary studies to address this.

An FOB has also been devised for use in dogs (111).

CNS Follow-Up and Supplemental Studies

In the preceding section it was explained that the multi-observational tests are fairly rudimentary and are made under suboptimal conditions for any given variable. Group sizes of 5 or 6 in these tests are a compromise between sufficient power for hazard identification and limiting the number of animals used. Some of the measures will be adequately powered to detect small changes (e.g., rectal temperature), whereas others (notably open field measures) may only detect large changes. Specific follow-up studies should be fully optimized and appropriately powered.

Locomotor Activity. For a specific study on locomotor activity, the rat would be left in a novel arena for 30 minutes and its activities tracked automatically, either using a videotracking system or an array of photobeams (112,113). The two types of systems have different advantages and disadvantages; videotracking systems measure distance traveled in centimetres and are adaptable to a wide range of apparatus. Photobeam systems give activity in counts and can only be used with the cages they were designed for (transparent, and of reasonably fixed dimensions) but are more reliable for measuring vertical activity (i.e., rearing). Rats tend to explore the novel environment initially, but their activity diminishes over time (114,115). The 3-minute open field test in the FOB is too brief to detect this habituation to the surroundings. Although even a brief exposure may detect the effects of a sedative drug compared to the vehicle-treated controls, depending on the baseline activity of the control group, a stimulant effect may not be detectable. However, rats treated with a stimulant drug will still be exploring the arena long after the controls have settled down to grooming. Therefore, a 30-minute locomotor test can detect both sedative and stimulant effects.

Locomotor activity testing does not require any training of animals, and several animals can be monitored simultaneously, allowing a typical locomotor activity study for one compound to be run in a day. Activity in rodents follows a circadian rhythm, with a noticeable decrease in activity midway through the light phase of the light-dark cycle (114). Therefore, most behavioral pharmacologists will tend to run their locomotor activity testing in the morning. It is also possible to conduct it during the dark phase, for example, by adjusting the light-dark cycle. Typically, group sizes of around 10 are used.

Motor Coordination Tests. The two tests most useful here are beam walking and rotarod (116–118). They can be applied together on the same animals; as the beam walking is less strenuous it is preferable to test the subjects on this first. Unlike the locomotor activity test, these tests require pretraining to achieve a reliable level of performance. The animals can then be assigned to treatment groups after the final predose assessment, in order to achieve a balance between the groups in terms of predose performance. Poor performers (according to preset criteria) can be eliminated from further testing prior to dosing.

Rats can be trained using three beams of gradually decreasing widths; rats weighing around 200–250 g are agile enough to walk along a narrow beam (approximately 120 cm in length) after minimal training. They require a motivation to do this, which is achieved by having a bright light near the starting point, and a goal box at the other end (painted black), with the beam fixed approximately 75 cm above the floor.

The rotarod task presents a subtly different challenge—dynamic balance and motor coordination. Rats are required to maintain balance on a turning spindle by walking forwards at the same speed. Large diameter lane dividers separate the rats and enable the testing of four rats simultaneously. Some laboratories use a fixed speed, whereas others use an accelerating rotarod. For the latter test, rats first have to be trained on the apparatus over 1–3 days, beginning with fixed-speed exposures at increasing rotation speeds, progressing to accelerating mode.

Both the beam walking and rotarod tests are susceptible to performance impairment by such drugs as clonidine and benzodiazepines. In mice, the beam-walking task has been reported to be more sensitive than the rotarod in detecting motor incoordination induced by benzodiazepines (119); whether this also applies to rats and to other classes of drug is unknown, so it is prudent to use both tests in tandem.

A relatively new method of assessing motor coordination in rats is quantitative gait analysis (120). It has been applied for functional assessment of experimental spinal cord injuries, (121) peripheral neuropathy (122), and arthritis models (123) and has obvious potential for assessing motor coordination in safety pharmacology studies. A rat traverses a walkway with a glass floor; light is passed though the glass and is entirely internally reflected. At those points where a paw touches the glass, light exits the floor and scatters, illuminating the points of contact. The glass floor is monitored by a closed-circuit television (CCTV), camera, and the footprint images are analysed by software.

Elevated Plus-Maze (X-Maze) Anxiety Test.   This is a simple, straightforward test that is capable of detecting anxiogenic activity from a wide variety of pharmacological classes (124–127). Viewed from above, the apparatus is essentially a large, horizontal plus-sign, comprising two open arms (facing each other) and two enclosed arms (i.e., "corridors") also facing each other. The surface of the apparatus is fixed 50 cm above the floor. A rat is placed in the centre of the apparatus, and monitored by CCTV (either manually or by a videotracking system). The number of entries onto each arm and the time spent on each arm are noted over a 5-minute period. Rats will naturally have a conflict between a motivation to explore the apparatus and an aversion to the open arms. Anxiogenic drugs (such as yohimbine and picrotoxin) reduce the proportion of open arm entries and the time spent on the open arms, whereas anxiolytic drugs (e.g., diazepam) have the opposite effect. As with the standard locomotor activity test, retesting on the same apparatus would result in habituation and reduced activity. Therefore, the plus-maze is generally used as a single-exposure test. It is important to get the baseline activity pattern right; this is achieved by appropriate habituation to handling, optimal lighting levels, a noise-free room, and the observer monitoring the behavior remotely.

Nociception.   Drugs can either reduce or increase sensitivity to noxious stimuli, which are generally divided into thermal and mechanical stimuli. Commonly used quantitative tests of nociception include the tail flick and hot-plate tests, involving a thermal stimulus applied to the tail or soles of the feet, either by irradiation or conduction.

Tests of hyperalgesia (increased sensitivity to noxious stimuli) include the above two tests, plus the plantar heat test, hind-paw mechanical pressure test (Randall-Sellito test), and Von Frey hair test (128). Some drug-induced sensory neuropathies can also result in allodynia, where normally nonnoxious stimuli (such as ice-cold water) can elicit a nociceptive response. Tests to assess this include application of an acetone drop to the plantar surface of the hind paw and immersion of the tail in ice-cold water (129).

All tests of nociception require some predose habituation and training of the animals to achieve optimal data. All such tests are affected by drug-induced changes in cutaneous blood flow in the hind paw or tail (leading to changes in tail skin temperature), and this should be evaluated in the event of a positive finding before concluding that there is an effect on nociception (130,131). Effects on tail skin temperature can be assessed using thermocouples applied to the surface of the tail (132), by thermographic imaging (133), or by application of thermosensitive liquid crystal paint (134). If there is an increase in tail skin temperature, the tail flick test can be re-run at a higher ambient temperature to raise tail skin temperature and thereby prevent further drug-induced increases.

Auditory Function. There are two main methods of assessment: electrophysiological recordings and motor (i.e., startle) responses. Both these methods are also used in humans. Electrophysiological recordings of brainstem auditory-evoked responses (BAER) can be made either in rodents or dogs in response to auditory stimuli (135). The characteristics of the response are well-defined, and it is possible to identify the location of any drug-induced effect (e.g., auditory apparatus or the central auditory pathways). This is achievable in unanaesthetised dogs, although anaesthesia is generally required for rats.

The auditory startle reflex involves placing a rat on a mechanical transducer in a sound-attenuated chamber, and applying a loud (e.g., 120 dB) startle stimulus. The motor response is fairly reproducible, but it can be attenuated if preceded by an audible tone. Once this "prepulse inhibition" has been established, the intensity of the tone can be varied until it is inaudible, and there is no prepulse inhibition of the startle response to the loud noise. This can be tested at different frequencies of the prepulse tone, a method known as reflex modification audiometry. In principle, this would be a very sensitive test for drug-induced effects on the auditory system. Such an approach has rarely been used in safety pharmacology laboratories, although it is used in neurotoxicology studies in the chemical and agrochemical industries (136).

Visual Function. Here again, the two main methods of assessment are electrophysiological recordings (electroretinogram; ERG) and visual function tests in conscious animals. Unlike the BAER, the ERG only measures the response of the retina, so drug effects in the CNS are not detected. It is however, useful as a second-tier test to home-in on the site of action of the drug. ERG studies are usually done on rats and generally require anaesthesia (137–139). ERGs are evoked responses recorded from the cornea in response to flash stimuli. Typically, the ERG comprises a negative a-wave, a positive b-wave, a late negativity, and a positive c-wave (137). The anatomical generators of these waves within the retina have been characterised (137). The ratio of rods to cones in the rat retina is approximately 100:1 (140); the contribution of cones to the ERG can be teased-out using a twin-flash paradigm (which isolates the cone response) rather than a single flash [which stimulates both rods and cones (140)]. The rat ERG has been analysed pharmacologically (141). ERGs have also been used in toxicology studies in dogs (142).

A long-established, semiquantitative behavioral method for assessing visual acuity in rats is the Lashley jumping stand (143). The test involves placing a rat on a raised platform, where the rat has to distinguish between visual cues to escape. However, this is of limited practicality in a safety pharmacology environment. Superior, quantitative tests of visual acuity in rodents have been developed relatively recently, including a trapezoid-shaped water maze, where the rat has to swim towards a fine grating to escape from the water, (144,145) and an optometry system where the animal (rat or mouse) is at the center of a "virtual cylinder" of a rotating vertical grating and is observed for head-tracking movements (146). The latter test appears to be suitable for safety pharmacology studies, as it is able to quantify both visual acuity and contrast sensitivity rapidly without prior habituation or training of the animal.

Another potential side effect related to visual function is raised intraocular pressure, leading to drug-induced glaucoma (147). Although invasive techniques have been used, including telemetry (148), it can also be measured noninvasively by tonometry, even in species as small as mice (149).

Proconvulsive Tests. For the purposes of safety pharmacology studies, convulsions can be elicited in rats or mice either by electrical current applied via ear electrodes [electroshock seizures; (150,151)] or by intravenous administration of a convulsant drug, such as pentylenetetrazol (PTZ) (103). Electroshock induces generalized tonic-clonic seizures, whereas PTZ initially produces myoclonic jerks, which lead to generalized tonic-clonic seizures (150,152). With the maximal electroshock method, the current intensity is adjusted until the convulsive threshold is reached; compounds with proconvulsant activity will reduce this threshold. With the chemical seizure method, proconvulsant compounds will increase the number of clonic convulsions and decrease the latency to onset of the tonic convulsions (103,152,153). Both the above methods have been around for more than 50 years.

Another approach is to apply in vitro techniques using hippocampal slice electrophysiology. This technique has been used since the 1970s, including for mechanistic investigation of convulsant and anticonvulsant drugs, (154) yet has not been widely applied to safety pharmacology investigations. The in vitro hippocampal seizure activity technique has been described for rat (154,155), guinea-pig (156), and mouse (157). In brief, transverse hippocampal slices (e.g., 500 μm thick) are maintained in aerated artificial CSF solution in a perfusion chamber. Extracellular recordings are made from the CA1 or CA3 cell field, and their afferent neuronal input (the Schaffer collateral/commissural pathway) is stimulated at a low frequency (e.g., 1–2 times per minute). Convulsant agents of various pharmacological classes induce epileptiform activity or will lower convulsive thresholds and exacerbate epileptiform activity induced by convulsant drugs such as PTZ.

Electroencephalography. Measurement of surface brain electrical activity is complementary to behavioral observations, in that neither approach could replace what the other one assesses. In safety pharmacology, electroencephalography (EEG) recordings can fulfil three main purposes. First, drug-induced changes in power spectra are detectable. In fact, it has been shown that different classes of centrally acting drugs have distinguishable EEG profiles (i.e., "signatures") in the rat, in terms of power spectra (158–161). Second, drug effects on sleep-wakefulness are detectable on the EEG (162,163). Third, the EEG can detect drug-induced seizure-like abnormalities that may not always translate into overt convulsive activity (164,165). The availability of modern data acquisition software with Fourier fast-transform analysis enables generation of power spectra.

EEGs can be measured from freely-moving rats (158–166), dogs (167), rabbits (168) and guinea-pigs (169). An elegant, nonsurgical technique has recently been described in guineapigs, using scalp electrodes attached to a telemetry transmitter that is housed in a jacket worn by the animal (170). This enables rapid preparation of the animals and is ideally suited for safety pharmacology purposes; presumably it could also be adapted for use in rats.

Cognitive Function. Cognitive functions are higher-level brain functions, which incorporate learning, memory, and problem-solving. There are many different types of learning and memory, and for each category there are several techniques to address it. The techniques fall into three main types: avoidance tasks, mazes, and operant procedures. The two species most commonly used are rats and monkeys; rats are used for each of these three types of technique, whereas monkeys are reserved for operant procedures.

Of the avoidance tasks, the most convenient starting point for safety pharmacology applications is *passive avoidance*, as it only requires 2 trials per animal and can be automated. The apparatus comprises a chamber with a grid floor. Depending on the specific design, a rat (or mouse) can either step down from a platform onto the grid floor or enter the chamber via a runway. Either way, on contact with the grid floor it immediately receives a brief (e.g., 2 s) foot-shock and is then removed. Twenty-four hours later the animal is retested in the same apparatus; the latency to enter the chamber/step onto the grid floor (now switched-off) is recorded. Test compounds can either be administered immediately after the training trial (to test effects on learning) or before the test trial (to test effects on memory) (103).

The most commonly-used mazes are watermazes (where an animal has to use navigational cues to locate a submerged platform), the radial maze, where food-deprived rats have to learn which arms contain hidden food, the Y-maze, and the T-maze. Of these, the *Morris watermaze* is probably the most suitable for safety pharmacology investigations, as it does not require the rats to be placed on a partial food deprivation schedule, rats rapidly learn the task, and there are no odor cues to clean-up between trials. It comprises a large-diameter circular tank (2 m diameter for rats) containing water (rendered opaque by adding either milk powder or vegetable dye), maintained at $\sim 25°C$. Approximately 2 cm beneath the surface there is a small "escape" platform (~ 11 cm diameter). Rats (or mice) learn to locate the platform using visual information from cues around the room. Their swim paths are recorded by videotracking equipment that calculates path length, swimming speed, time spent in each quadrant, and several other measures. There are two main protocols in the Morris watermaze: "place navigation," which uses a fixed platform position for each trial and assesses the development of long-term memory over ~ 5 days, and "short-term spatial memory," where the platform is moved to a new location each day (171–173).

In *operant procedures*, rats (or monkeys) are trained to perform tasks in response to specific stimuli in exchange for food rewards. Stimuli (visual or auditory) are presented, and the animal has to perform a function (e.g., press a lever) in response. In the rat version of the test, one of two retractable levers is inserted into the operant chamber as the "sample." When the rat presses the lever (indicating that it has registered the sample), the lever is immediately withdrawn. Then, after a variable delay (0 to 20 s), both levers are presented simultaneously, and the rat has to press the original "sample" lever to obtain a food reward ("delayed matching-to-sample"). Alternatively, rats can be trained to press the nonsample lever ("delayed nonmatching to sample"). Such paradigms require the rats to be placed on a partial food deprivation schedule, the rats have to be habituated to the test apparatus, and then trained until they attain a predetermined level of performance; together, this can amount to several weeks before testing a compound (174,175).

In all the above types of tests, drugs can have specific effects on mnemonic processes but can also have effects on performance by affecting the level of anxiety, attention, arousal, motor function, or visual function. Where food is used as a positive reinforcer (reward), test compounds may indirectly affect performance by effects on appetite; where foot shock is used as a negative reinforcer, test compounds that affect nociception may affect performance in the test. Although some of these confounding factors are accounted for within the test itself, the most pragmatic approach is to obtain an effect first before worrying about confounding factors. They can then be dissected out or eliminated subsequently.

Abuse/Dependence Liability. Several classes of therapeutically useful drugs are associated with abuse liability, others with dependence liability, and some with both. Abuse liability is largely, but not exclusively, confined to centrally acting drugs, whereas physical dependence can also occur with non-CNS agents (176). The first step in preclinical assessment of abuse/dependence liability is to consider the potential risk with that particular compound. Such an approach would take into account whether the compound entered the central nervous system, and if so, whether it interacted with molecular targets (either primary or secondary) associated with abuse/dependence potential, with potencies within a reasonable multiple of the expected brain concentration (177). There are four main approaches for evaluating abuse/dependence potential in animals: self-administration, conditioned place preference, drug discrimination, and withdrawal phenomena. *Self-administration* requires implantation of an intravenous catheter in either rodents or primates. Animals rapidly learn to press a lever to obtain an injection of the reinforcer (compound producing "drug-seeking" behavior), and will work harder (in terms of more lever presses) to obtain drugs of greater reinforcing efficacy (178). Interestingly, whereas both primates and rodents will self-administer various classes of drugs known to be abused by humans, animals will not self-administer hallucinogens (179). One drawback of the self-administration protocols is the use of intravenous administration, with the requirements to have an intravenous formulation and to maintain catheter patency. *Conditioned place preference* can be performed using any route of administration, including oral. This is an indirect method of assessing drug-seeking behavior in rodents (103,180,181). It involves pairing the administration of a reinforcer with a contextual cue (i.e., environmental surroundings), by use of a two-compartment box with different wall patterns or flooring surfaces. Rodents will select the compartment previously associated with administration of the positive reinforcer. *Drug discrimination paradigms* involve training animals in an operant procedure in which they have a choice of two levers to obtain a food reward. One lever is linked to a reward only when the animal has been dosed with a training drug (e.g., cocaine), whereas the other lever is matched to vehicle administration. Once trained, animals may be dosed with compounds having the potential for a similar pharmacological action as the training drug. If this is the case, the animal will tend to select the lever associated with the training drug, whereas if the compound does not produce a similar effect to the training drug the animal will select the other lever (103,182). The drug discrimination technique shows high pharmacological selectivity, in that the animal does not discriminate being in a "drugged state" per se (183). However, this is also its main drawback: the inherent specificity to the training drug precludes detection of abuse liability of compounds producing completely novel sensations (103).

Drug withdrawal assessment involves abrupt cessation of dosing following repeated administration of a compound. The withdrawal syndrome varies between different classes of agent, with some (e.g., anxiety) more subtle than others (e.g., convulsions). For compounds interacting with opiate receptors, the withdrawal syndrome can be precipitated with the antagonist naloxone. Compounds can also be assessed for their ability to alleviate withdrawal symptoms associated with a standard dependence-producing drug; such activity would imply dependence potential in the test compound. Whereas tests of abuse liability typically reveal a bell-shaped dose-response curve (with a narrow effective dose range), studies on dependence generally require administration of high doses for prolonged periods (103).

From a regulatory perspective, US and Japanese authorities ultimately require to see self-administration studies in primates for all CNS-active NCEs where there is a potential for abuse liability (178). Rodent studies are useful to companies as part of their initial evaluations. Whereas the FDA guidance on abuse/dependence liability has remained in draft form since 1990, (178) guidelines are emerging from the European Medicines Evaluation Agency (EMEA) on this topic (184).

Respiratory System

The respiratory system can be divided functionally into a pumping apparatus and a gas exchange unit, both of which are susceptible to the effects of drugs from a variety of different pharmacological classes (185,186). Whereas the incidence of respiratory side effects in clinical development is lower than those of gastrointestinal, cardiovascular, and CNS, such effects can occur suddenly and can be life threatening (185,186). Therefore, the respiratory system is included as one of the three vital organ functions by ICHS7A.

The *pumping apparatus* generates and regulates ventilation. Inspiration is active, being enacted by the diaphragm and intercostal muscles, whereas expiration is generally passive. The rate and depth of respiration are controlled by respiratory generators in the located in the ventral medulla of the brainstem (187), which are influenced by higher brain centres integrating cardiorespiratory responses to specific demands of the organism, as described earlier under the cardiovascular section of this chapter. These areas receive afferent input from arterial chemoreceptors, pulmonary chemo- and mechanoreceptors, and nasopharyngeal afferents (187). Therefore, ventilatory patterns can be affected by drugs acting at the level of the various integrative centers, the respiratory generators, or the chemo- and mechanoreceptors (185).

The *gas exchange unit* consists of the lungs, comprising the airways, alveoli, and interstitial area containing blood and lymph vessels and an elastic fibrous network (185). Drugs can reduce airflow by causing bronchoconstriction, excessive mucus secretion, oedema, or breakdown in elastic support tissue (185); drugs can also interfere with normal airflow by causing smooth muscle hyperplasia, reduction of ciliary beat frequency, and inhibition of mucus secretion. Functional changes such as these are termed obstructive disorders. On the other hand, restrictive disorders involve a reduction in the normal elasticity (compliance) of the lung, thereby increasing the pressure required to expand the lung. A decrease in lung compliance tends to produce a rapid-shallow breathing pattern that can ultimately lead to respiratory fatigue and failure (185). Restrictive disorders can be caused by interstitial thickening due to oedema, cellular infiltration, or abnormal surfactant production (185). They are defined functionally as a reduction in total lung capacity or lung compliance (185,188).

Respiratory Core Battery Studies

The most commonly-used method of measuring ventilatory patterns in rodents (generally rats) is the whole-body plethysmography chamber. The animal is confined (rather than restrained) within a plexiglass chamber. Small pressure changes occur within the chamber during inspiration and expiration and are detected by sensitive pressure transducers. Although the technique is susceptible to changes in temperature and humidity, the main advantage is minimal stress compared to "head-out" methods (see below) and relative simplicity compared to telemetry techniques (see below). Data acquisition software will derive the following parameters from the respiratory waveform: tidal volume, respiratory rate, minute volume (tidal volume multiplied by rate), peak inspiratory flow, peak expiratory flow, and fractional inspiratory time (time in inspiration divided by total cycle time). Some software packages for whole-body plethysmography also derive a parameter termed "enhanced pause" (Penh), which is presumed to correlate with changes in pulmonary resistance (189). However, Penh and respiratory resistance often do not correlate (190,191), and several authors have recommended restricting its use to that of a preliminary flag, rather than as a definitive indicator of airways dysfunction (192).

An alternative approach is to make respiratory recordings from a tracheal cannula in anaesthetized animals, for example, in dogs with simultaneous recording of haemodynamic parameters. This also enables "forced maneuvres" (i.e., mechanical lung inflation and deflation) to assess obstructive and restrictive effects. The presence of anaesthesia will tend to mask the effects of respiratory depressant and stimulant drugs, and so this would have to be supplemented by measurements of effects on rate in conscious animals. A selective decrease in airflow during inspiration generally indicates a decrease in respiratory drive, whereas a selective decrease in airflow during expiration is generally indicative of an obstructive disorder (185).

Respiratory Follow-Up Studies

More detailed tests of respiratory function should be performed to further investigate any indicators of dysfunction in the core battery test. Further investigation of ventilatory effects include measurement of arterial blood gases, responses to inhalation of CO_2 and to intravenous injection of NaCN to distinguish central from peripheral nervous system effects (193), denervation of carotid chemoreceptors with the same aim in mind (194), and cervical vagotomy to assess the involvement of pulmonary receptors in the drug response (185). Lung mechanics can be further investigated by forced maneuvres (see above) and diffusion of gases across the alveolar wall (185). Obstructive disorders can be assessed using dynamic measurements of airflow resistance. This can be done indirectly, by using a "head-out" plethysmography chamber, where the head and trunk are separated into two compartments, in order to measure the delay between thoracic and nasal airflows in unanesthetised animals (195). An increase in this delay reflects increased airway resistance. A more direct method of measuring airflow resistance in conscious rats and primates has been devised using telemetry (196,197). A pressure catheter (attached to a telemetry transducer in the abdomen) is passed through the diaphragm and positioned beneath the serosal layer of the esophagus within the thoracic cavity. By combining the telemetry measurements of intrapleural pressure with the use of a plethysmography chamber, dynamic measurements of airflow resistance can be measured repeatedly in conscious animals (185). This augmented evaluation of respiratory function has been recommended by some authorities for the core battery assessment (185).

Other follow-up studies in vitro might include tracheal rings to assess effects on smooth muscle (198), isolated lungs (199), isolated phrenic nerve-diaphragm preparation (200), mucus secretion (201), and ciliary beat frequency (202).

Gastrointestinal Tract

The majority of medicines are administered by oral ingestion, and therefore the gastrointestinal tract (particularly the stomach) is exposed to a far higher concentration of drug than any other organ system. It is therefore not surprising that the incidence of gastrointestinal side effects is relatively high. Although, with notable exceptions (e.g., gastric ulceration caused by nonsteroidal anti-inflammatory drugs), the severity of such side effects is rarely life threatening, it may be of a sufficient magnitude to impact on patient compliance and physician preference. In addition, gastrointestinal side effects, particularly inhibition of gastric emptying, can impede or delay drug absorption, which has implications both for nonclinical studies (pharmacokinetics, efficacy, and toxicology) and clinical development. Drugs can affect satiety, taste, salivation, gastric acid secretion, gastric emptying, intestinal peristalsis, electrolyte secretion into the intestinal lumen, bile secretion, gut flora, and anal sphincter tone. Consequences include changes in appetite, food unpalatability, nausea, gastric ulceration, vomiting, indigestion, constipation, flatulence, and diarrhea.

Gastrointestinal First-Tier Studies

The most commonly-used methods in rodent safety pharmacology studies are assessment of gastric emptying and intestinal transit using an inert marker (e.g., charcoal meal or phenol red) (203,204). Following an overnight fast, rats (or mice) are dosed with the test compound, either orally or by another route, and a suspension of the inert marker is administered orally at a predetermined time post-dose. Animals are killed 20–30 minutes later; the stomachs are weighed to give an index of gastric emptying (205), and the transit distance of the marker through the gut is expressed as a percentage of the total length of the small intestine. Although this is a crude method, and gastric emptying and intestinal transit are affected by food type and fasting, it is capable of detecting drug-induced effects that can be evaluated more thoroughly using more sophisticated techniques (206).

Gastrointestinal Investigative Studies

Imaging techniques offer a more sophisticated alternative to the charcoal meal. Scintigraphy using polystyrene pellets labeled with gamma-emitting isotopes, such as ^{99m}Tc or ^{111}In, has been used in conscious dogs (207,208) as well as rats (203). A gamma camera is used to take either still or moving images of the pellets exiting the stomach. Other in vivo techniques include myographic recordings by telemetry (209) and measurement of gastric acid secretion by catheterization of the pylorus in rats (210).

In vitro techniques useful either for frontloading or investigative follow-up studies include smooth muscle preparations that were once the mainstay of "classical pharmacology" (e.g., guinea-pig ileum, guinea-pig colon, isolated rat stomach), as well as more sophisticated preparations, such as perfused lumen of the guinea-pig ileum (211), recordings from enteric nerves controlling longitudinal and circular muscle in rat ileum (212), and other methods of studying drug effects on intestinal motility (213).

Renal Function

This is one organ function that has been relatively ignored by safety pharmacologists since the implementation of the ICHS7A guidelines. Prior to this, it was studied routinely as part of the "List A" assessment. Yet there are numerous drugs that can affect renal function, even acutely. Many drugs pass through the kidney unmetabolised, and so effects on renal function are always a potential concern with any new compound.

Traditionally in safety pharmacology assessments, renal function has tended to be assessed by collecting urine from either water-loaded or saline-loaded rats for 24 hours in metabolism cages (also referred to as metabolic cages or metabowls), with analysis of urine volume and sodium and potassium output (214). This only represents a cursory glance at renal function and is derived from methods used to screen for potential diuretic drugs. To address renal function adequately, measurements of glomerular filtration rate (GFR) and renal plasma flow (RPF) also have to be made, preferably under steady-state conditions with respect to arterial blood pressure and urine output. GFR can be estimated by measuring inulin clearance in rats, whereby inulin is infused intravenously and urine collected at intervals thereafter. Inulin is a polysaccharide that is freely filtered by the glomeruli and is not bound to plasma proteins nor secreted or metabolically altered in the renal tubules. An alternative to inulin is iothalamate (215,216). RPF can be estimated by clearance of p-aminohippurate (PAH), which is freely filtered and secreted but not metabolised by the tubules. Alternatively, renal arterial blood flow (RBF) can be recorded directly using a flow transducer (217). Such methods have generally required the use of anaesthesia, with blood collection from a cannulated artery and urine collection from a ureter or the bladder—all of which have their drawbacks (218). The above methods may also be applied during simultaneous assessment of cardiovascular parameters in anaesthetised dogs (219,220), minipigs (49), or cynomolgus monkeys (220,221).

Alternative methods of estimating GFR and RPF that do not require the collection and analysis of urine samples have been proposed for use in anaesthetised (215) and unanaesthetised rats (218). Other options include subcutaneous implantation of slow-release pellets for inulin and PAH (222). Baseline values for GFR, RPF, and RBF have been collated for this species from the literature (215). More recently there have been developments in the application of magnetic resonance imaging (MRI) techniques for non-invasive assessment of renal function in rats (223–225).

Bladder Function

The urinary bladder consists of a capsule of smooth muscle whose function is the storage and periodic evacuation of urine. Bladder emptying involves a relaxation of the internal bladder sphincter in conjunction with contraction of the detrusor muscle in the bladder wall, which are both under the control of the autonomic nervous system (226). Therefore, drugs can cause unwanted bladder retention, bladder incontinence, and urge incontinence. Side effects of drugs on bladder function can be investigated in anaesthetised rats by measuring internal bladder pressure by means of a catheter introduced into the bladder dome (227,228). It is also possible to measure responses to pelvic nerve stimulation (227) and to record afferent nerve activity (229). Bladder emptying can also be recorded continuously by telemetry in monkeys (230). Bladder function can also be assessed in vitro, either by using whole-bladder preparations, detrusor myography, or single cells (226).

ADVANCED TOPICS

Functional Measurements During Repeat-Dose Toxicity Studies

Although this is outside the scope of this chapter, it is worth making a few comments here. Pharmacologists view repeat-dose toxicity studies as a missed opportunity to obtain functional data during chronic dosing. Toxicologists on the other hand have to preserve the integrity of their studies, as the primary purpose is to use a well-established protocol that provides readouts of clinical observations, clinical chemistry and haematology, toxicokinetics, food and water consumption, body weights, limited functional measurements (e.g., ECG), and, ultimately and most importantly, histopathology. Calls to do more in the way of functional assessments date back to reviews by Zbinden and others (231–234). However, the toxicology environment and study design is not ideal for enabling optimal functional measurements, and so compromises have to be made. Nonetheless, some basic, noninvasive techniques, such as tail cuff blood pressure in rats, noninvasive ECG recording in dogs, whole-body plethysmography in rats, and behavioral techniques such as FOB (or elements thereof), rotarod, nociceptive assessment, and so on, are achievable within a repeat-dose toxicity study. The main issues are lack of incentive to do it (i.e., no regulatory requirement) and resource implications.

It should be stressed, however, that measurements on repeat-dose toxicity studies are not a replacement for studying pharmacological responses to compounds after single administration (4). First, higher doses can generally be achieved on acute administration compared to repeat-dose studies. Second, functional measurements during repeat-dose studies generally assess "effects" rather than "responses" to drugs in animals that may have some degree of multiple organ impairment due to repeated drug exposure. Third, the experimental conditions may be difficult to optimize for the variable being measured, there are a large number of animals to measure from in a short space of time, and other procedures (e.g., blood sampling) are being done. Finally, tolerance may develop to the drug response on repeated dosing (176), and so effects may be missed if evaluated several days into the dosing phase (4).

In summary, functional measurements on repeat-dose toxicity studies should be viewed as *complementary* to single-dose safety pharmacology studies. There is potentially much to gain in terms of predictive power from a relatively small increase in effort.

Risk Assessment Using Safety Pharmacology Data

Risk assessment with respect to protecting volunteers in Phase I clinical trials is relatively straightforward as it does not take into account the therapeutic target or the extent of the unmet medical need, given that there is no potential therapeutic benefit in the case of healthy volunteers (4). However, safety pharmacology data has potential value well beyond its primary remit of protecting clinical trials volunteers. It can be used to assess the risk of failure of a project during clinical development. A matrix can be used that rates different parameters using a "traffic lights" system (4). First are the outcomes of the safety pharmacology tests themselves, ranging from outcomes predictive of non-serious, reversible side effects (e.g., gastrointestinal) to those predictive of side effects impacting on quality of life (e.g., various CNS side effects), and ultimately to those predictive of potentially life-threatening effects (e.g., proarrhythmia, profound hypotension, broncho-constriction). Next would be the severity of the disease target, ranging from minor/moderate diseases (e.g., eczema, rhinitis, Raynaud's), to debilitating diseases (e.g., asthma, angina, arthritis, stroke, epilepsy, Parkinson's), through to diseases that are life threatening or even lethal if untreated (e.g., cancer, AIDS, myocardial infarction). Finally, the quality of the existing therapy (which the candidate drug is designed to surpass) should be rated, as being either "good," "partially effective/side-effects," or "poor/nonexistent." The target population should also be considered; for example, cognitive impairment may be more problematic in geriatric and paediatric patients, and hypotensive effects may be more pronounced with age. Risk assessment on safety pharmacology data is generally based on safety margins, calculated from plasma concentrations at which an effect is seen compared to the expected C_{max} in humans.

Special Cases

Primary Molecular Target Not Present in "Default" Species

This issue crops up fairly frequently: either the molecular target (e.g., a receptor subtype) is not present in one or more of the two commonest species used for safety pharmacology evaluations (rat and dog), or the equivalent molecular target in one or both of these species has different binding characteristics from the human equivalent, and the compound shows selectivity for the human target over the equivalent target in the species in question. When the primary molecular target is not present in the usual "default" species, the options are either to conduct the safety pharmacology tests in another suitable species (e.g., minipig or primate instead of dog for cardiovascular measurements; mouse instead of rat for CNS, respiratory, and GI measurements), or to use a transgenic knock-in mouse with the gene inserted for the human receptor (235,236). However, there are inherent drawbacks with the latter option, as the species may not accommodate functioning of the inserted receptor in a way analogous to its function in humans. For the less stringent issue (selectivity of the compound for the human receptor), the above options also apply, but it may also be possible to synthesize a compound selective for (say) the rat version of the receptor. In this case, the rodent safety pharmacology could comprise studies in (say) mouse with the development compound and studies in rat with a compound selective for the rat version of the receptor. Nonetheless, the conventional default species (rat and/or dog) would still be relevant for evaluation of the "nontarget" safety pharmacology of the development compound.

Although mice are suitable for various noninvasive assessments, including behavioral tests, whole-body plethysmography, tail-cuff blood pressure, renal function, and gastrointestinal function, the small size of their heart and blood vessels poses a major problem for cardiovascular assessments (237). Nonetheless, with the advent of transgenic mice (and the relative absence of transgenic rats!), various techniques have been developed to assess cardiovascular function in this species, including echocardiography (238,239), cardiac output (240), blood pressure by implantable telemetry (241,242), regional blood flow distribution using microspheres (243), and even arterial blood flow using pulsed-Doppler flowmetry (89,91,244).

Oncology Compounds

Little or no guidance exists on how much safety pharmacology evaluation is required for oncology compounds. Safety pharmacology is barely mentioned in recent reviews on nonclinical safety assessment of oncology drugs (245,246), and ICHS7A appears to exempt certain oncology products from nonclinical safety pharmacology evaluation (1). However, therapeutics in oncology has advanced significantly from the cytotoxic cancer chemotherapy compounds, and products are emerging that are safe enough to enable chronic, daily therapy to contain the condition (247–249). Such compounds may enter clinical development via the conventional starting point of testing in healthy volunteers, rather than fast-forwarding to terminally-ill patients. Therefore, a good rule of thumb is that if the compound is to be tested in healthy volunteers, then the nonclinical safety pharmacology evaluation should be as per all other therapeutic indications, whereas if the clinical trials begin and end with cancer patients, the safety pharmacology evaluation can be scaled-down on a case-by-case basis according to known risks associated with the compound. Nonetheless, even with these highly toxic compounds aimed at end-stage cancer patients, basic knowledge of the risks to vital organ functions is highly desirable, and therefore it would be prudent to apply the core battery safety pharmacology assessments even though regulatory requirement is a grey area.

Biotechnology-Derived Pharmaceuticals

New biological entities (NBEs) derived from pharma biotechnology include vaccines, gene therapy products, antisense oligonucleotides, monoclonal antibodies (mAbs), human cytokines, immune modulators, and miscellaneous large proteins. The regulatory requirements for preclinical safety testing (ICH S6) of NBEs are not so proscriptively defined as for small molecules, with even less guidance on requirements to address safety pharmacology. Thus for each NBE under development, a considered scientific approach needs to be undertaken to determine the applicability of meaningful safety pharmacology assessment.

Considering, for example, mAbs these are engineered specifically to interact with a single human target, typically a cytokine, growth factor, ligand-binding receptor, etc., that is considered causal in the initiation or exacerbation of an inappropriate immune-mediated response or disease-enhancing mechanism. mAbs are designed to have high specificity and avidity for the human target. This selectivity will preclude recognition of and binding to the cytokine/receptor target in other lower species, although some primate homology can usually be demonstrated, albeit often at reduced potency. A panel of tissues from different species can be used to determine specific binding, thus indicating the most suitable species for preclinical safety assessment, typically rhesus or cynomolgus monkeys. Rodents, which do not demonstrate any binding for the mAb, are thus inappropriate for the determination of potential functional changes to physiological systems. This limits the potential species for safety pharmacology testing to the primate displaying some homology of the human target.

Due to the specificity of molecular target for biologics, it may not be appropriate to perform any specific safety pharmacology tests (250). However, information on the potential role of the target molecule (or of normal physiological processes impacted on by neutralisation of the protein) needs to be considered. Information may be derived from published literature or from the study of the altered phenotypics of knockout or add-in mice. Thus, in the case of binding to and neutralization of raised levels of a specific immunocytokine or its receptor, in an autoimmune disease, safety pharmacology testing is unlikely to be required and may not be scientifically or ethically justifiable. However, for example, the targeting of a receptor modulating vascular endothelial functionality may suggest the need to determine cardiovascular safety.

Cardiovascular assessment can be incorporated into the primate single and multidose toxicity studies, recording blood pressure, heart rate, and multilead ECG at T_{max}. Any potential liability for QT prolongation should be made using appropriate correction for changes in heart rate, as discussed previously (see section Cardiovascular Core Battery Techniques). Should there be any additional concerns for potential cardiovascular effects, perhaps due to lack of information on the molecular target's role in cardiovascular homeostasis, primate telemetry methods can be used to supplement data from the toxicity studies. As with small molecules, if more detailed investigation is warranted, then conventional anaesthetised preparations can be studied to evaluate detailed haemodynamics combined with an assessment of effects on other organ functions (e.g., respiration).

The use of a single species (primate) limits the ability to perform specific evaluations of CNS effects; these can generally only be based on close observational monitoring during conventional toxicology studies. However, the potential of the NBE for brain penetration should aid the decision as to whether specific CNS studies are warranted; this is clearly the case for NBEs injected directly into the brain. Similarly, respiratory evaluations for general hazard identification can only be realistically based on observations of change(s) in the rate, depth and pattern of respiration. Such observations should be done at the time of peak plasma concentration. All safety physiological assessments should include the measurement of core temperature, as fever is commonly induced by cytokines, and by cytokine release (251).

Safety Pharmacology in Disease Models

Although the primary aim of safety pharmacology assessment is to protect volunteers from acute effects of new candidate drugs, if the drug progresses beyond Phase I clinical trials it will be tested (and ultimately used) in diseased patients. However, there is rarely any safety pharmacology evaluation in animal models of the target disease. Although this may appear to be a major oversight, it should be approached with caution. First, disease models often only "model" limited aspects of the human disease, usually for good reason and sometimes because of the inherent limitations of the model. Therefore, the aspect of altered physiology with which the drug may eventually interact adversely in diseased patients may not be present in the animal model. Secondly, animal disease models of chronic diseases tend to develop the disease very rapidly compared to the human equivalent. Here, aspects of compensatory mechanisms and chronic pathophysiology are not present in the disease model. Therefore, additional safety pharmacology evaluation in disease models should be applied on a case-by-case basis, where there is specific cause for concern. For example, candidate drugs for acute treatment of stroke should be assessed for effects on blood pressure and cerebral blood flow, both in normal animals and in stroke models, to ensure they do not compromise their potential efficacy or, worse still, exacerbate the condition. Similarly, proarrhythmic risk of candidate drugs targeted at ischaemic heart disease should probably also be assessed in relevant animal models of the disease, as the diseased heart is a major risk factor for torsade de pointes. The problem with this is knowing where to stop, particularly if the indication changes or there are multiple indications, or in the case of patients with more than one disease (e.g., an analgesic being taken by a patient with Parkinson's disease), so an intelligent, limited approach is preferable.

FUTURE TRENDS

The immediate future is likely to retain a combined approach towards safety pharmacology, including in silico, in vitro, and in vivo. In silico approaches can begin even prior to chemical synthesis, and are currently used to estimate binding affinities/potencies to secondary molecular targets such as hERG (45,252). This may be extended to a range of other nontarget receptors to assess potential adverse effects (253,254). In silico predictions of blood-brain barrier penetration (255) will also facilitate risk assessment of CNS side effects from known or predicted binding affinities/potencies at receptors in the CNS. At the level of organ function, in silico models have been developed to predict effects of multiple ion channel interactions on the cardiac action potential and on transmural dispersion (256,257). An additional challenge for in vivo work will be to obtain multiple endpoints from the same animals without compromising quality of the data or increasing the burden on the individual animals.

In the "QT" arena, the use of in vitro proarrhythmia models is likely to increase, particularly where safety margins with respect to hERG IC_{50} and effects on QT are low (e.g., <30-fold) (67). On the other hand, application of such models may reach a ceiling because of improvements in the aforementioned safety margins and lack of regulatory requirement and/or acceptance of them. Now that the safety pharmacology assessment of torsadogenic risk is addressed relatively comprehensively across the pharmaceutical industry (compared to pre-1997 QT risk evaluation and to non-QT aspects of safety pharmacology), there is likely to be a rebalancing of emphasis to address other areas of safety pharmacology. This will probably involve the application of techniques outside the mainstream of safety pharmacology, such as in vitro techniques (including electrophysiological recordings) to assess CNS, respiratory and gastrointestinal function (258), imaging techniques applied to gastrointestinal and cardiac function, quantification of receptor occupancy in the CNS, and in vivo neurophysiological recordings (such as EEG telemetry) to detect neurological effects. A major "blind spot" is likely to be recognized and addressed: detection of functional effects that only reveal themselves after repeat-dosing. Incorporation of functional measurements into repeat-dose toxicity studies looks increasingly likely, not as a replacement for traditional single-dose safety pharmacology studies but finally considered valuable in its own right.

The conventional target-based model of safety pharmacology (and indeed, of drug discovery in general) has been challenged recently by new technology that enables rapid

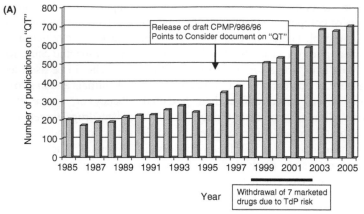

Data from MEDLINE using text search term "QT", plotted as publications per annum.

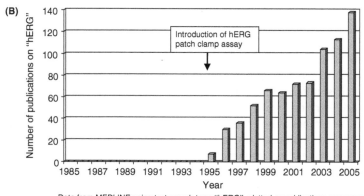

Data from MEDLINE using text search term "hERG", plotted as publications per annum.

Figure 2 (**A**) Growth in publications on "QT" from the mid-1990s onwards. (**B**) Growth in publications on "hERG" from the mid-1990s onwards.

in vivo screening using zebrafish embryos in multi-well plates (259–261). This phenotype-based model (which in previous times would have been referred to as a "black box" approach) may not replace the conventional approach to safety pharmacology but may offer an opportunity for frontloading and to plug various gaps that are currently being ignored due to the complexity and unknown predictive power of animal models, notably retinal toxicity (262) and ototoxicity (263). However, extensive pharmacological/toxicological validation is required before such models will gain credibility within the pharmaceutical industry, not to mention the regulatory authorities.

The primary drivers to safety pharmacology are likely to remain as being drug withdrawals involving a common safety pharmacology mechanism, emerging regulatory guidance documents based on safety concerns, and the development of new technologies useful to safety pharmacologists. Nowhere is the impact of these "combined stimuli" more evident, than on the resources applied to the 'hERG/QT' area of research (Fig. 2). In principle, this could happen again to any aspect of the discipline, most probably on a smaller scale.

CONCLUDING REMARKS

Safety pharmacology is a key discipline within pharmaceutical nonclinical safety assessment, which uses functional (i.e., physiological) data for risk assessment. Neglect of this discipline, both in terms of in-house expertise, resources, and influence, was a contributing factor to the "QT Crisis" of the late 1990s, where several marketed drugs were withdrawn from sale. This example should therefore underline the importance of all types of safety pharmacology data. In principle, the more that is known about the pharmacology of a new medical entity (primary, secondary, and safety pharmacology), the greater the chance of product success and the better-prepared a company is to deal with clinical adverse effects that arise during development and marketing.

ACKNOWLEDGMENTS

The authors wish to thank their colleagues in the Safety Pharmacology Departments within AstraZeneca, elsewhere in Safety Assessment within AstraZeneca, and in Preclinical Drug Safety at UCB-Celltech, for thought-provoking discussions on all aspects of safety pharmacology over several years, particularly Jean-Pierre Valentin, Tim Hammond, Chris Pollard, Nick McMahon, Isobel Strang, Sharon Storey, Silvana Lindgren, Mike Swedberg, Russ Bialecki and Lew Kinter (AstraZeneca), and Roly Foulkes, Michael Canning, and Deborah Harding (UCB-Celltech). We would also wish to express our gratitude to the Safety Pharmacology Society (www.safetypharmacology.org) for providing an international forum, enabling us to exchange ideas with colleagues in other companies.

REFERENCES

1. Anon. ICHS7A—Note for Guidance on Safety Pharmacology Studies for Human Pharmaceuticals. European Agency for the Evaluation of Medicinal Products, Committee for Proprietary Medicinal Products (CPMP), London, UK, 2000. Reference CPMP/ICH/539/00.
2. Sterner W, Korn WD. Zur Pharmakologie und Toxikologie von Etofyllinclofibrate. Arzneimittelforschung 1980; 30:2023–2031.
3. Anon. Japanese Guidelines for Nonclinical Studies of Drugs Manual, Pharmaceutical Affairs Bureau, Japanese Ministry of Health and Welfare, Yakugi Nippo 1995.
4. Redfern WS, Wakefield ID, Prior H, Pollard CE, Hammond TG, Valentin J-P. Safety pharmacology—a progressive approach. Fundam Clin Pharmacol 2002; 16:161–173.
5. Williams PD. The role of pharmacological profiling in safety assessment. Regul Toxicol Pharmacol 1990; 12:238–252.
6. Sullivan AT. Good laboratory practice and other regulatory issues: a European view. Drug Dev Res 1995; 35:145–149.
7. Kinter LB. General pharmacology/safety pharmacology: customers, biologics and GLPs. Drug Dev Res 1995; 35:142–144.
8. Sullivan AT, Kinter LB. Status of safety pharmacology in the pharmaceutical industry—1995. Drug Dev Res 1995; 35:166–172.
9. Kinter LB, Dixon LW. Safety pharmacology program for pharmaceuticals. Drug Dev Res 1995; 35:179–182.
10. Porsolt RD. Safety pharmacology—a critical perspective. Drug Dev Res 1997; 41:51–57.
11. Anon. Committee for Proprietary Medicinal Products (CPMP) Points to Consider: The assessment of QT interval prolongation by non-cardiovascular medicinal products, 1997. CPMP/986/96.
12. Laurence DR, Bennett PN. Clinical Pharmacology. Edinburgh: Churchill Livingstone, 1992; 121–122.
13. Lazarou J, Pomeranz BH, Corey PN. Incidence of adverse drug reactions in hospitalized patients: a meta-analysis of prospective studies. JAMA 1998; 279:1200–1205.
14. Editorial. SuperMAB on trial. Lancet 2006; 367:960.
15. Kennedy T. Maintaining the drug discovery/development interface. Drug Dis Today 1997; 2:436–444.

16. Pirmohamed M, James S, Meakin S, et al. Adverse drug reactions as cause of admission to hospital: prospective analysis of 18 820 ptients. BMJ 2004; 329:15–19.

17. Shah RR. Drug-induced prolongation of the QT interval: why the regulatory concern? Fund Clin Pharmacol 2002; 16:119–124.

18. Fung M, Thornton A, Mybeck K, Hsaio-Hui Wu J, Hornbuckle K, Muniz E. Evaluation of the characteristics of safety withdrawal of prescription drugs from worldwide pharmaceutical markets—1960 to 1999. Drug Inf J 2001; 35:293–317.

19. Goldstein A, Aronow L, Kalman SM. 2nd ed. Principles of Drug Action. New York: Wiley, 1974:569–621.

20. Maurissen JPJ. Neurobehavioural methods for the evaluation of sensory functions. In: Chang LW, Slikker W, eds. Neurotoxicology—Approaches and Methods. San Diego: Academic Press, 1995:239–264.

21. Burgen ASV, Mitchell JF. 7th ed. Gaddum's Pharmacology. Oxford: Oxford University Press, 1972:226.

22. Olson H, Betton G, Robinson D, et al. Concordance of the toxicity of pharmaceuticals in humans and animals. Regul Toxicol Pharmacol 2000; 32:56–67.

23. Igarashi T, Nakane S, Kitagawa T. Predictability of clinical adverse reactions of drugs by general pharmacology studies. J Toxicol Sci 1995; 20:77–92.

24. Webster R, Leishman D, Walker D. Towards a drug concentration effect relationship for QT prolongation and torsades de pointes. Curr Opin Drug Discov Devel 2002; 5:116–126.

25. Redfern WS, Carlsson L, Davis AS, et al. Relationships between preclinical cardiac electrophysiology, clinical QT interval prolongation and torsade de pointes for a broad range of drugs: evidence for a provisional safety margin in drug development. Cardiovasc Res 2003; 58:32–45.

26. De Bruin ML, Pettersson M, Meyboom RHB, Hoes AW, Leufkens HGM. Anti-HERG activity and the risk of drug-induced arrhythmias and sudden death. Eur Heart J 2005; 26:590–597.

27. Fuenmayor LD, Diaz S. The effect of fasting on the stereotyped behaviour induced by amphetamine and by apomorphine in the albino rat. Eur J Pharmacol 1984; 99:153–158.

28. Hammond TG, Carlsson L, Davis AS, et al. Methods of collecting and evaluating non-clinical cardiac electrophysiology data in the pharmaceutical industry: results of an international survey. Cardiovasc Res 2000; 49:741–750.

29. Valentin JP, Bass AS, Atrakchi A, Olejniczak K, Kannosuke F. Challenges and lessons learned since implementation of the safety pharmacology guidance ICH S7A. J Pharmacol Toxicol Methods 2005; 52:22–29.

30. Bass A, Lewis Kinter L, Williams P. Origins, practices and future of safety pharmacology. J Pharmacol Toxicol Methods 2004; 49:145–151.

31. Lees KR. Cerestat and other NMDA antagonists in ischemic stroke. Neurology 1997; 4:S66–S69.

32. Haverkamp W, Breithardt G, Camm AJ, et al. The potential for QT prolongation and proarrhythmia by non-antiarrhythmic drugs: clinical and regulatory implications. Cardiovasc Res 2000; 47:219–233 (published simultaneously in Eur Heart J 2000;21:1216-1231).

33. Cavero I, Mestre M, Guillon J-M, Crumb W. Drugs that prolong QT interval as an unwanted effect: assessing their likelihood of inducing hazardous cardiac dysrhythmias. Expert Opin Pharmacother 2000; 1:947–973.

34. Gralinski MR. The assessment of potential for QT interval prolongation with new pharmaceuticals: impact on drug development. J Pharmacol Toxicol Methods 2000; 43:91–99.

35. Fermini B, Fossa AA. The impact of drug-induced QT interval prolongation on drug discovery and development. Nature Reviews. Drug Discov 2003; 2:439–447.

36. Shah RR. Drug-induced QT interval prolongation: regulatory perspectives and drug development. Ann Med 2004; 36:47–52.

37. Fenichel RR, Malik M, Antzelevitch C, et al. Independent academic task force. Drug-induced torsades de pointes and implications for drug development. J Cardiovasc Electrophysiol 2004; 15:475–495.

38. Guth BD, Germeyer S, Kolb W, Markert M. Developing a strategy for the nonclinical assessment of proarrhythmic risk of pharmaceuticals due to prolonged ventricular repolarization. J Pharmacol Toxicol Methods 2004; 49:159–169.

39. Mitcheson JS, Chen J, Lin M, Culberson C, Sanguinetti MC. A structural basis for drug-induced long QT syndrome. Proc Natl Acad Sci USA 2000; 97:12329–12333.

40. Vandenberg JI, Walker BD, Campbell TJ. HERG K$^+$ channels: friend and foe. Trends Pharmacol Sci 2001; 22:240–246.

41. Bennett PB, Guthrie HR. Trends in ion channel drug discovery: advances in screening technologies. Trends Biotechnol 2003; 21:563–569.

42. Netzer R, Bischoff U, Ebneth A. HTS techniques to investigate the potential effects of compounds on cardiac ion channels at early-stages of drug discovery. Curr Opin Drug Discov Devel 2003; 6:462–469.

43. Brown AM. Drugs, hERG and sudden death. Cell Calcium 2004; 35:543–547.

44. Guthrie H, Livingston FS, Gubler U, Garippa R. A place for high-throughput electrophysiology in cardiac safety: screening hERG cell lines and novel compounds with the IonWorks HT™ system. J Biomol Screening, 2005; 10:832–840.

45. Aronov AM. Predictive in silico modelling for hERG channel blockers. Drug Discov Today Biosilico 2005; 10:149–155.

46. Brockway BP, Mills PA, Azar SH. A new method for continuous chronic measurement and recording of blood pressure, heart rate and activity in the rat via radio-telemetry. Clin Exp Hypertens 1991; 13:885–895.

47. Gras J, Llenas J, Palacios JM, Roberts DJ. The role of ketoconazole in the QTc interval prolonging effects of H$_1$-antihistamines in a guinea-pig model of arrhythmogenicity. Br J Pharmacol 1996; 119:187–188.

48. Carlsson L, Amos GJ, Andersson B, Drews L, Duker G, Wadstedt G. Electrophysiological characterization of the prokinetic agents cisapride and mosapride in vivo and in vitro: implications for proarrhythmic potential? J Pharmacol Exp Ther 1997; 282:220–227.

49. Bollen P, Ellegaard L. The Gottingen minipig in pharmacology and toxicology. Pharmacol Toxicol 1997; 2:3–4.

50. Meng H, McVey M, Perrone M, Clark KL. Intravenous AMP 579, a novel adenosine A(1)/A(2a) receptor agonist, induces a delayed protection against myocardial infarction in minipig. Eur J Pharmacol 2000; 387:101–105.

51. Oguchi Y, Hamlin RL. Rate of change of QT interval in response to a sudden change in the heart rate in dogs. Am J Vet Res 1994; 55:1618–1623.

52. Fridericia L. Dir Systolendaeur in elektrokardiogram bei normalen menchen und bei herzkranken. Acta Medica Scandinavica 1920; 53:469–486.

53. Van de Water A, Verheyen J, Xhonneux R, Reneman RS. An improved method to correct the QT interval of the electrocardiogram for changes in heart rate. J Pharmacol Methods 1989; 22:207–217.

54. Matsunaga T, Mitsui T, Harada T, et al. QT corrected for heart rate and relation between QT and RR intervals in beagle dogs. J Pharmacol Toxicol Methods 1997; 38:201–209.

55. Tattersall ML, Dymond M, Hammond T, Valentin J-P. Correction of QT values to allow for increases in heart rate in conscious Beagle dogs in toxicology assessment. J Pharmacol Toxicol Methods, 2006; 53:11–19.

56. Batey AJ, Doe CPA. A method for QT correction based on beat-to-beat analysis of the QT/RR interval relationship in conscious telemetered beagle dogs. J Pharmacol Toxicol Methods 2002; 48:11–19.

57. Fossa AA, Wisialowski T, Magnano A, et al. Dynamic beat-to-beat modeling of the QT-RR interval relationship: analysis of QT prolongation during alterations of autonomic state versus human ether a-go-go-related gene inhibition. J Pharmacol Exp Ther 2005; 312:1–11.

58. Schneider J, Hauser R, Andreas J-O, Linz K, Jahnel U. Differential effects of human ether-a-go-go-related gene (HERG) blocking agents on QT duration variability in conscious dogs. Eur J Pharmacol 2005; 512:53–60.

59. van der Linde H, Van de Water A, Loots W, et al. A new method to calculate the beat-to-beat instability of QT duration in drug-induced long QT in anesthetized dogs. J Pharmacol Toxicol Methods 2005; 52:168–177.

60. Bode G, Olejniczak K. ICH Expert Working Group, ICH topic: the draft ICH S7B step 2: note for guidance on safety pharmacology studies for human pharmaceuticals. Fund Clin Pharmacol 2002; 16:105–118.

61. Anon. Note for guidance on the nonclinical evaluation of the potential for delayed ventricular repolarization (QT interval prolongation) by human pharmaceuticals (CHMP/ICH/423/02). European Medicines Agency, Committee for Human Medicinal Products (CHMP), London, U.K., 2005. www.emea.eu.int/pdfs/human/ich/042302en.pdf.

62. Cavero I, Crumb W. ICH S7B draft guideline on the non-clinical strategy for testing delayed cardiac repolarisation risk of drugs: a critical analysis. Expert Opin Drug Saf 2005; 4:509–530.

63. Gintant GA, Limberis JT, McDermott JS, Wegner CD, Cox BF. The canine Purkinje fibre: an in vitro model system for acquired long QT syndrome and drug-induced arrythmogenesis. J Cardiovasc Pharmacol 2001; 37:607–618.

64. Guth BD, Germeyer S, Kolb W, Markert M. Developing a strategy for the nonclinical assessment of proarrhythmic risk of pharmaceuticals due to prolonged ventricular repolarization. J Pharmacol Toxicol Methods 2004; 49:159–169.

65. Abi-Gerges N, Small BG, Lawrence CL, Hammond TG, Valentin J-P. Evidence for gender differences in electrophysiological properties of canine Purkinje fibres. Br J Pharmacol 2004; 142:1255–1264.

66. Herron W, Towers C, Templeton A. Experiences in method development for the analysis of in vitro study solutions for content. J Pharmacol Toxicol Methods 2004; 49:211–216.

67. Lawrence CL, Pollard CE, Hammond TG, Valentin J-P. Nonclinical proarrhythmia models: Predicting Torsades de Pointes. J Pharmacol Toxicol Methods 2005; 52:46–59.

68. Wilson LD, Said T, Rosenbaum DS. Disease models for elucidation of mechanisms and prediction of drug-induced proarrhythmia. Drug Discov Today Dis Models 2005; 2:205–213.

69. Hondeghem LM, Carlsson L, Duker G. Instability and triangulation of the action potential predict serious proarrhythmia, but action potential duration prolongation is antiarrhythmic. Circulation 2001; 103:2004–2013.

70. Belardinelli L, Antzelevitch C, Vos MA. Assessing predictors of drug-induced torsade de pointes. Trends Pharmacol Sci 2003; 24:619–625.

71. Carlsson L, Almgren O, Duker G. QTU-prolongation and torsades de pointes induced by putative class III antiarrhythmic agents in the rabbit: etiology and interventions. J Cardiovasc Pharmacol 1990; 16:276–285.

72. Johansson M, Carlsson L. Female gender does not influence the magnitude of ibutilide-induced repolarization delay and incidence of torsades de pointes in an in vivo rabbit model of the acquired long QT syndrome. J Cardiovasc Pharmacol Ther 2001; 6:247–254.

73. Weissenburger J, Chezalviel F, Davy JM, et al. Methods and limitations of an experimental model of long QT syndrome. J Pharmacol Methods 1991; 26:23–42.

74. Sugiyama A, Satoh Y, Shiina H, Takeda S, Hashimoto K. Torsadegenic action of the antipsychotic drug sulpiride assessed using in vivo canine models. J Cardiovas Pharmacol 2002; 40:235–245.

75. Valentin JP, Hoffmann P, De Clerck F, Hammond TG, Hondeghem L. Review of the predictive value of the Langendorff heart model (Screenit system) in assessing the proarrhythmic potential of drugs. J Pharmacol Toxicol Methods 2004; 49:171–181.

76. Schram G, Zhang L, Derakhchan K, Ehrlich JR, Belardinelli L, Nattel S. Ranolazine: ion-channel-blocking actions and in vivo electrophysiological effects. Br J Pharmacol 2004; 142:1300–1308.

77. Fleming T, Nissen SE, Borer JS, Armstrong PW. Cardiovascular and Renal Drugs Advisory Committee: U.S. Food and Drug Administration. Report from the 100th Cardiovascular and Renal Drugs Advisory Committee meeting: U.S. Food and Drug Administration: December 8–9, 2003 Gaithersburg, MD. Circulation 2004; 109:e9004–e9005.

78. Antzelevitch C, Belardinelli L, Wu L, et al. Electrophysiologic properties and antiarrhythmic actions of a novel antianginal agent. J Cardiovasc Pharmacol Ther 2004; 9:S65–S83.

79. Antzelevitch C, Belardinelli L, Zygmunt AC, et al. Electrophysiological effects of ranolazine, a novel antianginal agent with antiarrhythmic properties. Circulation 2004; 110:904–910.

80. Wu L, Shryock JC, Song Y, Li Y, Antzelevitch C, Belardinelli L. Antiarrhythmic Effects of Ranolazine in a Guinea Pig in Vitro Model of Long-QT Syndrome. J Pharmacol Exp Ther 2004; 310:599–605.

81. Song Y, Shryock JC, Wu L, Belardinelli L. Antagonism by ranolazine of the pro-arrhythmic effects of increasing late INa in guinea pig ventricular myocytes. J Cardiovasc Pharmacol 2004; 44:192–199.
82. Boyett MR, Honjo H, Kodama I. The sinoatrial node, a heterogeneous pacemaker structure. Cardiovasc Res 2000; 47:658–687.
83. Cho HS, Takano M, Noma A. The electrophysiological properties of spontaneously beating pacemaker cells isolated from mouse sinoatrial node. J Physiol 2003; 550:169–180.
84. Gillespie JS, Muir TC. A method of stimulating the complete sympathetic outflow from the spinal cord to blood vessels in the pithed rat. Br J Pharmacol 1967; 30:78–87.
85. Grant TL, McGrath JC, O'Brien JW. The influence of blood gases on alpha 1- and alpha 2-adrenoceptor-mediated pressor responses in the pithed rat. Br J Pharmacol 1985; 86:69–77.
86. Brown CM, MacKinnon AC, Redfern WS, et al. The pharmacology of RS-15385-197, a potent and selective α_2-adrenoceptor antagonist. Br J Pharmacol 1993; 108:516–525.
87. Valentin JP, Bessac AM, Colpaert FC, John GW. Use of the pithed rat model to determine the relative potencies of 5-HT2A/2C receptor antagonists following acute intravenous and oral administration. Methods Find Expert Clin Pharmacol 1995; 17:267–271.
88. Zhuo J, Ohishi M, Mendelsohn FA. Roles of AT1 and AT2 receptors in the hypertensive Ren-2 gene transgenic rat kidney. Hypertension 1999; 33:347–353.
89. Van Dorpe J, Smeijers L, Dewachter I, et al. Prominent cerebral amyloid angiopathy in transgenic mice overexpressing the london mutant of human APP in neurons. Am J Pathol 2000; 157:1283–1298.
90. Tabrizchi R, Pugsley MK. Methods of blood flow measurement in the arterial circulatory system. J Pharmacol Toxicol Methods 2000; 44:375–384.
91. Koistinaho M, Kettunen MI, Goldsteins G, et al. Beta-amyloid precursor protein transgenic mice that harbor diffuse A beta deposits but do not form plaques show increased ischemic vulnerability: role of inflammation. Proc Nat Acad Sci USA 2002; 99:1610–1615.
92. Gardiner SM, Kemp PA, March JE, Woolley J, Bennett T. The influence of antibodies to TNF-alpha and IL-1beta on haemodynamic responses to the cytokines, and to lipopolysaccharide, in conscious rats. Br J Pharmacol 1998; 125:1543–1550.
93. Wakefield ID, March JE, Kemp PA, Valentin JP, Bennett T, Gardiner SM. Comparative regional haemodynamic effects of the nitric oxide synthase inhibitors, S-methyl-L-thiocitrulline and L-NAME, in conscious rats. Br J Pharmacol 2003; 139:1235–1243.
94. Prinzen FW, Glenny RW. Developments in non-radioactive microsphere techniques for blood flow measurement. Cardiovasc Res 1994; 28:1467–1475.
95. Takahara A, Dohmoto H, Yoshimoto R, Sugiyama A, Hashimoto K. Cardiovascular action of a cardioselective Ca(2+)channel blocker AH-1058 in conscious dogs assessed by telemetry. Eur J Pharmacol 2001; 413:101–108.
96. Little RA, Redfern WS. A method for studying baroreflex bradycardia in the unanaesthetized rat. Br J Pharmacol 1981; 74:308P–309P.
97. Kuwahara M, Yayou K, Ishii K, Hashimoto S, Tsubone H, Sugano S. Power spectral analysis of heart rate variability as a new method for assessing autonomic activity in the rat. J Electrocardiol 1994; 27:333–337.
98. Calvert CA. Heart rate variability. Vet Clin North Am Small Anim Pract 1998; 28:1409–1427 viii.
99. Irwin S. Comprehensive behavioural assessment: 1a A systematic quantitative procedure for assessing the behavioural and physiologic state of the mouse. Psychopharmacology 1968; 13:222–257.
100. Moser VC. Screening approaches to neurotoxicity: A functional observational battery. J Am Coll Toxicol 1989; 8:85–93.
101. Tilson HA, Moser VC. Comparison of screening approaches. NeuroToxicology 1992; 13:1–14.
102. Porsolt RD, McArthur RA, Lenègre A. Psychotropic screening procedures. In: van Haaren F, ed. Methods in Behavioral Pharmacology. Amsterdam: Elsevier, 1993:23–51.
103. Porsolt RD, Lemaire M, Dürkmüller N, Roux S. New perspectives in CNS safety pharmacology. Fundam Clin Pharmacol 2002; 16:197–207.
104. Trabace L, Cassano T, Steardo L, et al. Biochemical and neurobehavioral profile of CHF2819, a novel, orally active acetylcholinesterase inhibitor for Alzheimer's disease. J Pharmacol Exp Ther 2000; 294:187–194.

105. Redfern WS, Strang I, Storey S, et al. Spectrum of effects detected in the rat Functional Observational Battery following oral administration of non-CNS targeted compounds. J Pharmacol Toxicol Methods 2005; 52:77–82.

106. Haggerty GC. Development of Tier I neurobehavioral testing capabilities for incorporation into pivotal rodent safety assessment studies. J Am Coll Toxicol 1989; 8:53–69.

107. Mattson JL, Spencer PJ, Albee RR. A performance standard for clinical and Functional Observational Battery examination of rats. J Am Coll Toxicol 1996; 15:239–250.

108. Moser VC, Becking GC, MacPhail RC, Kulig BM. The IPCS collaborative study on neurobehavioral screening methods. Fundam Appl Toxicol 1997; 35:143–151.

109. Baird SJS, Catalano PJ, Ryan LM, Evans JS. Evaluation of effect profiles: Functional Observational Battery Outcomes. Fundam Appl Toxicol 1997; 40:37–51.

110. Moser VC. The functional observational battery in adult and developing rats. Neurotoxicology 2000; 21:989–996.

111. Gad SC, Gad SE. A functional observational battery for use in canine toxicity studies: development and validation. Int J Toxicol 2003; 22:415–422.

112. Patterson JP, Markgraf CG, Cirino M, Bass AS. Validation of a motor activity system by a robotically controlled vehicle and using standard reference compounds. J Pharmacol Toxicol Methods 2005; 52:159–167.

113. Vorhees CV, Acuff-Smith KD, Minck DR, Butcher RE. A method for measuring locomotor activity in rodents: contrast-sensitive computer-controlled video tracking activity assessment in rats. Neurotoxicol Teratol 1992; 14:43–49.

114. Kelley AE. Locomotor activity and exploration. In: van Haaren F, ed. Methods in Behavioral Pharmacology. Amsterdam: Elsevier, 1993:499–518.

115. Kelley AE. Locomotor activity and exploration. In: Sahgal A, ed. In: Behavioural Neuroscience: A Practical Approach, Vol. II. Oxford: IRL Press, 1993:1–21.

116. Bogo V, Hill TA, Young RW. Comparison of accelerod and rotarod sensitivity in detecting ethanol- and acrylamide-induced performance decrement in rats: review of experimental considerations of rotating rod systems. Neurotoxicology 1981; 2:765–787.

117. Hamm RJ, Pike BR, O'Dell DM, Lyeth BG, Jenkins LW. The rotarod test: an evaluation of its effectiveness in assessing motor deficits following traumatic brain injury. J Neurotrauma 1994; 11:187–196.

118. Piot-Grosjean O, Wahl F, Gobbo O, Stutzmann J-M. Assessment of sensorimotor and cognitive deficits induced by a moderate traumatic injury in the right parietal cortex of the rat. Neurobiol Dis 2001; 8:1082–1093.

119. Stanley JL, Lincoln RJ, Brown TA, McDonald LM, Dawson GR, Reynolds DS. The mouse beam walking assay offers improved sensitivity over the mouse rotarod in determining motor coordination deficits induced by benzodiazepines. J Psychopharmacol 2005; 19:221–227.

120. Clarke KA. A technique for the study of spatiotemporal aspects of paw contact patterns, applied to rats treated with a TRH analogue. Behav Res Methods Instrum Comput 1992; 24:407–411.

121. Hamers FPT, Lankhorst AJ, Van Laar TJ, Veldhuis WB, Gispen WH. Automated quantitative gait analysis during overground locomotion in the rat: Its application to spinal cord contusion and transaction injuries. J Neurotrauma 2001; 18:187–201.

122. Artur SP, Varejão DVM, Cabrita AM, et al. Functional assessment of peripheral nerve recovery in the rat: gait kinematics. Microsurgery 2001; 21:383–388.

123. Coulthard P, Pleuvry P, Brewster M, Wilson KL, Macfarlane TV. Gait analysis as an objective measure in a chronic pain model. J Neurosci Methods 2002; 116:197–213.

124. Handley SL, Mithani S. Effects of alpha-adrenoceptor agonists and antagonists in a maze-exploration model of "fear"-motivated behaviour. Naunyn-Schmied. Arch Pharmacol 1984; 327:1–5.

125. Pellow S, Chopin P, File SE, Briley M. Validation of open:closed arm entries in an elevated plus-maze as a measure of anxiety in the rat. J Neurosci Methods 1985; 14:149–167.

126. Handley SL, McBlane JW. An assessment of the elevated X-maze for studying anxiety and anxiety-modulating drugs. J Pharmacol Toxicol Methods 1993; 29:129–133.

127. Redfern WS, Williams A. A re-evaluation of the role of α_2-adrenoceptors in the anxiogenic effects of yohimbine, using the selective antagonist delequamine in the rat. Br J Phamacol 1996; 116:2081–2089.

128. Authier N, Gillet J-P, Fialip J, Eschalier A, Coudore F. Description of a short-term Taxol®-induced nociceptive neuropathy in rats. Brain Res 2000; 887:239–249.

129. Polomano RC, Mannes AJ, Clark US, Bennett GJ. A painful peripheral neuropathy in the rat produced by the chemotherapeutic drug, paclitaxel. Pain 2001; 94:293–304.

130. Hole K, Tjølsen A. The tail-flick and formalin tests in rodents: changes in skin temperature as a confounding factor. Pain 1993; 53:247–254.

131. Sawamura S, Tomioka T, Hanaoka K. The importance of tail temperature monitoring during tail-flick test in evaluating the antinociceptive action of volatile anesthetics. Acta Anaesthesiol Scand 2002; 46:451–454.

132. Redfern WS, MacLean MR, Clague RU, McGrath JC. The role of α_2-adrenoceptors in the vasculature of the rat tail. Br J Pharmacol 1995; 114:1724–1730.

133. Sotgiu ML, Castagna A, Lacerenza M, Marchettini P. Pre-injury lidocaine treatment prevents thermal hyperalgesia and cutaneous thermal abnormalities in a rat model of peripheral neuropathy. Pain 1995; 61:3–10.

134. Romanovsky AA, Ivanov AI, Shimansky YP. Selected contribution: ambient temperature for experiments in rats: a new method for determining the zone of thermal neutrality. J Appl Physiol 2002; 92:2667–2679.

135. Dyer RS. The use of sensory evoked potentials in toxicology. Fund Appl Toxicol 1984; 5:24–40.

136. Herr DW, Graff JE, Derr-Yellin EC, Crofton KM, Kodavanti PRS. Flash-, somatosensory-, and peripheral nerve-evoked potentials in rats perinatally exposed to Aroclor 1254. Neurotoxicol Teratol 2001; 23:591–601.

137. Herr DW, Boyes WK. Electrophysiological analysis of complex brain systems: sensory-evoked potentials and their generators. In: Chang LW, Slikker W, eds. Neurotoxicology: Approaches and Methods. San Diego: Academic Press, 1995:205–221.

138. Melena J, Safa R, Graham M, Casson RJ, Osborne NN. The monocarboxylate transport inhibitor, alpha-cyano-4-hydroxycinnamate, has no effect on retinal ischemia. Brain Res 2003; 989:128–134.

139. Pinilla I, Lund RD, Sauve Y. Contribution of rod and cone pathways to the dark-adapted electroretinogram (ERG) b-wave following retinal degeneration in RCS rats. Vision Res 2004; 44:2467–2474.

140. Nixon PJ, Bui BV, Armitage JA, Vingrys AJ. The contribution of cone responses to rat electroretinograms. Clin Exp Ophthalmol 2001; 29:193–196.

141. Xu L, Ball SL, Alexander KR, Peachey NS. Pharmacological analysis of the rat cone electroretinogram. Vis Neurosci 2003; 20:297–306.

142. Jones RD, Brenneke CJ, Hoss HE, Loney ML. An electroretinogram protocol for toxicological screening in the canine model. Toxicol Lett 1994; 70:223–234.

143. Lashley KS. The mechanism of vision: I. A method for rapid analysis of pattern vision in the rat. J Gen Psychol 1930; 37:453–460.

144. Prusky GT, West PW, Douglas RM. Behavioral assessment of visual acuity in mice and rats. Vis Res 2000; 40:2201–2209.

145. Prusky GT, Harker KT, Douglas RM, Whishaw IQ. Variation in visual acuity within pigmented, and between pigmented and albino rat strains. Behav Brain Res 2002; 136:339–348.

146. Prusky GT, Alam NM, Beekman S, Douglas RM. Rapid quantification of adult and developing mouse spatial vision using a virtual optomotor system. Invest Ophthalmol Vis Sci 2004; 45:4611–4616.

147. Tripathi RC, Tripathi B, Haggerty C. Drug-induced glaucomas: mechanism and management. Drug Saf 2003; 26:749–767.

148. Schnell CR, Debon C, Percicot CL. Measurement of intraocular pressure by telemetry in conscious, unrestrained rabbits. Invest Ophthalmol Vis Sci 1996; 37:958–965.

149. Reitsamer HA, Kiel JW, Harrison JM, Ransom NL, McKinnon SJ. Tonopen measurement of intraocular pressure in mice. Exp Eye Res 2004; 78:799–804.

150. Löscher W, Fassbender CP, Nolting B. The role of technical, biological and pharmacological factors in the laboratory evaluation of anticonvulsant drugs II. Maximal electroshock seizure models. Epilepsy Res 1991; 8:79–94.

151. Kitano Y, Usui C, Takasuna K, Hirohashi M, Nomura M. Increasing-current electroshock seizure test: a new method for assessment of anti- and pro-convulsant activities of drugs in mice. J Pharmacol Toxicol Methods 1996; 35:25–29.

152. De Deyn PP, D'Hooge RD, Marescau B, Pei Y-Q. Chemical models of epilepsy with some reference to their applicability in the development of anticonvulsants. Epilepsy Res 1992; 12:87–110.
153. Krall RL, Penry JK, White BG, Kupferberg HJ, Swinyard EA. Antiepileptic drug development: II. Anticonvulsant drug screening. Epilepsia 1978; 19:404–428.
154. Oliver AP, Hoffer BJ, Wyatt RJ. The hippocampal slice: a system for studying the pharmacology of seizures and for screening anticonvulsant drugs. Epilepsia 1977; 18:543–548.
155. Salazar P, Tapia R, Rogawski MA. Effects of neurosteroids on epileptiform activity induced by picrotoxin and 4-aminopyridine in the rat hippocampal slice. Epilepsy Res 2003; 55:71–82.
156. Harrison PK, Sheridan RD, Green AC, Scott IR, Tattersall JE. A guinea pig hippocampal slice model of organophosphate-induced seizure activity. J Pharmacol Exp Ther 2004; 310:678–686.
157. Freund RK, Marley RJ, Wehner JM. Differential sensitivity to bicuculline in three inbred mouse strains. Brain Res Bull 1987; 18:657–662.
158. Sebban C, Zhang XQ, Tesolin-Decros B, Millan MJ, Spedding M. Changes in EEG spectral power in the prefrontal cortex of conscious rats elicited by drugs interacting with dopaminergic and noradrenergic transmission. Br J Pharmacol 1999; 128:1045–1054.
159. Sebban C, Tesolin-Decros B, Millan MJ, Spedding M. Contrasting EEG profiles elicited by antipsychotic agents in the prefrontal cortex of the conscious rat: antagonism of the effects of clozapine by modafinil. Br J Pharmacol 1999; 128:1055–1063.
160. Dringenberg HC, Diavolitsis P, Noseworthy PA. Effect of tacrine on EEG slowing in the rat: enhancement by concurrent monoamine therapy. Neurobiol Aging 2000; 21:135–143.
161. Dimpfel W. Preclinical data base of pharmaco-specific rat EEG fingerprints (tele-stereo-EEG). Eur J Med Res 2003; 8:199–207.
162. Edgar DM, Seidel WF. Modafinil induces wakefulness without intensifying motor activity or subsequent rebound hypersomnolence in the rat. J Pharmacol Exp Ther 1997; 283:757–769.
163. Lancel M, Faulhaber J, Deisz RA. Effect of the GABA uptake inhibitor tiagabine on sleep and EEG power spectra in the rat. Br J Pharmacol 1998; 123:1471–1477.
164. Tortella FC, Hill RG. EEG seizure activity and behavioral neurotoxicity produced by (+)-MK801, but not the glycine site antagonist L-687,414, in the rat. Neuropharmacology 1996; 35:441–448.
165. Mackenzie L, Medvedev A, Hiscock JJ, Pope KJ, Willoughby JO. Picrotoxin-induced generalised convulsive seizure in rat: changes in regional distribution and frequency of the power of electroencephalogram rhythms. Clin Neurophysiology 2002; 113:586–596.
166. Maloney KJ, Cape EG, Gotman J, Jones BE. High-frequency gamma electroencephalogram activity in association with sleep-wake states and spontaneous behaviors in the rat. Neuroscience 1997; 76:541–555.
167. Takeuchi T, Harada E. Age-related changes in sleep-wake rhythm in dog. Behav Brain Res 2002; 136:193–199.
168. Pietrzak B, Czarnecka E. The effect of combined administration of ethanol and sertraline, fluoxetine and citalopram on rabbit EEG. Pharmacol Res 2003; 47:527–534.
169. Tobler I, Franken P, Jaggi K. Vigilance states, EEG spectra, and cortical temperature in the guinea pig. Am J Physiol 1993; 264:R1125–R1132.
170. Mumford H, Wetherell JR. A simple method for measuring EEG in freely moving guinea pigs. J Neurosci Methods 2001; 107:125–130.
171. McNamara RK, Skelton RW. The neuropharmacological and neurochemical basis of place learning in the Morris water maze. Brain Res Rev 1993; 18:33–49.
172. D'Hooge R, De Deyn PP. Applications of the Morris water maze in the study of learning and memory. Res Brain Res Rev 2001; 36:60–90.
173. Myhrer T. Neurotransmitter systems involved in learning and memory in the rat: a meta-analysis based on studies of four behavioural tasks. Brain Res Rev 2003; 41:268–287.
174. Slikker W, Beck BD, Cory-slechta DA, Paule M, Anger WK, Bellinger D. Cognitive tests: interpretation for neurotoxicity? (Workshop summary) Toxicol Sci 2000; 58:222–234.
175. Paule MG, Fogle CM, Allen RR, Pearson EC, Hammond TG, Popke EJ. Chronic exposure to NMDA receptor and sodium channel blockers during development in monkeys and rats: long-term effects on cognitive function. Ann NY Acad Sci 2002; 993:116–122.
176. Haefely W. Biological basis of drug-induced tolerance, rebound and dependence. Contribution of recent research on benzodiazepines. Pharmacopsychiatry 1986; 19:353–361.

177. Mansbach RS, Feltner DE, Gold LH, Schnoll SH. Incorporating the assessment of abuse liability into the drug discovery and development process. Drug Alcohol Depend 2003; 70:S73–S85.

178. Balster RL, Bigelow GE. Guidelines and methodological reviews concerning drug abuse liability assessment. Drug Alcohol Depend 2003; 70:S13–S40.

179. Ator NA, Griffiths RR. Principles of drug abuse liability assessment in laboratory animals. Drug Alcohol Depend 2003; 70:S55–S72.

180. Tzschentke TM. Measuring reward with the conditioned place preference paradigm: a comprehensive review of drug effects, recent progress and new issues. Prog Neurobiol 1998; 56:613–672.

181. Bardo MT, Bevins RA. Conditioned place preference: what does it add to our preclinical understanding of drug reward? Psychopharmacol 2000; 153:31–43.

182. Colpaert FC. Drug discrimination in neurobiology. Pharmacol Biochem Behav 1999; 64:337–345.

183. Ator NA. Contributions of GABAA receptor subtype selectivity to abuse liability and dependence potential of pharmacological treatments for anxiety and sleep disorders. CNS Spectr 2005; 10:31–39.

184. Committee for Medicinal Products for Human Use Guideline on the non-clinical investigation of the dependence potential of medicinal products 2005. EMEA/CHMP/SWP/94227/2004.

185. Murphy DJ. Assessment of respiratory function in safety pharmacology. Fund Clin Pharmacol 2002; 16:183–196.

186. Ben-Noun L. Drug-induced respiratory disorders: incidence, prevention and management. Drug Saf 2000; 23:143–164.

187. Feldman JL, Mitchell GS, Nattie EE. Breathing: rhythmicity, plasticity, chemosensitivity. Ann Rev Neurosci 2003; 26:239–266.

188. American Thoracic Society. Lung function testing: selection of reference values and interpretive strategies. Am Rev Resp Dis 1991; 144:1202–1218.

189. Chong BT, Agrawal DK, Romero FA, Townley RG. Measurement of bronchoconstriction using whole-body plethysmograph: comparison of freely-moving versus restrained guinea-pigs. J Pharmacol Toxicol Methods 1998; 39:163–168.

190. DeLorme MP, Moss OR. Pulmonary function assessment by whole-body plethysmography in restrained versus unrestrained mice. J Pharmacol Toxicol Methods 2002; 47:1–10.

191. Mitzner W, Tankersley C, Lundblad LK, Adler A, Irvin CG, Bates JH. Interpreting Penh in mice. J Appl Physiol 2003; 94:828–832.

192. Bates J, Irvin C, Brusasco V, et al. The use and misuse of Penh in animal models of lung disease. Am J Respir Cell Mol Biol 2004; 32:373–374.

193. Murphy DJ, Joran ME, Grando JC. A non-invasive method for distinguishing central from peripheral nervous system effect of respiratory depressant drugs in conscious rats. Gen Pharmacol 1995; 26:569–575.

194. Ide T, Shirahata M, Chou CL, Fitzgerald RS. Effects of a continuous infusion of dopamine on the ventilatory and carotid body responses to hypoxia in cats. Clin Exp Pharmacol Physiol 1995; 22:658–664.

195. Pennock BE, Cox CP, Rogers RM, Cain WA, Wells JH. A non-invasive technique for measurement of changes in specific airway resistance. J Appl Physiol 1979; 46:39–406.

196. Murphy DJ, Renninger JP, Gossett KA. A novel method for chronic measurement of pleural pressure in conscious rats. J Pharmacol Toxicol Methods 1998; 39:137–141.

197. Murphy DJ, Renninger JP, Coatney RW. A novel method for chronic measurement of respiratory function in the conscious monkey. J Pharmacol Toxicol Methods 2001; 46:13–20.

198. Kanairo M, Shibata O, Saito M, Yoshimura M, Makita T, Sumikawa K. Effects of vasopressors on contractile and phosphatidylinositol responses of rat trachea. J Anesthesia 2002; 16:289–293.

199. Nyhlen K, Rippe B, Hultkvist-Bengtsson U. An isolated blood-perfused guinea-pig lung model for simultaneous registration of haemodynamic, microvascular and respiratory variables. Acta Physiol Scand 1997; 159:293–302.

200. Tsai MC. Effect of neomycin on post-tetanic twitch tension of the mouse diaphragm preparation. Br J Pharmacol 1987; 90:625–633.

201. Ramnarine SI, Liu YC, Rogers DF. Neuroregulation of mucus secretion by opioid receptors and K(ATP) and BK(Ca) channels in ferret trachea in vitro. Br J Pharmacol 1998; 123:1631–1638.

202. Dimova S, Maes F, Brewster ME, Jorissen M, Noppe M, Augustijns P. High-speed digital imaging method for ciliary beat frequency measurement. J Pharm Pharmacol 2005; 57:521–526.
203. Harrison AP, Erlwanger KH, Elbrønd, Anderson NK, Unmack MA. Gastrointestinal-tract models and techniques for use in safety pharmacology. J Pharmacol Toxicol Methods 2004; 49:187–199.
204. Mittelstadt SW, Hemenway CL, Spruell RD. Effects of fasting on evaluation of gastrointestinal transit with charcoal meal. J Pharmacol Toxicol Methods 2005; 52:154–158.
205. Yeung CK, McCurrie JR, Wood D. A simple method to investigate the inhibitory effects of drugs on gastric emptying in the mouse in vivo. J Pharmacol Toxicol Methods 2001; 45:235–240.
206. Papasouliotis K, Gruffydd-Jones TJ, Sparkes AH, Cripps PJ. A comparison of orocaecal transit times assessed by the breath hydrogen test and the sulphasalazine/sulphapyridine method in healthy beagle dogs. Res Vet Sci 1995; 58:263–267.
207. Nguyen A, Camilleri M, Kost LJ, et al. SDZ HTF 919 stimulates canine colonic motility and transit in vivo. J Pharmacol Exp Ther 1997; 280:1270–1276.
208. Iwanaga Y, Wen J, Thollander MS, et al. Scintigraphic measurement of regional gastrointestinal transit in the dog. Am J Physiol 1998; 275:G904–G910.
209. Gacsalyi U, Zabielski R, Pierzynowski SG. Telemetry facilitates long-term recording of gastrointestinal myoelectrical activity in pigs. Exp Physiol 2000; 85:239–241.
210. Chiu PJ, Barnett A, Tetzloff G, Kaminski J. Gastric antisecretory properties of SCH 32651. Arch Int Pharmacodyn Ther 1984; 270:116–127.
211. Patten GS, Head RJ, Abeywardena MY, McMurchie EJ. An apparatus to assay opioid activity in the infused lumen of the intact isolated guinea-pig ileum. J Pharmacol Toxicol Methods 2001; 45:39–46.
212. Coupar IM, Lu L. A simple method for measuring the effects of drugs on intestinal longitudinal and circular muscle. J Pharmacol Toxicol Methods 1996; 36:147–154.
213. Percy WH. In vitro techniques for the study of gastrointestinal motility. In: Gaginella TS, ed. Handbook of Methods in Gastrointestinal Pharmacology. New York: CRC Press, 1996:189–224.
214. Ichihara K, Okumura K, Kamei H, et al. Renal effects of the calcium channel blocker aranidipine and its active metabolite in anesthetized dogs and conscious spontaneously hypertensive rats. J Cardiovasc Pharmacol 1998; 31:277–285.
215. Ronnhedh C, Jaquenod M, Mather LE. Urineless estimation of glomerular filtration rate and renal plasma flow in the rat. J Pharmacol Toxicol Methods 1996; 36:123–129.
216. Valentin JP, Mazbar SA, Humphreys MH. Long-term captopril treatment restores natriuresis after carotid baroreceptor activation in the SHR. Am J Physiol 1997; 273:R70–R79.
217. Neylon M, Marshall JM, Johns EJ. The effects of chronic hypoxia on renal function in the rat. J Physiol 1997; 501:243–250.
218. Fischer PA, Bogoliuk CB, Ramirez AJ, Sanchez RA, Masnatta LD. A new procedure for evaluation of renal function without urine collection in rat. Kidney Int 2000; 58:1336–1341.
219. Cambridge D, Whiting MV, Allan G. Cardiac and renovascular effects in the anaesthetized dog of BW A575C: a novel angiotensin converting enzyme inhibitor with beta-adrenoceptor blocking properties. Br J Pharmacol 1988; 93:165–175.
220. Brooks DP, Edwards RM, Depalma PD, Fredrickson TA, Hieble JP, Gellai M. The water diuretic effect of the alpha-2 adrenoceptor agonist, AGN 190851, is species-dependent. J Pharmacol Exp Ther 1991; 259:1277–1282.
221. Lenz T, Sealey JE, Maack T, et al. Half-life, hemodynamic, renal, and hormonal effects of prorenin in cynomolgus monkeys. Am J Physiol 1991; 260:R804–R810.
222. Supanz S, Sadjak A, Fellier H, Eidenberger T. Effects of the novel thromboxane (TXA2) receptor antagonist linotroban on inulin and para-aminohippuric acid clearances in the conscious male and female rat. ArzneimForsch 1997; 47:1026–1030.
223. Laurent D, Poirier K, Wasvary J, Rudin M. Effect of essential hypertension on kidney function as measured in rat by dynamic MRI. Magn Reson Med 2002; 47:127–134.
224. Pedersen M, Shi Y, Anderson P, et al. Quantitation of differential renal blood flow and renal function using dynamic contrast-enhanced MRI in rats. Magn Reson Med 2004; 51:510–517.
225. Maril N, Margalit R, Mispelter J, Degani H. Functional sodium magnetic resonance imaging of the intact rat kidney. Kidney Int 2004; 65:927–935.
226. Fry CH. Experimental models to study the physiology, pathophysiology, and pharmacology of the lower urinary tract. J Pharmacol Toxicol Methods 2004; 49:201–210.

227. Vera PL, Nadelhaft I. Effects of the atypical neuroleptic clozapine on micturition parameters in anesthetized rats. Neurourol Urodynamics 2001; 20:623–639.

228. Myers RA, Plym MJ, Signor LJ, Lodge NJ. 1-(2-pyrimidinyl)-piperazine, a buspirone metabolite, modulates bladder function in the anesthetized rat. Neurourol Urodynamics 2004; 23:709–715.

229. le Feber J, van Asselt E, van Mastrigt R. Afferent bladder nerve activity in the rat: a mechanism for starting and stopping voiding contractions. Urol Res 2004; 32:395–405.

230. Ghoniem GM, Aertker MW, Sakr MA, Shaaban AM, Shoukry MS. A telemetric multichannel computer-based system for monitoring urodynamic parameters in awake rhesus monkeys. J Urol 1997; 157:704–709.

231. Zbinden G. Predictive value of animal studies in toxicology. Regul Toxicol Pharmacol 1991; 14:167–177.

232. Zbinden G. Neglect of function and obsession with structure in toxicity testing. Proceedings of 9th International Congress Pharmacology. Vol. 1. New York: Macmillan, 1984:43–49.

233. Matsuzawa T, Hashimoto M, Nara N, Yoshida M, Tamura S, Igarashi T. Current status of conducting function tests in repeated dose toxicity studies in Japan. J Toxicol Sci 1997; 22:375–382.

234. Luft J, Bode G. Integration of safety pharmacology endpoints into toxicology studies. Fund Clin Pharmacol 2002; 16:91–103.

235. Vicini S, Ortinski P. Genetic manipulations of GABAA receptor in mice make inhibition exciting. Pharmacol Ther 2004; 103:109–120.

236. Roselt P, Meikle S, Kassiou M. The role of positron emission tomography in the discovery and development of new drugs; as studied in laboratory animals. Eur J Drug Metab Pharmacokinetics 2004; 29:1–6.

237. Lorenz JN. A practical guide to evaluating cardiovascular, renal, and pulmonary function in mice. Am J Physiol Regul Integr Comp Physiol 2002; 282:R1565–R1582.

238. Yang XP, Liu YH, Rhaleb NE, Kurihara N, Kim HE, Carretero OA. Echocardiographic assessment of cardiac function in conscious and anesthetized mice. Am J Physiol 1999; 277:H1967–H1974.

239. Collins KA, Korcarz CE, Lang RM. Use of echocardiography for the phenotypic assessment of genetically altered mice. Physiol Genomics 2003; 13:227–239.

240. Badea CT, Fubara B, Hedlund LW, Johnson GA. 4-D micro-CT of the mouse heart. Mol Imaging 2005; 4:110–116.

241. Kramer K, Kinter L, Brockway BP, Voss HP, Remie R, Van Zutphen BL. The use of radiotelemetry in small laboratory animals: recent advances. Contemp Top Lab Anim Sci 2001; 40:8–16.

242. Kramer K, Kinter LB. Evaluation and applications of radiotelemetry in small laboratory animals. Physiol Genomics 2003; 13:197–205.

243. Prinzen FW, Bassingthwaighte JB. Blood flow distributions by microsphere deposition methods. Cardiovasc Res 2000; 45:13–21.

244. Aristizabal O, Turnbull DH. 44-MHz LiNbO3 transducers for UBM-guided Doppler ultrasound. IEEE Transactions on Ultrasonics Ferroelectrics & Frequency Control 2003; 50:623–630.

245. DeGeorge JD, Ahn C-H, Andrews PA, et al. Regulatory considerations for preclinical development of anticancer drugs. Cancer Chemother Pharmacol 1998; 41:173–185.

246. Tomaszewski JE. Multi-species toxicology approaches for oncology drugs: the U.S. perspective. Eur J Cancer 2004; 40:907–913.

247. Lallana EC, Abrey LE. Update on the therapeutic approaches to brain tumors. Expert Rev Anticancer Ther 2003; 3:655–670.

248. Wiedmann MW, Caca K. Molecularly targeted therapy for gastrointestinal cancer. Curr Cancer Drug Targets 2005; 5:171–193.

249. Isobe T, Herbst RS, Onn A. Current management of advanced non-small cell lung cancer: targeted therapy. Semin Oncol 2005; 32:315–328.

250. Foulkes R. Preclinical safety evaluation of monoclonal antibodies. Toxicology 2002; 174:21–26.

251. Yang H, Hang H, Czura CJ, Tracey KJ. The cytokine activity of HMGB1. J Leukocyte Biol 2005; 78:1–8.

252. Aptula AO, Cronin MTD. Prediction of herg K^+ blocking potency: application of structural knowledge. SAR and QSAR Environ Res 2004; 15:399–411.

253. Krejsa CM, Horvath D, Rogalski SL, et al. Predicting ADME properties and side effects: the BioPrint approach. Curr Opin Drug Discov Dev 2003; 6:470–480.
254. Engelberg A. Iconix Pharmaceuticals. Inc.—removing barriers to efficient drug discovery through chemogenomics. Pharmacogenomics 2004; 5:741–744.
255. Norinder U, Haeberlein M. Computational approaches to prediction of the blood-brain distribution. Adv Drug Deliv Rev 2002; 54:291–313.
256. Noble D, Levin J, Scott W. Biological simulations in drug discovery. Drug Discov Today 1999; 4:10–16.
257. Bottino D, Penland RC, Stamps A, et al. Preclinical cardiac safety assessment of pharmaceutical compounds using an integrated systems-based computer model of the heart. Prog Biophysics Mol Biol 2006; 90:414–443.
258. Wakefield ID, Pollard CE, Redfern WS, Hammond TG, Valentin J-P. The application of in vitro methods to safety pharmacology. Fund Clin Pharmacol 2002; 16:209–218.
259. Rubinstein AL. Zebrafish: from disease modelling to drug discovery. Curr Opin Drug Discov Dev 2003; 6:218–223.
260. Parng C. In vivo zebrafish assays for toxicity testing. Curr Opin Drug Discov Dev 2005; 8:100–106.
261. Zon LI, Peterson RT. In vivo drug discovery in the zebrafish. Nature Rev Drug Discov 2005; 4:35–44.
262. Neuhauss SCF. Behavioural genetic approaches to visual system development and function in zebrafish. J Neurobiol 2003; 54:148–160.
263. Bang PI, Yelick PC, Malicki JJ, Sewell WF. High-throughput behavioural screening method for detecting auditory response defects in zebrafish. J Neurosci Methods 2002; 118:177–187.
264. www.biologicsconsulting.com/Preclinical_PharmTox.htm.
265. Porsolt RD, Picard S, Lacroix P. International Safety Pharmacology Guidelines (ICH S7A and S7B): Where Do We Go from Here? Drug Dev Res 2005; 64:83–89.
266. Kinter LB, Siegl PK, Bass AS. New preclinical guidelines on drug effects on ventricular repolarization: safety pharmacology comes of age. J Pharmacol Toxicol Methods 2004; 49:153–158.
267. Morganroth J. Design and Conduct of the Thorough Phase I ECG Trial for New Bioactive Drugs. In: Morganroth J, Gussak I, eds. Cardiac Safety of Noncardiac Drugs: Practical Guidelines for Clinical research and Drug Development. New Jersey: Humana Press, 2005:205–222.
268. Shah RR. Drugs, QT interval prolongation and ICH E14: the need to get it right. Drug Safety 2005; 28:115–125.

Appendix 1 Current and Emerging Regulatory Documents Impacting on Safety Pharmacology Studies

Document	Topic	Territory	Status	Main Implication	Commentary
ICHS6 (www.ich.org/Media Server.jser?@_ID = 503&@_MODE=GLB)	Biotechnology-derived pharmaceuticals: nonclinical evaluations	EU, FDA, JMHW	Adopted 1997	Safety pharmacology endpoints required either as separate studies (in vivo and/or in vitro) or incorporated into the toxicity studies	(264)
ICHM3(M) (www.emea.eu.int/ pdfs/human/ich/028695en. pdf)	Nonclinical safety studies for the conduct of human clinical trials for pharmaceuticals	EU, FDA, JMHW	Adopted 2000	Safety pharmacology evaluations required prior to human exposure; may be additions to toxicity studies or as separate studies	(None)
ICHS7A (www.fda.gov/cber/ gdlns/ichs7a071201.pdf)	All safety pharmacology (except proarrhythmia): nonclinical evaluations	EU, FDA, JMHW	Adopted 2001	All NCEs to be evaluated in safety pharmacology tests prior to human exposure	(29,265)
CPMP/SWP/2599/02/Rev 1 (www.emea.eu.int/pdfs/ human/swp/259902en.pdf)	Nonclinical studies to support single micro-dose clinical trials	EU	Adopted 2004	Safety pharmacology studies may be replaced by an extended single-dose toxicity study in one species	(None)
ICHS7B (www.emea.eu.int/ pdfs/human/ich/042302en. pdf)	Proarrhythmic risk: nonclinical evaluation	EU, FDA, JMHW	Adopted 2005	All NCEs to be tested in vitro and in vivo to assess torsadogenic risk prior to human exposure	(30,62,266)

(continued)

Appendix 1 Current and Emerging Regulatory Documents Impacting on Safety Pharmacology Studies (*Continued*)

Document	Topic	Territory	Status	Main Implication	Commentary
ICHE14 (www.nihs.go.jp/dig/ich/efficacy/e14/e14_040610_e.pdf)	Proarrhythmic risk: clinical evaluation	EU, FDA, JMHW	Adopted 2005	All NCEs to undergo a "Thorough Phase I ECG Trial"—regardless of preclinical risk assessment	(62,267,268)
Drug Abuse Advisory Committee, FDA (appended to review in Ref. 178)	Guidelines for Abuse Liability Assessment (draft; unpublished)	FDA	Draft issued 1990	Risk-assessment of abuse liability (clinical and non-clinical)	(178)
EMEA/CHMP/SWP/94227/2004 (www.emea.eu.int/pdfs/human/swp/9422704en.pdf)	Nonclinical evaluation of dependence potential	EU	Draft issued 2005	All new CNS-active NCEs require assessment for dependence potential	(None)
FDA-CDER G:\6384dft.doc 04/07/05 (www.fda.gov/cder/guidance/6384dft.pdf)	Nonclinical studies to support exploratory IND studies (clinical trials of limited exposure on NCEs for which there is no therapeutic intent)	FDA	Draft issued 2005	Safety pharmacology endpoints can be incorporated into toxicology studies	(None)

Safety pharmacology position papers and guidance documents withdrawn or superseded are not listed here; refer to Bass et al. 2004.
Abbreviations: CNS, central nervous system; ECG, electrocardiogram; EU, European Union; FDA, food and drug administration; IND, Investigational New Drug; JMHW, Japanese Ministry of Health & Welfare; NCEs, new chemical entities.
Source: From Ref. 29.

4

Metabolism and Toxicokinetics

J. Caroline English
*Health and Environment Laboratories, Eastman Kodak Company, Rochester,
New York, U.S.A.*

INTRODUCTION

Definitions and Scope

Metabolism (M) and toxicokinetic studies constitute a part of the overall toxicological evaluation of chemicals. Studies are designed to obtain information on the fate of the compound in the organism; therefore, they focus more on the *behavior* and less on the *effect* of the compound. The information developed permits a more complete understanding of the relationship between chemical exposure and toxicity. The focus of this chapter is toxicokinetic study design, data analysis, and data interpretation, as applied to the understanding of health effects, with particular reference to regulatory guidelines.

The term "toxicokinetics" has emerged to describe the generation of pharmacokinetic data in toxicity studies or separate studies patterned after toxicity study design. The overarching goal is to evaluate internal (i.e., systemic) exposure to a compound over time and relate that exposure to toxicity. Toxicokinetics encompasses the rate and extent of four processes that act on a compound in a biological system, collectively referred to as ADME. They include, uptake into the blood stream and lymphatic system [absorption, (A)], distribution (D) within the body, conversion to new entities (biotransformation or M), and excretion (E) of the compound and its biotransformation products. Toxicity is often associated with metabolic conversion of the compound to a more toxic metabolite or reactive intermediate. For this reason, M and toxicokinetic studies are inextricably linked, and characterizing exposure to metabolites might be equally or more important than characterizing exposure to the original compound.

The specific objectives of toxicokinetic studies depend upon the specific regulatory or safety need, but they typically involve determining the magnitude, rate, and duration of the internal dose and its relationship to administered dose level. As the dose level is increased, the ability of the body to eliminate the compound can become overwhelmed. This occurs because most processes that govern chemical disposition (e.g., extraction from blood by organs, M, biliary, and urinary E) have a finite capacity. When this capacity is saturated or exceeded, as frequently occurs at high dose levels, accumulation to toxic levels might result. The relationship between toxicokinetics and toxicodynamics is critical for limiting extrapolation from high experimental dose levels to those levels encountered by people; it is the most important determinant for moving a drug candidate into phase I human trials.

Guidance and Tier Approaches

Guidance in study design and conduct for M and toxicokinetic studies has been provided by several regulatory agencies and international organizations. For the testing of chemicals according to internationally accepted protocols, the Organisation for Economic Cooperation and Development (OECD) has published *417 Toxicokinetics*, (1), *427* In vivo *skin A* (2), and *428* In vitro *skin A*, (3), available for purchase at (4).

For testing food ingredients, the United States Food and Drug Administration (USFDA) published *Redbook I* (5), and *Redbook 2000* (6); located online at (7). For assessment of compounds to be used in food-producing animals, guidance is found in the USFDA Center for Veterinary Medicine's *Guideline for M Studies and for Selection of Residues for Toxicological Testing* (8). For human pharmaceuticals, USFDA published guidance for industry on drug M and drug interactions in vitro (9), located at (10), and in vivo (11), located online at (12). Also for human drugs, the International Conference on Harmonization (ICH) published two safety guidelines in the areas of toxicokinetics and pharmacokinetics: S3A, for assessment of systemic exposure in toxicity studies (13), and S3B, for repeated dose tissue D studies (14), located online at (15). The United States Environmental Protection Agency (USEPA) guidelines for testing of industrial chemicals or agrochemicals include M and pharmacokinetics (16) and dermal penetration (17), found online at *Environmental Protection Agency, Office of Prevention, Pesticides, and Toxic Substances: Test Methods and Guidelines, Series 870 Health Effects Test Guidelines.* For toxicokinetic studies conducted within the National Toxicology Program (NTP), a paper describing the purpose and guidelines was published by Buchanan et al. (18). Some examples of data sought from these studies include the extent and rate of A by relevant routes of exposure, the biological half-life of the compound; the D pattern in organs and tissues; routes and rates of elimination; and amount and nature of metabolites. The extent to which the above-mentioned parameters are dependent upon sex, species, dose level, route of administration, and repeated versus single administration may also be explored. Comprehensive guidelines address these multiple aspects of toxicokinetic investigation, but rarely are all elements necessary for the evaluation of a given compound. For this reason, toxicokinetic data development is especially conducive to tiered or staged testing, and various approaches that incorporate this philosophy have been devised (16,18–20).

In a tiered testing approach, a minimal data set is first acquired and evaluated. Ideally, a set of criteria is defined that triggers the next tier or stage of testing, and several factors might influence the need for information beyond a minimal data set. These factors include the need for toxicokinetic data to help design or interpret a toxicity study; the commercial use of the product and extent of consumer exposure; and the significance of findings related to A, M, or persistence revealed by the first-tier studies. The need for additional data can be determined as the data unfold. Tiered approaches require that the expertise for data evaluation and final decision making is available to the regulatory authority and the industry responsible for performing studies. However, staging the acquisition of toxicokinetic data might significantly reduce animal use, product development cycle time, and study costs.

An alternative, or complementary approach, to the generation of in vivo toxicokinetic data, is the development of physiologically based toxicokinetic (PBTK) models, also known as physiologically based pharmacokinetic (PBPK) or dosimetry models. These models are based on actual anatomical (e.g., tissue volumes) and physiological (e.g., cardiac output) characteristics combined with biochemical characteristics (e.g., metabolic rates, partition coefficients) of the compound under study. They can predict the toxicokinetic behavior of the compound under a variety of exposure conditions. Such models take advantage of existing data available for human and animal physiology (21), in vitro, in vivo, and in silico methods for estimating chemical-specific parameters, and additional in vivo data to test or refine the model. A particular advantage of PBTK models is their potential for predicting the impact of human variables, such as age, disease state, or genetic polymorphisms, on toxicokinetic behavior. Although no regulatory guidance is available, PBTK models are currently the most accurate means for extrapolation between exposure routes and species, and their uses in chemical risk assessment and drug research have been widely endorsed (22–30). Some recent modeling applications are described at the end of this chapter.

Selected guidelines currently in use for toxicokinetic and M are presented and compared in Table 1. The remainder of this chapter focuses on the development of basic toxicokinetic data and, where applicable, outline first-stage or "Tier 1" studies. It should be noted that, prior to any toxicokinetic study, an initial assessment of a chemical's toxicokinetic behavior should be made based on physicochemical properties, knowledge of the toxicokinetic behavior of structurally similar substances, or information gleaned from basic toxicity studies (19,31,32).

STUDY DESIGN AND STUDY PARAMETERS

Test Substance and Carrier

The test substance and any carrier used for administration should be comparable to that used in toxicity studies and resemble the substance encountered by humans. Consistency with toxicity studies is also important for volume administered and formulation, both of which can influence A. Appropriate characterization (e.g., purity, identity, stability, homogeneity) should be performed. The objectives of toxicokinetic studies are facilitated with the use of radiolabeled test substances. The principle underlying the use of radiolabeled material is that a substance possessing a radionuclide will behave identically to its corresponding "cold" compound, and it will not influence the behavior of the unlabeled compound in any way. Radiolabeled test substances facilitate the determination of a mass balance and allow for a more complete accounting of the fate of all test substance–related material at the end of the study. Radiolabeling might afford greater analytical sensitivity and specificity than can often be attained with unlabeled material. Carbon-14 is commonly used for organic materials, but other moderately energetic beta-emitting isotopes having appropriate decay rates may be used. When the radiochemical synthesis is performed, the label should be placed within a metabolically stable position of the molecule. Dual-labeling with two different isotopes may be performed when a compound is known to undergo hydrolysis, and both portions of the molecule need to be tracked. If, however, one portion of the molecule is of greatest concern from a structure-activity standpoint, then labeling of this portion alone might be adequate. The radiochemical purity of the test substance should typically be high (e.g., >95%) and significant impurities (e.g., ≥2%) need to be identified.

Unlabeled test substances are, in most guidelines, allowed as an alternative to radiolabeled ones, provided the objectives of the study can be met. Indeed, use of unlabeled compounds may be preferred in some circumstances. If the synthesis of radiolabeled test substance is unfeasible from an economic or technical standpoint,

Table 1   Guidelines for Metabolism and Toxicokinetic Studies

	Organization for Economic Cooperation and Development Toxicokinetics Guideline for Testing Chemicals	International Conference on Harmonization (13,14) Toxicokinetics Guideline for Human Drugs	United States Environmental Protection Agency (16,17) Metabolism and Pharmacokinetics Guideline for Pesticides and Toxic Substances (Tier 1)	Buchanan et al. (18) guidelines for toxicokinetic studies within the national toxicology program (minimal study design)
Study design				
Species	One or more appropriate animal species	Same as toxicity test	Rat; other, or additional species if significant toxicity	Same as toxicity studies
Number of animals	Four per group. Where sexual dimorphism exists, use four animals of each sex.	Appropriate number to provide basis for risk assessment	At least four males: both sexes, if evidence of sex difference in toxicity.	Ensure three samples per time point of analysis. Initially, one sex of one species.
Dose levels	At least two for single-dose studies. No observed toxic effect level and high level at which TK parameters change or toxic effect occurs.	The same three dose levels used in toxicity study	Single nontoxic dose for each route of exposure	Same used or anticipated in toxicity studies. Three levels recommended as minimum (e.g., 0.1, 0.01, and 0.001 of LD50).
Route of administration	Same as used in toxicity studies. Intravenous for absorption or distribution useful.	Same as route(s) intended for product	Oral gavage is customary method: other routes might be required	Same used in toxicity study or most common route of human exposure and IV
Observations				
Absorption/ systemic exposure	Measure amount of test substance and/or metabolites in excreta and carcass or compare with reference group amount of dose excreted renally,	Measure parent compound and/or metabolite in plasma, serum, or whole blood, ideally the same as used in clinical studies.	Determine percent of dose in excreta and, as necessary, tissues and residual carcass.	Assay blood or plasma at 812 time points for parent compound (major metabolite if rapid metabolism).

	area under plasma level vs. time curve of parent or metabolites, or biological response.	As needed, assay genotoxicity indicator tissue, pregnant or lactating animals, embryos, fetuses, or newborns.		
Distribution	Whole-body autoradiography and/or serial sacrifices with analysis of tissues and organs for test substance and/or metabolites	Tissue distribution should be determined in some circumstances, especially for potential sites of action.	Collect liver, fat kidney, spleen, blood, target organ, portal of entry for nonoral study, residual carcass at sacrifice; store frozen. Assay for radioactivity if significant amount of dose unaccounted for in excreta.	Tissue(s) other than plasma may be analyzed to assess systemic exposure. Tissue distribution not included in minimal study design.
Metabolism	Elucidate structures of measured metabolites. Propose metabolic pathways. In vitro studies helpful to elucidate pathways. Other biochemical studies may be performed.	Measure metabolite levels in plasma or other body fluid when compound is prodrug, metabolized to active form, or is extensively metabolized and measurement of parent is impractical.	Identify and quantitate unchanged test substance and metabolites comprising >5% of the dose in excreta. Provide metabolic scheme.	Limited metabolism knowledge assumed, e.g., when major metabolite is measured instead of parent. Metabolite identification not included in minimal study design.
Excretion	Assay urine, feces, expired air, (sometimes bile) at intervals until 95% excreted or for seven days.	Excreta measurements not included in standard study design.	Assay urine, feces, expired air as appropriate for radioactivity at intervals until 90% recovered or for seven days.	Excreta measurements not included in minimal study design.

Abbreviation: TK, toxicokinetic.

analytical methods should be developed for measuring stable isotopes of the test substance and key metabolites in appropriate biological matrices (e.g., excreta and tissues). Such methods may also be needed if the animals to be used for toxicokinetic measurements are also involved in a toxicity study. This latter approach, also referred to as concomitant toxicokinetics, represents the ultimate integration of toxicokinetic and toxicity studies and can provide the most useful information for design and interpretation of toxicity studies (33).

Probe Studies

The investigator charged with designing a toxicokinetic study needs to select appropriate sampling times, sampling matrices, and analytical methods. Often, little or no information is available to guide the investigator beforehand, and probe or pilot studies are therefore recommended. Specimens collected during the probe will be of value in developing analytical methods for separating and quantitating parent compound and metabolites and for determining which biological matrices are most appropriate to collect during the definitive study.

Test System

Selection and Justification

Toxicokinetic studies are performed primarily to assist in the interpretation of toxicity studies, and, as such, the test system selected will necessarily be the same as that used for the toxicity study. Most basic toxicokinetic studies are performed with young adult male and/or female rats of the appropriate strain. Weight variation of animals used should not exceed $\pm 20\%$ of the mean weight (1). The use of one sex in initial toxicokinetic studies may suffice. If there is evidence of a sex-related difference in toxicity, studies may be confined to the more sensitive sex. Additional test systems might be needed to address compound-specific objectives, for example: (1) an additional species for interspecies comparisons, (2) animals of different ages to examine age-dependent changes in toxicokinetic parameters, and (3) animals in a particular physiological state (i.e., pregnancy, diabetic, inborn metabolic errors, etc.) to examine susceptibility issues. Special considerations for conducting toxicokinetic studies in support of reproductive toxicology studies have been reviewed elsewhere (34).

Animal Number

The conventional approach to the evaluation and interpretation of toxicokinetic data involves the collection of a sufficient number of serial samples to allow the time course of the chemical to be fully described in each individual. Guidelines that specify the number of animals to be used typically indicate three or four of each sex per group. Enough animals should be used such that data are obtained for no fewer than three animals per dose level (18). Four or more animals might therefore be needed in anticipation of the occasional lost sample or analytical mishap. Where a high degree of interindividual variation in toxicokinetic behavior is displayed, more animals per group might be justified. An alternative study design that addresses variability within the group of animals tested (35), involves the use of composite, rather than serial, sampling for the collection of data. This technique, which borrows from population pharmacokinetics (36), is used especially during drug development to estimate pharmacokinetic parameter probability Ds when sample numbers are limited. As a rule, samples are obtained from more animals using fewer sampling times. Advantages cited for this approach include reduced sampling-related stress to animals and, when toxicokinetic studies are concomitant with toxicity studies, lower total animal use. The interested reader is referred to Vozeh et al. (37) for a comprehensive review and perspective on this subject.

Test Substance Administration

Routes

The routes of test substance administration used for toxicokinetic studies are generally those of common human exposure (i.e., oral, inhalation, and cutaneous). The route should be the same as that used in toxicity studies to aid in their interpretation. Although drinking water or feed exposure is commonly chosen for toxicity studies, the gavage method is often preferred for estimating A from the gastrointestinal tract. The toxicokinetic behavior of a chemical given in the feed or drinking water is likely to differ from that given by bolus administration; however, the latter offers advantages in ease of quantitative dose recovery for material balance studies as well as in simplifying the analysis and interpretation of toxicokinetic data. A common strategy is to perform toxicity studies principally with one route and method of administration, while conducting toxicokinetic studies via the same and other relevant routes/methods to obtain systemic (internal) exposure data for making route comparisons. Such data might be useful for supporting route-dependent extrapolations in risk assessment.

When the cutaneous route is studied, animals are prepared 16 to 24 hours prior to dose administration by clipping the skin of hair in the region of the shoulders and back. The test substance is applied evenly to the skin and protected with a suitable covering (2,16,38). For the inhalation route, exposures are usually accomplished with a nose-cone or head-only apparatus. Finally, some designs might warrant the inclusion of the intravenous (IV) route of administration. By definition, A following IV injection is considered to be complete, i.e., 100%, making it useful both for defining important toxicokinetic parameters and as a reference dose (RfD) route for determining extent of A via other routes. Typical plasma concentration versus time profiles for bolus and nonbolus methods of administration are shown in (Fig. 1). The IV route alone has no A phase that is seen with the other routes, because the test substance is introduced directly into the circulatory system. Intravenous dosing may be accomplished via a lateral tail vein injection or an implanted venous cannula, commonly within the jugular or femoral vein.

Dose Levels

Guidelines vary in the number of dose levels required (one to three) and the criteria to be used in their selection. Examples cited in Table 1 include a single nontoxic dose level; a minimum of two dose levels that include a minimally toxic one [e.g., lowest observed effect level (LOEL)] and a nontoxic level [e.g., no observable effect level (NOEL)]; and three levels anticipated, or used, in toxicity studies and selected on the basis of potency and slope factors. More dose levels allow better characterization of the dose-dependent behavior of a chemical; in particular, dose ranges of proportional toxicokinetic behavior (Fig. 2, curves A and B), and dose region where kinetics shift from linear to nonlinear (Fig. 2, curves C and D). By displaying the curves in log-linear format, the regions where elimination is proportional to concentration remaining (first-order) is readily observed as linear. The nonlinear regions of curves c and d reflect concentration-independent elimination (zero-order).

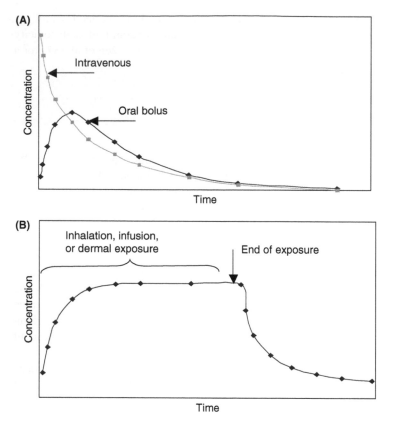

Figure 1 Analyte concentration (linear scale) versus time obtained for different routes and methods of test substance administration. (**A**) Intravenous and oral bolus dosing. (**B**) Inhalation or dermal exposure or IV infusion.

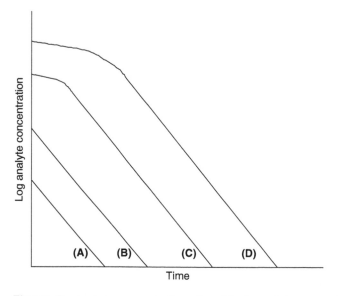

Figure 2 Analyte concentration (logarithmic scale) versus time for intravascularly dosed compound. Curves (**A**), (**B**), (**C**), and (**D**) represent increasing dose levels. Saturation is evident at dose level (**C**).

When a radiolabeled test substance is administered for the purpose of determining a mass balance (generally, a bolus dose), gravimetric determination of the administered dose (dpm or μCi) is recommended. This is accomplished by determining the radioactivity in weighed aliquots of the dose preparation to obtain a mean concentration (e.g., dpm/mg), and measuring the weight of the administered dose preparation. Multiplication of the above mean concentration by weight of dose administered will yield the dose administered in dpm that becomes the denominator in later calculations of the fraction or percent of dose.

Dose Regimen

Single exposures are generally used for basic toxicokinetic studies. For the oral or intravenous routes, a single bolus administration is used. Where the inhalation or cutaneous route is needed, a single exposure of a defined period is typical. Other factors to be considered in the design of inhalation or dermal toxicokinetic studies are the length of time needed to attain steady-state concentrations in the body, the expected duration of relevant human exposure, and the need to minimize any discomfort or stress experienced by the animals. Guidelines (2,16) recommend a minimum dermal exposure period of 6 hours and a cleansing step at the end of the exposure period to recover unabsorbed test substance from the skin. For inhalation studies, a 4- to 6-hour exposure using a nose-cone or head-only apparatus is specified (16). This specialized apparatus prevents deposition of the test substance on the animal's coat, which could, in turn, result in ingestion during grooming or dermal uptake, confounding the interpretation of the results. However, if dermal penetration is sufficiently slow and grooming of the coat is curtailed by the use of Elizabethan-style collars, the use of whole-body inhalation chambers might be justifiable. A single administration of test substance at specified dose levels is usually adequate when evaluating dose level-, route-, sex- or species-dependent toxicokinetic behavior and meets the basic requirements of most guidelines. Repeated dose or infusion studies, although not routinely required, might yield important additional information. If repeated dose toxicokinetic data are called for, the regimen should consist of daily exposures over a period ranging from five days to three weeks. Circumstances where such studies might be warranted have been well described (14,18,39) and include the following. Interpretation of a repeated dose toxicity study might require a repeated dose toxicokinetic study, particularly when biochemical, morphological, or functional changes occur relative to the single dose situation. If the test substance causes enzyme induction or inactivation, changes will generally be manifested within several days of repeated dosing and commonly will be accompanied by changes in toxicokinetic behavior. Substances that display long elimination half-lives from plasma or other tissues after a single dose might require repeated dose toxicokinetic studies to accurately determine the extent of tissue accumulation or the potential for persistence within the body.

Sample Collection

Matrices

The types of excreta and tissue specimens that should be collected can best be determined with the help of information obtained in probe studies. Guidelines generally address the collection of excreta and blood or plasma but differ with respect to how collection of those matrices should be prioritized in a testing scheme. For example, ICH, and NTP guidelines do not call for routine E and mass balance data, whereas first-level studies required under OECD guidelines and EPA generally do require such data.

Analysis of excreta at several postexposure time points is required to gather information on extent of A and biotransformation and routes and rates of E. Quantitative analysis of excreta is also needed to account for the entire mass of the dose and thereby the complete disposition of the test substance, as required in a mass balance study. The separate collection of urine and feces can be accomplished with M chambers specially designed for this purpose (Fig. 3). Expired air may be directed through traps suitable for the collection of exhaled volatile test substance and metabolites (e.g., activated charcoal) as well as carbon dioxide (e.g., 2.5 M potassium hydroxide) that is derived from test substance M. Determination of the extent of A and the calculation of mass balance invariably requires analysis of the carcass, and separate analysis of specified tissues is usually desirable. For a dermal exposure, recovery of the test substance washed from the skin and that associated with any containment devices or protective coverings must also be assayed. Mass balance information is not routinely obtained following inhalation studies because the dose absorbed from the lung is not known. When feasible, however, recovery data provide a good measure of the total inhalation dose.

To assess systemic exposure, collection of blood or plasma at several time points is usually required. Blood is chosen over plasma if the analyte possesses a high affinity for the cellular fraction. Collection of the target tissue for the measurement of analyte levels can also be done, and values might correlate better with organ-specific toxicity findings. Blood collection might be preferred; however, because it allows for serial measurements to be made within the same animal, thereby reducing interindividual variation. The simplifying assumption is that the concentration of toxic substance in blood (or plasma) is a function of the concentration in target tissue(s). The use of microdialysis systems can

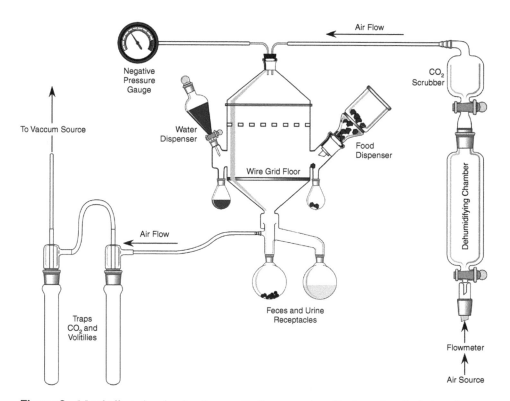

Figure 3   Metabolism chamber for the quantitative, separate collection of expired air and excreta.

overcome many of the limitations of blood or tissue sampling and enables continuous in vivo monitoring for a compound in any number of matrices, for example, tissue extracellular fluid, plasma, bile, or cerebrospinal fluid. This technique, reviewed elsewhere (40), involves the insertion of a probe containing a dialysis membrane into the matrix of interest. Small molecules diffuse into the probe and can be collected, whereas larger molecules, including protein-bound chemicals, are excluded by the membrane. The collected fluid consequently requires no further clean-up processing prior to analysis. Concentrations of analytes can be precisely measured directly within the tissue of interest or close surrogate, and microdialysis places fewer restrictions on the selection of sampling times (see below).

When study objectives require a determination of tissue D of the test substance, whole-body autoradiography is a valuable tool for examining changes in radiolabel D within the same animal, over a specified period of time. The alternative method for assessing tissue D is collection of appropriate tissues at serial times after dose administration. Collection and storage (frozen) of tissues and the residual carcass at terminal sacrifice is required in one guideline (16) and helps ensure a complete material balance. Although tissue D studies might be required for providing information on accumulation of the parent compound or metabolites, especially in relation to potential sites of action, views are split on the necessity of acquiring this information as a part of an initial data set. Tissue D studies will typically include known or suspected target tissues, organs of M and E, site of action for therapeutics, and tissues associated with the accumulation of tested chemicals that are structurally related to the test substance.

Sampling Times

The quantitative collection of excreta and expired air specimens requires monitoring to begin immediately after administration of the test substance, or for inhalation exposure, at the end of the exposure period. The period of collection continues for seven days or until 90% (16) or 95% (1) of the administered dose is recovered, whichever occurs first. Percentage of dose recovered is generally determined by assay for the cumulative total radioactivity in excreta, including expired air when needed. Daily specimen collection is typically performed; however, several appropriate interim collections might also be required immediately following treatment. Many chemicals are excreted primarily by the kidneys into the urine, following M, to water-soluble conjugates. Hence, protocols will commonly specify more frequent collection of urine (e.g., 0–6, 6–12, and 12–24 hours) within the first day of dose administration.

Sampling times also need to be chosen for serial sampling of body fluids, usually blood or plasma and occasionally bile, urine, or milk from lactating animals. The goal is to define the concentration versus time relationship for the parent compound and/or specific metabolites from the beginning of exposure through elimination (Fig. 1). Therefore, sampling must be started at an appropriate interval after bolus administration—during, and after infusion, dermal, or inhalation exposure—and should continue until the detection limit is reached. The number and frequency of sampling times should be sufficient to define this concentration-time relationship, and the times will vary depending upon the route and method of administration, as well as number of phases associated with the compound's kinetic behavior. The kinetic profile of substances given via the route, for example, will lack an A phase. Likewise, substances may be eliminated from the body in one, two, or more distinct phases, each with its own half-life. Each phase should ideally be described by a minimum of three time points, which should be chosen with the help of pilot study data. For blood or plasma, Buchanan et al. (18) specifies collection of 8 to 12 samples within a 24-hour period of bolus administration. For some compounds, as few as 5 samples within a 24-hour period (31) might provide reasonable estimates of two important toxicokinetic parameters, the maximum concentration (Cmax) and the area under the concentration-versus-time curve (Fig. 4). Where the test substance is administered via feed or water, diurnal behavior patterns will influence systemic exposure, and 4 to 8 evenly spaced samples should be obtained over 24 hours for derivation of the daily average level (41). If excessive blood withdrawal is a concern because of the frequency or size of samples required, periodic monitoring of the hematocrit is advisable because both the health of the animal and the toxicokinetics can be impacted by excessive removal of blood from the body. For protocols that specify the determination of tissue D over time, whether by autoradiography or serial sacrifices, sampling times may be chosen using the same considerations described above for body fluids. As described above, microdialysis sampling may be used in place of blood or tissue sampling without requiring excessive removal of blood or serial sacrifices. Small sample volumes obtained with microdialysis require sensitive analytical methods, but because the animal loses essentially no fluid, more frequent samples can be obtained, and fewer animals can be used.

Analytical Methods

Selection of Analytes

Analytes to be measured in blood and other serial samples should include the test substance itself and/or one or more metabolites, especially those metabolites in the pathway leading to toxicity. Test substances might not be readily detectable if they undergo very rapid biotransformation, such as hydrolysis in the bloodstream or first-pass M in the liver or portal of entry. In this situation, analysis for an early metabolite as a substitute for the parent compound might be necessary. An understanding of the likely routes of M for the compound under study is useful for predicting metabolites and developing analytical methods. Information on common metabolic pathways can be found in toxicology textbooks (42) and from commercial M databases that enable searches by chemical structure, substructure, and similarity features.

Developing an analytical method for selected analytes also requires some knowledge regarding the expected behavior of those compounds in the biological matrix.

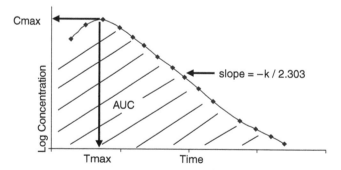

Figure 4 Analyte concentration (logarithmic scale) versus time following test substance administration, illustrating basic toxicokinetic parameters: maximum analyte concentration (Cmax), time of maximum analyte concentration (Tmax), area under the curve, and relationship between slope and elimination rate constant (k). *Abbreviation*: AUC, area under the curve.

Substances that are too reactive to measure directly may be determined indirectly by trapping the metabolite or reactive intermediate to form a stable reaction product. Endogenous molecules, such as hemoglobin or glutathione, have been used effectively for this purpose.

The tendency of a compound to bind reversibly to plasma and tissue proteins should also be considered during analytical method development. In general, the concentration of unbound or free compound in the plasma should be determined because it is this unbound fraction that is available for tissue uptake and biological activity. The analytical method used should distinguish unbound fraction from total compound in the sample where extensive protein binding occurs. Where little protein binding occurs, measurement of total compound in the sample is a reasonable indicator of free compound.

Analytes to be measured in excreta include the test substance itself and any appreciable metabolites or breakdown products of the parent compound. For test substances containing a radiolabel, the total radioactivity in the specimen should also be determined. Specific kinetic parameters should not be calculated from total radioactivity data unless it is known that the substance does not undergo biotransformation (43). Where a radiolabeled test substance has been used, tissue D can be determined by whole-body autoradiography or by preparation of collected tissue samples, as appropriate (e.g., combustion, digestion, decolorization), for liquid scintillation spectrometry or other suitable method.

Metabolite Measurement and Identification

For the quantitative determination of parent compound and metabolites in biological specimens, high performance liquid chromatography (HPLC) or gas chromatography (GC), with mass spectrometry or other suitable detection methods, are commonly used. Useful detection methods include radioisotope methods for radiolabeled compounds; electrochemical techniques for redox active compounds; and atomic A spectroscopy for metals. Prior to the assay, sample preparation procedures, such as protein precipitation, extraction, or another technique, are often needed to remove background interferences. In the case of protein or biotechnology-derived compounds, immunoassay methods, including radioimmunoassay (RIA) and enzyme immunoassay (EIA), are highly sensitive and specific.

For the identification of parent compound and metabolites in excreta, a combination of methodologies may be used. Metabolite identification is commonly required for each metabolite that comprises >5% (16) to >10% (18) of the administered dose. Mass spectrometry is an analytical technique for identifying compounds based on their molecular mass, thus it has broad applicability. When combined with chromatography, it becomes a powerful method for rapid identification, sensitive measurement, and structural elucidation. Consequently, liquid chromatography-tandem mass spectrometry (LC-MS/MS) has become the method of choice for quantitation and identification of analytes. Alternatively, cochromatography or coelution of known material (authentic standard) and unknown analyte can provide a first level of metabolite characterization using HPLC or GC. Specifically, chromatographic retention time of an unknown substance (e.g., a radiolabeled component of urine) can be compared with the retention time for authentic standards. In a similar fashion, evidence for the presence of conjugated metabolites can be provided by chromatographic retention time shifts occurring after hydrolytic treatment of the sample with either specific enzymes for cleavage of phase II conjugates, (e.g., β-glucuronidase, sulfatase) or nonspecific hydrolysis treatments (e.g., dilute HCl).

Definitive structural confirmation is accomplished using nuclear magnetic resonance spectroscopy.

Specificity, Sensitivity, Precision

Methods used for the quantitative and qualitative analyses of all analytes need to be fully validated (44). The method should be specific for the compound, and any interference by endogenous components should be investigated. Stability of the analyte under experimental and storage conditions, as well as recovery of the analyte from the biological matrix, should be addressed as a part of the validation. The method should be appropriately sensitive, with the lower limits of detection and quantification specifically defined. The precision of the method should be determined by examining the reproducibility of results over a suitable period of time.

DATA EVALUATION AND INTERPRETATION

Data and Statistical Analyses

The primary goal of toxicokinetic studies is to characterize the systemic exposure to a test substance, with respect to both magnitude and duration. As described in the preceding section, the concentration of analyte, generally parent compound or specific metabolite(s), is measured over time in one or more matrices consisting of a body fluid or tissue. The following section is subdivided into three parts that address data analysis for (1) systemic A and elimination, (2) disposition, and (3) statistical summary. The presented stepwise approach was devised as a practical introduction for handling basic toxicokinetic data obtained from guideline studies. The reader is referred elsewhere for introductions to the basic concepts of toxicokinetics (45–47), and to Gibaldi and Perrier (48) for a comprehensive presentation of the mathematical framework for this discipline.

Systemic Data Analysis

The first step recommended for data analysis is to graphically examine the analyte concentration data obtained from each individual animal, against time, on log-linear axes. Visual inspection of this curve can provide useful toxicokinetic information, in particular, the number of phases associated with the elimination, the maximum concentration achieved (Cmax), and the time of maximum concentration (Tmax) (Fig. 4). Many computer software programs are now available for the graphing and analysis of toxicokinetic data that will compute the parameters discussed in this section. The vast majority of elimination curves will possess a linear terminal portion, regardless of test substance, route, or dose level. The slope of this terminal linear segment of the curve (Fig. 4) is generally used to estimate the elimination rate constant, k, by the relationship:

$$k = -2.303/\text{terminal slope}$$

This relationship assumes that, for extravascular (ex) routes of administration, the A rate is substantially faster than the elimination rate. Alternatively, for metabolites, the rate of formation must be greater than the rate of elimination. Where the A rate is slower than the elimination rate, as perhaps occurs with sustained-release formulations of drugs or with slow percutaneous penetration, the terminal slope actually reflects the A rate; thus, the A rate constant, k_a is estimated by:

$$k_a = -2.303/\text{terminal slope}$$

Whether the A or elimination rate term is defined by the terminal slope is not necessarily evident from the data set, unless the administration or other route known to result in rapid A was used to clearly define the elimination rate constant. Alternatively, an independent estimation of A rate or rate of metabolite formation might need to be made; in vitro systems can often be used for this purpose (49–51).

The elimination half-life $(t_{1/2})$ is the time required to decrease the analyte concentration by one-half and is related to the elimination rate constant by the following relationship:

$$t_{1/2} = \ln 2/k$$

Ideally, data will be available for a period of time equivalent to four or five half-lives postexposure, which is the time it takes for about 94% or 97%, respectively, of the elimination to occur.

Virtually all concentration-versus-time curves will have, at least, a terminal log-linear segment reflecting first-order behavior. For intravascularly dosed substances, the slope of this linear phase might describe the entire curve (Fig. 2A, B), and a first-order mathematical expression of the concentration at time t (C_t) can be readily obtained by determining the elimination rate constant and the ordinate intercept (C_0), which become exponent and coefficient, respectively, in the following equation:

$$C_t = C_0 e^{-kt}$$

For curves having additional phases approximating first-order behavior, such as two elimination phases or an A phase, the rate constants (and half-lives) associated with each phase may be estimated by the method of residuals or by linear regression analysis, and comparable first-order expressions for C_t obtained (46,48). When the capacity of first-order processes governing toxicokinetic behavior is exceeded, as might occur at high exposure levels, curves will show systematic deviations from these linear mathematical expressions (Fig. 2C, D).

Another parameter derived from the concentration-versus-time curve is the area under the curve (AUC) (Fig. 4). The AUC may be measured by the trapezoidal rule, for example:

$$\text{AUC} = \Sigma[(t_2 - t_1)/2](C_1 + C_2), \text{etc.}$$

where t_1 and t_2 are the first two time points, C_1 and C_2 are the corresponding analyte concentrations, and areas are calculated and summed through the last sampling time and respective concentration (C_{last}). For calculation of an AUC that includes the triangular area beyond the last sampling time, (i.e., extrapolated to infinity), the term C_{last}/k is added to the sum, thus:

$$\text{AUC}_{0-\infty} = \text{AUC} + C_{last}/k$$

Systemic clearance (Cl) (also referred to as total Cl, and usually blood or plasma Cl) represents the volume of blood or plasma that is cleared of compound-per-unit time and is a favored descriptor of the body's efficiency for elimination of a substance. Cl is given by the relationship:

$$\text{Cl} = \text{dose} \times \text{F/AUC}_{0-\infty}$$

where F is the fraction of the dose that is absorbed, and by definition, is equal to 1 for studies done by the IV route. "F" is sometimes referred to as bioavailability, and for studies performed using an ex route, it is calculated as:

$$F = (AUC_{ex} \times dose_{iv})/(AUC_{iv} \times dose_{ex})$$

where AUC and dose are known for the IV and ex routes.

A parameter that conveys information on the extent of D of the analyte is the apparent volume of distribution (V_d), which can be readily determined for parent compound from an IV dose study. The V_d represents the ratio of the amount of analyte in the body (i.e., $dose_{iv}$) to a theoretical analyte concentration (C_0) obtained by extrapolation of the concentration curve to the time of dose administration, i.e., the ordinate intercept. Thus:

$$V_d = dose_{iv}/C_0$$

For studies done by an ex route, the appropriate equation is:

$$V_d = (dose_{ex} \times F)/(AUC \times k).$$

Disposition Data Analysis

Because of the intervals separating the collection periods, studies requiring the collection and analysis of excreta are not generally useful for derivation of the above-described kinetic parameters. Their purpose is more often to determine the routes and rates of E of total test substance equivalents, the extent of biotransformation, and for the identification of end products of biotransformation. A, defined as the amount or mass of test substance-related material transferred into the body (52), may also be obtained from disposition data. Disposition analysis may include the analysis of tissues for concentration of the test substance, specific metabolites, or total radiolabel. In addition, reversible, and irreversible protein binding in plasma or other tissue may be evaluated.

Excreta, tissue, and carcass measurements are of value for accounting for the entire administered dose at the end of the study, i.e., obtaining a mass balance, which in turn, strengthens conclusions related to the compound's disposition. The use of a radiolabeled test substance makes mass balance determinations relatively straightforward. Briefly, all excreta collected during the study are weighed, as are traps for expired air, any tissues collected, and the residual carcass. M chambers are rinsed during and after the study, and rinsings are quantitatively collected and weighed. For dermal route studies, containment devices, protective coverings, and postexposure skin washings are similarly collected. Aliquots of liquid matrices are weighed and analyzed directly by liquid scintillation counting; solid matrices are homogenized, extracted, or combusted, as needed, prior to liquid scintillation counting. Each resultant liquid scintillation count value (lsc) is converted to disintegrations per minute (dpm) after correction for combustion efficiency, as necessary. Table 2 provides an example for the collation of mass balance data for a tissue matrix, in this case, the liver. The activity in dpm is divided by the aliquot weight, and the average dpm/weight of replicate aliquots is determined. The average dpm/weight is multiplied by the corresponding total weight of the matrix (e.g., excreta or tissue) to obtain the total associated activity. Finally, the total dpm associated with each matrix are added together to obtain total recovered dose for each animal. A summary table showing total dose recovered is shown in Table 3. Total recovered dose will ideally be equal to $100 \pm 5\%$ of the administered dose, and the percentage of the administered dose in each matrix can be readily determined. The amount of dose absorbed is obtained from the total amount of radioactivity recovered from excreta, tissues, and carcass. Radioactivity data can

Table 2 Example Mass Balance Data Table for the Liver

Sample number	Animal number	Sample time (hour)	Tare weight (g)	Tare + sample (g)	Total sample (g)	Tare+D H$_2$O+ sample (g)	Total weight homogo- nato (g)	LSC ali- quot (g)	DPMc[a]	Activity conc. (DPM/g)	Mean activity conc. (DPM/g)	Total activity (DPM)	Percent of dose
1269	9	168	76.84	88.27	11.43	111.27	34.43	0.251	688	8252	8072	92263	0.33
1270	9	168	76.84	88.27	11.43	111.27	34.43	0.285	747	7892			
1271	10	168	76.65	87.02	10.37	107.73	31.08	0.252	622	7400	7305	75755	0.30
1272	10	168	76.65	87.02	10.37	107.73	31.08	0.258	621	7210			
1273	11	168	76.93	87.36	10.43	108.38	31.45	0.266	555	6324	6311	65825	0.27
1274	11	168	76.93	87.36	10.43	108.38	31.45	0.290	606	6298			
1275	12	166	76.96	87.07	10.11	107.34	30.38	0.229	524	6869	6862	69371	0.28
1276	12	166	76.96	87.07	10.11	107.34	30.38	0.251	573	6854			

Test substance, [2-^{14}C]; nominal dose concentration, 20 mg/g; dose volume, 5 mL/kg body weight; notebook source, In-244.
[a] DPMc = [DPM (sample)-DPM (blank background)] factor used to correct for combustion efficiency for oxidized samples.

Table 3 Example Summary Table for Mass Balance Data

Rat #	Urine % Dose	Urine μCi	Cage wash D-1-120 and Acetone % Dose	Cage wash D-1-120 and Acetone μCi	CO_2 Traps 1 and 2 % Dose	CO_2 Traps 1 and 2 μCi	Feces % Dose	Feces μCi	Blood % Dose	Blood μCi	Tissue Liver and kidney % Dose	Tissue Liver and kidney μCi	Tissue Carcass % Dose	Tissue Carcass μCi	Total % Dose	Total μCi
9	21.06	2.64	16.30	2.05	52.88	6.64	1.06	0.13	0.10	0.01	0.38	0.05	4.66	0.59	96.45	12.11
10	15.85	1.82	14.95	1.72	57.80	6.85	1.26	0.14	0.11	0.01	0.37	0.04	5.12	0.59	95.45	10.98
11	22.62	2.52	7.15	0.80	57.48	6.41	1.11	0.12	0.10	0.01	0.34	0.04	5.53	0.62	94.33	10.53
12	27.46	3.01	5.05	0.55	57.35	6.29	1.11	0.12	0.10	0.01	0.35	0.04	4.25	0.47	95.67	10.50
Total recovered % dose and activity															381.90	44.11
Mean	21.75	2.50	10.86	1.28	56.38	8.50	1.13	0.13	0.10	0.01	0.36	0.04	4.89	0.66	95.47	11.03
SD	4.79	0.50	5.59	0.72	2.34	0.17	0.06	0.01	0.01	0.00	0.02	0.00	0.68	0.07	0.67	0.75

Summary of sample analysis: Test substance, [2-^{14}C]; nominal dose level, 100 mg/kg; nominal dose concentration, 20 mg/g; dose volume, 5 mL/kg body weight; notebook source, LN-244.
Abbreviation: SD, standard deviation.

alternatively be expressed as μg- or μmole-equivalents by conversion of dpm using the specific radioactivity of the dose preparation. The presence of metabolites in urine and other excreta is typically determined by chromatography, with radiochemical or other method of detection used for quantification. The extent of test substance M can be determined for each metabolite or for total M by adding the amounts in each E matrix.

Statistical Analysis

Data evaluation typically involves the calculation of the mean and standard deviation of group data. Analysis of variance and log transformation of concentration data might be useful, as discussed by Igarashi et al. (41). Computer mathematical curve-fitting programs can be used to derive toxicokinetic parameters, providing the "best fit" of a given equation or model to a given data set. Some specialized programs additionally provide information about the "goodness of fit" (e.g., how closely observed and calculated values compare, whether deviations are systematic or random), and how well parameters are estimated. Statistical tests (e.g., F test, Akaike criterion) can be used to choose between models.

A confidence interval method is recommended when toxicokinetic parameters obtained for different treatment groups (e.g., treatment routes or formulations) need to be compared (48). When statistical comparisons are required, the use of an adequate number of animals and consideration of interindividual variability become critical for the detection of differences that are both statistically and biologically significant. More recently, population approaches have been applied to data analysis and estimation of parameters, using a statistical methodology commonly known as nonlinear mixed-effects modeling (36,53). The software available for data analysis has become increasingly user friendly, and population modeling has enjoyed a corresponding gain in popularity (32).

Interpretation and Use of Data

Toxicokinetic parameters are critical determinants of a toxic response. Knowledge of the amount of chemical and the manner in which it exists in the test animal during a given interval allows a more meaningful correlation between dosage and effects observed. Studies describing the time course of systemic exposure to the compound and its metabolites also can be used to test any presumed association between a toxic chemical and a toxic outcome. Most importantly perhaps, toxicokinetic descriptions help predict under what circumstances toxicity is likely to occur, thereby improving the reliability of the safety evaluation or risk assessment for a given chemical.

Systemic Exposure

Systemic exposure is usually expressed as AUC and/or Cmax (Fig. 4). If a test substance is associated with a lack of toxicity, it might be important to demonstrate that systemic exposure has, in fact, occurred. This is particularly true for pharmaceutical agents, where showing systemic exposure is a validation of the toxicity test. Application of toxicokinetic data can help to ensure that all potential toxicities of a compound have been identified. This occurs by ensuring that the systemic levels of the test substance in animals under study are appreciably higher than systemic levels of the substance anticipated or measured in humans. On the other hand, demonstrating a lack of appreciable systemic exposure might be desirable for chemicals associated with nonintentional exposure. In this case, slow or minimal A, accompanied by rapid, efficient elimination are favorable attributes.

If systemic exposure is sufficiently low, it might be reasonable to limit or forgo certain longer-term toxicity studies or modify uncertainty factors used in the derivation of a RfD.

Systemic exposure information should be used in establishing dose levels for subsequent toxicity studies (33). When the high dose level is selected, based solely on clinical or pathological endpoints, a dosage might result that saturates A, M, or E of the compound. The resulting data will rarely be of any relevance to exposure of humans and, therefore, of little value in safety evaluation or risk assessment. Dose selection does not lend itself to a standard formula or approach, but the reader is referred to Morgan et al. (54) for an excellent discussion of the factors that should be considered in applying toxicokinetic data to dosage selection in toxicity studies. Systemic exposure data is similarly useful for selecting initial human doses and for escalating doses in drug clinical trials (55).

Elimination

This term is used to describe the removal of a compound from the body, whether by M or E. The overall rate can be expressed as either the Cl or the elimination half-life in plasma or alternative matrix, and terms can be derived for parent compound or specific metabolites. Persistent substances have relatively low Cls and long half-lives and might be associated with bioaccumulation, depending upon the duration and frequency of exposure. For therapeutics, rapid Cl from the circulation might indicate a need for more frequent dosing in repeat-dose toxicity studies.

Cl and elimination half-life are useful for making predictions concerning steady state. When an organism is exposed to a chemical, steady state in the body is reached when the rate of chemical uptake is equivalent to its rate of elimination. In other words, for a given level of continuous exposure, the steady-state concentration (C_{ss}) in a given matrix represents the maximum level that the chemical can attain, and will attain, given a sufficient length of exposure. If a rate of uptake or input (k_0) is available (e.g., infusion rate, inhalation uptake rate, dermal penetration rate), the average steady-state concentration can be predicted as:

$$C_{ss} = k_0/Cl$$

assuming Cl is unchanged by continuous exposure. Similarly, elimination half-life can be used to predict the time required to approach steady state upon repeated exposure. The time to reach 95% of average steady-state concentrations is given by the formula:

$$t_{95\% \text{ ss}} = -3.32 \times t_{1/2} \log(1 - 0.95).$$

Dose-Dependent Kinetics

Several processes contribute to the removal of a compound from the body, including active transport into the renal tubule, M, and protein binding. These processes involve the occupation of a limited number of binding sites. Increasing concentrations of a substance will occupy a proportionately increasing number of available binding sites until all sites are occupied, i.e., saturation occurs. Still higher concentrations of the substance beyond saturation will result in a disproportionate increase in the concentration of free compound. When systemic exposure has been determined over the range of toxicity study dose levels, graphical representation of the data (i.e., AUC or Cmax versus dose level) will reveal important information (Fig. 5):

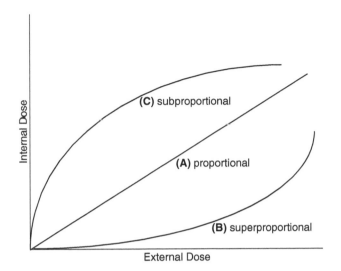

Figure 5 Relationships between external and internal doses. (**A**) A linear relationship results when internal dose is proportional to external dose; (**B**) a superproportional relationship results when elimination processes become saturated as dose level increases; (**C**) a subproportional relationship results when uptake processes become saturated or other shifts in toxicokinetic behavior occur as dose level increases.

- a linear relationship indicates dose proportionality (linear kinetics),
- a super-proportional increase in AUC or Cmax with dose level indicates nonlinear kinetics (e.g., saturation of M or E), and
- a subproportional increase in AUC or Cmax with dose level might indicate poor A, autoinduction of M, or other adaptive or high dosage shifts in toxicokinetic behavior.

Two of the more sensitive parameters for detecting nonlinear or saturation kinetics are Cl and dose-normalized AUC (i.e., AUC/dose). These parameters remain constant across the dose range of linear kinetics but change at dose levels that exceed the linear range. Revealing nonlinear toxicokinetics has important implications for the interpretation of toxicity studies (56). Toxicity data obtained at dose levels that fall outside the linear or proportional range will be of limited use for extrapolation to low dose levels.

Absorption

The method used to determine the extent and rate of A of a test substance depends upon the route of administration of the test substance and the type of data acquired. Bolus IV injection results in complete (100%) A of the parent compound; uptake is nearly instantaneous. When use of an IV reference group is specified, either the amount of dose excreted or an AUC should be determined for comparison with the tested route. For oral and dermal administration, the fraction (F), or percentage (F×100), of the parent compound absorbed can be determined by relating AUCs determined by the IV and ex routes (see Systemic data analysis). Without a RfD, oral or dermal A may be expressed as a fraction or percent of the dose administered, (calculated from the total amount of dose-related material recovered from excreta, expired air, and carcass) divided by the dose administered. Analysis of the parent compound concentration versus time curve, as described (see Systemic data analysis), might allow a determination of the A rate constant for oral, dermal, or inhalation A. For the cutaneous route of exposure, it might be appropriate to calculate an A rate for substances penetrating at a relatively constant rate. This often occurs when an excess of the test substance is applied to the skin for the entire exposure duration.

Extent of cutaneous A can be calculated by subtracting the dose recovered from the skin surface from the dose administered. Similarly, rate of A following an inhalation exposure might be equivalent to the rate of loss of test substance from a static exposure system (57–59). For inhalation exposures, extent of A is not routinely calculated because of the difficulty of determining dose administered. However, the experimentally determined ratio of inhalation and IV parent compound AUCs (first-order conditions) might provide an estimate of the inhalation dose ($dose_{inh}$):

$$dose_{inh} = AUC_{inh} \times dose_{iv}/AUC_{iv}$$

Distribution

The apparent V_d provides an indication of the extent of a compound's D out of the analyzed matrix (usually plasma). The V_d is larger for substances that are more extensively distributed to tissues. It is common practice to relate apparent volume of D to known volumes of body fluids. Thus, a V_d equal to 580 ml/kg body weight (bw) is suggestive of a D restricted to total body water (body water accounts for 58% of bw) (46) and a lack of D to ex tissues. Conversely, V_d can exceed 1000 ml/kg (i.e., 100%) for substances that have a high affinity for certain tissues relative to plasma. A high V_d generally reflects some degree of tissue concentration. Tissue to plasma concentration ratios can be used to indicate the extent of tissue D or accumulation; a time-independent alternative is the relative residence, R_R, which is calculated by determining the ratio of tissue to plasma AUCs (47). When tissue D is determined by the measurement of total radioactivity as a surrogate for test substance and related metabolites, it should be recognized that radiolabel might become incorporated into endogenous biomolecules through normal catabolism. This conversion of a test substance and incorporation into the carbon pool represents an innocuous situation, in contrast with the irreversible binding of reactive metabolites to critical biomolecules that is often responsible for toxicity.

Biotransformation and Bioactivation

M studies reveal what substances, in addition to the original (parent) compound, the organism is exposed to in a toxicity study. Excreted metabolites represent the end products of biotransformation; their measurement provides information on the extent of biotransformation and the number and relative amounts of different end products formed. In some cases, additional information can be inferred regarding the metabolic pathways and bioactivated intermediates that are involved in the conversion of parent compound to end products. Toxicity of a compound might be associated with M, or with one or more metabolites. When this is the case, the onset of toxicity can often be correlated with a certain concentration of metabolite in blood or target tissue. Dose-related comparisons are useful, because toxicity can arise from routes of M that are minor at lower doses but become significant at dose levels that saturate competing elimination pathways. Comparing metabolite profiles across a range of dose levels sometimes provides evidence that a specific metabolite or pathway is associated with toxicity. Thus, the presence of a new or disproportionate increase in a specific metabolite as the dose level is increased to toxic levels would suggest a role for the metabolite in toxicity. Differences in metabolite profiles observed after single and repeated dosing might also be indicative of enzyme induction or inhibition and might contribute to differences in acute and chronic toxicities.

Single vs. Repeat-Dose Comparisons

Repetitive dosing frequently alters a chemical's toxicokinetic behavior, with implications for drug, environmental, or workplace exposure. Changes in some measures of systemic exposure, such as AUC or Cmax, might occur following repetitive dosing as a result of induction or inhibition of the compound's own M or changes in extent of A. Enzyme induction and inhibition can be examined by comparison of metabolite profile after single and repeated treatment. More direct evaluation of enzymology might include measurements of enzyme activities in vitro or product formation rates using the tissues from exposed and naive animals.

Repeated dose studies are also useful for determining the extent and tissue(s) of bioaccumulation. Bioaccumulation potential is higher for compounds having a low systemic Cl or long elimination half-life, and an accurate description of these parameters requires a well-defined terminal slope of the concentration versus time curve. The potential for bioaccumulation might be difficult to detect in single dose studies if systemic concentrations drop quickly below limits of analytical sensitivity. Repeated dose studies should focus on systemic measurements using an analytical method that is specific for the active form of the chemical found in target tissues or tissues suspected of the greatest degree of accumulation (e.g., fat).

Route and Species Comparisons

Route-dependent differences in A, D, biotransformation, and associated kinetics are well known and important modifiers of a chemical's toxic potential. The oral route, in particular, can result in a "first-pass effect" where extensive M by the liver modifies the systemic delivery of the compound. If hepatic M serves to detoxify the compound, the inhalation route will deliver a greater dose of the toxicant relative to the oral route. On the other hand, if bioactivation occurs in the liver, hepatic toxicity might be more prevalent with an oral versus alternate exposure route. In selecting the route of exposure for toxicity studies, primary consideration should be given to those routes expected in humans potentially exposed during the manufacture or use of the chemical. Route-dependent differences in toxicokinetics can explain route differences in toxicity and can have a significant impact on risk assessment (60).

Cross-species extrapolation from experimental animals to humans is a fundamental problem faced by toxicologists. Species-related differences in toxic response can result from species-specific toxicokinetic differences (e.g., extent of A, degree of metabolic activation) and might also result from intrinsic species differences in sensitivity, sometimes referred to as toxicodynamic differences (61). Certain modes and mechanisms of toxicity are not applicable to human safety evaluation or risk assessment. Data that elucidate the mode of toxic action of a chemical, and the relative sensitivities of humans and test animals, are needed to avoid false predictions of toxicity or safety in humans. In addition, humans are highly heterogenous when it comes to traits that can modify toxicity. Toxicokinetics, along with toxicodynamics and exposure factors, can contribute to special sensitivity of children when compared with adults. The importance of toxicokinetic factors is greatest at the newborn stage but can also be significant at later stages of maturation. Within the first few days of life, certain barriers, such as the skin and the blood-brain barrier, are more permeable. Elimination of compounds is generally lower during the first few months of life, based on lower activities of metabolizing enzymes and lower renal glomerular filtration rates (62). Thus, the traits of the human population of interest must all be considered when extrapolating from animals to humans. To improve the reliability of toxicokinetic extrapolation, it is recommended that PBTK models be developed for the test animal and humans, relating exposure dose to internal tissue dose. An understanding of the mechanism of toxic action in the test species, and the potential for this mechanism to operate in humans, will further strengthen predictions of human toxicity based on toxicological data. In vitro determination of biotransformation and relative sensitivities of humans and test animals can help ensure that the test species is an appropriate model. Comparative data showing significant species differences might help preserve a viable new product or prevent undue restriction of an existing product where its toxic effects are irrelevant to humans.

Reporting

Reporting requirements for toxicokinetic studies, such as the guidance provided, tend to be flexible and dependent upon the type(s) of study performed. They range from the most basic of instructions, as the following from ICH (13):

A comprehensive account of the toxicokinetic data generated, together with an evaluation of the results and of the implications for the interpretation of the toxicology findings, should be given. An outline of the analytical method should be reported or referenced. In addition, a rationale for the choice of the matrix analyzed and the analyte measured should be given to a comprehensive list of specifications for the body of the report (16), as summarized below:

- Summary: a summarized analysis of results and conclusions drawn
- Introduction: objectives, guideline references, regulatory history, if any, and rationale
- Materials and methods: test substance identification: physico-chemical properties, vehicles or carriers, identification of radiolabeled material; test system: species, strain, age, sex, bw, health status and husbandry; study design and methodology; statistical analysis
- Results: tabulated radioactivity analysis results (typically dpm and µg equivalents), graphs, representative chromatograms and spectrometric data, proposed metabolic pathways and molecular structure of metabolites. If applicable, justification of exposure conditions, dose levels; description of pilot studies; quantity and percent recovery of radioactivity in urine, feces, and expired air, and other matrices as appropriate; tissue D (% dose and µg equivalents per g tissue); material balance; plasma concentrations and pharmacokinetic parameters; rate and extent of A; quantities of test substance and metabolites (% dose) in excreta; individual animal data
- Discussion and conclusions: provide a plausible explanation of the metabolic pathway for the test substance; emphasize species and sex differences whenever possible; discuss the nature and magnitude of metabolites, rates of Cl, bioaccumulation potential, and level of tissue residues, as appropriate; concise conclusion.

CURRENT APPLICATIONS

Data developed in toxicokinetic and associated M and mechanistic studies have improved human health risk estimates and reduced their uncertainty (63–66). Dosimetry models (e.g., PBTK or PBPK, nasal air flow, dermal, and pulmonary uptake) are increasingly being used to estimate human kinetic parameters. These models incorporate the principal biological factors governing the disposition of the compound in the body, including blood flow rates, organ volumes, intrinsic tissue solubility of the compound, protein binding, and metabolic rate constants. These models enable a chemical's disposition to be simulated and provide estimates of the dose delivered to a target tissue. The behavior of the compound can also be predicted under varying conditions, making possible high-to-low dose, cross-species, and route-to-route extrapolations.

Toxicokinetic models can also be developed for groups of compounds that are metabolically related, in which the model consists of linked submodels for each compound (67). Models developed for such "families" of compounds quantify the internal dose for the parent compound as well as internal doses for each metabolite. When such models are used in conjunction with parent compound toxicity studies, it is possible to estimate potentially toxic levels for each of the metabolites. This approach to risk assessment, named the family approach, has been recommended as an efficient method for determining acceptable exposure limits for metabolically related compounds.

Quantitative risk assessments rely on the knowledge or expectation that the response to the chemical is related to its concentration, but this is not universally the case, as discussed in Route and Species Comparisons and elsewhere (68–70). Although there are limits to the valid application of tissue concentration data in quantitative risk assessment, its use as a measure of exposure is preferable to the use of administered dose, which is standard practice in the absence of toxicokinetic data. The dosimetry model can be extended by incorporating mechanistic data, as it becomes available, thus building a risk assessment model that uses available knowledge of a compound's kinetics and dynamics. A recent application is the modeling of inhaled chemical vapors that cause a toxic response at the portal of entry, the respiratory tract. Respiratory tract toxicity is an area where dosimetry models have greatly improved extrapolation between test species and humans. Such factors as regional airflow delivery, water solubility, reactivity, and local M can all be integrated quantitatively into a PBTK model, yielding reliable estimates of dose across species whose anatomies and physiologies are distinctly different (71).

When dosimetry models are not available for determining human kinetic parameters, certain parameters can be estimated by a method known as interspecies allometric scaling (72,73). In this method, a parameter determined for the experimental animal is adjusted to human proportions, usually by a power function x of the bw, thus:

Parameter α bw^x

AUC and Cl are useful parameters for making species comparisons and can assist in the determination of appropriate allometric scaling factors. Allometry is not generally useful for extrapolating metabolic parameters across species, but other parameters in humans, such as the apparent volume of D and half-life, have been successfully predicted from similar parameters in rats (74).

In determining acceptable human exposure levels for chemicals, the use of 10-fold safety factors, each for interspecies differences and human variability, is common practice. These safety factors, also called uncertainty factors, and more recently, chemical-specific adjustment factors (CSAF) reflect both the kinetic and dynamic aspects of interspecies differences and human variability (75). Renwick (76) has described a mechanism by which the usual 100-fold safety factor used for food additives could be modified by known or predicted differences in toxicokinetics between experimental animals and humans. The safety factor could be significantly reduced, for example, if a compound was shown to undergo complete M (detoxication) prior to A. Toxicokinetic data have been applied to the derivation of safety factors used to set occupational exposure limits (77) and to establish acceptable or tolerable daily intakes (78,79). For the reader interested in development of CSAFs for interspecies differences and human variability, guidance is available at (80,81).

This section has introduced several applications of toxicokinetic data for improving extrapolation to humans, risk assessment, and modifying safety factors. Besides these quantitative applications, toxicokinetic data have practical utility in the qualitative understanding of a compound's behavior, as described throughout the chapter. The identification of key toxicokinetic characteristics, such as elimination half-life, first-pass M, bioactivation, and dose saturation, are invaluable to understanding circumstances under which toxicity is likely to be expressed.

REFERENCES

1. OECD. OECD Guideline for testing of chemicals, "417: Toxicokinetics" (updated guideline, adopted 4th April 1984).
2. OECD. OECD Guideline for the testing of chemicals, "427 skin absorption: In vivo method" (original guideline, adopted 13th April 2004).
3. OECD. OECD Guideline for the testing of chemicals, "428 skin absorption: In vitro method" (original guideline, adopted 13th April 2004).
4. http://www.oecd.org/findDocument/0,2350,en_2649_34377_1_1_1_1_1,00.html.
5. USFDA 1982. Toxicological principles for the safety assessment of direct food additives and color additives used in food (Redbook I). Bureau of foods, FDA, 1986.
6. USFDA 2000. Toxicological principles for the safety of food ingredients (Redbook 2000); Updated October 2001 & November 2003.
7. http://vm.cfsan.fda.gov/~redbook/red-toca.html.
8. USFDA 1994. Guideline for metabolism studies and for selection of residues for toxicological testing In: General principles for evaluating the safety of compounds used in food-producing animals. Revised July 1994, FDA Center for Veterinary Medicine.
9. USFDA 1997. Drug metabolism/drug interaction studies in the drug development process: Studies in vitro. Center for Drug Evaluation and Research.
10. http://www.fda.gov/cder/guidance/clin3.pdf.
11. USFDA 1999. In Vivo Drug metabolism/drug interaction studies—study design, data analysis, and recommendations for dosing and labeling. Center for Drug Evaluation and Research.
12. http://www.fda.gov/cber/gdlns/metabol.pdf.
13. ICH 1995. Toxicokinetics: the assessment of systemic exposure in toxicity studies. Guideline for industry S3A, March 1995.
14. ICH 1995. Pharmacokinetics: guidance for repeated dose tissue distribution studies. Guideline for Industry S3B, March 1995.
15. http://www.ich.org/UrlGrpServer.jser?@_ID=276&@_TEMPLATE=254.
16. USEPA 1998. Health effects test guidelines OPPTS 870.7485 metabolism and pharmacokinetics.
17. USEPA 1998. Health effects test guidelines OPPTS 870.7600 dermal.
18. Buchanan JR, Burka LT, Melnick RL. Purpose and guidelines for toxicokinetic studies within the national toxicology program. Environ Health Perspect 1997; 105:468–471.
19. ECETOC 1992. EC 7th Amendment: role of mammalian toxicokinetic and metabolic studies in the toxicological assessment of industrial chemical. Technical report no. 46.
20. Wilson AGE, Frantz SW, Keifer LC. A tiered approach to pharmacokinetic studies. Environ Health Perspect 1994; 102:5–11.
21. Arms & Travis 1988. Reference physiological parameters in pharmacokinetic modelling, office of health and environmental assessment, EPA, EPA/600/6-88/004, 1-1-7, 16. Washington, DC.

22. Clewell HJ, Andersen ME. Dose, species, and route extrapolation using physiologically based pharmacokinetic models. Toxicol Ind Health 1985; 1:111–131.

23. Blancato JN. Physiologically-based pharmacokinetic models in risk and exposure assessment. Ann Ist Super Sanitá 1991; 27:601–608.

24. Leung HW. Development and utilization of physiologically based pharmacokinetic models for toxicological applications. J Toxicol Environ Health 1991; 32:247–267.

25. Andersen ME, Clewell HJ, III, Frederick CB. Applying simulation modeling to problems in toxicology and risk assessment-a short perspective. Toxicol Appl Pharmacol 1995; 133:181–187.

26. Charnick SB, Kawai R, Nedelman JR, Lemaire M, Niederberger W, Sato H. Perspectives in pharmacokinetics. Physiologically based pharmacokinetic modeling as a tool for drug development. J Pharmacokinet Biopharm 1995; 23:217–229.

27. Molen GWVD, Kooijman SALM, Slob W. A generic toxicokinetic model for persistent lipophilic compounds in humans: an application to TCDD. Fundam Appl Toxicol 1996; 31:83–94.

28. Poulin P, Theil FP. Prediction of Pharmacokinetics prior to in vivo studies II. Generic physiologically based pharmacokinetic models of drug disposition. J Pharm Sci 2002; 91:1358–1370.

29. Dixit R, Riviere J, Krishnan K, Andersen ME. Toxicokinetics PBTK in toxicology and risk assessment. J Toxicol Environ Health B 2003; 6:1–40.

30. Andersen ME. Toxicokinetic modeling and its applications in chemical risk assessment. Toxicol Lett 2003; 138:9–27.

31. Smith DA, Humphrey MJ, Charuel C. Design of toxicokinetic studies. Xenobiotica 1990; 20:1187–1199.

32. Campbell DB. Are we doing too many animal biodisposition investigations before phase I studies in man? A re-evaluation of the timing and extent of ADME studies Eur J Drug Metab Pharmacokinet 1994; 19:283–293.

33. Spurling NW, Carey PF. Dose selection for toxicity studies: a protocol for determining the maximum repeatable dose. Hum Exp Toxicol 1992; 11:449–457.

34. Schwartz S. Providing toxicokinetic support for reproductive toxicology studies in pharmaceutical development. Arch Toxicol 2001; 75:381–387.

35. Van Bree J, Nedelman J, Steimer JL. Application of sparse sampling approaches in rodent toxicokinetics: a prospective view. Drug Inferm J 1994; 28:263–279.

36. Steimer JL, Ebelin ME, Van Bree J. Pharmacokinetic and pharmacodynamic data and models in clinical trials. Eur J Drug Metab Pharmacokinet 1993; 18:61–76.

37. Vozeh S, Steimer JL, Rowland M, et al. The use of population pharmacokinetics in drug development. Clin Pharmacokinet 1996; 30:81–93.

38. Boatman RJ, Perry LG, Fiorica LA, et al. Wright, dermal absorption and pharmacokinetics of isopropanol in the male and female F-344 rat. Drug Metab Dispos 1998; 26:197–202.

39. Frantz SW, Beatty PW, English JC, Hundley SG, Wilson AGE. The use of pharmacokinetics as an interpretive and predictive tool in chemical toxicology testing and risk assessment: a position paper on the appropriate use of pharmacokinetics in chemical toxicology. Regul Toxicol Pharmacol 1994; 19:317–337.

40. Weiss DJ, Lunte CE, Lunte SM. In vivo microdialysis as a tool for monitoring pharmacokinetics. Trends Anal Chem 2000; 19:606–616.

41. Igarashi T, Yabe T, Noda K. Study design and statistical analysis of toxicokinetics: a report of JPMA investigation of case studies. J Toxicol Sci 1996; 21:497–504.

42. A Parkinson. Biotransformation of xenobiotics, Casarett & Doull's toxicology, the basic science of poisons 5th ed. C.D Klaassen. McGraw-Hill, ed., 1996.

43. Sweatman TW, Renwick AG. The tissue distribution and pharmacokinetics of saccharin in the rat. Toxicol Appl Pharmacol 1980; 55:18–31.

44. Shah VP, Midha KK, Dighe S, et al. Analytical methods validation: vioavailability, bioequivalence and pharmacokinetic studies. Pharm Res 1992; 9:588–592.

45. Clark B, Smith DA. An Introduction to Phamacokinetics. Boston, Massachusetts: Blackwell Scientific Publications, 1981.

46. Renwick AG. Toxicokinetics—pharmacokinetics in toxicology. In: Hayes AW, ed. Principles and Methods of Toxicology. New York: Raven Press, 1994.

47. Abou-donia MB. Metabolism and toxicokinetics of xenobiotics. In: Derelanko M, Hollinger M, eds. CRC Handbook of Toxicology. Boca Raton, FL, CRC Press, Inc., 1995.

48. Gibaldi A, Perrier D. Pharmacokinetics. In: Swarbrick J, ed. Revised and Expanded. 2nd ed. New York: Dekker, 1982.

49. Silber PM, Myslinski NR, Ruegg CE. In vitro methods for predicting human pharmacokinetics. Lab Anim 1995;36–38.

50. Obach SR, Baxter JG, Liston TE, et al. The prediction of human pharmacokinetic parameters from preclinical and in vitro metabolism data. J Pharmacol Exp Ther 1997; 283:46–58.

51. Li AP. In vitro approaches to evaluate ADMET drug properties. Curr Top Med Chem 2004; 4:701–706.

52. Dain JG, Collins JM, Robinson WT. A regulatory and industrial perspective of the use of carbon-14 and tritium isotopes in human ADME studies. Pharm Res 1994; 1:925–928.

53. Ette EI, Kelman AW, Howie CA, Whiting B. Analysis of animal pharmacokinetic data: performance of the one point per animal design. J Pharmacokinet Biopharm 1995; 23:551–566.

54. Morgan DG, Kelvin AS, Kinter LB, Fish CJ, Kerns WD, Rhodes G. The application of toxicokinetic data to dosage selection in toxicology studies. Toxicol Pathol 1994; 22:112–123.

55. Piantadosi S, Liu G. Improved designs for dose escalation studies using pharmacokinetic measurements. Stat Med 1996; 15:1605–1618.

56. Lin JH. Dose-dependent pharmacokinetics: experimental observations and theoretical considerations. Biopharm Drug Dispos 1994; 15:1–31.

57. Filser JG, Bolt HM. Pharmacokinetics of halogenated ethylenes in rats. Arch Toxicol 1979; 42:123–136.

58. Andersen ME. Recent advances in methodology and concepts for characterizing inhalation pharmacokinetic parameters in animals and man. Drug Metab Rev 1982; 13:799–826.

59. Andersen ME. Inhalation pharmacokinetics: evaluating systemic extraction, total in vivo metabolism, and the time course of enzyme induction for inhaled styrene in rats based on arterial blood: inhaled air concentration ratios. Toxicol Appl Pharmacol 1984; 73:176–187.

60. Doe JE, Hoffmann HD. Toluene diisocyanate: an assessment of carcinogenic risk following oral and inhalation exposure. Toxicol Ind Health 1995; 11:13–32.

61. Eason CT, Bonner FW, Parke DV. The importance of pharmacokinetic and receptor studies in drug safety evaluation. Regul Toxicol Pharmacol 1990; 11:288–307.

62. Schwenk M, Gundert-Remy U, Heinemeyer G, et al. Children as a sensitive subgroup and their role in regulatory toxicology: DGPT workshop report. Arch Toxicol 2003; 77:2–6.

63. Beliles RP, Totman LC. Pharmacokinetically based risk assessment of workplace exposure to benzene. Regul Toxicol Pharmacol 1989; 9:186–195.

64. Frederick CB, Wilson AGE. Comments on incorporating mechanistic data into quantitative risk assessment. Risk Anal 1991; 11:581–582.

65. Meek ME, Hughes K. Approach to health risk determination for metals and their compounds under the Canadian environmental protection act. Regul Toxicol Pharmacol 1995; 22:206–212.

66. Bond JA, Himmelstein MW, Medinsky MA. The use of toxicologic data in mechanistic risk assessment: 1,3-butadiene as a case study. Int Arch Occup Environ Health 1996; 68:415–420.

67. Barton HA, Deisinger PJ, English JC, et al. Family approach for estimating reference concentrations/doses for series of related organic chemicals. Toxicol Sci 2000; 54:251–261.

68. Monro A. What is an appropriate measure of exposure when testing drugs for carcinogenicity in rodents? Toxicol Appl Pharmacol 1992; 112:171–181.

69. Monro A. The paradoxical lack of interspecies correlation between plasma concentrations and chemical carcinogenicity. Regul Toxicol Pharmacol 1993; 18:115–135.

70. Monro A. Drug toxicokinetics: scope and limitations that arise from species differences in phamacodynamic and carcinogenic responses. J Pharmacokinet Biopharm 1994; 22:41–57.

71. Bogdanffy MS, Sarangapani R. Physically based kinetic modeling of vapors toxic to the respiratory tract. Toxicol Lett 2003; 138:103–107.
72. D'Souza RW, Boxenbaum H. Physiological pharmacokinetic models: some aspects of theory, practice, and potential. Toxicol Ind Health 1988; 4:151–171.
73. Ings RMJ. Interspecies scaling and comparisons in drug development and toxicokinetics. Xenobiotica 1990; 20:1201–1231.
74. Bachmann K, Pardoe D, White D. Scaling basic toxicokinetic parameters from rat to man. Environ Health Perspect 1996; 104:400–407.
75. Renwick AG. Safety factors and establishment of acceptable daily intakes. Food Addit Contam 1991; 8:135–150.
76. Renwick AG. Data-derived safety factors for the evaluation of food additives and environmental contaminants. Food Addit Contam 1993; 10:275–305.
77. Naumann BD, Weideman PA. Scientific basis for uncertainty factors used to establish occupational exposure limits for pharmaceutical active ingredients. Hum Ecol Risk Assess 1995; 1:590–613.
78. Morgenroth V, III. Scientific evaluation of the data-derived safety factors for the acceptable daily intake. Case study: diethylhexylphthalate. Food Addit Contam 1993; 10:363–373.
79. Würtzen G. Scientific evaluation of the safety factor for the acceptable daily intake (ADI). Case study: butylated hydroxyanisole (BHA). Food Addit Contam 1993; 10:307–314.
80. http://www.who.int/ipcs/publications/methods/harmonization/en/csafs_guidance_doc.pdf.
81. I.P.C.S., 2001. Guidance document for the use of data in development of chemical-specific adjustment factors (CSAFs) for interspecies differences and human variability in dose/concentration-response assessment. International programme on chemical safety, World Health Organization, Geneva, Switzerland.

5

Toxicologic Pathology Assessment

Lynda L. Lanning
Otsuka Maryland Research Institute, Rockville, Maryland, U.S.A.

INTRODUCTION

Anatomic pathology, microscopic pathology, and clinical pathology evaluations in toxicology studies generate an enormous amount of critical data. The anatomic and microscopic pathologist(s) and clinical pathologist form the link between in-life data and postlife data. Data interpretations must be done as a part of the whole study picture, including clinical observations, various in-life measurements, such as food or water consumption and body weights, necropsy and histopathology findings, clinical pathology findings, and organ weight data. Pertinent factors in hematological, hemostasis, and clinical chemistry test selection, methodology, and interpretation include, but are not limited to, animal data (including species, strain, and age) and test material data (known toxic effects, chemical interactions). In addition, appropriate specimen collection and handling are critical to the validity, reliability, and consistency of test results. Clinical pathology data are generally subjected to statistical analysis; however, care should be taken to establish the difference between statistical significance and biological or toxicological significance of any changes observed. The clinical pathologist utilizes the review of concurrent control data, historical control data, and individual animal data versus group means when evaluating the relative biological significance of changes. The anatomic and microscopic pathologist(s) take(s) into account both the recognition of injury to tissue and its biological or toxicological significance based on the nature of the injury in conjunction with other available data. Assessment of altered gross and cellular morphology depends on the ability of the pathologist to discriminate between test material-induced changes, secondary changes, regenerative changes, spontaneous disease, postmortem changes, iatrogenic changes, and normal biologic/physiologic variations. Accuracy and clarity of the pathology data and report are key to the usefulness and validity of the study. The clinical pathologist and the anatomic and microscopic pathologist(s) can and should be an integral part of the toxicology team providing input from study design through final study report.

CLINICAL PATHOLOGY

General Considerations

Proper specimen collection and handling are critical for accurate hematological and clinical chemistry evaluation. Collection sites vary with the species, the volume of specimen required, the necessity for anesthesia, and the number of collection time points required by the study protocol (1,2). Table 1 describes the suggested sample volumes for rats and mice by age. The minimum amounts required for routine hematology and clinical chemistry assays are dependent on the type of equipment used in the clinical laboratory; however, in general, these amounts are 0.5 ml of whole blood [ethylenediaminetetraacetic acid (EDTA) anticoagulant] for hematology and 0.5 ml of serum for a routine clinical chemistry panel. Standard operating procedures (SOPs) should be in place for all blood sampling techniques. Only those staff members trained and proficient in the blood collection technique required by the study protocol should perform the collection.

In rodents, anesthetics, when required, should be chosen carefully (3). Clinical pathology parameters may be affected by these agents, many of which are known microsomal protein inducers and/or may cause splenic sequestration of peripheral blood cells. Alternately, stress during blood collection without anesthetics is known to result in marked alteration in cellular values (4,5). The anesthetic of choice for laboratory rodents is a 70% carbon dioxide (CO_2)/30% oxygen mixture. This agent is relatively safe, nontoxic, and readily available, does not induce microsomal proteins, does not alter cardiac function/output, and is accepted by the American Veterinary Medical Association (6). Anesthetics are rarely used in rabbits, dogs, and nonhuman primates because appropriate restraint is achievable without their use.

Hematology

The importance of appropriate hematological assessment in toxicology studies has been recognized for many years. In elucidating toxic effects through hematology, the investigator must be aware of the appropriate methods of blood collection and handling, sampling times, testing selection, quality control (QC) evaluation, and test

Table 1 Suggested Sample Volumes from Mice and Rats

Species	Volume in mL		
	Age 6 weeks	Age 17 weeks	Age 6 months
Mouse (nonsacrificial)			
Whole blood	0.5	0.75	1.0
Plasma	0.25	0.37	0.5
Serum	0.25	0.37	0.5
Mouse (terminal)			
Whole blood	1.0	1.5	1.75
Plasma	0.5	0.75	0.87
Serum	0.5	0.75	0.87
Rat (nonsacrificial)			
Whole blood	1.0	1.5	3.0
Plasma	0.5	0.75	1.5
Serum	0.5	0.75	1.5
Rat (terminal)			
Whole blood	3.0	4.0	5.0
Plasma	1.5	2.0	2.5
Serum	1.5	2.0	2.5

result interpretation. One should remain aware that the test substance might affect stem cell health, maturation, and/or release, or peripheral blood cell distribution, function, and/or use. In addition, the role of normal animal species physiology and its impact on hematological parameters cannot be overlooked when interpreting test results.

Selection of Parameters

The investigator should consider several points when selecting the appropriate hematological parameters for evaluation. These items include sample volume requirements, information desired, time points for evaluation, and route of sample collection. "Routine" hematological evaluation in toxicity testing is generally used in those studies where hematological effects are not expected based on the known structure and/or function of the test material. The parameters measured include white blood cell (WBC) count, red blood cell (RBC) count, hematocrit (HCT), hemoglobin (HGB), mean corpuscular hemoglobin (MCH), mean corpuscular hemoglobin concentration (MCHC), and platelet count (PLT). Blood smears should be prepared at sample collection for the WBC differential/cellular morphology evaluation (one slide) and reticulocyte count (one slide prepared after staining the reticulocytes). Some hematology analyzers today can perform WBC differential counts specific for each species however, the slide should be available in case suspicious/inaccurate counts are produced by the analyzer. If the investigator suspects test material-related hematological changes may occur during the study, the use of more specialized tests or techniques may be warranted and should be included in the study protocol. For example, if a test material is a suspected bone marrow toxicant, a bone marrow smear should be prepared at necropsy and evaluated for potential stem cell damage or maturation/release effects. Determination of methemoglobin (metHb) concentrations is helpful if the test material is a known or suspected oxidizing agent.

Specimen Collection and Quality

For routine hematological measurements, which require whole, uncoagulated blood, the anticoagulant of choice is the potassium salt of EDTA. This product is available as either a powder or liquid in a variety of commercial blood collection tubes of varing volumes, however the liquid EDTA is preferable for adequate mixing. It is important to include the appropriate amount of blood for the volume of anticoagulant present in the tube to minimize volume effects, such as erythrocyte shrinkage, that will result in artifactual changes in the HCT, mean corpuscular volume (MCV), and MCHC. Other, less commonly used anticoagulants include heparin, sodium fluoride, sodium citrate (used for coagulation measurements), and potassium oxalate.

After the specimen is collected from the animal and placed into the collection tube, the blood and anticoagulant should be *gently* mixed by hand for 30 seconds to 60 seconds. The specimen should then be placed on a mechanical rocker prior to analysis. The WBC differential smears should be prepared from EDTA-anticoagulated whole blood within 2 hours of sample collection. The smears should be allowed to air dry and then fixed with absolute methanol. These smears are typically stained with Wright-Giemsa stain in preparation for microscopic evaluation. The WBC differential and platelet and erythrocyte morphological assessment are conducted concurrently from this smear. Reticulocytes should be vitally stained for 10 minutes within 2 hours of sample collection and a thin-thin smear prepared.

Common Parameters—Methodology and Interpretation

White Blood Cell Count. The term WBC (leukocyte) pertains to all types of leukocytes, including granulocytes (neutrophils, eosinophils, basophils), lymphocytes, and monocytes. WBCs in the peripheral blood are in transit from sites of production (i.e., bone marrow, thymus) to sites of function or destruction. Each type of WBC has distinct morphological and functional features. The WBC count is usually reported in units of thousands per cubic millimeter.

Automated instruments have virtually replaced performance of WBC counts by manual methods, however the WBC count may be obtained by use of a specialized type of microscopic slide called a hemocytometer. The manual method requires mixing the whole blood in a special white cell dilution pipette containing a red cell lysing solution. After the RBCs are lysed, the specimen is placed on a hemocytometer, and the cells are counted under $100\times$ magnification.

Automated WBC counts may be measured by either laser light scatter or, more commonly, by impedance particle counting. The laser light scatter method uses a focused light beam. As the cells travel through the light beam, the amount of light scattered at different angles is measured. Impedance particle counting involves suspension of an aliquot of the specimen in isotonic saline that flows through a narrow aperture across which a direct current (DC) is maintained (7,8). The while blood cells are differentiated from RBCs by diameter (in rats, RBC diameter is 5.9 µm, compared with 10 to 12 µm for neutrophils; in mice, the RBC diameter is 5.5 µm, compared with 10 to 12 µm for neutrophils) (9), and lysing of the erythrocytes. A significant advantage of impedance cell counters in laboratory animal testing is the ability to adjust the discriminators to the specific cell size(s) of various species (10).

Caution should be used when evaluating the WBC data since several common mistakes in blood collection and analysis may result in erroneous data and confound the results. Nucleated RBCs (NRBC) cannot be distinguished from WBCs by most automated analyzers. This will artificially increase the WBC count produced by these analyzers. After the WBC differential count is completed, the automated WBC count should be corrected for the number of NRBCs (see discussion below) as needed. Platelet clumps may also artificially produce high WBC counts. This becomes a problem when the specimens are not mixed adequately with the anticoagulant.

Leukocytosis is indicated by a WBC count that is higher than the normal value for that species and age animal. Diseases and conditions that can cause leukocytosis include, but are not limited to, inflammatory conditions conditions (i.e., infections, immune mediated anemia, necrosis), glucocorticoid-associated conditions (i.e., stress, hyperadrenocorticism), physiologic shift (i.e., fight or flight response), neoplasia (i.e., leukemia, lymphoma), estrogen toxicosis (early), parasitism, hypersensitivity disorders/reactions, and leukocyte adhesion deficiencies. Conversely, leukopenia may be the result of overwhelming inflammation, peripheral leukocyte destruction, bone marrow toxicity, loss of lymph, and stress. Determination of the cause of the WBC count change may be difficult; however, leukogram patterns derived from the WBC differential will provide important clues. For example, an acute inflammatory leukogram would show an increase in total WBC, segmented, and nonsegmented neutrophils, and a decrease in lymphocytes. Physiologic leukocytosis would show an increase in total WBC, segmented neutrophils, and lymphocytes with no increase in nonsegmented neutrophils.

Hematocrit. The HCT (packed cell volume) is the quantitative measurement of erythrocyte concentration after optimal packing of erythrocytes in a commercially available microhematocrit capillary tube. A manual measurement of the HCT is performed by centrifugation of anticoagulated whole blood in a microhematocrit centrifuge. The packed red cell column in the microhematocrit capillary tube is then measured using a microhematocrit reader. Visual inspection of the centrifuged specimen may provide additional information, such as evidence of hemolysis, icterus, lipemia, and leukocytosis.

The HCT can also be calculated on automated hematology instruments by multiplying the RBC count and the MCV. This automated method avoids technical such errors as the presence of trapped plasma and reading errors. HCT is expressed as a percentage.

An increased HCT is indicated by a HCT value that is higher than the normal value for that species and age animal. Increased HCT values can be due to either an increase in the circulating RBC mass or by a decrease in plasma volume (dehydration).

Red Blood Cell Count.   The RBC, or erythrocyte, is a nonnucleated biconcave disk derived from bone marrow stem cells under the influence of erythropoietin. Erythropoietin is produced by the kidneys, and its production is stimulated by hypoxia and/or stem cell turnover. The maturation time from stem cell to RBC in the peripheral circulation is approximately five days. The RBC transports oxygen, CO_2, and nutrients. The average life span of the RBC varies by species (mouse 20–45 days, rat 50–65 days, rabbit 45–70 days, dog 100–120 days).

Although automated instruments have replaced performance of RBC counts by manual methods, the RBC count may be obtained by use of a hemocytometer. Automated RBC counts may be measured by either laser light scatter or, more commonly, by impedance particle counting as discussed in the WBC section. The RBC is usually reported in units of millions per cubic millimeter.

Anemia, the term used to describe a decreased RBC count, is indicated by a RBC count that is lower than the normal values for that species and age animal. Anemias are classified on the basis of responsiveness (i.e., regenerative or nonregenerative), cell size (i.e., normocytic, macrocytic, microcytic), HGB content (i.e., normochromic, hypochromic) and/or pathophysiology (i.e., blood-loss, hemolysis). The red cell indices, such as MCV, HGB, MCHC, are the critical endpoints to evaluate when determining the anemia classification. Causes of anemia include, but are not limited to, inflammatory diseases, chronic renal disease, chemotherapeutic agent toxicosis, plant toxicosis (Bracken fern), nutritional factors (i.e., iron, copper, folate, or vitamin B_{12} deficiency), liver disease, and drug-induced immune hemolytic disorders (10).

Erythrocytosis, the term used to describe an increased RBC count, is indicated by a RBC count that is higher than the normal values for that species and age animal. Conditions that may result in erythrocytosis include, but are not limited to, dehydration (the most common cause of erythrocytosis in mammals), chronic pulmonary disease, hyperthyroidism, renal neoplasms/cysts, and polycythemia vera.

Hemoglobin.   HGB is the oxygen-carrying pigment of the erythrocyte. It is an oligomeric protein containing four separate globin peptide chains, each of which is noncovalently bound to a porphyrinic heme group. Each heme group has a central iron atom that is reversibly bound with molecular oxygen. The International Committee for Standardization in Hematology recommends the cyanomethemoglobin method for HGB measurement. This reaction converts HGB to cyanomethemoglobin following the addition of potassium ferricyanide to the specimen. All HGB derivatives except sulfhemoglobin are converted to cyanomethemoglobin, which is a stable pigment with an absorption at 540 nm. The HGB concentration is calculated by comparison of the unknown solution to a standard solution of HGB and is usually expressed in units of grams per deciliter.

The HGB should be approximately one-third of the HCT if the RBCs are of normal size. The HGB value is used to determine several of the red cell indices that are used in characterizing anemias.

Mean Corpuscular Volume.   The MCV measurement is the volume of the average red cell calculated from the number of RBCs and HCT as described below:

$$MCV = \frac{\text{Hematocrit } (\%) \times 10}{\text{RBC count } (10^6/\mu L)}$$

The MCV is generally higher in young animals due to the presence of more immature RBCs, which are larger and have not yet taken the biconcave shape. RBCs with increased MCV values are referred to as macrocytic. Those with decreased MCV values are microcytic. The MCV is usually expressed as femtoliters or cubic micrometers.

Mean Corpuscular Hemoglobin.   The MCH measurement is the concentration of HGB by weight in the average RBC (expressed in units of picograms or micromicrograms) and is calculated as described below:

$$MCH = \frac{\text{Hemoglobin concentration } (g/dL) \times 10}{\text{Hematocrit } (\%)}$$

Mean Corpuscular Hemoglobin Concentration.   The MCHC is the ratio of the HGB concentration to HCT (expressed as a percentage) and is calculated as described below:

$$MCHC = \frac{\text{Hemoglobin concentration } (g/dL) \times 100}{\text{Hematocrit } (\%)}$$

This measurement is considered to be the most constant erythrocyte index, providing that the HGB and HCT measurements are accurate (12). RBCs with normal MCHC values are referred to as normochromic. Those with decreased MCHC values are hypochromic. It is not physiologically possible to produce hyperchromic erythrocytes (increased MCHC) because HGB synthesis stops when an optimal HGB is reached within the red cell precursor's cytoplasm. Most increased MCHC values are falsely increased due to hemoglobinemia, in vitro hemolysis, spectral interference in the assay, and cell shrinkage related to in vivo hypoosmolal states followed by cell contact with a relatively hyperosmolar diluent in the analyzer.

Platelet   Count.   The PLT is an automated direct count determined by impedance, as described in the section on WBC count, and is usually expressed in units of thousands per cubic millimeter. In addition, pulse editing is used to discriminate between RBCs and platelets. Because of their small size, wide size range, aggregation, and difficulty in distinguishing between platelets from debris or microcytic red cells, PLTs are measured less precisely than other components of the blood count (expected variability of approximately 22%) (13). Automated measurements deal with these issues by mathematically analysis of the platelet volume distribution to ensure that it represents the lognormal distribution expected. An estimate of platelet numbers should be done on the WBC differential slide, particularly if the PLT, and/or histogram are outside the expected range. This visual inspection will allow for exclusion of spurious PLTs caused by the presence of platelet clumps, debris, microcytic RBCs, or cellular fragments (14). The significance of the PLT is discussed in the later section concerning coagulation/hemostasis.

Mean Platelet Volume.   The mean platelet volume (MPV) is an automated direct measurement of platelet size and is usually expressed in units of femtoliters. It has been documented that the MPV is inversely correlated with the PLT (15,16). Significant changes in size will alter the platelet biomass, which, in turn, determines hemostatic ability as long as platelet function is not impaired. Therefore, in evaluating platelet hemostatic function, the circulating platelet biomass is a more meaningful indication than MPV or PLT alone. The following platelet volumes have been reported: dog, nonhuman primate, pig, and human, 7.6 to 8.3 fl; and rate guinea pig and mouse, 3.2 to 5.4 fl (17). In general, it is considered that larger platelets are metabolically and functionally more active than smaller platelets (18).

Reticulocyte Count.   The reticulocyte is an immature erythrocyte that is not nucleated but contains some ribosomal or mitochondrial material. When whole, anticoagulated blood is incubated in a solution of new methylene blue, and the ribonucleic acid is precipitated as a dye-ribonucleoprotein complex. This complex appears as a dark blue network or dark blue granules that allows the reticulocyte in a smear to be readily identified and counted. The reticulocyte count is usually expressed as a percentage. The reticulocyte smear must be prepared within 2 hours of specimen collection. Care must be taken to store the slides in the dark, away from fluorescent light.

Methemoglobin Concentration.   Methemoglobin (metHb) is formed when the heme irons of HGB are oxidized. It is usually expressed as a percentage of total HGB concentration. metHb cannot combine reversibly with oxygen or carbon monoxide and is a dark, greenish brown color that does not revert to red upon exposure to oxygen. Because metHb is readily reduced by normal intraerythrocytic mechanisms (metHb reductase enzyme system), it should be measured within 30 minutes of sample collection. The four-wave-length spectrophotometric method based on the work of Evelyn and Malloy (19) is commonly used for metHb measurements. There are species differences in metHb formation (20) that should be considered when evaluating metHb data.

Differential (Cellular Elements)—Peripheral Blood.   Several commonly used automated hematology analyzers are capable of performing a WBC differential specific for various species. These analyzers, if appropriately programmed, are capable of accurate differential counts. This does not, however, preclude the necessity of preparing a well-made thin-film peripheral blood smear for evaluation of the WBC differential if suspicious results are obtained from the automated counts and for cellular morphology of WBCs, RBCs, and platelets. The slides must be made in such a manner as to create the appropriate areas on the slide necessary for evaluation. A monolayer of cells at the feathered edge of the slide is required for cellular morphology assessment. A slightly thicker area is desirable for WBC differential counts and platelet estimates. The slide should look similar to a thumbprint, with the edges of the smear approaching but not touching the edges of the slide. The end of the smear should feather out to a rounded edge.

WBC differential smears should be prepared from room temperature, EDTA-anticoagulated whole blood within 2 hours of sample collection. The specimen should be mixed on a rocker for 5 minutes prior to smear preparation in order to ensure homogeneity. Once prepared, the smear should be allowed to air-dry and then stained with Wright-Giemsa stain for microscopic evaluation. In addition to the WBC differential, WBC, platelet, and erythrocyte morphologic assessment are conducted using this same smear.

The systematic microscopic evaluation of the smear should begin with the high dry objective and then under oil immersion at 50× to evaluate the smear for general impression of numbers of cells and morphology and to locate the monolayer of the smear for the differential count. The 100× objective is then used to perform the differential and morphology assessments. Upon examination, typically, a differential contains five types of mature WBCs: neutrophils, lymphocytes, monocytes, eosinophils, and basophils. Small numbers (<3.0%) of immature WBCs may also be present in the smear. Complete descriptions of various cell type characteristics are found in numerous texts (10,21).

The differential is a count of 100 WBCs. The constituents are reported as a percentage of the 100 cells counted. For interpretation, it is also useful to report results in absolute numbers of individual cell types. Absolute counts are calculated using the following formula:

Absolute count = % cell count (expressed as a decimal) × cWBC

where cWBC=WBC count corrected for the presence of NRBCs (see below).

Occasionally, NRBCs will appear in the smear. When present, these cells must be counted and reported as: number of NRBCs/100 WBCs. If three or more NRBCs are counted per 100 WBCs, the automated WBCF must be corrected and reported to account for the inability of the automated impedance cell counter to distinguish between a NRBC and a WBC. This correction is calculated using the following formula:

$$\text{Corrected WBC} = \frac{\text{Total WBC} \times 100}{100 + \text{Number of NRBC per 100 WBC}}$$

Differential (Cellular Elements)—Bone Marrow. The quality of the bone marrow smear or cytospin preparation is absolutely critical to evaluation. For rodents and rabbits, bone marrow smears should be prepared from femoral marrow. Typically smears are prepared using a size 000 paintbrush moistened with physiologic phosphate-buffered saline. For larger species, imprints of sternal marrow (at necropsy), marrow aspirates and/or core biopsies may be used. If smears are made, ensure that an adequate smear is prepared by making at least two slides from each animal. Care must be taken to avoid exposure of the bone marrow to formalin before, during, and after slide preparation. After the slides are allowed to air-dry, they should be fixed in absolute methanol for 5 minutes and air-dried. The typical stain used for smears is a modified Wright-Giemsa stain. Core biopsies should be processed as other tissues for histopathologic evaluation. Microscopic evaluation of the bone marrow should include characterization of the tissue architecture (difficult to do in smears), differentiation, and counting of cells, and evaluation of individual cell morphology. Bone marrow differential counts should be performed on at least 500 cells and should be reported by cell lineage and stage of maturation. A myeloid/erythroid (M:E) ratio is often calculated from differentiation of 500 or 1000 precursors of the myeloid and erythroid series cells and then dividing the number of myeloid cells by the number of erythroid cells.

Another method of bone marrow assessment utilizes flow cytometry. This method is a better tool for estimating total cellularity than is smear evaluation because in smears only a limited number of cells are evaluated and only semiquantitative morphologic information is obtained. Flow cytometry can assess phenotype and function at the single cell level in a rapid manner. Species-specific monoclonal antibodies may be used to phenotype bone marrow progenitors of the lymphoid, myeloid, and erythroid series, and stem cells. Bone marrow cells can be uniquely identified on a cytogram of fluorescence plotted against forward angle scatter. The maturity and lineage characteristics of these discrete areas can then be determined by electronic gating and evaluation for the presence or absence of antibodies with and without lineage markers.

Regardless of the method of bone marrow evaluation, it is important that interpretation of the bone marrow evaluation results be performed in conjunction with the peripheral blood picture and histopathological evaluation of the hematopoietic organs.

Coagulation/Hemostasis. Evaluation of hemostasis in the toxicology study includes an assessment of both plasma coagulation factors and platelets (22). The prothrombin time (PT) and activated partial thromboplastin time (PTT) assays are utilized to assess the function of the plasma coagulation factors, with the exception of Factor XIII. The thrombin time (TT) assay is utilized to assess the presence of functional fibrinogen. Plasma coagulation reactions are divided into the extrinsic, intrinsic, and common pathways. The extrinsic system involves the reactions of tissue factor and Factor VII that result in the conversion of Factor X to Factor Xa. The intrinsic system is composed of Factors VIII, IX, XI, and XII, prekallikrein, and kininogen. The common pathway includes Factors V, X, and XIII, prothrombin, and fibrinogen. The coagulation cascade begins with the activation of the extrinsic or the intrinsic pathways, both of which, through an interconnected series of enzyme-activating steps, result in the formation of Factor IIa and the conversion of soluble fibrinogen (Factor I) into an insoluble fibrin plug through the common pathway.

Coagulation assays require the use of whole blood collected using trisodium citrate as the anticoagulant. The ratio of anticoagulant to whole blood is critical.

The PT assay is a nonspecific test that measures the functional ability of the extrinsic coagulation system. The PT assay measures plasma clotting time in seconds after the addition of tissue thromboplastin (Factor III) and calcium chloride to the specimen. To ensure accuracy, the assay is performed in duplicate. The difference between the duplicate measurements should not exceed 5%. A prolonged PT is indicative of abnormalities of Factors V, VII or X, prothrombin or fibrinogen. It may also be prolonged due to the presence of an inhibitor.

The activated PTT (APTT) assay is a nonspecific test that measures the functional ability of the intrinsic and common coagulation systems. The assay measures plasma clotting time in seconds after the specimen is incubated with a surface activating agent (Factor VII activator), partial thromboplastin, and calcium chloride. To ensure accuracy, the assay is performed in duplicate. The difference between the duplicated measurements should not exceed 5%. A prolonged PTT may be due to abnormalities of Factors V, VII, IX, X, XI, or XII. It may also be due to the presence of an inhibitor.

The TT assay is a specific test that estimates the quantity of functionally active fibrinogen. The assay measures plasma clotting time in seconds after the specimen is incubated with thrombin and calcium chloride. The assay is performed in duplicate. The difference between the duplicated measurements should not exceed 5%. TT prolongation may be due to reduced functional fibrinogen (dysfibrinogenemia), reduced fibrinogen (hypofibrinogenemia), the presence of fibrinogen degradation products, heparin, and antibody to thrombin or amyloidosis.

Platelets are measured as described previously. Megakaryopoiesis (proliferation and maturation of megakaryocytes, which occurs mostly in the bone marrow) is regulated by the number of circulating platelets under the influence of a cytokine, thrombopoietin (18). Thrombopoietin influences platelet production by stimulating committed stem cells, inducing additional endomitosis in immature megakaryocytes and shortening the megakaryocyte maturation time (23,24). Platelet functions include: (1) adhesion to exposed subendothelium, (2) aggregation in response to activated platelet membrane $\alpha_{IIb}\beta_3$ on neighboring platelets, (3) secretion of preformed fibrinogen, Factor V, adenosine diphosphate (ADP), newly formed thromboxane and arachidonic acid, (4) facilitation/maintenance of coagulation by providing high affinity binding sites for coagulation enzymes and cofactors, and (5) clot retraction using the platelet actin and myosin.

There are numerous specialized in vitro assays for assessment of platelet adhesion, aggregation, and secretion that may be utilized when platelet function abnormalities are suspected. The typical assessment of platelets in a toxicology study includes only the PLT. Thrombocytopenia is defined as a PLT below normal limits established for a specific species. It should be noted that there are significant differences in platelet number, function, and induced changes between species (10,25). In animals, it is reported that petechial or ecchymotic hemorrhage does not occur until the PLT is $<100\times10^9$/liter (26). Thrombocytopenia should be confirmed by a review of the peripheral blood smear. Thrombocytopenia may occur due to increased platelet removal/destruction (i.e., autoimmune thrombocytopenia, disseminated intravascular coagulation, exposure to sulfonamides), platelet sequestration (i.e., splenomegaly, endotoxemia), hemodilution (i.e., following instillation of colloids, plasma or crystalloids) or impaired platelet production due to megakaryocyte injury from pharmaceuticals (i.e., chemotherapeutics), toxicants (i.e., Bracken fern), radiation, viruses, or neoplasia. Thrombocytosis is defined as a PLT above normal limits established for a specific species. Thrombocytosis may occur with myeloproliferative disease (i.e., primary thrombocythemia or acute megakaryocytic leukemia), or it may occur as a secondary reaction to such conditions as inflammation or nonhemic malignant neoplasia.

Clinical Chemistry

The importance of appropriate clinical chemistry assessment in toxicology studies has been recognized for many years. Just as with hematological parameter assessment, in elucidating toxic effects through clinical chemistry analysis, the investigator must be aware of the appropriate methods of blood collection, specimen handling, sampling times, testing selection, QC evaluation, and test result interpretation. In addition, one must be aware of normal animal species physiology and its impact on clinical chemistry parameters when interpreting assay results.

Selection of Parameters

The investigator should consider several points when selecting clinical chemistry parameters for evaluation (27). These items include sample volume requirements, information desired, time points for evaluation, and route of sample collection. A 'routine' clinical chemistry evaluation in toxicity testing is generally used in those studies where clinical chemistry effects are not expected based on the known structure and/or function of the test material. The parameters measured would include those that would assess changes in all major organ systems. For example, a routine panel of assays would include alkaline phosphatase (ALP), alanine aminotransferase (ALT), aspartate aminotransferase (AST), and bilirubin to assess liver damage; creatine kinase (CK) for muscle damage; creatinine (CRT) and blood urea nitrogen (BUN) to assess kidney damage; and sodium, potassium, and chloride to assess the electrolyte status of the animal. If the investigator suspects that a particular test material will cause insult to a specific organ/tissue, the use of more specialized assays may be warranted and would be included in the study protocol.

Specimen Collection and Quality

Specimen collection for clinical chemistry analysis requires the use of serum collection tubes (no anticoagulant) with or without a gel for ease of separation of the serum from the cellular components. Blood collected into serum separator tubes must be allowed to clot at room temperature for 30 minutes to minimize residual fibrin. Tubes are then centrifuged pursuant to conditions specified by the manufacturer of the tube. The serum is then removed and placed into a prelabeled screw-cap polypropylene tube. Serum specimens should be kept cool prior to analysis. If the serum specimen is to be stored or shipped for later analysis, the specimen should be frozen immediately at $< -15°C$ and held for a limited period of time. It should be noted that there are many potentially interfering substances sometimes present in serum, which can have an effect on clinical chemistry analyses. These include, but are not limited to, lipemia, hemolysis, and jaundice.

Common Parameters—Methodology and Interpretation

Enzymes (List Is Not Complete but Represents Most Commonly Used Assays).

Alkaline phosphatase. ALP is composed of several isoenzymes that are present in practically all tissues of the body, especially at or in the cell membranes. These enzymes catalyze the hydrolysis of monophosphate esters and have a wide substrate specificity (28). The actual natural substrates upon which they act in the body are not known. There are specific forms of ALP in liver, bone, intestine, placenta, and kidney; however, the predominant forms present in normal serum are the liver and bone forms. It appears that the enzyme is associated with lipid transport in the intestine and liver and calcification in the bone. The preferred methods for analysis of serum ALP is the adenosine monophosphate-utilizing 4-nitrophenyl phosphate method that measures the 4-nitrophen-oxide ion produced by removal of the phosphate group from 4-nitrophenyl phosphate by ALP.

The three major causes of high serum ALP activity are induction of hepatic ALP (i.e., intrahepatic or posthepatic cholestasis), induction of hepatic ALP release (i.e., iatrogenic corticosteroids, phenobarbital, hyperadrenocorticism), and increased osteo-blastic activity (i.e., osterosarcoma, fractures). In addition, normal young growing animals have serum ALP activities up to 3 times higher than those in normal mature animals (10). Hepatic ALP production is induced by increased intracanalicular hydrostatic pressure. It is a microsomal membrane-bound enzyme that does not leak during altered hepatocellular permeability. It is the most sensitive indicator of cholestasis and will be high prior to increases in total bilirubin. The magnitude of the ALP increases observed due to other causes will not be as great as that produced by cholestasis. Exposure to numerous chemicals/pharmaceuticals (i.e., acetaminophen, allopurinol, antifungal agents, halothane, clofibrate) is also reported to cause increases in ALP (29).

Aminotransferases. The aminotransferases, including ALT, and AST, are indicators of hepatocyte damage (30). These enzymes are present in hepatocyte cytosol, and during episodes of altered plasma membrane permeability, they leak into the extracellular fluid. ALT is an enzyme that catalyzes the transfer of an amino group from alanine to oxoglutarate to produce glutamate. AST catalyzes the transfer of an amino group from aspartate to oxoglutarate to form L-glutamate. The preferred methods for analysis of serum ALT and AST are the International Federation of Clinical Chemistry reference methods.

In laboratory animal species, ALT is specific for liver damage or disease, whereas AST is found in liver and muscle tissue. As described above, these enzymes leak out of the hepatocyte cytosol when the plasma membrane permeability is altered. Leakage occurs due to the high concentration gradient between the intra- and extracellular compartments. In general, the magnitude of ALT increases in liver damage or disease is greater than that of AST. This is due, in part, to the presence of some AST in hepatocyte mitochondria that are less likely to leak. Additionally, elevations of ALT activity persist longer than do those of AST (the plasma half-life of both is approximately 2 to 4 days). The cause of hepatic enzyme leakage is increased plasma membrane permeability, which may result from a reduced oxygen supply to the liver, direct effects of toxins, pharmaceuticals or chemicals, inflammation, and/or fatty change. Although the magnitude of the increase of ALT/AST is directly proportional to the number of hepatocytes affected (28), it is not related to the reversibility/irreversibility of the change. This is also true of increased AST as a result of muscle damage or disease (i.e., myocardial infarction).

Creatine kinase. CK catalyzes the reversible phosphorylation of creatine by adenosine triphosphate (ATP). When muscle contracts, ATP is used (forming ADP), and CK catalyzes the rephosphorylation of ADP (forming ATP) using creatine phosphate, the major phosphorylated compound in muscle as the phosphorylation reservoir (31). Three isoenzymes of CK have been described: MM, which is found in skeletal and cardiac muscle; MB, which is also found in skeletal and cardiac muscle; and BB, which is found primarily in the brain but is also present in the prostate, gut, lung, urinary bladder, uterus, placenta, and thyroid gland. All of these are found in the cytosol or associated with myofibrillar structures. The preferred method for analysis of serum CK is the enzymatic N-acetyl cysteine (NAC) method as recommended by the Scandinavian Society of Clinical Chemistry and Clinical Physiology and optimized by Szasz et al. (32).

CK is a leakage enzyme and increased serum values occur with reversible and irreversible damage. CK values increase within hours of muscle injury and reach maximum values by approximately 12 hours postinjury. CK has a relatively short half-life in serum and will return to normal levels at 24 hours to 48 hours after muscle damage from a single insult occurs. Therefore, high serum CK values are indicative of active or recent muscle injury or damage (including rigorous exercise).

Lactate dehydrogenase. Lactate dehydrogenase (LDH) is a hydrogen transfer enzyme that is found in the cytoplasm of most of the cells of the body. Tissue levels of LDH are approximately 500 times greater than normal serum levels, so leakage from a small number of cells can result in significant increases in the serum values of LDH. The peak of the increase in serum LDH values is usually observed within 48 hours to 72 hours after the insult. Causes of increased serum LDH include muscle damage or necrosis, hemolysis, liver disease, renal tubular necrosis, pyelonephritis, and malignant neoplasia.

Bilirubin. Total bilirubin is derived primarily from the heme moiety of the HGB released from senescent erythrocytes destroyed in the reticuloendothelial cells of the liver, spleen, and bone marrow. It is produced in peripheral tissues from protoporphyrin IX by microsomal heme oxygenase, transported to the liver in association with albumin, and transported across the sinusoidal membrane by carrier-mediated active transport. In the hepatocyte cytosol, bilirubin is bound primarily to ligandin and Z protein and rapidly conjugated with glucuronic acid to produce bilirubin mono- and diglucruonide, which are excreted into bile via an energy-dependent, active-transport process. The preferred method for analysis of serum bilirubin is the Jendrassik-Grof method, which measures the azobilirubin solution formed by the reaction of total bilirubin with a caffeine reagent followed by the addition of diazotized sufanilic acid.

Increases in serum total bilirubin may be due to increased HGB destruction (i.e., hemolytic hyperbilirubinemia) or liver damage (i.e., obstructive hyperbilirubinemia). Increased serum total bilirubin is an early indicator of cholestasis. Hyperbilirubinuria (only conjugated bilirubin is found in the urine) is often observed prior to increases in serum total bilirubin. Typically, increased total bilirubinemia is accompanied by increased ALP (10).

Creatinine. CRT is derived from the nonenzymatic, spontaneous conversion of free creatine in the muscle. Approximately 1% to 2% of muscle creatine is converted to CRT daily (33), and the amount of endogenous CRT produced is proportional to muscle mass. The excretion rate is also constant and parallels production. The preferred method for analysis of serum CRT is the Jaffe reaction, which measure the red-orange adduct formed during the reaction between CRT and the picrate ion in alkaline media. There are several noncreatinine Jaffe-reacting chromogens [i.e., protein, glucose, guanidine, acetone (34)], however, that may slightly increase the measurements using this method. The definitive method for CRT in serum utilizes isotope-dilution mass spectrometry (35).

CRT can provide similar information to BUN in renal disease or postrenal obstruction or leakage. It is freely filtered through the glomerulus; however, small amounts are reabsorbed by the renal tubules as well as secreted by the proximal tubules. Increased serum CRT levels occur when glomerular filtration is decreased. CRT levels are also increase by reduced renal perfusion. CRT clearance may also be measured and is considered to be an accurate index of glomerular filtration rate.

Electrolytes. The major electrolytes (sodium, potassium, chloride) are primarily free charged ions that have diverse roles in the body, including, but not limited to, the following: maintenance of osmotic pressure and waster distribution, maintenance of pH, regulation of muscle contraction, involvement in oxidation/reduction reactions, and serving as enzyme cofactors. Analysis for the presence and quantity of these electrolytes uses ion-selective electrodes that are highly selective and accurate. Electrolyte gain or loss can occur in the gastrointestinal tract (dietary intake, loss of saliva, gut stasis, diarrhea, vomiting), kidney (lack of antidiuretic hormone, excess or lack of aldosterone, tubular disease), lung (hyperventilation, febrile episodes), and skin (sweat, febrile episodes).

Sodium. Sodium is the major cation of extracellular fluid and is central in the maintenance of water distribution and osmotic pressure. Serum sodium is an indicator of total body sodium if the animal is appropriately hydrated. Common causes of hyponatremia include prolonged vomiting, persistent diarrhea, salt-losing enteropathies, glycosuria (solute diuresis), diminished tubular reabsorption, aldosterone deficiency, severe polyuria, metabolic acidosis, and severe edema and ascites. Hypernatremia occurs with excessive loss of sodium-poor body fluids, such as with profuse sweating, prolonged hyperpnea, vomiting diarrhea, polyuria, decreased antidiuretic hormone, hyperadrenocorticism, and brain injury. Hypernatremia in association with hypokalemia and hypercalcemia may be seen in hepatic disease, cardiac failure, burns, and osmotic diuresis (36).

Potassium. Potassium is the major intracellular cation and is the critical ion in maintaining ionic gradients for neural impulse transmission. Because approximately 90% of serum potassium is intracellular, serum potassium concentration is not an indicator of total body potassium. Serum potassium abnormalities are commonly a result of acid-base imbalances and have serious consequences, such as muscle weakness or paralysis and cardiac conduction abnormalities leading to cardiac arrest. Hypokalemia can result from decreased intake, redistribution of extracellular potassium into intracellular fluid (as seen with alkalosis or acidosis), and increased loss of potassium-rich fluids (i.e., renal tubular acidosis, vomiting, diarrhea). Causes of hyperkalemia include redistribution of potassium into extracellular fluid (i.e., massive tissue necrosis, dehydration, acidosis, hemolysis, leukocytosis, thrombocytosis) and decreased excretion (i.e., acute renal failure, renal tubular acidosis, adrenocortical insufficiency).

Chloride. Chloride is the major extracellular anion and is regulated passively by gradients derived from active sodium transport across cell membranes. Like sodium, chloride is involved in water distribution, osmotic pressure, and anion-cation balance in the extracellular fluid compartment. The serum chloride concentration is directly proportional to the sodium concentration. Hypochloremia is primarily seen with chronic pyelonephritis, metabolic acidosis, persistent gastric secretion, and prolonged vomiting. Dehydration, renal tubular acidosis, and metabolic acidosis with prolonged diarrhea result in hyperchloremia.

Glucose.   The serum concentration of glucose is regulated by a complex interaction of hormones, such as glucagon, insulin, cortisol, and epinephrine. Glucose should ideally be measured in a fasting animal. The causes of increased serum glucose concentrations include postprandial blood collection, diabetes mellitus, hyperadrenocorticism, moribundity, exogenous glucocorticoids, and morphine. Decreased serum glucose concentrations can result from ethanol ingestion, liver failure, and deficiency of growth hormone, glucocorticoids, and glucagon. Severe and possibly irreversible central nervous system dysfunction can result from hypoglycemia. Clinical signs of hypoglycemia include confusion, lethargy, ataxia, and seizure, which may progress to loss of consciousness and death.

Proteins.   The body contains a multitude of different proteins, of which approximately three hundred can be identified in the plasma alone (37). With the exception of the protein hormones and immunoglobulins, the majority of the plasma proteins are synthesized in the liver. They are constantly undergoing catabolism, primarily in the liver, and replacement with each plasma protein having its own specific turnover rate. The different functions of proteins are as numerous as the proteins themselves. These functions include serving as complement factors, coagulation factors, anions in acid-base balance, and carriers for vitamins, hormones, fats, free HGB, and unconjugated bilirubin. Commonly, serum total protein and albumin are measured. Albumin is the most abundant protein in plasma and is the major determinant of plasma oncotic pressure. Normally, serum total protein concentration is in direct proportion to the serum albumin concentration. Although hyperalbuminemia is only seen in dehydration, hypergammaglobulinemia, and hyperfibrinogenemia, hypoalbuminemia (and hyproteinemia) are common in many diseases states and may result form impaired synthesis (liver disease), increased catabolism (tissue damage), reduced absorption (malnutrition), protein loss (glomerulonephritis, protein-losing enteropathy, burned skin) or altered distribution (ascites). The preferred method for analysis of serum total protein is the biuret reaction method, which measures the amount of a colored product that is formed from the reaction of peptide bonds of proteins with copper (II) (Cu[II]) ions in alkaline solution. The preferred method for analysis of serum albumin, in all species except rabbits, is the bromocresol green-albumin complex after allowing albumin and bromocresol green to bind at pH 4.2. The preferred method for analysis of serum albumin in rabbits is the bromocresol purple method, which measures the bromocresol purple-albumin complex after allowing albumin and bromocresol purple to bind at pH 5.2 with acetate.

Urea.   Urea, the major nitrogen-containing metabolic product of protein catabolism, is synthesized in the liver from aminonitrogen-derived ammonia. A small amount of urea is also absorbed from the large intestine. Urea is found throughout the total body water compartment due to passive diffusion, and renal excretion is the most important route of excretion. It is removed in the glomerulus by simple filtration and is found in the same concentration in the glomerular filtrate as in the blood. Based on the rate of urine flow (directly proportional), urea will passively diffuse with water from the tubular lumen back into the blood. The preferred method for analysis of urea nitrogen in the serum (BUN) is the urease with glutamate dehydrogenase (coupled-enzyme system) method, which measures the decreased in absorbance resulting form the glutamate dehydrogenase reaction.

Assessment of increases in BUN are categorized as prerenal azotemia, renal azotemia, and postrenal azotemia. Prerenal azotemia is an increase in BUN concentration due to increased protein catabolism (i.e., tissue damage, febrile episodes) or decreased renal perfusion (i.e., dehydration, shock, cardiovascular compromise). A high BUN with a normal serum CRT level is indicative of prerenal azotemia. Renal azotemia results when approximately 75% of the nephrons are nonfunctional. Both serum CRT and BUN are increased similarly in renal azotemia. Obstruction to urinary outflow results in postrenal azotemia. Serum CRT and BUN are increased with postrenal azotemia; however, there is a disproportionately greater increase in the BUN level as compared with the CRT level (10,27,28).

Urinalysis

Urinalysis should be performed in any toxicology studies when the test material is suspected to be a renal toxicant. Although urinalysis techniques utilized in toxicity testing, particularly in rodents, are relatively primitive and the reliability of the results corresponds with the methods employed, the results (interpreted along with histopathology results) can be effective in determining whether the kidney is functioning properly or if it is being overwhelmed beyond its capacity. In general, however, five animals per sex per group may not provide the consistency necessary to characterize changes successfully.

Selection of Parameters

As a minimum, the general appearance, specific gravity, acidity, protein, glucose, ketones, bilirubin, urobilinogen, and cellular content/morphology (microscopic) should be determined. In general, the protein, glucose, ketones, bilirubin, and urobilinogen are determined qualitatively using reagent strips. For more specific measurements, clinical chemistry analysis can be performed on urine to quantitate analytes, such as total protein, glucose, bilirubin, and urobilinogen.

Specimen Collection and Quality

The collection techniques employed in most toxicological studies are primitive. Urine is generally collected in metabolism cages that collect the urine in a container below the cage. For the best results, the collection container is surrounded by a wet ice bath. Typically, for rodents, urine is collected over a 12-hour period. The urine is evaluated for total volume, color, cloudiness, pH, and specific gravity immediately after the collection period.

Common Parameters—Methodology and Interpretation

Ketones. The ketones measured in the urine qualitatively usually include acetone and acetoacetate. Increased ketones in the urine may be due to diabetes mellitus, prolonged fasting, persistent vomiting or very low carbohydrate diets.

Glucose. Increased glucose in the urine may be due to diabetes mellitus, major trauma, exogenous steroids, infection or pheochromocytoma (adrenal gland tumor).

pH. Values of urinary pH will not reflect the normal physiological situation because the dissolved CO_2 dissipates during the collection period, which results in an elevated pH. Unless the pH is outside the range of 6.0 to 7.0, changes are most likely incidental to the collection technique.

Specific Gravity. Hair, dander, excrement, and dust, which are common contaminants in metabolism cage-collected urine samples, will falsely elevate the specific gravity. This is a crude measurement of the concentrating ability of the kidney (osmolality) and may be altered in some types of nephrotoxicity.

Microscopic Evaluation. Microscopic evaluation of the urine sediment allows for the detection of epithelial cells, bacteria, casts, RBCs, WBCs, and crystals. It should be remembered that some bacteria will grow in the urine during the collection period. Casts in the sediment are indicative or renal tubular damage. Crystals are often precursors to renal and/or urinary bladder stones. RBCs are typically seen in conjunction with urinary bladder or urethral mucosal damage. The presence of WBCs is indicative of infectious changes in the kidney, urinary bladder, ureter, and/or urethra.

Quality Control

To ensure the reliability of the data generated, it is important for the clinical laboratory to participate in an interlaboratory comparison program, such as the College of American Pathologists (CAP) Interlaboratory Comparison Program for Proficiency Testing, for all assays performed in the laboratory. In addition, the laboratory may subscribe to the CAP Quality Assurance Service (QAS). QC data generated in the clinical laboratory are transferred monthly, via modem, to the service for evaluation against the previous monthly data and for comparison with other laboratories. This service allows the clinical laboratory to ensure that the QC data generated by the laboratory are accurate and conform to the data generated by other participating laboratories. The CAPQAS provides participants with a computer software package that allows them to maintain QC records on computer for quick and accurate evaluation using the Westgard rules and for transmission of data directly to CAP. The clinical laboratory may participate in hematology, clinical microscopy (urinalysis), and clinical chemistry surveys with a minimum of two specimens per interval for "regulated" analytes. Successful participation in these surveys is required by law for medical clinical laboratories under the Clinical Laboratory Improvement Amendments guidelines (42 CFR 493).

To ensure the highest quality results, a veterinary clinical pathologist should review data at the end of each day and prior to discarding or freezing any unused samples. Any questionable results should be dealt with at that time. In all cases, documentation of rejection and repeated sample runs must be made along with the possible source of variation and any corrective action taken.

The clinical laboratory must have written QC procedures that are followed. A subset of the Westgard rules are typically used as criteria for acceptance or rejection of the test data. The initial rule selected for use is the 1:2S-"warning" rule, a violation of which should trigger a close inspection of the control data. The following rules are commonly selected to determine rejection or acceptance of the run: 1:3S, 2:2S, and R:4S. When three levels of control are used (hematology) the following rules are used:

1:2S—One point falls outside 2 standard deviations (SD) (Warning Rule)
1:3S—One point falls outside 3SD
2:2S—Two consecutive points for the same control value fall outside 2SD
R:4S—In one run, one control value exceeds the mean +2SD and another control value exceeds the mean—2SD.

When two levels of control are used, as with many chemistry analyzers, all points must be within 2SD for acceptance. These parameters have 'target' values assigned for the specific analyzer using specific reagents.

Specific to hematology analyses, assayed control material must be analyzed prior to use, and the mean and standard deviation will be calculated by the instrument microprocessor. The QC material should be analyzed prior to, during, and after each automated hematology experimental run. Normal and abnormal controls should be used to determine the precision, accuracy, and reproducibility of the eight parameters measured by the instrument. Hematology QC data may be stored in most instruments and printed monthly. Upon receipt of new lot numbers of control materials, the previous month's data must be printed for archiving purposes and deleted from the instrument. For clinical chemistry analyses, assayed normal, and abnormal QC materials must be included at the beginning and end of each clinical chemistry experimental test run. All control materials should be assayed prior to use, and the mean and standard deviation calculated for each level.

Equipment maintenance records (scheduled and unscheduled), calibration records, and cumulative QC data must be maintained for all laboratory equipment.

MORPHOLOGIC PATHOLOGY

In toxicology studies, clinical pathology is accompanied by gross and microscopic pathology at study termination. Together, these endpoints are used in not only identifying organ or tissue injury but also in evaluating their biologic, and toxicologic significance. Assessment of altered gross and cellular morphology depends on the ability of the pathologist to discriminate between test material-induced changes, secondary changes, changes associated with methodology of specimen preparation, spontaneous disease, postmortem changes, iatrogenic changes, and normal physiologic variations.

Collection Methodology for Routine and Special Histology

The selection of tissues for collection and histopathological evaluation should be made in accordance with appropriate regulatory guidelines. A general tissue list is found in Table 2.

Necropsy Techniques

Good necropsy techniques are critical to the histopathological evaluation process. At necropsy, specific attention is placed on the following items: (1) animal identification, (2) tissue accountability, (3) lesion recognition and accountability, (4) accurate recording of gross findings/appropriate descriptions and required entries on the individual animal necropsy form, (5) proper gross trimming of the wet tissues and tissue fixation, and (6) weighing each protocol-specified tissue. The necropsy must be performed by necropsy prosectors trained and proficient in the necropsy procedure, lesion recognition, and documentation of findings. Ideally, the pathologist will systematically examine each tissue prior to placing it in the fixative container. This enables the pathologist to ensure maximum accountability of tissues, to verify all gross findings noted by the prosector and to identify any additional changes that the pathologist deems significant.

Scheduled necropsies for routine histopathology should be initiated within 5 minutes after the animal is euthanized. All tissues and organs are examined in situ,

Table 2   General Tissue Collection List

Adrenal glands	Peripheral nerve (i.e., sciatic nerve)
Aorta	Pituitary gland
Bone (sternum and femur)	Prostate (ventral and dorsal)
Bone marrow	Rectum
Brain	Representative lymph nodes (i.e., mandibular, mesenteric)
Cecum	Salivary glands
Colon	Seminal vesicles
Duodenum	Skeletal muscle
Esophagus	Skin
Eyes with optic nerve	Spinal cord (cervical, thoracic, lumbar)
Gallbladder (if applicable)	Spleen
Heart	Stomach (glandular and nonglandular)
Harderian glands	Testes
Ileum	Thymus
Jejunum	Thyroid glands/parathyroid glands
Kidneys	Trachea
Lungs w/mainstem bronchi	Urinary bladder
Mammary glands	Uterus
Nasal mucosa	Vagina
Ovaries	Gross lesions
Pancreas	

dissected from the carcass, reexamined, including cut surfaces, and fixed in 10% neutral buffered formalin or other appropriate fixative. All tissues and organs specified in the protocol are saved and fixed in their entirety. Tissues saved for histopathology should be fixed at a thickness not to exceed 0.5 cm. The animal identification (i.e., tail tattoo, ear tag) should also be saved in the formalin jar with the wet tissues. The trachea and lungs should be perfused by introducing 10% neutral buffered formalin (approximately 4–8 mL for rats) into the trachea until the lungs are completely filled to normal inspiratory volume. The kidneys should be sliced so that the cut surfaces can be examined. Typically the left kidney is sliced longitudinally, and the right kidney is sliced transversely (slightly off-center to preserve quality sections for histopathology). This also ensures identification of right versus left kidneys throughout processing and evaluation. The entire gastrointestinal tract, including the stomach, should be perfused with 10% neutral buffered formalin to fix the mucosal surface quickly.

Fixatives and Fixation

Proper fixation of tissues is another critical aspect of necropsy that is often overlooked. Utilization of inadequate amounts of fixative and inappropriate tissue handling are the most common mistakes made during routine rodent necropsy. When using formalin fixation, it is recommended that at least a 10:1 formalin to tissue ratio be used. Sections from solid tissues, such as liver and spleen, should not exceed 0.5 cm in order to assure complete fixation. Special fixatives are recommended for certain tissues, such as Davidson's fixative for the eyes, freshly made 4% paraformaldehyde for testes, and Bouin's fixative for ovaries. If fresh frozen sections are needed for immunostaining, they may be prepared at 3-mm thickness and placed face down in a cryomold with O.C.T. embedding medium completely encasing it. Once the mold is removed from the embedding ring, the rings should be carefully wrapped, preferably with parafilm and aluminum foil. Careful wrapping prevents desiccation of the specimens during storage at $-80°C$, and they can be maintained in this manner for months without degradation of enzyme activity. Fixation procedures of tissues for electron microscopy are varied and critical to the quality of the image produced (38).

Histology Techniques

There are numerous texts that provide extensive information on histological and histochemical techniques (39–44). Wet tissues are trimmed according to specific protocol guidelines and established histology laboratory SOPs. An excellent guide for tissue trimming and orientation is found in the "Registry of Industrial Toxicology Animal Guides for Organ Sampling and Trimming Procedures in Rats" (45).

Gross lesions or abnormal tissue changes recorded on the necropsy section of the individual animal necropsy form are verified during trimming. Any additional lesions or abnormalities found during trimming are recorded in the necropsy observation section, noting that it was found at trimming, and processed accordingly. Tissues should be trimmed at a maximum thickness of 0.4 cm for processing. The trimmed specimens are placed in cassettes prelabeled with the study number, group number, animal number, and block number. Any residual tissue remaining after tissue trimming should be wrapped in gauze, and double-bagged in labeled, sealed polyethylene bags containing a sufficient amount of fixative to keep the tissues moist.

For paraffin-embedded tissues, fully automated tissue processing units are commonly used in histology laboratories. The processing schedule should be specific for the species and type of tissue. Paraffin temperatures, reagent rotation/changes, study number, number of cassettes, processor identification, processing technician, and date should be documented for each processing run. Prior to activation of the processor, the maintenance schedule program, paraffin temperatures, and reagent rotation/change documentation should be checked for completeness and accuracy. Processed tissues are embedded according to specific protocol guidelines and established histology laboratory SOPs. The embedding scheme should take tissue size and consistency into consideration, and the tissues should be assigned to the blocks to maximize tissue recovery for subsequent microscopic evaluation.

After the tissues are embedded in paraffin, tissue sections are routinely cut at 4 microns to 6 microns. The slides should be labeled with the study number, group number, animal number, special stain (if applicable), and slide number using an indelible marker or, if available, automated slide etching. After the slides are dried, they are placed in staining racks and typically stained with hematoxylin and eosin (H&E). Reagents and staining solutions used during staining should be rotated and changed on a regular schedule. Stained slides are coverslipped with an appropriate size coverslip and placed on slide trays for drying and labeling. If the slides were originally labeled with marker, they should at this point be labeled with a computer-generated label. After the slides are dried and labeled, they are evaluated by a QC histology technician for slide quality (i.e., air bubbles, knife marks in tissue). In addition, the technician should also perform a random 'slide-block' match to ensure accuracy.

Another option for embedding tissues is embedding in such plastics as 2-hydroxyethylmethacrylate (GMA). Plastic embedding has some advantages over paraffin processing, such as less shrinkage of tissues, because no clearing agent or heat is required. During polymerization, GMA does not react with any tissue group of importance in staining, so GMA sections bind stain similarly to paraffin sections. Cellular morphology and tissue relationships are better preserved in GMA sections making this a better choice for critical evaluation of tissues, such as the testes and neural tissues. Sections can also be cut at 1 micron to 2 microns, which is much thinner than sections available from paraffin blocks. One of the most significant advantages of GMA over other epoxy methods is the water solubility of its monomer and the hydrophilic property of its polymer. The disadvantages of GMA techniques are cost of the reagents (higher than paraffin embedding) and the range of special stains that can be used (less that paraffin sections).

Microscopic Evaluation by Light Microscopy

Despite advances in many areas of molecular science, altered cellular morphology remains the hallmark of toxicity. Histopathology is a descriptive and interpretive science, and there are many variables affecting the complex two-dimensional images that are evaluated by the pathologist. Microscopic evaluation of tissues for toxicological changes takes into account both the recognition of tissue changes and the biological significance of those changes. Assessment of altered gross and cellular morphology depends on the ability of the pathologist to discriminate between test material-induced changes, secondary changes, spontaneous disease, postmortem changes, iatrogenic changes, and normal physiologic variations. In addition, the pathologist must employ a consistent descriptive "dictionary" when describing these changes. This allows the identified changes to be tabulated, categorized, and quantitated. Thus, a relationship between test material exposure and a biologic change can be revealed and evaluated. The recognition and appropriate classification of relevant changes is the science of histopathology. It is the study pathologist that must also associate altered structure with the possibility of altered function. Many texts are available for further reading on the interpretation of microscopic tissue changes (46–49). In addition, pathology peer reviews are commonly performed for many toxicology and carcinogenicity studies. The purpose of the pathology peer review is to ensure consistency and accuracy of the pathology findings and interpretation by reaching consensus between the study pathologist and either an internal or external reviewing pathologist with regard to microscopic changes in the tissues.

Special Techniques

Although standard histopathology procedures are the backbone of the accurate assessment of tissue change, the development, and application of a wide variety of special techniques have greatly advanced the pathologist's ability to ascertain mechanistic data as part of the overall tissue response evaluation.

One such technique provides information on the proliferation of cells within a tissue. This technique can either use 5-bromo-2$'$-deoxyuridine (BrDU) to label cells in S phase or monoclonal antibodies to proteins involved in cell division [i.e., proliferating cell nuclear antigen (PCNA)]. BrDU is the most commonly used label in cell proliferation studies (50,51). It is incorporated into the DNA of cells undergoing replicative DNA synthesis and then revealed at the cellular level using immunostaining. BrDU immunostaining is fairly robust with successful staining using various combinations of different fixatives, embedding mixtures, and section thicknesses. Immunostaining for PCNA is capable of identifying proliferating cells in vitro as well as in alcohol-fixed or formalin-fixed, paraffin-embedded tissue. PCNA is a highly conserved protein expressed during the late G_1/S phases of the cell cycle (52). The advantages of PCNA immunostaining over BrDU staining are the lack of a need for prior administration of a DNA precursor label to the animal and the ability to stain archival formalin-fixed, paraffin-embedded material. BrDU staining is considered to be more sensitive since all cells that have replicated during the

BrDU exposure period are evident. PCNA staining gives a snapshot of the replicating cells at a given moment in time.

Another powerful tool available to pathologists is morphometrics (53,54). Morphometrics is the measurement of appearance/biological shape and uses the application of superimposition algorithms to coordinate data collected at anatomical landmarks. Geometric morphometric methods can be applied to two- and three-dimensional coordinate data sets and have relevance to applications in medical imaging, microscopic evaluation, and other studies of biological shape. The technical aspects of morphometry can be complex and involve computer-based acquisition of images, editing and analysis of the collected images, and production of high quality hardcopy and film-based output. In addition, morphometrics can provide quantitative measurements that can be used to support interpretation of the more subjective findings from routine microscopic evaluation.

Confocal laser scanning microscopy (CLSM) is a relatively new generation of instruments for microscopic examination that utilizes advances in computer technology and the sensitivity of optical imaging devices (55–59). CLSM utilizes a gas laser, conventional microscope, confocal optics, extremely sensitive light sensors, and state-of-the-art computer hardware and software to produce crisp images of thick specimens at various depths. Therefore, by moving the focal plane of the instrument step by step through the depth of the specimen, a series of optical sections can be recorded (60). As a valuable by-product, the computer-controlled CLSM produces digital images that are amenable to image analysis and processing (i.e., particle counting, measurements, and pixel intensity analysis) and that can also be used to compute surface- or volume-rendered 3-D reconstructions of the specimen.

Routine Immunohistochemistry

Immunohistochemical methods utilize the specificity of antibodies as diagnostic reagents for the direct visualization of a variety of cell- and tissue-bound antigens, including enzymes, oncodevelopmental antigens, tissue-specific proteins, immunoglobulins, polypeptide and steroid hormones, bacterial and viral antigens, and the unique biochemistry of the 10-nm intermediate filaments specific for general cell categories and tumor types. These highly specific methods allow the pathologist to take into consideration the function, secretion, and physiology of a cell in determining the tumor cell type (61).

Of the different immunohistochemical methods, immunoperoxidase has developed into the most commonly used technique. The most sensitive immunoperoxidase procedure for localizing a variety of histologically significant antigens and other markers employs primary antibody, biotinylated secondary antibody, and a preformed avidin-biotinylated horseradish peroxidase complex. It has been termed the ABC technique. Uses of the ABC technique include, but are not limited to:

- Measurement of antigen concentration on a single cell
- Amplification of antibody titers
- Radio-, enzyme, and fluorescent immunoassays
- Coupling of antibodies and antigens to agarose
- Immunohistochemical staining
- Multiple labels in tissues
- Purification of cell surface antigens
- Localization of hormone binding sites

- Examination of membrane vesicle orientation
- Cytofluorometric separation of cells
- Nitrocellulose and nylon transfer blot detection
- In-situ hybridization and blot techniques with biotinylated nucleotides
- Genetic mapping
- Hybridoma screening

Electron Microscopy

The electron microscope (EM) is a tool utilized to extend the information gained through light microscopy (62). It can provide unique and valuable information, suggesting actual mechanisms of toxicity in local tissue and intracellular sites. There are two basic types of EM, Scanning EM (SEM) and Transmission EM (TEM). In SEM, the specimen is scanned with a focused beam of electrons that produce "secondary" electrons as the beam hits the specimen. These are detected and converted into an image on a computer screen, and a three-dimensional image of the surface of the specimen is produced. The SEM allows a greater depth of focus than the optical microscope. For this reason the SEM can produce an image that is a good representation of the three-dimensional sample. In TEM, specimens are examined by passing the electron beam through them, revealing more information of the internal structure of specimens. The image produced is a two-dimensional representation.

It is generally accepted that EM should not be performed in routine toxicology studies unless there are specific reasons to suspect the presence of significant ultrastructural abnormalities. The electron microscopist should have some knowledge of the light microscopic pathology in general and, specifically, should know the histopathological findings in each sample being evaluated. Light and ultrastructural abnormalities are usually present in a graded continuum. In a toxicology study setting, significant ultrastructural pathology is only rarely seen in a tissue or organ in the absence of some type of corresponding light microscopic change. There are two basic reasons for performing EM in association with a toxicology study. The first is to characterize or to confirm the nature of a given lesion as observed by light microscopy. Second in the absence of light microscopic findings in a study where changes were predicted, EM can support the conclusion of the absence of changes within a tissue.

REFERENCES

1. Adams RJ. Techniques of experimentation—blood collection. In: Fox JG, Anderson LC, Loew FM, Quimby FW, eds. Laboratory Animal Medicine. 2nd ed. Philadelphia, Pennsylvania: Elsevier, 2002:1008–1013.
2. Hrapkiewicz K, Medina L, Holmes DD, eds. Clinical Laboratory Medicine. In: an introduction. Ames, Iowa: Iowa State Press, 1998.
3. Walter GL. Effects of carbon dioxide inhalation on hematology, coagulation, and serum clinical chemistry values in rats. Toxicol Pathol 1999; 27:217.
4. Payne BJ, Lewis HB, Murchison TE, et al. Hematology of laboratory animals. In: Melby EC, Jr., Altman NH, eds. Handbook of Laboratory Animal Science. Boca Raton, Florida: CRC Press, 1976:382–461.
5. Bickhardt K, Buttner D, Muschen U, et al. Influence of bleeding procedures and some experimental conditions on stress-dependent blood constituents of laboratory rats. Lab Anim 1983; 17:61–165.

6. Report of the AVMA Panel on Euthanasia, J Am Vet Med Assoc, 2001; 218:669–696.

7. Coulter WH. High speed automatic blood cell counter and cell size analyzer. Proc Natl Elect Conf 1956; 12:1034.

8. Sellers TS, Bloom JC. Hematologic evaluation of laboratory animals. Lab Anim 1982; 11:43–51.

9. Sanderson JH, Phillips CE. An Atlas of Laboratory Animal Haematology. Oxford, England: Clarendon Press, 1981.

10. Stockham SL, Scott MA. Fundamentals of Veterinary Clinical Pathology. Ames, Iowa: Iowa State Press, 2002.

11. Hardy RM. Hypoadrenal gland disease. In: Ettinger SJ, Feldman EC, eds. Textbook of Veterinary Internal Medicine. Philadelphia, Pennsylvania: Saunders, 1995:1584.

12. Zawidzka ZZ. Hematology evaluation. In: Arnodl DL, ed. Handbook of In vivo Toxicity Testing. San Diego, California: Academic Press, 1990:463–508.

13. Klee GG. Performance goals for internal quality control of multichanneled hematology analyzers. Clin Lab Haematol 1990; 1:65.

14. Dumoulin-Lagrange M, Capelle C. Evaluation of automated platelet counters for the enumeration and sizing of platelets in the diagnosis and management of hemostatic problems. Semin Thromb Hemost 1983; 9:235–244.

15. Bessman JD, Williams LF, Gilmer PR. Mean platelet volume: the inverse relation of platelet size and count in normal subjects and an artifact of other particles. Am J Clin Pathol 1981; 76:289.

16. Corash L. Platelet sizing: Techniques, biological significance, and clinical applications, Curr. Top Hematol 1983; 4:99–122.

17. Prost-Dvojakovic RJ. Study of platelet volumes and diameter in 11 mammals. In: Ulutin ON, ed. Platelets: Recent Advances in Basic Research and Clinical Aspects. New York: American Elsevier, 1975:30.

18. Thompson CB. Size dependent platelet subpopulations: Relationship of platelet volume to ultrastructure enzyme activity and function. Br J Haematol 1982; 50:509.

19. Evelyn KA, Malloy HT. Micro-determination of oxyhemoglobin, methemoglobin and sulfhemoglobin in a single sample of blood. J Biol Chem 1938; 126:655.

20. Clark DA, de la Garza M. Species differences in methemoglobin levels produced by administration of monomethylhydrazine. Proc Soc Exp Biol Med 1967; 125:912–916.

21. Jain N. 4th ed. Schalm's Veterinary Hematology. Philadelphia, Pennsylvania: Lea and Fibiger, 1986.

22. Kurata M, Hurii I. Blood coagulation tests in toxicological studies—review of methods and their significance for drug safety assessment. J Toxicol Sci 2004; 29:13–32.

23. McDonald TP. Array and site of production of thrombopoietin. Br J Haematol 1981; 49:493.

24. Odell TT. Megakaryopoiesis and its response to stimulated suppression. In: Baldini MG, Effe S, eds. Platelets: Production, Function, Transfusion, and Storage. New York: Grune and Stratton, 1974:11–20.

25. Dodds WJ. Platelet function in animals: species specificities. In: DeGaetano G, Garattini S, eds. Platelets: A Multidisciplinary Approach. New York: Raven, 1978:45–59.

26. Dodds WJ, Blood coagulation: hemostasis and thrombosis. In: Melby EC, Jr., Altman NH, eds. Handbook of Laboratory Animal Science, Boca Raton, Florida: CRC Press, 1974; 2:85–116.

27. Loeb WF, Quimby FW, eds. The Clinical Chemistry of Laboratory Animals. 2nd ed. Philadelphia, Pennsylvania: Taylor & Francis, 1999.

28. Latimer KS, Prasse KW, Mahaffey EA, Duncan KW, eds. Prasse's Veterinary Laboratory Medicine-Clinical Pathology. 4th ed. Ames Iowa: Blackwell Publishing (formerly Iowa State University Press), 2003.

29. Young DS, Pestaner LC, Gibberman V. Effects of drugs on clinical laboratory tests. Clin Chem 1975; 21:1–431.

30. Travlos GS. Frequency and relationships of clinical chemistry and liver and kidney histopathology findings in 13-week toxicity studies in rats. Toxicology 1996; 107:17–29.

31. Moss DW, Henderson AR. In: Burtis CA, Ashwood ER, eds. Enzymes. In: Tietz Textbook of Clinical Chemistry. Philadelphia, Pennsylvania: Saunders, 1994.

32. Committee on Enzymes of The Scandinavian Society for Clinical Chemistry and Clinical Physiology. Recommended method for the determination of creatine kinase in blood modified by the inclusion of EDTA. Scand J Clin Lab Invest 1979; 39:1–5.

33. Whelton A, Watson AJ, Rock RC. Nitrogen metabolites and renal function. In: Burtis CA, Ashwood ER, eds. Tietz Textbook of Clinical Chemistry. 2nd ed. Philadelphia, Pennsylvania: Saunders, 1994.

34. Soldin SH, Henderson L, Hill JG. The effect of bilirubin and ketones on reaction rate methods for the measurement of creatinine. Clin Biochem 1978; 11:82–86.

35. Welch MJ, Cohen A, Hertz HS. Determination of serum creatinine by isotope dilution mass spectrometry as a candidate definitive method. Anal Chem 1986; 58:1681–1685.

36. Kleinman LI, Lorenz JM. Physiology and pathophysiology of body water and electrolytes. In: Kaplan LA, Pesce AJ, eds. Clinical Chemistry: Theory, Analysis, and Correlation. St Louis, Missouri: Mosby, 1989.

37. Anderson RNL, Tracey P, Anderson NG. High resolution electrophoretic mapping of human plasma proteins. In: Putnam C, ed. The Plasma Proteins. 2nd ed. New York: Academic Press, 1984:4.

38. Hayat MA. Fixation for Electron Microscopy. New York: Academic Press, 1982.

39. Pearse AGE. 4th ed. Histochemistry—Theoretical and Applied. Philadelphia, Pennsylvania: Churchill-Livingstone, 1980.

40. Kiernan JA. Histological and Histochemical Methods—Theory and Practice. Philadelphia, Pennsylvania: Elsevier Science, 1990.

41. Sheehan D, Hrapchak B. Theory and Practice of Histotechnology. 2nd ed. Richmond, Washington: Battelle Press, 1980.

42. Luna LG. Histopathologic Methods and Color Atlas of Special Stains and Tissue Artifacts; American HistoLabs. Maryland: Gaithersburg, 1993.

43. Vacca L. Laboratory Manual of Histochemistry. Philadelphia, Pennsylvania: Lippincott-Williams-Wilkins, 1985.

44. Bancroft J, Gamble M. 5th ed. Theory and Practice of Histological Techniques. Philadelphia, Pennsylvania: Lippincott-Williams-Wilkins, 2001.

45. Bahnemann R, Jacobs M, Karbe E, et al. RITA—Registry of Industrial Toxicology Animal-data—Guides for organ sampling and trimming procedures in rats. Exp Toxicol Pathol 1995; 47:247–266.

46. Haschek WM, Rousseaux CG, Wallig MA, eds. Handbook of Toxicologic Pathology. 2nd ed. New York: Academic Press, 2002.

47. Turton J, Hooson J, eds. Target Organ Pathology. Philadelphia, Pennsylvania: Taylor and Francis, 1998.

48. Greaves P. Histopathology of Preclinical Toxicity Studies. Philadelphia, Pennsylvania: Elsevier, 2000.

49. Haschek WM, Rousseaux CG. Fundamentals of Toxicologic Pathology. New York: Academic Press, 1998.

50. Eldridge SR, Tillbury LF, Goldsworthy TL, et al. Measurement of chemically-induced cell proliferation in rodent liver and kidney: a comparison of 5-bromo-2'-deoxyuridine and [^{3}H]thymidine administration by injection or osmotic pump. Carcinogenesis 1990; 12:2245–2251.

51. Goldsworthy TL. Cell Proliferation, and Chemical Carcinogenesis, National Institute of Environmental Health Sciences (NIEHS) Workshop, Research Triangle Park, NC 1992.

52. Galand P, Degraef C. Cyclin/PCNA immunostaining as an alternative to tritiated thymidine pulse labeling for marking S phase cells in paraffin sections from animal and human tissues. Cell Tissue Kin 1989; 22:383–392.

53. Marcus LF. Advances in Morphometrics. New York: Plenum Press, 1996.

54. Bookstein FL. Morphometric Tools for Landmark Data. Oxford, England: Cambridge Press, 1991.

55. Beltrame F, Tagliasco V. Confocal microscopy and cellular bioinformatics. Cytotechnology 1993; 11:72–74.
56. Boyde A. Bibliography on confocal microscopy and its applications. Scanning 1994; 16:33–56.
57. Cox G. Trends in confocal microscopy. Sci Am 1993; 24:237–247.
58. Ockleford C. The confocal laser scanning microscope (CLSM). J Pathol 1995; 176:1–2.
59. Wright SJ, Centonze VE, Stricker SA, et al. Introduction to confocal microscopy and three-dimensional reconstruction. Methods Cell Biol 1993;38.
60. Lichtman JW. Confocal microscopy. Sci Am 1994; 271:40–45.
61. Elias JM. Immunohistopathology: a practical approach to diagnosis. Philadelphia, Pennsylvania: ASCP Press, 1990.
62. Cheville N. Ultrastructural Pathology: an introduction to interpretation. Ames, Iowa: Iowa State Press, 1994.

6

Acute Toxicology

Elmer J. Rauckman
Toxicology and Regulatory Affairs, Freeburg, Illinois, U.S.A.

Andrew I. Soiefer
North Jersey Toxicology Associates LLC, Randolph, New Jersey, U.S.A.

ACUTE TOXICITY STUDIES

Acute exposure may be defined as exposure to a toxicant for a short period, usually less than 24 hours. Toxicity tests designed to explore adverse chemical effects following brief exposures are useful in classifying toxic agents, protecting workers, safeguarding the community against accidental chemical release, and selecting appropriate doses for longer-term toxicity testing.

Study Objectives

The general goal of acute toxicity tests is to determine the toxic potential of a test chemical following a single exposure. A single dose of the chemical under study is administered to groups of laboratory animals that are then held and observed for a defined period to access adverse outcomes of exposure.

Routes of Exposure

Laboratory animals may be exposed to chemicals in a variety of ways. The route of exposure is usually chosen to reflect conditions under which humans may encounter the chemical under study. Exposure by the oral route is common and generally the default exposure route when it is not known how or if humans will be exposed. In addition, data from acute oral toxicity studies often forms the basis by which chemicals are compared to each other. In the workplace, humans are more likely to be exposed to chemicals through skin contact or by inhalation. Therefore, acute toxicity tests by the dermal and inhalation routes of exposure provide the safety information most critical to the occupational environment. For many chemicals, acute toxicity data by the dermal or inhalation routes are not available. Several possible explanations may account for this. For one, dermal studies are somewhat more labor intensive than oral studies, increasing the cost. Second, special equipment is required to expose laboratory animals to chemicals by the inhalation route, greatly increasing the cost and limiting the number of studies that can be conducted.

Finally, oral testing may have been performed early in the development of a material, prior to determination of how humans may become exposed, and route-specific testing was never conducted for a variety of reasons.

Animal Species

A wide variety of animal species may be handled in the laboratory and utilized in acute toxicity testing. Generally, tests include male and female animals to insure that gender-specific adverse effects are recognized. Rodents are the most commonly utilized animals for acute toxicity testing due to considerations of size, cost, and relevance of results. Testing guidelines for the United States and other international regulatory agencies routinely recommend the rat as the preferred species for acute oral and inhalation toxicity tests (1). Rabbits and rats are often recommended for dermal studies (2). Because these animal species are commonly chosen for human safety assessment, a large historical information base exists with governmental agencies, contract laboratories, animal suppliers, and in the published scientific literature.

Animals for acute toxicity testing are healthy, outbred strains obtained from United States Department of Agriculture approved and regulated suppliers. Upon receipt at the laboratory, animals are usually quarantined for seven days to fourteen days. Holding test animals for this period of time allows test animals to become acclimated to the laboratory. During this time any stress from transport should resolve and careful observation should reveal any unwanted and confounding disease states. Test animals are usually housed individually in suspended stainless steel cages or other suitable housing. Animal room temperature and humidity are carefully controlled within standard ranges to ensure animal health and comfort. Temperature is maintained at 72°F and humidity ranges from 40 to 60%. Room lighting is controlled to maintain a 12 hr light/12 hr dark cycle, and room ventilation is adjusted to produce a minimum of 10 air changes per hour. Standards for animal care are specified in the *Guide for the Care and Use of Laboratory Animals* (3).

Animals are selected for study and assigned to test groups in a strictly random manner to avoid introducing potential bias. The stock of available animals is culled to include only healthy animals that have passed a detailed pretest evaluation. All female animals are nulliparous and nonpregnant.

Experimental Design

Acute toxicology tests have undergone significant design changes in recent years. Although the output of these tests is somewhat the same, an attempt has been made to derive the key data set using as few animals as possible. In many cases where full dose-response evaluations might have been conducted in the past, current designs provide limit data that only establish a rough range of effect. In current test designs, materials that show little acute toxicity would not generally be tested above 2,000 mg/kg unless there was a regulatory requirement to go up to 5,000 mg/kg.

Estimation of acute oral toxicity evolved into what is known as the LD_{50} Test, which was codified by the Organization for Economic Cooperation and Development (OECD) as the 401 Guideline and by the Environmental Protection Agency (EPA) as the 798.1175 guideline. These guidelines required that animals of each sex be treated and recommended a minimum group size of five animals (in the case of rats) per sex and per dose level. Although many companies were using alternative testing procedures with fewer animals, regulatory requirements dictated that a full LD_{50} test be conducted on many regulated chemicals.

Animal rights activists and logic prevailed, and the OECD 401 guideline was deleted in 2001 after it was established that alternative protocols, using fewer animals and only one sex (usually females), provided toxicity information comparable to the OECD 401. Botham gives a short historical perspective of the process in a 2002 article (4).

Three OECD guidelines are available to estimate the acute oral toxicity of a material, these are:

- OECD Guideline 420: Acute Oral Toxicity—Fixed Dose Method (5)
- OECD Guideline 423: Acute Oral Toxicity—Acute Toxic Class Method (6)
- OECD Guideline 425: Acute Oral Toxicity—Up and Down Procedure (7)

The EPA also replaced its LD_{50} test procedures with a new harmonized guideline that follows the Up and Down Procedure.

- OPPTS 870.1100: Acute Oral Toxicity (8)

As the EPA requires a point estimate of the LD_{50} with confidence intervals for regulation of pesticides (4) and the up-and-down procedure is the only one of these three procedures that can provide this quantitative data, it forms the basis of the updated EPA testing guideline.

The fixed dose method uses a range-finding phase with single animals prior to dosing of five animals at a fixed dose of 5, 50, 300, or 2000 mg/kg (with a 5000 mg/kg option) and uses "evident toxicity" as an endpoint rather than just mortality. As this endpoint is not as objective or familiar as mortality and the LD_{50} range must be inferred, there can be less confidence in the results. In addition, information on toxic effects seen at dose levels near the lethal dose may not be obtained (9).

The acute toxic class (ATC) method is perhaps the most intuitive of these three procedures and uses sequential dosing of three animals of the same sex at doses of 5, 50, 300, or 2000 mg/kg (with a 5000 mg/kg option). The starting dose is selected to produce some mortality in the three animal group and is set using any relevant information about the chemical or similar chemicals. Depending on the outcome of the first group, additional group(s) are dosed at higher or lower fixed doses until the study objective is reached. A detailed flow-chart is available in the OECD 423 guideline (6). The current dose levels are designed to allow optimal integration with the Globally Harmonized Classification System (GHS), but guidance has been published on classification using other systems depending on the exact outcome of the study (10).

In principle any of these three methods will produce results satisfactory for classification of a chemical; however, it appears that the acute toxic class method is the procedure that is most commonly used in Germany, where it comprised 89% of reported acute oral toxicity tests in 2003 (11). In situations where the regulatory requirements mandate a point estimate of the LD_{50} with confidence interval, the only choice among these three tests is the up-and-down procedure.

The savings in animal usage and animal deaths on test was examined in the EU for the years 2001 through 2003, and it was reported that the average number of animals used for a full LD_{50} test was 38.5, and only an average of 10.5 animals were used in studies run using the ATC procedure. The average number of animal deaths on test was 14.5 for the LD_{50} test and only 2.4 for the ATC test (11).

The up-and-down procedure starts with the dosing of a single animal at a dose level estimated to be just below the lethal dose. The next animal is dosed at a higher or lower dose, depending on the outcome of the previous animal and this sequence is continued until there is a reversal of the outcome. After that, additional animals are dosed (usually four) until the criteria for stopping are met. The maximum likelihood method is used to estimate the LD_{50} and confidence interval using a computer program (7).

Similar to the situation with the acute oral test, acute dermal and acute inhalation test guidelines are undergoing a similar modernization. In principle the three alternative procedures for the acute oral study can be applied to dermal and inhalation studies. In practice, protocol development and validation requires considerable time and effort. As of this writing, OECD 433 acute inhalation testing is in draft form. This method is similar to the fixed dose method in that the primary endpoint for Guideline 433 is the observation of clear clinical signs of toxicity, or evident toxicity. Female animals are exposed for four hours or more to graduated concentrations of the test substance. A sighting study is recommended to select an appropriate starting concentration for the main study and to reduce animal usage. Fixed concentrations of 0.5, 2, 10, and 20 mg/L for vapors, 0.05, 0.5, 1, and 5 mg/L for dusts/mists, and 100, 500, 2500, and 5000 ppm for gases are used in both the sighting study and the definitive study. Animal welfare concerns dictate that testing of animals in GHS category 5 ($>$ 20 mg/L, vapor; $>$ 5 mg/L dusts/mists and $>$ 5000 ppm gases) not be conducted without adequate rationale. A stepwise procedure is used to expose groups of animals with the initial concentration selected to produce some signs of evident toxicity. Additional groups of animals may then be exposed at higher or lower fixed concentrations until the test substance classification is achieved.

In addition to OECD 433, an acute toxic class method for inhalation toxicity has been presented and commented upon as a draft guideline (OECD-GD39B). A complete description of the procedure, its modification to the GHS, and biometric evaluation of the procedure had been published (12). Similar to the oral ATC test, the inhalation test uses groups of three animals treated in a sequential manner until classification is achieved. It is anticipated that both of these alternative methods will gain acceptance and that the inhalation toxic class method will soon become the method of choice for classification of inhalation hazards.

Estimation of acute dermal toxicity is an important step in hazard identification of materials where industrial and consumer exposure occurs. Two points should be brought out regarding acute dermal toxicity: (1) For many low volatility industrial compounds, dermal exposure is the most prevalent form of exposure, and (2) Some compounds are much more systemically toxic by the dermal route than by the oral route. Formerly, the rabbit was the species of choice for acute dermal toxicity, but the rat has become the main species used in acute dermal testing in the EU and is becoming the species of choice in the rest of the world.

The current EPA acute dermal test guideline OPPTS 870.1200 requires three groups of five animals of one sex be tested to establish a range of effects, such that a point estimate of the LD_{50} can be calculated unless the toxicity is so low that significant mortality is not observed in a limit test at 2000 mg/kg. Following this, one group of animals of the other sex is to be dosed to assure there is no significant sex difference. Exposure is for 24 hours with a 14-day observation period (13). The current OECD dermal toxicity guideline, OECD 402, describes essentially the same protocol as the EPA guidance. The major difference is that the EPA guidance states that rabbits are preferred over rats and guinea pigs (although any of these may be used), whereas the OECD guidance gives no preference among these three species. In practice, most of the acute dermal studies in the EU are conducted using rats, while the use of rabbits as the preferred species has persisted longer in the U.S. Harmonization to utilize rats as the species of choice globally in acute dermal testing seems inevitable.

Alternative codified procedures for dermal acute testing are on the horizon as a formal proposal for a fixed dose test to be known as the OECD 434 has been put forward and formally received comments. At this point the procedures is analogous to the acute oral fixed dose procedure using five animals per dose, with dose levels set to optimize classification using the GHS. As this is only in first draft form, the reader is referred to the OECD website for details about the next draft and the final guideline. Relative to an acute toxic class method being codified, the procedure has already been published and undergone biometric validation (1).

All of these acute tests use a single dose of test material, followed by a 14-day observation period and a necropsy. Clinical signs observed during the observation period can provide important information about the biological targets of the test substance and the probable cause of death if there are mortalities. The OECD has published a monograph on the use of clinical signs as endpoints in toxicity testing (14). Likewise, information from a necropsy may reveal target organs and other information useful in the extrapolation of animal data to humans. Thus it is incumbent on the testing laboratory other information useful to have trained individuals recording the clinical signs and conducting necropsies and incumbent upon the laboratory and the sponsor to take account of the totality of data from a study and integrate it with other information about a test material and its analogs to inform the hazard evaluation and provide appropriate warnings to workers and consumers.

EYE IRRITATION STUDIES

These safety tests are critical for chemicals that may be accidentally or intentionally introduced into the eye. In the workplace, accidental ocular exposure by chemical splash can occur leading to serious and irreversible injury. Components of cosmetic and shampoo formulations frequently contact the eye in the course of everyday use.

Study Objective

The goal of the primary eye irritation safety test is to determine the irritant or corrosive potential of a chemical following a single application to the mammalian eye. Information derived from this study may be used as the basis for classification and labeling the test material. On rare occasions a material may be so toxic that systemic effects, including death, may result following a single ocular exposure.

Toxicology of the Eye

Humans and selected members of the animal kingdom are principally visual creatures. That is to say, sight or sightedness is our dominant sensory modality. Irreversible loss of vision in one or both eyes is a crippling injury, one that leaves the organism impaired and unable to efficiently respond to the environment that surrounds it. The visual apparatus is complex, containing peripheral and central elements. The eye is the critical sensory end organ of the visual system, and the cornea and conjunctiva are the structures that are directly exposed to external insults. The surface of the eye is bathed in fluid to protect it, and reflexive blinking acts to maintain this liquid coating. The cornea has special features that increase its vulnerability and susceptibility to irreversible injury. For one, unlike other parts of the body, the cornea must maintain transparency to remain functional. Whereas other parts of the body may be restored by the mechanisms of wound healing, the cornea will be functionally destroyed by vascularization and scar formation.

Safety Testing in Animals

The New Zealand white rabbit is the most commonly used animal species for eye irritation studies. Trained personnel may handle rabbits safely in the laboratory, and the albino rabbit eye is nonpigmented making adverse change easy to observe. Historical data demonstrates that the New Zealand White rabbit is sensitive to a wide variety of ocular irritants and is a suitable model for human safety assessment. The New Zealand White rabbit is recommended as the test species for eye irritation studies by a number of U.S. and international regulatory agencies (15).

Rabbits for study are chosen randomly from healthy, acclimated stock animals to avoid any unintentional selection bias. Males or females may be used because chemically initiated irritant or corrosive eye injury shows no relationship to gender. Stock females are nulliparous and nonpregnant. All animals chosen for study receive a baseline eye exam to ensure normal ocular health prior to test chemical exposure. The rabbit eye is typically evaluated macroscopically with indirect light and with long-wave UV for fluorescein dye retention.

Experimental designs of eye irritation studies vary. Current research protocols test fewer animals than in the past, and test compounds are screened to eliminate materials with very high (>11.5) or low (<2.0) pH. These chemicals can be assumed corrosive based on chemical properties and may be labeled without subjecting animals to irreversible eye injury. Buffering capacity, however, should be taken into consideration as a very dilute solution of a strong acid or base may exceed the pH limits but may be effectively neutralized by buffers in the eye and result in no significant irritation. Similarly, materials that produced severe irritation in a dermal study may be presumed to be severe eye irritants; however, exceptions are known where materials are severe skin irritants and very mild eye irritants. In general, unless there is some reason to believe a severe skin irritant will not be a severe eye irritant or there is some specific need for eye irritation data, severe skin irritants should be presumed to be severe eye irritants. With this in mind, skin irritation studies should be conducted prior to eye irritation studies.

Materials of unknown eye irritancy may be tested with and without a rinse procedure. Three animals are usually used for each treatment group (no rinse, rinse). For liquids, gels, and pastes, a volume of 0.1 ml is instilled into the conjunctival sac of one eye. The eyelid is then gently held shut for 1 or 2 seconds to limit test article loss. The contralateral eye is not treated and serves as a control. Powders and other solids are administered at a weight equivalent of 0.1 ml. For animals in a rinse group, the test and control eyes are rinsed with 0.9% physiological saline 30 seconds after test chemical administration. This rinsing procedure provides information on the time-course of irreversibility and/or the ability of a rinsing procedure to effectively remove a substance and may be useful in first aid recommendations and protective eyewear recommendations. Animals must be carefully observed following ocular exposure to an unknown chemical. In the event a severe local reaction takes place, the animal may experience pain and should be humanely euthanized.

In a standard eye irritation study design, the treated eyes will be evaluated macroscopically by indirect light at 1, 24, 48, and 72 hours postexposure. Ocular change is graded based on a scoring system developed by Draize (16). Scores for corneal opacity ("O," 0–4), area of corneal involvement ("A," 0–4), iritis ("I," 0–2), conjunctival redness ("R," 0–3), conjunctival swelling ("S," 0–4) and conjunctival discharge ("D," 0–3) are combined to yield a maximum score of 110. The mathematical equation to calculate the

Draize ocular score is as follows:

$$(O \times A \times 5) + (I \times 5) + 2(R + S + D) = \text{Ocular Score}$$

At 24 hours, all treated eyes are also routinely evaluated using fluorescein dye retention to access corneal damage. If ocular irritation is observed at any time point, the test may be extended to up to 21 days to record recovery, should it occur. If no treatment-associated irritation is observed by 72 hours, the chemical is judged nonirritating, and the test is ended.

Descriptive ratings for eye irritation based on the ocular score were suggested in the original test method (16). A chemical was described as a "nonirritant" if its maximum mean irritation score was less than or equal to 1.0. A chemical producing a mean irritation score less than or equal to 6.0 at 24 hours, without corneal or iridal involvement and reversible by day 7, was described as a "slight irritant." A "moderate irritant" produced an ocular score greater than 6.0 at 24 hours but less than 30.0 at maximum, and irritation was reversible by day 14. A maximum mean irritation score greater than 30.0 with corneal or iridal findings that persist beyond day 14 was described as a "severe irritant." "Corrosive" was reserved for chemicals that produced irreversible eye injury.

Another useful set of criteria for evaluating ocular irritation has been described by Kay and Calandra (17). In this scheme, descriptive rating and class are assigned based on the maximum mean ocular score over the first 4 days, the time to reach maximum, and score persistence. Using eye irritation data from tests with standard Draize design, one can assign up to eight levels of irritation from "nonirritating" to "extremely severe irritant" using this set of criteria.

Sensible modifications of the standard eye irritation test exist and offer several advantages. Alternate protocols may be employed to reduce animal usage, and some may even more accurately predict irritant effects to the human eye. In most situations a screening approach is appropriate, and the irritation test is initiated with a single animal. If the material produces severe irritation, no more animals are tested, and the material is labeled a severe eye irritant. If the screening test results indicate moderate or slight irritation, additional animals are tested to confirm the result, thereby reducing the possibility of underclassifying the material. Used in this manner, the screening approach is conservative, in that if an error is made it tends to be in the direction of over-classification rather than underclassification. The downside of any overclassification that results from using this conservative screening protocol is considered to be outweighed by the gains made in reducing animal discomfort and usage.

A low-volume eye test (LVET) has also been described and validated (18). This procedure uses only one-tenth the material of the standard Draize protocol, and the test substance is applied directly to the cornea. Data show that the LVET is actually more predictive of human response (19), and it generally produces less irritation and hence discomfort. Because the irritation scores are lower, the classification scheme is shifted in order to produce results comparable to the Draize test. Research has shown that the number of animals necessary to produce reasonably dependable results from the LVET can be reduced from six to three (20).

In situations where legal requirements do not specify the exact protocol or required number of animals, the use of these types of alternative protocols should be considered.

Alternatives to Animal Testing

Chemical manufacturers, consumer product producers, and others have the responsibility of identifying chemicals that have the potential to induce severe eye irritation or irreversible eye injury. Incidents involving chemicals hazardous to visual function are greatly reduced by the proper use of the information developed in the basic ocular irritation test. Despite the utility of this information, the ocular irritation test has become the focal point of considerable controversy because it is viewed by some as inhumane. No one disputes that introducing an irritating chemical into the eye of a laboratory animal produces a significant amount of distress. Although there are numerous reasons for developing a sensitive and reliable in vitro test as an alternative to using live animals, it is pressure from society, that has put the development of alternative procedures on the fast track.

The complex structure of the eye makes finding and validating an in vitro alternative for the rabbit ocular irritancy test challenging. One approach to this problem is to consider the various steps by which chemicals cause corrosive damage to the eye at a cellular and subcellular level. Regardless of the precise molecular mechanism, chemicals that can disrupt the physical structure of the eye do so by killing cells and disrupting membranes. In an attempt to model corrosivity, chemical effects on isolated cells and membranes have been explored and compared to the available literature on ocular corrosion. Measures of cell viability include growth inhibition, colony forming efficiency, cell detachment, total protein, and dye binding studies. Chemical effects on membrane integrity have been assessed by isotope release, dye release, and other assays that measure membrane breakthrough. Ocular irritation has been more difficult to model in vitro because it involves a cellular response from the immune system with the induction of inflammation. One of the more successful model systems to observe this effect is the chorioallantoic membrane of the chick embryo. Although many methods have shown potential, only a few have been validated across more than one class of chemical. The Interagency Coordinating Committee on the Validation of Alternative Methods (ICCVAM) compiled a review of the performance of four alternative methods to estimate eye irritation (21). Although this report shows that much progress has been made, at present, no single in vitro test captures all aspects of the whole animal response to an ocular irritant. For the classes of chemicals that can be adequately predicted using in vitro test methods, these alternative tests can be recommended to aid in hazard identification and classification

DERMAL IRRITATION STUDIES

Our skin is our boundary with the environment, and the environment is composed of chemicals. Dermal contact with chemicals occurs on a daily basis in the home, workplace, and everywhere in between. Dermal irritation studies are safety tests that predict the irritant and/or corrosive effects of chemicals that may accidentally or intentionally contact the skin. In the workplace, accidental dermal exposure can lead to serious and irreversible injury. In the home, chemicals used in a wide variety of common consumer products contact the skin in the course of everyday use.

Study Objectives

The goal of the primary skin irritation safety test is to determine the irritant and/or corrosive potential of a chemical following a single application to mammalian skin. Information derived from this study may be used as the basis for classification and labeling the test material. Some chemicals may be rapidly absorbed across the dermis producing systemic poisoning following a single dermal exposure. On these rare occasions, information regarding adverse systemic effects may be identified from a primary skin irritation test.

Toxicology of the Skin

Our skin covers the surface of our body and provides a boundary between our internal structures and the environment. Skin is a unique structure meeting the criteria of a specialized organ system. As such, our skin is one of the largest organs of the body, constituting as much as 10% of total body weight. In addition to protection from the environment, our skin provides other important physiological functions, including the regulation of body temperature and water retention. The skin is also metabolically active and can be an important site for the biotransformation of chemicals.

The skin is multilayered in structure with each of two main layers arising from different embryological cell masses. The thinner outer layer is called the epidermis, which as indicated by its name, has epithelial characteristics. The thicker inner layer is composed of connective tissue and is called the dermis. The thickness of the skin varies in different regions of the body. The palms of the hand and the soles of the feet are areas where the skin is relatively thick. The skin covering the scrotum is relatively thin. Skin thickness is an important variable, particularly in relation to chemical absorption across the dermal layer.

Safety Tests in Animals

The New Zealand White rabbit is the most commonly used animal species and strain for skin irritation testing. The New Zealand White rabbit has no dermal pigment and, due to its size and proportions, the dorsal surface of its back is relatively large. With these characteristics, dermal application of test materials is accurate, and adverse chemical effects may be easily observed. In a standard laboratory setting, rabbits may be handled easily and safely by trained personnel. Also, the New Zealand White rabbit has been shown to be sensitive to the irritant/corrosive effects of a wide range of chemicals. This combination of properties make the New Zealand White rabbit a rational alternative to larger mammals, providing a suitable dermal model for human safety assessment. The New Zealand White rabbit is recommended as the test species of choice for primary irritation testing by a number of U.S. and international regulatory agencies (22). The current OECD 404 guideline is comparable to the EPA 870.2500 guideline, with the exception of more guidance in the OECD concerning alternatives to actual skin testing. The OECD 404 recommends a sequential testing strategy in which all available information should be evaluated to determine the need for in vivo skin testing. This sequence has several formal steps, including structure-activity relationship (SARs), human experience with the material, consideration of physicochemical properties in vitro and ex vivo testing and finally in vivo testing.

As in ocular irritation testing, rabbits for study are chosen randomly from healthy, acclimated stock animals to avoid selection bias. Male and females may be used; females are nulliparous and nonpregnant. All selected animals receive a detailed pretest observation prior to dosing. Animals with preexisting skin irregularities are identified and removed from the study group.

Experimental design of skin irritation tests is based on the work of Draize (23). As in ocular testing, current protocols test fewer animals than in the past, and test compounds are screened to eliminate materials with very high or low pH. Strong acids or bases are assumed to be corrosive and may be labeled without subjecting animals to irreversible dermal injury. Test materials with structural similarities to chemicals known to be damaging to skin may be screened using one or two animals in a pilot test. Materials of unknown irritancy are typically tested using six animals, three male and three female. On the day prior to testing, animals selected for skin irritancy studies have the fur clipped from the dorsal surface of their backs. Care is taken to avoid abrading the skin with the animal clipper. The next day the test is initiated by applying the test material to the dorsal skin surface. For liquids, gels or pastes a 0.5 ml dose of test material is administered. Powdered test materials are similarly applied at a dose of 0.5 g and are moistened with 0.5 ml of distilled water. After administration of the test material, the test area is covered with a 1×1 inch, square, 4-ply gauze held in place with nonirritating tape. To prevent removal and ingestion of the test material, the test area is further covered with a semiocclusive elastic bandage. The elastic bandage is wrapped around the trunk of the rabbit and the ends are secured with adhesive tape. Specially designed animal collars may also be utilized to prevent treated animals from removing the bandage coverings and disturbing the test site. In the standard test design, the test material is allowed to remain in contact with the skin for four hours. After this exposure period the elastic bandage and gauze are removed. The boundary of the test site is marked, and any residual test material is gently wiped from the test site. The condition of test animals exposed to a chemical of undefined dermal irritancy must be carefully monitored. Should the test material produce severe injury to the skin, exposed animals may experience unacceptable levels of discomfort and should be humanely euthanized.

In the standard dermal irritation design, treated animals are evaluated for erythema and edema at 1, 24, 48, and 72 hours postexposure. In situations where irritation is still present at the 72-hour examination interval, observations may be extended for up to 7 days postexposure. Dermal irritation is graded based on a scoring system developed by Draize (23). Scores for erythema ("E," 0–4) and edema ("Ed," 0–4) are combined at each evaluation interval to yield a maximum score of 8. The primary irritation index is then calculated using the following equation:

$$\Sigma(E + Ed) \div (\text{No. of test sites} \times 4) = \text{Primary Irritation Index}$$

Descriptive ratings for skin irritation based on the primary irritation index have been described. Materials producing a primary irritation index of 0.00 are classified as nonirritating. Scores from 0.01 to 2.00 are rated as slightly irritating. Scores from 2.01 to 5.00 are rated as moderately irritating, and scores above 5.01 are classified as severely irritating.

In addition to erythema and edema, the following descriptors of dermal injury may be recognized and reported with or without an associated severity: beet redness, desquamation, fissuring, blanching, eschar formation, eschar exfoliation, ulceration, and necrosis.

Alternatives to Animal Testing

In the last 15 years, significant effort has been directed towards developing in vitro alternatives to Draize-type irritation tests. Development of methods for in vitro skin testing have progressed on a parallel track to ocular irritation screening (see above) but are more advanced. Some of the more successful techniques have employed coculture of relevant cell types on various support matrices and artificial membrane systems that develop color upon test material breakthrough. These test systems have been validated in discrete classes of chemicals and are useful for R & D applications and some regulatory classification. At present, the information provided by these techniques can be extremely useful but cannot completely substitute for whole animal testing.

TESTING STRATEGIES

Policies vary considerably between companies regarding toxicology testing of new and existing materials. New and existing substances in the United States are regulated under the Toxic Substances Control Act (TSCA). There are no specific data requirements specified under this act; thus, decisions concerning acquisition of toxicity data are generally left up to the producer/importer/user. A good testing strategy will protect workers, customers, and the business. The studies will be custom-tailored for each test material such that the maximum amount of information is obtained at the lowest cost and using the smallest number of animals. Testing prior to significant production has several advantages:

- Allows for proper hazard communication
- Allows proper classification for shipping
- Supports recommendations for engineering controls and personal protective equipment
- Establishes safety of the product relative to competitive materials
- Permits early identification of unacceptable chemicals
- Speeds the premanufacture notification process (PMN) for new materials.

Likewise, testing presents some challenges:

- Can be expensive
- Can slow product development if in critical path
- May be perceived as unnecessary by business interests
- Can result in TSCA Section 8(e) notifications.

Cost of testing for new products is often the factor that determines how much testing can be conducted. New product development teams are often working on a limited budget, and testing costs must compete with other development costs.

Why Do Safety Testing?

Safety testing is conducted for both moral-ethical reasons and for regulatory compliance. Although the United States does not have a minimum dataset requirement under TSCA, the EPA can and will use structural alerts and SAR data to argue that a material presents an unreasonable risk. In the absence of test data, it is reasonable to assume that a material is as, or more, toxic than materials with a similar structure. The EPA has the responsibility to protect public health, and conservative estimates of toxicity are reasonable and justifiable. Actual animal test data provide a realistic basis from which to estimate human hazard.

It is important to have enough information to be confident that a new material does not pose an unreasonable health risk. All available information should be used in hazard evaluation of a new material and in design of the appropriate testing program. Information from known toxicity of similar chemicals (i.e., SAR), knowledge of likely metabolic pathways, physical properties of the test material, in vitro data, proposed manufacturing procedures, and potential end uses should all be used to design a testing program that gives the most information possible using the smallest feasible number of animals.

Phasing

Phasing refers to implementing a testing program in a time and cost-effective manner. When considering acute tests, there is no obvious sequence, such as subacute prior to subchronic. However, logical considerations are potential human exposure and "knock-out" effects based on structural alerts. In addition, limitations of resources, including test material availability, can be a reason for the phasing of acute tests. For example, if one were in the early stages of compound development with limited sample, it might make sense to conduct an acute oral toxicity study in rats and a single irritation test in rabbits (skin or eye). These two studies together would give a good indication of the potential of a material to cause fatalities or severe irritant effects. The oral study in rats is sensitive and will generally be required for a PMN or standard classification schemes. The eye or skin test will also show if the material happens to be unusually toxic by the dermal route of exposure and, thus, gives limited, but possibly important, systemic toxicity data in a second species. Completion of the remainder of the standard series of acute tests could be logically postponed until more material is available or the material was found to be acceptable by these two initial tests.

Communications

Rapid communication of test results that suggest high hazard is required if current activity with the material could result in worker or customer harm. There are both legal and ethical issues involved in the decisions of what, when, and to whom test results are communicated. Legal communication requirements exist under EPA's TSCA Section 8(e) and the Occupational Safety and Health Administration's regulations. EPA's TSCA Section 8(e) requires that information be provided to the agency for any material that is considered a "substantial risk" within 30 calendar days after the information is known by a company manufacturing or distributing the material (including research and development work prior to actual manufacture). There have been many debates over the TSCA Section 8(e) regulation, and most companies have developed their own set of reporting criteria. EPA has issued more specific guidance, and most companies use criteria for deciding when to report a low LD_{50} value. There is a wider range of opinions regarding when to report strong irritants and sensitizers to the EPA. If the effect noted in animals could result in an irreversible loss of a bodily function or death, it is clearly reportable under TSCA Section 8(e). Thus, irritants that may cause loss of vision or sensitizers that may cause anaphylactic shock can be considered reportable. Hazard communication under OSHA regulations stipulate that results of new toxicity tests appear on the material safety data sheet for the material within 90 days of test report receipt. Practically, however, if test results are received indicating that a material presents an unusual hazard, immediate, and appropriate notification of potentially affected persons is encouraged. Notification should be made in clear language explaining what was found and how it might affect someone. Occupational health professionals should be closely involved and should determine if the handling procedures and personal protective equipment are adequate. Follow-up notification should be made if additional information is obtained showing that the material is more or less hazardous than indicated by the preliminary data.

REFERENCES

1. Health effects test guidelines, OTS, 870.1100 & 870.1300; OECD Guideline 401 (deleted), 420, 423, 425, and 434 (draft).
2. Health Effects Test Guidelines, OTS, 870.1200; OECD Guideline 402.

3. National Research Council, Guide for the Care and Use of Laboratory Animals, National Center for Research Resources, Bethesda MD, Report No.: ISBN-0-309-05377-3, 1996: 141 pages.
4. Botham P. Acute systemic toxicity. ILAR J 2002; 43:S27–S30.
5. Organization for Economic Cooperation and Development. OECD Guidelines for Testing of Chemicals. Guideline 420: Acute Oral Toxicity —Fixed Dose Method, Adopted:1992; update of 17 December 2001.
6. Organization for Economic Cooperation and Development. OECD Guidelines for Testing of Chemicals. Guideline 423: Acute Oral Toxicity—Acute Toxic Class Method, Adopted:1996, update of 17 December 2001.
7. Organization for Economic Cooperation and Development. OECD Guidelines for the Testing of Chemicals. OECD Guideline 425: Acute Oral Toxicity: Up-and-Down Procedure, Approved:2001; update of 17 December 2001.
8. EPA Harmonized Health Effects Test Guidelines, OPPTS, 870.1100 August 1999.
9. Lipnick RL, Cotruvo JA, Hill RN, et al. Comparison of the up-and-down, conventional LD50, and fixed-dose acute toxicity procedures. Food Chem Toxicol 1995; 33:223–231.
10. OECD Environment, Health, and Safety Publications Series on Testing and Assessment No. 24, Guidance Document on Acute Oral Toxicity Testing (2001).
11. Schlede E, Genschow E, Spielmann H, Stropp G, Kayser D. Oral acute toxic class method: a successful alternative to the oral LD_{50} test. Regul Toxicol Pharmacol 2005; 42:15–23.
12. Holzhütter H-G, Genschow E, Diener W, Schlede E. Dermal and inhalation acute toxicity class methods: Test procedures and biometric evaluations for the globally harmonized classification system. Arch Toxicol 2002; 77:243–254.
13. U.S. EPA, Health Effects Test Guideline, OPPTS. 1998: 780.1200.
14. OECD Environment, Health, and Safety Publications Series on Testing and Assessment No. 19, Guidance Document on the Recognition, Assessment and Use of Clinical Signs as Humane Endpoints for Experimental Animals used in Safety Evaluation (November 1999).
15. Health Effects Test Guidelines, OPPTS, 870.2400; OECD Guideline 405.
16. Draize JH, Woodward G, Calvery HO. Methods for the study of irritation and toxicity of substances applied topically to the skin and mucous membranes. J Pharmacol Exp Ther 1944; 82:377.
17. Kay JH, Calandra JC. Interpretation of Eye Irritation Tests. J Soc Cosmet Chem 1962; 13:281.
18. Griffith JF, Nixon GA, Bruce RD, Reer PJ, Bannan EA. Dose-response studies with chemical irritants in the albino rabbit eye as a basis for selecting optimum testing conditions for predicting hazard to the human eye. Toxicol Appl Pharmacol 1980; 55:501.
19. Freeberg FE, Hooker DT, Griffith JF. Correlation of animal eye test data with human experience for household products: an update. J Toxicol Cut Ocul Toxicol 1986; 5:115.
20. Bruner LH, Parker RD, Bruce RD. Reducing the number of rabbits in the low-volume eye test. Fundam Appl Toxicol 1992; 19:330.
21. The Interagency Coordinating Committee on the Validation of Alternative Methods. Background Review Document (BRD) "Current Status of In Vitro Test Methods for Identifying Ocular Corrosives and Severe Irritants: (1) The Bovine Corneal Opacity and Permeability (BCOP) test; (2) the Hen's Egg Test—Chorion Allantoic Membrane (HET-CAM); (3) the Isolated Rabbit Eye (IRE) test; and (4) the Isolated Chicken Eye (ICE) test. Notice of availability: Federal Register, Vol. 69, No. 212, pp 64081-64082, November 1, 2004. Documents located on the ICCVAM website: iccvam.niehs.nih.gov.
22. Health Effects Test Guidelines, OPPTS, 870.2500, 1998; OECD Guideline 2002:404.
23. Draize JH, Dermal toxicity. Assoc. Food and Drug Officials, U.S. Appraisal of the Safety of Chemicals in Food, Drugs and Cosmetics, Texas State Dept. of Health, Austin, Texas 1959: 46–59.

7

Multidose General Toxicology Studies

Kit A. Keller
Toxicology Consultant, Washington, D.C., U.S.A.

Christopher Banks
CTBR Bio-Research, Inc., Senneville, Quebec, Canada

INTRODUCTION

Whereas acute toxicity studies are generally performed to identify lethal doses and to demonstrate toxic effects at high dose levels associated with a single administration of an agent, multidose studies, often referred to as subacute, subchronic, and chronic studies, are performed to provide information on the effects of repeated lower-dose administration of a compound. The major endpoints in multiple dose studies are used to evaluate the cumulative and latent toxicity potential of a chemical including potential functional, biochemical, physiological and/or pathological changes. Such nonlethal effects may often be repairable over time, and a recovery phase is often added to repeat dose studies to identify reversibility.

The distinction between subacute and subchronic may sometimes be unclear, but it is generally accepted that subacute studies are of 28 days (1 month) duration or less, and subchronic studies are classically 13 weeks (3 months). A study duration of 13 weeks is considered to approximate 10% of the lifespan of a rodent. Longer duration toxicology studies are classed as chronic studies with a duration of 26 weeks (6 months), 39 weeks (9 months), or 52 weeks (1 year), allowing investigation of test article related effects over a larger proportion of the animal's lifespan. Carcinogenicity studies (discussed in Chapter 9) are performed almost exclusively in rats and mice and assess the tumorigenic potential of an agent over the majority of the rodent lifespan (1.5–2 years).

Distinctions in the types of subacute or subchronic studies required can be made according to the type of agent to be tested. Usually repeated dose studies of varying duration are carried out in sequence. The shorter studies generally aid in proper dose selection for the longer studies and may also identify possible adverse effects that should be monitored for. Table 1 lists some examples of subchronic and chronic testing requirements for various types of chemicals. When performed as part of the preclinical safety assessment of a pharmaceutical product by the international harmonization guidelines, the general toxicity studies are usually performed in one rodent species and a second nonrodent species such as dogs or non-human primates. When performed for the Environmental Protection Agency (EPA) according to the new harmonized guidelines

Table 1 Regulatory Agencies Requiring Multidose Toxicity Testing

Agency	Multidose studies
Industrial chemicals[a]	
EEC directives; dangerous substance directive (67/548; 79/831; 92/32)	New chemicals from 10–1000 tons/year require base set of studies from 28 days (rodent) up to chronic repeated dose toxicity studies (rodent and nonrodent)
OECD guidelines for testing of chemicals (407, 408, 409, 410, 411, 412, 413, 451, 452, 453)	Tier testing: multidose studies from 21–28 days up to chronic and carcinogenicity studies (rodents and nonrodents)
U.S. EPA: toxic substance control act (TSCA, 409A)	Specific studies requested on a case-by-case basis
Japan law 44 (jointly by MITI, MHW, and MOL)	New chemicals must undergo biodegradation studies; if bioaccumulation potential, then up to 28-day repeated dose toxicity studies required
Agrochemicals[a]	
EEC directives (79/117; 91/414)	Tier testing. May require up to a 3-month dietary or inhalation study
U.S. EPA: FIFRA (40 CFR 158)	
Human pharmaceuticals	
International Committee on Harmonization (ICH) Guidelines (Guideline Nos. M3, S6, S4)	Requires 2-week to 9-month studies in rodent and nonrodent depending upon the duration of human therapy required; some studies also may be required for excipients, impurities, or degradants
Veterinary pharmaceuticals	
EEC Directive (81/851 as amended by 92/18) Part III	Up to 90 days in rodent and nonrodent
U.S. FDA (Fed. Reg. 52;49572)	Up to 90-day feeding study in rodent and nonrodent; residue in animal products require further 6-month study in nonrodent
Food additives	
U.S. FDA (Redbook)	Up to 90-day study in two species; 2-year feeding study in two species for new additives

[a]Harmonized guidelines can be found at www.EPA.gov/OPPTS.
Abbreviations: EEC, European Economic Community; OECD, Organization for the Economic Cooperation and Development; US EPA, United States Environmental Protection Agency; TSCA, Toxic Substance Control Act; US FDA, United State Food and Drug Administration; MHW, Ministry of Health and Welfare; MAFF, Ministry of Agriculture, Forestry and Fisheries; MOL, Ministry of Labor; MITI, Ministry of International Trade and Industry.

from the Office of Prevention, Pesticides, and Toxic Substances (OPPTS) to investigate the effects of chemicals or pesticides, the studies are predominantly performed in rodents only. However, for the registration of pesticides, a chronic study in beagle dogs, which may be preceded by a subchronic study, will be required. Europe, Canada, and Japan generally follow these same guidelines.

The historical emphasis in multidose studies has been on defining a "no-observed-effect level" (NOEL) or "no-observed-adverse-effect-level" (NOAEL) and identifying potential target organs and systems. These are usually qualified in more than one species and for different durations.

STUDY DESIGN AND STUDY PARAMETERS

Repeat-dose general toxicity studies in laboratory animals are designed to monitor as many bodily functions as possible to maximize the potential for identifying adverse effects and target organs. Although there are some differences between the conduct of rodent and nonrodent studies, these are largely the consequence of practical considerations in handling of the different species. In general, the study designs have become standardized to a considerable degree irrespective of the species, the treatment duration, or the regulatory agency for which it is conducted such that a regular set of measured parameter are routinely included (Table 2). This standardization allows for objective comparison of different test materials in similar studies and also aids in species to species extrapolation. However, one must be careful that this same standardization does not lead to the mechanical design of studies without regard to the known or projected activity of a test material or to the species under study. The preclinical evaluation of novel biotechnology products can be a particular challenge in designing appropriate studies (1–3). Some possible additional endpoints to add to a basic study design are discussed in the "target organ" section at the end of this chapter, but these suggestions are by no means a complete listing of possible markers or assays that could be considered.

Table 2 Basic Multidose Study Design in Rodents and Nonrodents

	Rodent	Nonrodent
Number of animals	10–15/sex/group	3–4/sex/group
Number of PK satellites	3–25/sex/group	Not needed
Age at initiation	~6 weeks	~4–6 months
Common dosing methods	Oral gavage, diet, iv, inhalation	Oral capsule, oral intubation, iv
Common blood sampling methods	Retro-orbital, cardiac puncture, lateral tail vein, jugular, posterior vena cava	Posterior vena cava, saphenous, cephalic and femoral vein
Parameters measured		
Clinical observations	At least weekly	At least weekly
Body weight	At least weekly	At least weekly
Food consumption	At least weekly for the 1st month	At least weekly for the 1st month
Ophthalmosopic exam	Pretest, end of treatment	Pretest, end of treatment
Electrocardiographic exam	Not routine	Pretest, end of treatment
Hematology	At least once	Pretest, at least once during treatment
Clinical chemistry	At least once	Pretest, at least once during treatment
Urinalysis	Metabolism cage, at least once	Metabolism cage or catherization, pretest, at least once during treatment or at necropsy
Gross necropsy	Standard	Standard
Organ weight	At least liver and kidney	At least liver and kidney
Histopathology	At least high dose and control, target organs	At least high dose and control, target organs
Statistics	Various methods applicable	Very limited due to small group size

Abbreviation: PK, pharmacokinetics.

Study Basics

All good laboratory practices (GLP) studies require a signed and dated protocol. The protocol is the unique driving document for a study and is required by regulatory agencies to itemize all specifications and endpoints for a toxicology study. This is usually an extremely detailed document and is supplemented by standard operating procedures. This combination ensures that variation in procedures and endpoints are kept to minimum, and there is a high level of confidence in the accuracy and consistency of any results. The requirements for a protocol are specified in GLP regulations (see Chapter 1), together with the procedures to be followed for changing or amending the document during a study.

There are generally two key personnel responsible for a study, usually a toxicologist (who acts as the official study director and has final oversight of the study) and a veterinary pathologist.

Test Material Formulation and Administration

When embarking upon a series of toxicity studies, whenever possible, the test article to be investigated should be "technical grade" material or of similar composition to what humans are expected to be exposed to. The material should be well characterized with respect to purity, stability, and contaminant profile. The carrier or vehicle used in formulation of the test material should also be as well characterized as the test article, and any separate preparation processes should be clearly documented with expiration dates as appropriate. Dietary studies also require characterization of the vehicle. Not only must the diet be certified, but also lot numbers and expiration dates must be recorded.

It is essential that a clear chain of custody is established for the test material at the testing facility and that all activities involving the material are unambiguously documented. A material safety data sheet (MSDS) should accompany the compound on arrival, a description of the material should be recorded and matched to that documented by the supplier, storage conditions, and expiration date should be recorded and, all usage monitored by weighing containers before and after use. In addition to the prestudy characterization mentioned above, the test article should be analyzed by the test facility or supplier, on completion of the study, to confirm stability during storage over the duration of use.

Routinely, the vehicle used in formulating the test article is also appropriate for use as the control. A solution for intravenous administration should ideally be prepared in physiological saline; however, a more complex buffered vehicle containing preservatives may also be used, and this should also be used for administration to the control group, at the same dose volume and concentration as used in the high dose group. This is also true for gavage solutions or suspensions, dietary preparations, dermal formulations, and liquids to be nebulized for inhalation exposure. In the latter case, should the inhalation study be an investigation of a chemical or pesticide (for the EPA), then the entire formulation is considered to be the test article, and an air control (breathing room air) would be appropriate.

If the test material is insoluble in regular vehicles, there is a range of materials that can be used as vehicles or carriers to create suspensions. The most commonly used are methylcellulose and carboxymethylcellulose at concentrations of 0.1% to 1.0%, corn oil or polyethylene glycol (commonly a molecular weight of 400 is used and designated as PEG 400). Tween 80 can be used at low concentrations in combination with polymers as a surfactant to improve dispersion. However, adverse effects, especially in the gastrointestinal (GI) tract (diarrhea or soft stool), are associated with these vehicles. In addition, care must be taken during administration, as aspiration of the vehicle into the lungs can be fatal for the animal.

Analytical assessment of all formulations (solutions, suspensions, and diets) should be made during the study. Solutions should be checked for concentration and stability. Suspensions and diets also require a check for homogeneity. Capsule dosing (usually in dogs and occasionally in primates) requires confirmation of the concentration and stability of the test article in the gelatin capsule. Inhalation studies require an initial check of dosing solutions prior to atmosphere generation as well as frequent checks of the concentration of the test material in the generated atmosphere. As a minimum, for a subacute study, a check at the start and end of treatment is recommended. For subchronic and chronic studies, a check at the start, middle, and end of treatment is the usually accepted minimum.

Studies can be performed using a variety of dose routes to accommodate various formulation types and exposure scenarios. Wherever possible, the intended route of administration or potential exposure in humans should be mimicked in these safety studies. Routes of administration that are frequently used include oral, intravenous, subcutaneous, inhalation, intramuscular, and dermal, with, less often, intrarectal, intranasal, intravaginal or ocular. The oral route can be subdivided into active administration (i.e., gavage, intubation, or capsule) and passive dosing (i.e., adding the test article to the animal's food or water).

The formulation type, the dose route and dose regimen should be as close as possible to those expected for human exposure but should also take into account practical limitations of bioavailability or humane considerations. For example, pharmaceuticals are dosed according the expected clinical dosing regimen, and chemicals being safety tested for occupational exposure are usually administered five days per week. Such routes as intravenous, dermal, and inhalation are relatively easy to transfer from the animal studies to human risk assessment if toxicokinetic data are available. Oral gavage and dietary administration in rodents offer two widely differing oral presentations of the test article. The gavage route is a rapid, accurate way to deliver a bolus dose of an agent similar to that when administering solutions, suspensions, or tablets to humans. Incorporation of the test article into the diet offers a slower rate of absorption, better mimics unintentional human exposure to some chemicals, such as pesticides or food additives, and helps avoid peak plasma effects associated with bolus dose administration.

Test System

The various global regulatory testing guidelines generally require rodent studies as a minimum and in many cases also require nonrodent studies. The rat is considered the rodent species of choice for routine multidose toxicology studies (see Chapter 2). It's compact but practical size and relatively consistent genetic profile have encouraged its use and provide a comprehensive background database. Although mice offer economies of scale for test article use, their small size can render some routine procedures impractical. Thus, mice are usually limited to use in the carcinogenicity study and accompanying range-finding type studies. Procedures requiring extensive handling and biologic sampling are more suited to larger nonrodent species; the beagle dog is the most common choice. The dog provides a consistent, docile, and relatively cheap model to work with. However, under select circumstances the dog is an unsuitable nonrodent model, and primate studies are usually conducted in their place. Primates (cynomolgus monkey, rhesus monkey, baboon, or marmoset) offer a species genetically closer to humans and therefore theoretically more likely to identify potential hazards of some compounds to humans. Substitution of a more unusual species as the second nonrodent test model may be appropriate in some instances, though a justification must be given.

Preclinical evaluation of biotechnology products requires additional considerations for the selection of the appropriate species (2,3). Justification must be provided for the pharmacological relevance of the proposed species according to drug action or tissue specificity. Wherever possible, the testing program should include at least one species that demonstrates this specificity, and the use of transgenic animals or models of the disease should be considered when no cross reactivity can be demonstrated in common laboratory species. In practice, the majority of biologics are tested in rats and beagle dogs or non-human primates, but sometimes in only one species depending upon the specificity, clinical indication, and the stage of compound development.

Generally, purpose bred and "disease-free" animals are preferred. The study is initiated using young, growing animals, equal numbers of males and females per group (rats commonly 10–20/sex/group; dogs 3–8/sex/group), and usually three treated groups and one vehicle control group.

Most general toxicity studies utilize *ad libitum* fed rodents. However, for chronic studies, including carcinogenicity studies, the use of diet restriction has been shown to increase general health and life expectancy and may become the norm for these types of studies (4,5).

It is important that the allocation of animals to the study groups results in only healthy animals being used on the study and that body weights at the start of the treatment period are similar (not statistically significantly different). For rodent studies, a subpopulation of the animals intended for the study may have clinical pathology and postmortem examinations performed to ensure suitable health status. Suppliers of rodents should provide regular results of viral health screens from representative batches of animals.

Dogs and primates should undergo a range of in life examinations, including clinical pathology, to ensure suitability for use on the study. Animals should be allocated randomly to groups after exclusion of any animals considered unsuitable.

Number and Size of Treatment Groups

A standard study includes a vehicle control group and three test material treated groups. This concurrent control group is used for comparative purposes against the treatment groups for statistical analyses and may also indicate any adverse vehicle or environmental influences in the study. If the test material vehicle to be used in a study is of unknown potential toxicity or if there is the potential for adverse effects due to physical methods used in the study, it is may also be necessary to include a second "untreated" control group. A minimum of three treatment groups is generally required for identification of test material-related dose-response relationships, although additional treatment groups can be added as necessary.

The number of animals to be used on subacute and subchronic studies is a balance between ensuring a statistically meaningful population size and ethical considerations to use the minimum numbers of animals. Range-finding studies commonly use as little as 1–5 animals/sex/group. Subacute studies generally employ 10 rodents/sex/group or 2–3 dogs/sex/group, when the studies are to be submitted to the regulatory agencies. Subchronic studies performed using rodents usually employ 10–20/sex/group rats or mice of each sex. Dog studies can range from dogs 3–8/sex/group.

These minimum numbers are increased if one wants to include interim sacrifice periods, recovery animals, or satellite animals for biological sampling. In addition, when gavage dosing is initiated in young rodents it can be wise to allow for replacement animals for accidental deaths due to gavage accidents during the initial phase of the study.

The recovery or reversibility phase of a study follows the completion of the dosing period, and a number of the animals are retained from the control and one or more of the treated groups to assess any changes in the toxicologically relevant findings. It may not be necessary to add a recovery component to each of the treated groups. Sufficient information may be obtained from the examination of recovery animals in the high dose group alone. Nonetheless, it is important that the recovery animals are also included in the control group for comparative purposes. The need for a recovery period may only be ascertained from the results of prior repeat dose studies. For biological response modifiers, a period to assess recovery of normal physiological function is almost mandatory. For chemical entities, recovery periods are most often used to determine reversal of pharmacological effects rather than target organ toxicity. Clinical pathology and postmortem data at the end of the treatment period can give an indication of the endpoints that should be examined during the recovery phase. As stated earlier, the requirement for a recovery component increases the number of animals required on study. For rodent studies an additional five animals of each sex in each recovery group is normal. For studies using dogs or primates, one or two animals of each sex per group would suffice.

Dosage Selection

Appropriate dosage selection is one of the hardest components of study design. In general, data gathered from acute single dose studies will provide information to select appropriate dosages for a subacute study, the subacute study will provide data to select appropriate dosages for a subchronic study, and, finally, the subchronic data will aid in dosage selection for chronic studies. Key data points, from each study, that aid in dosage selection include the lowest-observed-effect level (LOEL) and the maximum tolerated dose (MTD).

To start the whole process, the current approach to acute range-finding studies uses a flexible protocol; either up and down for rodents or ascending for larger animals. This nomenclature refers to the regimen whereby the dose level is selected according to the signs of reaction at the previous dose level. The LOEL is identified as the lowest dosage producing the minimum adverse drug-related activities, whereas the MTD would be considered that dose of the agent that elicits clear evidence of toxicity but allows the animal to survive without undue distress. It is necessary to avoid the use of severely toxic doses in order to prevent unnecessary suffering in animals and to eliminate confounding factors introduced by stressed or moribund animals.

The goal is to establish a quantitative relationship between toxicity in the animals and exposure to the test material. In the ideal study, the low-dose group is equal to or a small multiple of expected human exposures and is associated with no toxicity. The mid-dose group should be conducted at the expected LOEL. However, in practice, many investigators, particularly those in industry, prefer the mid-dose to be a NOEL for risk assessment purposes because the difference between the NOEL and the expected human exposure is considered the margin of safety. Finally, the high dose should show toxicity but not enough to result in the death of more than 10% of the group. Many investigators target a 10% reduction in body weight gain as a marker of sufficient toxicity in the high dosage group. Dosage selection is most accurate for risk assessment purposes when based on plasma exposure levels. If this is not possible, extrapolation is best calculated based on surface area (mg/m^2) rather than just body weight mg/kg.

Acute studies should investigate high dose toxicity and the subsequent subacute, and subchronic studies should also yield some expression of toxic effect. However, there will be some instances where a demonstration of toxic effect requires extremely high doses that are many orders of magnitude above the expected human exposure and may require quantities of test article far beyond what is reasonable or financially justifiable. In these cases, alternative factors should be considered. For example, the U.S. EPA already imposes a "limit" to the dose levels required when testing innocuous materials (2 g/kg body weight when dosing orally and 2 mg/L of atmosphere when dosing rats by the inhalation route). There may also be physical limitations to the highest dose, such as test material solubility or saturation of kinetics that define the highest exposures possible. Many pharmaceuticals, especially protein-based drugs, have no apparent high-dose limit of toxicity and therefore cannot be evaluated in the usual way (i.e., the high-dose level would represent the "MTD"). In this case the highest dose is usually justified on the basis of plasma levels, multiples of the intended maximum clinical dose or on the establishment of the maximum pharmacological effect (provided that a sensitive species is identified). For any of these strategies it is important that the regulatory agency is consulted prior to the start of the preclinical program.

Toxicokinetics

Toxicokinetic data are required in toxicology studies used in the development of pharmaceuticals. Such systemic exposure data is less often collected for toxicity studies used for other regulatory submission. The relationship between exposure (plasma drug levels) and toxicity allows interpretation and extrapolation of the findings in different species and to relate these to potential or actual adverse effects.

The intravenous dose route represents 100% bioavailability. This reference point is used in bioavailability studies in pharmaceutical development and provides worse case toxicity for exposure by other routes. For example, if dermal exposure is one of the expected routes of human exposure, then the intravenous route mimics the increased uptake potential for damaged or diseased skin. If inhalation exposure is expected, again the intravenous route can represent a worst case scenario of diseased or damaged lungs. Such comparative data can be very useful for risk assessment analyses.

Blood analysis for the test material was initially included in toxicology studies merely to provide proof of exposure. Blood samples would be taken immediately after dosing to confirm the presence of test article and once again, immediately prior to the next dose, to assess potential for accumulation. It is now accepted that it is necessary to provide a much more complete picture of the behavior of the test article in the body. On a two-week subacute study, multiple samples should be taken after the first dose and again after the final dose. Ideally, five or more samples are taken in the 24 hours after dosing to follow the absorption and elimination of the test article. Consideration has to be given to the route of administration and the likely speed of absorption and hence the rapidity with which the maximal concentration (C_{max}) is reached (see Chapter 4).

Toxicokinetics for rats or mice on dietary studies presents specific problems. Because rodents are nocturnal they feed during the night, and diurnal fluctuations in systemic levels of the test material can be expected. It is important to determine the magnitude of these variations to assess the overall systemic exposure.

Obtaining multiple blood samples on large animal studies is relatively simple. A 10 kg beagle has approximately 750 to 1000 mL of circulating blood, of which 15% can be safely withdrawn in a single day, in any seven-day period. Therefore, more than 100 mL of blood can be taken for analysis. However, a 300 g rat has only 25 to 30 mL of circulating blood, and therefore only 2–3 mL of blood that can be taken for analysis. In addition, repeat blood sampling is difficult in rats and almost impossible in mice without compromising the animals.

It is important that the blood sampling does not compromise the primary objective of the study: to assess toxic potential of the test compound. Animals should not be lost prematurely during sampling, and the condition of the animal should not be affected by the sampling or anesthetic procedures. For these reasons, satellite animals are often included in rodent toxicity studies. These animals are treated identically to the main study animals, but no toxicology endpoints (i.e., clinical pathology, histopathology) are recorded. They are on the study solely to provide blood samples. It is usually possible to obtain three blood samples from each rat; the first two samples from the orbital sinus, under anesthetic, and the last taken from the abdominal aorta at euthanasia. An experienced technician could also obtain serial blood samples from the jugular vein, although an alternative method may be to catheterize the animals to obtain a greater number of serial samples. Mice are usually sacrificed at each blood sampling time point and sampled from the abdominal aorta.

Blood drug levels in dogs and primates are more prone to individual variability than rodents, and the use of serial blood sampling for these animals is valuable. The standard group size of three or four animals of each sex provides sufficient values at each time point to evaluate group effects.

Parameters to Be Measured

Clinical Signs

The examination of animals for ill-health and morbidity (referred to as clinical signs or clinical observations) is routinely performed on all toxicology studies. This usually entails at least a twice-daily check for mortality or overt clinical signs (at the beginning and the end of the working day). It is not normally necessary to remove the animal from the cage for this examination, but it should be sufficiently detailed to identify animals that are in distress or are showing apparently treatment-related signs. This AM/PM check minimizes unnecessary loss of data due to autolysis of animals that have died or loss due to cannibalism in gang-housed animals.

In addition, a more detailed examination is performed less often, usually at a stated time after dosing, and involves removing the animal from the cage and performing a full examination of the entire animal, including palpation for masses. In most cases, the examination can be performed by adequately trained technical staff. However, a veterinarian may be able to provide a more thorough assessment, especially in dogs and primates. Examinations should include assessment of the skin, fur condition, eyes, mucosa, gait and posture, respiratory, circulatory, and nervous system functions, and general behavior. Some laboratories now include use of functional observational battery as a screen for potential neurotoxicity.

The observation of the animals before, during, and/or following the dosing procedures makes it more likely to identify transient effects, particularly secondary pharmacologically related events. It may also document findings related to the particular dosing procedure and help in the interpretation of findings at the end of the study. An attempt should be made to ascertain the onset of the adverse event as well as the recovery time, as appropriate.

Body Weights

The body weight measurements before and during the treatment period are an integral part of all toxicology studies. Body weight is most often evaluated as changes in body weight gain because most toxicology studies are conducted with young adult animals, which are still in their growth phase. The body weights are used in the allocation of animals to dose groups, pretreatment health screening and the monitoring of the animal's condition throughout the dosing period. Body weight values are necessary for the prediction of diet concentrations, for dose per kg calculations in capsule studies, and calculation of dose volumes for gavage or injection studies. Body weights should be recorded on a weekly basis at a minimum for studies up to 13 weeks. After 13 weeks on longer-term chronic studies, body weights may be recorded less often. More frequent measurements may be necessary to monitor treatment-related effects or the health of a particular animal.

Food and Water Consumption

This should be monitored at least weekly on subacute and subchronic studies and, in conjunction with body weights, is a sensitive indicator of ill health or treatment-related effects. The measurement of food consumption can be complicated in rodent studies when animals are gang housed. Weekly food consumption values are divided by the number of individuals in the cage to estimate individual food consumption. However, this calculated number gives no indication of individual food consumption status. Thus the values may need to be adjusted or excluded from the report when animals are moribund or die during any particular week.

In studies where the test material is admixed with diet, it is important not only to monitor dietary intake to calculate exposure to the test material but also to document possible palatability problems. Food spillage should also be recorded (this is the amount that is discarded or dropped as the animal feeds and may be an indication of palatability problems) and taken into account when calculating dietary concentrations of test articles to avoid underdosing. Spillage may be measured or visually assessed from the food scattered on the tray paper under the cage.

Water consumption measurements are no longer standard on many toxicology studies. This measurement requires the filling and weighing of water bottles on a regular basis, and thus can be labor intensive in these days of available automatic watering system. On rodent and dog studies where the data are considered necessary, it is usually sufficient to measure intake for one week every six to eight weeks. It can often be difficult to generate accurate data as the animals frequently play with the drinking tubes causing considerable spillage.

Ophthalmoscopic Examination

Examination of the eye and adjacent structures for abnormalities or treatment-related effects by a trained ophthalmologist should be a routine assessment on multidose toxicology studies. The examination is performed in both the rodent and nonrodent, although the pigmented dog eye is generally considered a better model than the eye of the albino rat. This is of particular importance when testing substances known to bind to melanin. The examinations should be performed prior to treatment and again prior to termination of the study as a minimum. Interim examinations should be considered, especially if the compound may accumulate in the retina or is known to affect blood pressure. The examination should include indirect and slit lamp examinations. All regions of the eye should be included (cornea, lens, retina, conjunctiva, sclera, iris, and fundus) (6). Prior to examination, a mydriatic can be administered to allow visualization of the deeper structures without pupillary constriction.

Cardiovascular Assessments

Electrocardiography and measurement of blood pressure are generally confined to nonrodents but can, when necessary, be assessed during rodent studies as well. Similar to ophthalmic examination, this procedure should be performed prior to the study start to establish individual baselines and again before termination, with interim assessments if appropriate. It is important that measurements are performed at similar times of day and, ideally, prior to dosing, to avoid transient pharmacological effects that can be assessed by additional measurements following dosing.

Each species has different requirements for the placement and even the type of electrode employed. In busy laboratory settings, electrocardiograms (ECGs) are often recorded using limb leads alone. Although additional information can be obtained by the use of chest leads, the time involved in preparing the animal often makes it impractical.

Systolic blood pressure can be measured indirectly by using a pediatric cuff, and systemic blood pressure can be measured directly in dogs by an arterial catheter in the ear artery. It is not feasible to measure systemic pressure in rats in standard toxicity studies.

Clinical Pathology

All multidose toxicity studies should include hematology, blood biochemistry, and urinalysis at least once during the study, usually near the end of treatment. Studies longer than 13 weeks also usually include one or two interim samples. In addition, prior to treatment, all nonrodents should be sampled and analyzed to ensure suitability for testing and to establish baseline values. For rodent studies, a subpopulation can be sampled prior to initiation of dosing as a general health screen.

As discussed in the Toxicokinetic section above, it is important that the blood sampling methodology and the volume of blood taken does not compromise the health status of the animals. Blood samples are usually obtained from the jugular vein or femoral vein of conscious dogs or primates, respectively. Rodents may be sampled by a variety of methods, depending on the blood volumes required. During the study, rodents can be lightly anesthetized and sampled via the jugular vein or orbital sinus, and conscious rodents can be restrained and bled from the lateral tail vein. At termination of the study, rodents can be anesthetized and blood obtained from the abdominal aorta or by cardiac puncture. However, both the sampling method and fasting state of the animal needs to be factored in when interpreting the data. For example, blood samples from tail cuts can result in anomalous results due to the extrusion of extracellular fluids and damaged cell constituents into the samples. It is also important that the blood be sampled at approximately the same time of day and that the sampling be randomized among the treatment groups to avoid confounding changes in blood constituents due to circadian rhythms.

Urine samples are obtained passively by housing the animals in metabolism cages over a given period of time. Dogs and primate urine can also be collected by catheterization of the urinary bladder.

Table 3 presents a list of clinical pathology parameters often measured in multidose studies (see also Chapter 5 for more details). Specific parameters for analysis may differ slightly according to the regulatory agency and type of compound being tested. These parameters can be considered a basic screen, and additional analyses should be considered when investigating specific pharmacological effects or concerns.

An analysis of the hematopoietic system provides an overall assessment of the circulating blood, focusing primarily on the erythrocytes, the leukocytes, and clotting ability. Parameters associated with the status of erythron include the erythrocyte (red blood cell) count, hematocrit, and hemoglobin concentration, complimented by the morphology assessment and the erythrocyte indices.

For standard clinical pathology assessments, the total number of leukocytes are counted, a blood smear prepared, and a white cell differential count performed, including identification of any abnormal morphology. The leukocytes are categorized into lymphocytes, neutrophils, eosinophils, basophils, and monocytes as a percentage of the total leukocyte count. Absolute values for the leukocytes should be calculated routinely to evaluate changes in cell numbers. In carcinogenicity studies, red, and white blood cell counts are used primarily as a tool for identifying hematopoietic cancers (e.g., leukemia).

The blood clotting system is the third part of the hematopoietic system to be evaluated (7). A platelet count may be the only measurement possible when the relatively large blood volumes for clotting time assessments cannot be obtained. Any reduction in platelet numbers (thrombocytopenia) can have significant effects on the well-being of the animal. The total bleeding time is a means of assessing overall coagulation efficiency that

Table 3 Standard Hematology, Clinical Chemistry, and Urinalysis Parameters

Hematology	Clinical chemistry	Urinalysis
Hemoglobin	Urea nitrogen	Color and turbidity
Hematocrit or packed cell volume	Creatinine	Specific gravity
Red blood cell count	Electrolytes (Na, K, Cl)	Osmolality
Reticulocyte count	Calcium phosphorus	pH
Erythocytic indices (MCV, MCH,	Total CO_2	Protein
MCHC, RDW)	Alanine aminotransferase	Urobilinogen
White blood cell count	Aspartate aminotransferase	Bilirubin
Differential white blood cell count	Gamma glutamyl transferase	Electrolytes (Na, K, Cl)
Platelet count	Alkaline phosphatase	Nitrites
Mean platelet volume	Lactate dehydrogenase	Glucose
Prothrombin time	Total protein	Ketones
Activated partial thromboplastin time	Albumin	Occult blood
	Globulin (calculated)	Creatinine
	Total bilirubin	Microscopic sediment
	Cholesterol	
	Triglycerides	
	Glucose	
	Bile acids	

Abbreviations: MCV, mean corpuscular volume; MCH, mean corpuscular hemoglobin; MCHC, mean corpuscular hemoglobin concentration; RDW, red cell distribution width; Na, sodium; K, potassium; Cl, chloride; CO_2, carbon dioxide.

can be applied to a range of species. It requires the production of a standardized incision and the monitoring of the subsequent bleeding time. When samples can be taken into citrate anticoagulant, further investigation can be performed on activated partial thromboplastin times or prothrombin times, assessing the intrinsic and extrinsic coagulation pathways, respectively.

Blood chemistry analysis can be especially useful to help identify target organs of toxicity as well as the general health status of the animal. It is important that animals are fasted prior to sampling to prevent dietary influences on glucose levels and, to a lesser extent, potassium or phosphorus concentrations. In addition, an assessment of the degree of hemolysis in the sample should be made as potassium concentration and lactate dehydrogenase (LDH) activity may be affected and assays employing colorimetric endpoints, such as bilirubin, may be compromised.

Urinalysis is easy to perform, but interpretation is fraught with difficulty due to the crude procedures often used in collection. Possible contamination of the samples with hair, dust, bacteria, and food should be taken into account as well.

Postlife Observations—Necropsy and Pathology

On completion of the dosing and/or recovery period the animals are euthanized, and a postmortem (necropsy) examination performed. The primary purpose is to obtain tissue samples for histopathological examination. Significant information can also be obtained from gross observations and organ weights. If animals are killed before the scheduled study termination or die unexpectedly, a postmortem examination should be performed and tissues retained. Organ weights are usually not recorded for animals that die on study due to inherent inaccuracies induced by autolysis.

A number of methods can be used for euthanasia, including lethal chemical injection and asphyxiation. The selection of a particular method can be dependent on the type of postlife parameters needed. For example, an injectable anesthetic is more suitable for inhalation studies so that there is no interference in lung histopathology assessment. The order of necropsy should be randomized to minimize variations in the data related to individuals or the time of sacrifice. Immediately after euthanasia, any blood samples and/or urine samples should be taken for clinical pathology, and a bone marrow smear prepared. For animals dying on study, blood samples should be taken whenever possible as they may provide valuable information for the interpretation of the cause of death. However, such data are not included in the statistical analyses for the treatment group. Following euthanasia and fluid sampling, the animals are usually exsanguinated, which helps reduce the variability in subsequent organ weights.

A proper necropsy should include a gross evaluation of all major organ systems. Examination should also include an external evaluation of body condition, such as staining or hair loss, and should correlate with any in-life findings. Even on short-term studies the animals should be palpated for subcutaneous masses. All findings should be recorded in a precise, descriptive, and consistent manner, indicating location, size, shape, color, and type of change or lesion. It is important that descriptive terms rather than diagnostic or interpretive terms be included in the raw data. Any possible artifacts induced by the method of euthanasia or method of prosection (i.e., incision, cutting, removal, and trimming of tissues) should be noted.

A full list of tissues together with any macroscopic abnormalities should be placed into fixative for future processing and examination. The list of tissues retained on completion of toxicity studies is variable according to species and regulatory authority. Table 4 presents a generic list that satisfies the majority of cases.

Organ Weights. Some regulatory guidelines require that key organs be weighed during the necropsy of each animal in standard multidose toxicology studies. Regardless of requirements, most laboratories make this a routine part of their necropsy procedures because organ weight changes can be very sensitive indicators in many toxic events (8). However, variability in organ weights of rodents in studies of greater than one-year duration indicate little scientific rationale for recording organ weights in these studies (9). The most commonly weighed organs are the liver, lungs, kidneys, spleen, and gonads, as well as suspected or known target organs.

Calculations generally include organ weight to body weight ratios. However, if body weight changes occur on study, such ratios can often be misleading. Therefore, it is also customary to include organ weight to brain weight ratios, which are generally less variable because test-material-associated body weight changes do not generally affect brain weight.

In order to minimize spurious variation in organ weights, it is important to use consistent and careful dissection techniques. Common confounding factors include remaining tissue or fat adhering to the organ, entrapped blood, and variations in cutting (e.g., where the spinal cord is cut when weighing the brain). Careful technique is also necessary for insuring the integrity and quality of the tissue for subsequent histopathologic evaluation. Other experimental factors that can influence organ weights that often are overlooked include local environmental conditions affecting organ hydration, the method of euthanasia, the extent of time between death and necropsy, the fasting state of the animal, and exsanguination state.

Most organ weights are recorded to the nearest 1 mg. Smaller organs, such as the thyroid, adrenal, and pituitary, are weighed to the nearest 0.1 mg. An evaluation of the accuracy of organ weights revealed that reporting too many significant figures tends to limit their interpretive usefulness, whereas recording the weights with too few figures can also limit their usefulness (9,10).

Table 4 Tissues for Histopathological Processing and Examination

Abnormalities observed at necropsy	Mammary gland (inguinal)
Animal identification (not processed)	Optic nerves
Adrenals	Ovaries
Aorta (thoracic)	Pancreas
Bone and marrow (sternum)	Pituitary
Brain (cerebrum, cerebellum, midbrain, and medulla oblongata)	Prostate
Cecum	Rectum
Cervix	Salivary gland
Colon	Sciatic nerve
Duodenum	Seminal vesicles
Epididymides	Skeletal muscle
Esophagus	Skin
Eyes	Spinal cord
Harderian glands	Spleen
Heart (including section of aorta)	Stomach
Ileum	Testes
Jejunum	Thymus
Kidneys	Thyroid lobes (and parathyroids)
Lacrimal glands	Tongue
Liver (sample of 2 lobes)	Trachea
Lungs (all lobes)	Urinary bladder
Lymph nodes (mandibular and mesenteric)	Uterine horns
	Uterus
	Vagina

Histopathology. The list of tissues that should be examined is variable according to species and the regulatory agency. The site from which some tissue samples are taken can be critical to accurate interpretation of histopathology data. For example, it is important to select the same site for bone sampling in all animals within a particular study because it is known that even minor differences can influence histomorphologic variables.

For dog or primate studies, tissues from all groups are usually processed and examined (this corresponds to approximately 1500 tissues). Due to the larger number of rodents per group, the initial examination normally comprises all tissues from the control and high-dose groups and any animals that died prematurely, plus any abnormal tissues from the intermediate and low-dose groups. If any treatment-related changes are identified in the high dose group, these target organs in the low and intermediate groups or recovery animals should then be examined. A valid histopathologic evaluation should always include a peer review process for any study conducted for regulatory submission. This involves a check of a percentage of the diagnoses in a particular study by a second pathologist.

The proper fixation, slide preparation, and staining of individual organs or tissues are critical to accurate interpretation of any histopathologic finding. The majority of tissues are fixed in neutral buffered 10% formalin. The lungs should be infused with fixative after weighing. Tissues, such as eyes, testes, and epididymides, that possess a thick capsule and are preserved whole, require a faster penetrating fixative to avoid degradation during the fixation process. Commonly used fixatives for these organs include Bouin's, Davidson's, or Zenker's solutions. Tissues are routinely prepared for histopathological examination by embedding in paraffin wax, sectioning onto slides and stained. Hematoxylin and eosin stain is used routinely for tissues from toxicity studies and requires considerable experience to produce consistently stained sections. The hematoxylin serves as a powerful nuclear stain (blue), and the counter stain (or secondary stain) eosin differentiates the cytoplasm into various shades of pink. In addition to the routine staining, specialized staining methods can provide help in discerning specific compound-related changes in particular organs.

On GLP studies, histopathologic evaluations should entail proper peer review and quality assurance audit of the process to ensure the integrity and consistency of any findings.

Additional Endpoints

In some studies additional "nonstandard" endpoints may be warranted based on known pharmacological or toxicological findings in earlier studies. Early in vivo and in vitro pharmacological screens can also help identify possible unwanted receptor binding and other biochemical targets that may lead to specific toxicity (11). With the advent of new immunology and safety pharmacology testing guidelines, some investigators suggest adding additional functional testing into their protocols (12,13). However, it is important that any additional endpoints not interfere with the conduct and interpretation of the general study; otherwise a separate study to investigate such additional endpoints would be necessary. Some additional tests and markers that may be added to identify specific organ toxicity are discussed in the "Target organ" section at the end of this chapter.

DATA REPORTING, ANALYSIS, INTERPRETATION, AND RISK ASSESSMENT

Documentation and Reporting

A study report written for submission to regulatory agencies must contain at a minimum: the title and purpose of the study, the facility performing the experiment, the key personnel involved in the study, and details of the timing of various study activities. All data collected data should be included in the report in the form of individual data tables and summary data tables with the results of any statistical analysis. The bulk of the report text is divided between a description of the study design and the experimental methods used and the presentation and interpretation of the data. The experimental methods section is usually a reflection the study protocol. All protocol amendments and deviations form the original protocol or SOPs should be identified. Standard subacute or subchronic toxicity tests should present detailed results and discussion sections as well as an outline of the study in the form of a summary. The summary or study abstract should be an independent document that provides critical details of the methods and results. It should include only those findings considered related to treatment, and it is important that the conclusion reflects the purpose of the study as defined in the protocol.

Data Analysis and Interpretation

The use of statistical tests on data from studies with group sizes of at least 10 animals is routine and a valuable tool in data interpretation. Statistical analysis almost always uses comparison to concurrent control data (and/or positive control data, if included). Numerous different methods of statistical analyses can be used. It is common to follows a decision tree with the data first assessed for homogeneity of variance, followed by an appropriate analysis of variance, such as in the example shown below:

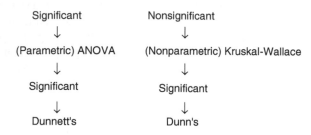

Bartlett's Homogeneity of Variance

Significant	Nonsignificant
↓	↓
(Parametric) ANOVA	(Nonparametric) Kruskal-Wallace
↓	↓
Significant	Significant
↓	↓
Dunnett's	Dunn's

Although statistical analysis is an effective way of assessing large amounts of data, it is just as important to consider the biological significance of the effect, along with an understanding of the limitations of the study design. The biologic, toxicologic, and statistical significance of a particular effect are often interpreted differently. The use of compiled data from the control groups of previous studies (historical control data) can be useful when trying to ascertain whether any particular data point is within expected biological variation.

The presence or lack of a dose-response can also be a useful tool in deciding whether an effect is test material related. Generally, if an effect occurs in several test groups without a dose relationship, the same effect is usually found in the control group as well. This is a strong indication that the effect is not caused by the test material. Trend analysis is useful in evaluating dose-responses.

For nonrodent species, the use of statistical analysis is usually not appropriate, due to the small group sizes. Therefore, findings in nonrodent studies tend to be viewed on an individual basis rather than relying on group results. Most often the test values obtained during the treatment period are compared with individual pretreatment values or the laboratory background data. In this way the individual animal becomes its own control. Baseline data is particularly useful when assessing the results of hematological and clinical chemistry data. The toxicologist gives as much weight to comparison of clinical data from a dog during treatment with that of the same animal before treatment started, as they do with comparing the results of treated animals with the controls.

This approach is more difficult for the rat, mainly because it is not practical to take the pretreatment samples for the large number of animals on study. In rodent studies, it is more common to give more weight to group findings than to individual findings, because it is possible to apply appropriate statistical methods to large group size rodent data. For many endpoints, the number of affected animals versus the number of unaffected animals in each group can also be a measure of severity.

Target organs or systems are identified using all of the measured parameters on the study (i.e., clinical chemistry, ECG, ophthalmologic examination, organ weights, and histopathology). When possible the latency to onset of a finding should be identified and any reversibility of a toxic effect determined in recovery animals when included. Distinctions of the findings are also often qualified as expected pharmaceutical effects, secondary pharmaceutical effects, adaptive or regenerative effects, probable or possible direct toxic effects, or probable effect secondary to other perturbations (14,15).

In long-term studies tolerance may develop, such as seen with anticholinesterases, where an initial toxic effect is reduced over time due to adaptation of the biological system. Another factor to consider in interpretation of findings in longer-term studies is the potential for possible induction of the metabolic system responsible for a test materials metabolism. This could lead to decreased or increased toxicity over time, depending on whether the parent chemical or a metabolite is the responsible chemical toxin.

Interpretation of Specific Study Parameters

Clinical Signs. Clinical signs are most often thought of as a gross indication of an animal's general health. These findings are often overlooked as an important component in identifying target organ effects, and more care needs to be taken when reviewing these data. Changes, such as cyanosis, flushing, and weakness, are often the first indication of cardiotoxic effects. Piloerection of the fur and/or lacrymation (tearing of the eyes) can be indicative of disturbances of the autonomic nervous system. Discharges from the nostril can be a sign of pulmonary edema. Changes in the normal glossy coat can be indicative of effects on sebaceous glands or on grooming behavior. In some instances clinical signs can help identify very specific targets. For example, agents adversely affecting the cellular division of skin cells have been shown to cause abnormally high incidences of ulceration and inflammation in areas subjected to minor trauma of everyday life, such as the feet and tail.

Body Weights and Food Consumption. Body weight and food consumption data are considered gross indicators of general systemic toxicity. Test material–related food and body weight effects will most often demonstrate a dose-response pattern. As a general rule most investigators consider reduced body weight gain or body weight losses of toxicological significance if the reduction is at least 10% less than the mean control value. In some studies, reduction in body weight may be directly related to reductions in food consumption. The role that reduced food consumption may have played in reducing body weights may be assessed by calculating a "food efficiency index" (i.e., food consumed/body weight gained). Reduced food intake is not considered a main factor in body weight reductions if the food efficiency index is similar between the treated and control groups.

Evaluation of body weights on rodent studies can use group mean values supplemented by a statistical assessment. In larger toxicology studies, body weight and food consumption changes will most often demonstrate a dose response. Preliminary interpretation of body weight effects on studies using dogs or primates can also be performed using the group mean data but should include a review of the individual data as interindividual variation is more common in nonrodents. It is often helpful to calculate weekly and total body weight gains or changes and compare the treated and control groups. This is especially helpful in large animal studies showing greater individual variation in body weights at the start of treatment.

Ophthalmologic Examination. A trained veterinary ophthalmologist may be necessary for proper analysis of the data. Ophthalmologic findings in treated animals should be compared to possible findings from the preexposure examination for that same individual before concluding that there is a chemical effect. Microscopic examination can also confirm the findings seen with gross examination. In many instances, the interpretation of findings in some structures of the eye in terms of human risk assessment may be unclear because of the species specificity of many eye structures.

Cardiovascular Assessment. Properly employed and analyzed, ECGs can be one of the most sensitive indicators of cardiovascular dysfunction. There are marked differences between species and between sedated and nonsedated animals. The proper interpretation of ECGs usually requires a trained veterinary cardiologist. Computer assisted analyses programs are available that function in data extraction and calculation of the necessary quantitative data. However, a significant amount of information from ECGs is qualitative rather than quantitative, such as pattern recognition, and requires extensive experience in cardiac pathophysiology to identify (16–18). A typical ECG is represented in Figure 1. The amplitude and configuration of the various waves and peaks can vary by method (i.e., placement of the electrodes) and species, but all will display this general pattern. The P wave is produced by atrial depolarization, the QRS complex by biventricular depolarization and the S-T segment and T wave by ventricular repolarization. Atrial repolarization is masked by the QRS complex. Under ischemic conditions the T wave is characteristically inverted. Pathological injury to the myocardium is often manifested by elevation of the S-T segment. Hypercalcemia or hypocalcemia can result in early or late ventricular repolarization characterized by shortened or prolonged Q-T intervals, respectively.

Although blood pressure and heart rate measures are noninvasive, do not require sedation, and are easy to perform, they can be subject to significant short-term variability, greatly reducing both their sensitivity and reliability. Any interpretation of these data needs to keep such considerations in mind. Electrolyte balance and nutritional status can confound data interpretation as well.

Clinical Pathology. There are major differences between species for clinical chemistry values in healthy laboratory animals that need to be considered in any cross-species extrapolation (19–21). Significant differences can also occur based on strain, sex, and age of the animal (19,22,23).

It is important to compare any clinical pathology changes in treated animals to those values in concurrent controls for which blood was collected by identical methods and study conditions. Significant differences are observed between fasted and nonfasted laboratory animals (24). Even small differences in the collection method can influence individual clinical pathology values (25,26). For example, a small but statistically significant difference in a number of clinical pathology parameters have been reported for orbital sinus blood samples following 100% CO_2 versus 34%/66% O_2/CO_2 anesthesia in rats.

In studies where chemical pathology findings are borderline, equivocal, or inexplicable, especially in large animal studies with small group numbers, comparison with historical control values from the laboratory or animal supplier can greatly aid in data interpretation and toxicological relevance. However, such comparisons must take into account any differences in sampling methods, study conditions, and analytical methodology used in the historical control database used for comparison.

Hematology. The most common hematology change, observed across species in safety testing, is reduction in red blood cells (anemia). An increase in reticulocytes (reticulocytosis) and in severe cases erythroblasts (erythroblastemia) are an indication of accelerated production in the bone marrow following injury or hypoxic conditions. Splenic enlargement is another sign of hematopoietic injury, although spleen weight in dogs is not considered a reliable indicator of blood cellularity. Increases in blood components can also

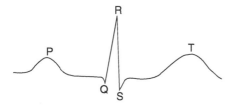

Figure 1   Typical electrocardiogram.

be a manifestation of injury, such as an increase in red blood elements (polycythemia), and is often interpreted as a regenerative overcompensation to injury.

Identification of chemical injury to the hematopoietic system is complicated by the constant cell turnover and production of new cellular components. Each cell type has a particular life span within the system, and species differences in the life spans further complicates risk assessment. In most instances, the sequence of cells disappearing from the peripheral blood will be consistent with known transit time and origin of the cell. For example in rodents, neutrophils (originating in the bone marrow with a lifespan of ~ 10 hours) are the first to decrease in the event of myeloid injury. On the other hand, reductions in thrombocytes after bone marrow injury generally take much longer to appear due to their relatively long life spans in the circulation. Lymphocytes are less affected by bone marrow injury because they predominately originate in lymphoid tissues. The amount and timing of blood sampling and fasting can also have a marked impact on reticulocyte count and hemoconcentration. In addition, there are many confounding factors to consider when interpreting changes in blood elements. Mild exercise, stress, inflammation, nutritional status, anorexia, large infusion volumes, and hemorrhage can all influence blood components. A range of historical control values for selected hematology parameters in common laboratory animals are given in Table 5. However, for specific interpretive purposes historical control data from similar strain, age, and supplier should be used.

Clinical Chemistry. When interpreting clinical chemistry data, the distinction between a chemically induced change and natural variation needs to include consideration of the species, strain, gender, age, study conditions, the time of sampling (cyclic biorhythms), diet and water intake, stress, and the route of administration of the test compound. Several environmental factors, including caging density, lighting, room temperature, humidity, and even cage bedding can influence study results. Circadian variations for some parameters, such as hormones and blood glucose levels, can be dramatic and need to be factored in to any data interpretation. One of the easiest controlled factors is diet. Fasting prior to sample collection can produce marked differences in plasma enzymes, urea, creatinine, and glucose. Biochemical changes associated with stress (caging, restraint, handling, and invasive measurements) include changes in plasma corticosterone/cortisol, catecholamines, and electrolytes. A range of historical control values for selected clinical chemistry parameters in common laboratory animals are given

Table 5 Historical Control Ranges for Selected Hematological Parameters in Laboratory Animals

	Mouse	Rat	Rabbit	Dog	Monkey
Erythrocyte count (10^6/mm^3) (RBC)	6.9–11.7	6.0–11.4	5.1–7.9	5.7–8.2	3.1–8.6
Hematocrit (mL%)	33.0–49.9	35.0–52.0	31.0–48.6	41.5–59.4	31.5–50.0
Hemoglobin (g/dL)	11.5–16.5	11.5–18.5	9.8–17.4	14.5–18.9	9.0–16.5
Mean corpuscular volume (μ^3)	45.4–53.6	45.1–65.5	57.8–68.6	64.0–86.4	57.1–90.0
Mean corpuscular hemoglobin (pg)	12.7–20.2	14.3–23.3	17.1–24.5	21.5–27.9	18.0–35.4
Leukocyte count (10^3/mm^3) (WBC)	2.0–17.1	3.0–19.0	5.2–12.5	5.5–17.7	4.5–21.6
Platelet count (10^3/mm^3)	400–1200	350–1200	175–650	150–600	100–600
Reticulocyte counts (%RBC)	0.2–3.9	0.2–2.0	0–2.0	0–0.7	0–1.4

Values collected from a wide range of published data and reviews; ranges may vary according to strain, supplier, sampling methods, anesthesia used, fasted/fed stated, gender, and age.
Abbreviations: RBC, red blood cells; WBC, white blood cells.

Table 6 Historical Control Ranges for Selected Clinical Chemistry Parameters in
Laboratory Animals

	Mouse	Rat	Rabbit	Dog	Monkey
Calcium (mg/dL)	3.2–11.8	7.2–13.9	5.6–14	9.0–11.7	8.2–12
Magnesium (mg/dL)	0.8–3.9	1.6–4.4	2.0–5.4	1.5–2.8	1.0–2.7
Phosphorus, inorganic (mg/dL)	2.3–11	3.1–11	2.3–7.8	2.7–5.7	2.8–7
Sodium (mEq/L)	128–163	140–156	132–155	139–153	143–164
Potassium (mEq/L)	3.6–9	4.0–8	3.6–6.9	3.6–5.2	3.8–6.7
Chloride (mEq/L)	105–128	97–110	92–116	100–121	100–118
Total protein (g/dL)	4.0–8.6	4.7–8.5	5.3–8.3	5.1–8.6	5.9–8.7
Albumin (g/dL)	2.3–4.8	2.7–5.1	2.4–5.0	2.5–3.5	1.8–4.8
Total bilirubin (mg/dL)	0.1–0.9	0–0.5	0–0.7	0–0.7	0.1–1.3
Total cholesterol (mg/dL)	26–170	10–100	10–83	125–275	90–220
Creatinine (mg/dL)	0.2–1	0.2–0.9	0.5–2.6	0.7–2.1	0.5–2
Glucose (mg/dL)	62.8–200	50–175	50–175	80–165	43–148
Urea nitrogen (BUN) (mg/dL)	12–40	5–29	9.2–31.7	5–24	7–26
Alanine aminotransferase (IU/L)	23.8–250	17.5–50	25–78.9	20–60	20–60
Alkaline phosphatase (IU/L)	10–180	25–300	40–120	60–260	200–800
Aspartate aminotransferase (IU/L)	20–300	45–100	10–113	30–78	12.5–60
Creatinine kinase (IU/L)	50–680	50–400	200–1000	20–400	33–1000
Lactate dehydrogenase (IU/L)	750–185	61–121	30–300	30–112	30–320

Values collected from a wide range of published data and reviews; ranges may vary according to strain, supplier,
sampling methods, anesthesia used, fasted/fed stated, gender, and age.
Abbreviation: IU, international unit.

in Table 6. However, for specific interpretive purposes historical control data from similar
strain, age, and supplier should be used.

ELECTROLYTES.   Electrolyte levels may be affected by species, gender, and age of the
animal (22). Many other, study related confounding factors, also need to be taken into
account when interpreting changes in plasma electrolyte levels. Excessive stress and use of
restraining procedures during blood collection can markedly affect potassium, calcium,
and magnesium levels. In rodents, the blood collection site and anesthesia method can also
influence electrolyte values. In many instances, the electrolyte changes are secondary to
adverse effects on renal function, dehydration and/or anorexia.

Changes in electrolytes, especially magnesium and calcium, may in turn also cause
secondary effects, such as increased cardiac tissue sensitivity, arrhythmias, or significant
changes in vascular permeability. Changes in plasma anion concentrations (chloride,
bicarbonate, and inorganic phosphate) are of lesser significance for cardiac function.

Calcium and magnesium: When considering any possible effects that increases in
calcium and magnesium may have caused in cardiac function, the concentration not bound
to proteins (free concentrations) are more important than total plasma concentrations.
Depending on the species, approximately 40% calcium and 30% magnesium are bound.
Hypercalcemia may be masked, if there is a concomitant reduction of plasma albumin, as
often seen in renal injury. Decreased magnesium can also sometimes be evident with
liver cirrhosis.

Sodium and chloride: Hypernatremia (excess sodium) or hyponatremia (deficient
sodium) may be observed in cardiac failure, depending on the volemic (i.e., hydration)
state of the animal. Decreases can also be indicative of possible adrenal or renal
insufficiency. Increased chloride can be associated with hyperventilation, renal tubular

acidosis, severe dehydration, and uremia. Decreased chloride has been observed in congestive heart failure and pyloric obstructive disease. Changes in plasma chloride levels without changes in sodium are usually associated with disturbances in the acid-base balance.

Potassium: Increases in serum potassium levels can be indicative of adrenal insufficiency, diabetic ketosis or renal injury. Reductions are often observed with excess vomiting, diarrhea, or starvation.

OSMOLALITY AND ACID-BASE BALANCE. Plasma osmolality and acid-base measurements generally have limited use in standard in toxicology studies. Although there are several formulas for the calculation of osmolality from plasma concentrations of sodium, urea, and glucose that can be used with humans blood samples, these formulas have limited applicability with other species, due to the variability of these components. In addition, these parameters should be interpreted with caution for small laboratory animals because of a high variability due to blood collection procedures.

Plasma osmolality changes can be indicative, for example, of such cardiac conditions as congestive heart failure, which can be manifested as an increase in plasma sodium levels and extracellular fluid volume with evidence of hyponatremia.

ENZYMES. When tissues are injured, damaged cells leak intracellular enzymes into the systemic circulation and/or urine. Changes in specific enzyme levels are one of the most common markers of target organ toxicity used in general toxicology studies (27). Commonly measured enzymes include aspartate animotransaminase (AST, formerly SGOT), alanine animotransaminase (ALT, formerly SGTP), alkaline phosphatase (ALP), gamma glutamyl transferase (GGT), glutamate dehydrogenase (GLDH), LDH, sorbital dehydrogenase (SDH), creatinine kinase (CK or CPK), and N-acetylglucosamidase (NAG). These enzymes are differentiated by not only what cells they can come from but also by where they are normally located in the cell (i.e., brush border membrane, lysosomes, mitochondria, cytoplasm).

As with other endpoints, certain methodological considerations need to be taken into account when interpreting any changes. Many investigators do not realize that these enzymes have a relatively short half-life in the blood as well as differing rates of clearance. In addition, different dosages of an agent can cause damage and subsequent enzyme release at different time intervals. Thus, the presence of enzymes in the blood can often be a hit-or-miss proposition, and the absence of marker enzymes should not be considered an indication that organ damage has not occurred. Chemical-induced organ dysfunction that is not associated with morphologic damage to the organ will not be detected by the presence of serum enzymes, because these enzymes are released only by dead or dying cells. Finally, some enzyme changes may be due to enzyme induction rather than morphological injury, such as in the increase in ALP that occurs with glucocorticosteroids.

The identification of toxicity-related increases in enzyme levels can be confounded by the normal presence of these enzymes in blood components. For example, both CPK and LDH should be measured in plasma rather than serum, due to the relatively high concentrations of these enzymes in platelets. Blood samples with visible signs of hemolysis should not be used, again due to extraneous enzymes from the various damaged blood cells. Damaged tissue at the site of blood collection can also lead to erroneous enzyme levels.

Creatinine phosphokinase: Creatinine phosphokinase (CK) is a cytosolic enzyme with three major isozymes: CK-MM is the muscle type isoenzyme, CK-MB is the myocardial type isoenzyme, and the third dimer, CK-BB, is the brain type isoenzyme. Confounding factors include administration route, study conditions, and animal age. Intramuscular injections cause increased plasma CK. CK values may also be affected by stress and heavy exercise. Age of an animal also affect plasma CK, with activities generally being higher in younger animals. Changes in CK are observed with muscle, cardiovascular and, pulmonary injuries and in some cerebral diseases.

Lactate dehydrogenase: LDH is a cytosolic enzyme with five major isoenzymes. The distribution of LDH in various tissues is generally ubiquitous, with large variations in normal levels between and within species. Due to the broad range of normal plasma LDH levels in laboratory animals, especially in rats and monkeys, significant changes in LDH levels are often difficult to detect and to interpret. This enzyme has a greater predictive value in humans, where there is less variability. Increases have been observed in hemolytic diseases, liver, muscle, and heart damage, pancreatitis, and anemia. When necessary, electrophorectic identification and quantification of the various isoenzymes can aid in interpretation. Although, some drugs, have been shown to modify the electorphoretic mobility of some LDH isoenzymes.

Aspartate aminotransaminase (formerly SGOT) and alanine aminotransaminase (formerly SGTP): Each of these enzymes has two isoenzymes (cytosolic and mitochondrial). These enzymes are often altered following hepatic and myocardial damage. AST and ALT are not tissue specific. However, in many laboratory animals, cardiac AST levels are higher than in most major tissues, whereas cardiac tissue ALT levels usually vary between species. In the rat, mouse, and dog, ALT levels are highest in liver. In primates, hepatic, and cardiac levels are similar.

Alkaline phosphatase: There are two major isoenzymes, osseous and intestinal. The high variability in laboratory animals, especially rats and monkeys, compared to human limits the predictive value. In young animals the osseous ALP predominates; in older animals intestinal ALP is highest. Increased ALP is generally associated with liver injury and osteoblastic bone disease.

γ-Glutamyl transferase: This enzyme is a good marker for chemically induced cholestasis in humans but less so in laboratory animals. In the rat, kidney GGT levels are 200 times higher than in the liver.

Amylase: Serum levels of this enzyme are generally elevated when pancreatitis or renal insufficiency are present. Reduction in amylase levels can be indicative of hepatobiliary toxicity.

LIPIDS. Adverse effects on lipid metabolism can be manifested as changes in plasma cholesterol, triglycerides, plasma lipoproteins, total lipids, phospholipids, apoplipoproteins, and nonesterified fatty acids. The plasma lipid pattern can vary with animal age, sex, diet, and period of food withdrawal prior to sample collection. There are both qualitative and quantitative differences in lipid metabolism in the most commonly used laboratory animals. This is due to differences in rates and routes of absorption, synthesis, metabolism, and excretion (28,29). In rat, mouse, rabbit, guinea pig, ferret, and dog, the major plasma lipoprotein classes are the high-density lipoproteins (HDL). In contrast, the major classes in primates, including humans, are LDHs. This factor has a significant impact on interpretation and extrapolation of lipid data from common toxicology test species to human risk. Plasma lipid changes are most often associated with hepatoxicity, although hypo- or hyperthyroidism is also associated with changes.

GLUCOSE. Changes in glucose concentrations are most often associated with renal injury. However, stress, including restraint, can cause marked elevations in plasma glucose levels as well. In addition, nutritional status can have a marked influence on glucose levels. Neonates are more susceptible than adults to fasting (anorexic) induced hypoglycemia due their relatively small store of glycogen. Decreases have also been reported in adrenal, thyroid or pituitary hormone deficiencies, liver disease and pancreatic tumors.

BLOOD UREA NITROGEN, CREATININE, AND BILIRUBIN. Increases in urea nitrogen, often accompanied by increased protein, can be indicative of renal injury but is not considered the most sensitive indicator (i.e., renal function can be reduced by 50% before levels are changed). On the other hand, increases in creatinine levels are considered a much more sensitive indicator of renal injury. Urea nitrogen levels are often reduced in animals with severe liver injury and overhydration conditions. Increases in total bilirubin can be indicative of excessive heme turnover by the reticulo-endotheolial system or obstruction of the bile duct (cholestatis), but the low renal threshold in rats and dogs reduces the usefulness of the marker in borderline cases.

PROTEIN AND ALBUMIN. Hypoproteinemias are usually characterized by decreases in albumin and/or globulin fractions. Possible causes include reduced hepatic synthesis, increased renal excretion, impaired nutritional status, infection, hemorrhage, and impaired intestinal and/or pancreatic function. Hyperproteinemia is most often due to dehydration. Few protein changes are pathognomonic (i.e., indicative of a specific disease or pathology).

Urinalysis. Urinalysis is the most useful noninvasive measure of kidney function. The conditions under which samples are collected are critical and must be considered when interpreting data. Reduced water consumption as well as severe emesis or diarrhea will affect urine output. A range of historical control values for selected urine parameters in common laboratory animals are given in Table 7. However, for specific interpretive purposes historical control data from similar strain, age, and supplier should be used.

VOLUME AND OSMOLALITY. If carefully collected over a specific period of time, the volume of urine may be useful for fluid balance assessments (e.g., diuresis, dehydration, etc.). Osmolality is an indicator of the ability of the kidney to concentrate urine.

pH. The pH is meaningless, unless urine is collected directly from the bladder. This is due to the quick dissipation of dissolved CO_2 after urination. Fasting, ketosis, and/or tubular dysfunction can increase the acidity of urine.

ELECTROLYTES. Electrolyte balance in the urine is highly dependent on water and food intake and other extrarenal factors (e.g., vomiting or diarrhea). They are not sensitive indicators of organ toxicity.

KETONES. Increases of ketones in the urine indicate disturbances in carbohydrate metabolism.

Table 7 Historical Control Ranges for Selected Urine Parameters in Laboratory Animals

	Rat	Rabbit	Dog	Monkey
Volume (mL/kg/day)	134–350	20–362	20–167	70–80
Specific gravity	1.039–1.078	1.003–1.036	1.015–1.050	1.015–1.065
pH	7.3–8.5	7.6–8.8	6.2–7.0	5.5–7.4
Calcium	3–9	12.1–19	1–3	10–20
Chloride	50–75	190–300	5–15	80–120
Magnesium	0.2–1.9	0.65–4.2	1.7–3	3.2–7.1
Phosphorous	20–40	10–60	20–50	9–20.6
Potassium	50–60	40–55	40–100	160–245
Sodium	90–110	50–70	20–189	NA
Total protein	1.2–6.5	0.7–1.9	1.6–5.0	0.87–2.48
Creatinine	24–40	20–80	15–80	20–60
Urea nitrogen	1–1.6	1.2–1.5	0.3–0.5	0.2–0.7

Values collected from a wide range of published data and reviews; ranges may vary according to strain, supplier, sampling methods, fasted/fed stated, gender, and age.

GLUCOSE.   Elevated glucose levels are either the result of increased blood glucose, which can be confirmed in the clinical chemistry testing, or an indication of damage to the proximal tubules. In tubular injury, changes in glucose can be a sensitive and early marker of injury.

PROTEIN.   Increased total urinary protein may indicate renal injury or extrarenal hemorrhage or inflammation. Increased proteins may also be seen with urinary tract infections. If renal injury is suspected, the ratio of high to low molecular weight proteins may differentiate tubular versus glomerular injury. A concomitant drop in albumin concentrations in the plasma may occur in cases of marked increases in urinary proteins.

ENZYMES.   Urinary enzymes are not standard in most studies because they have proven to be difficult to analyze properly and are often less sensitive than other markers of renal toxicity. However, a few enzymes can provide useful information on the site of renal injury (30,31). Urine ALP, GGT, and alanine aminopeptidase (AAP) have been used as indicators of tubule damage, and NAG has proven a reliable indicator of damage to the papilla.

SEDIMENT.   The sediment is examined microscopically for the presence of erythrocytes, leukocytes, renal epithelial cells, bladder cells, crystals, and spermatozoa. The presence of erythrocytes is indicative of hemoglobinuria, hematuria, or hepatic porphyria. Leukocytes may indicate renal or bladder bacterial infection. Crystalluria may be due to pH-dependent precipitation of urates or phosphates or may reflect high urinary concentrations of the test material and/or a metabolite. Urinary spermatozoa indicate male ejaculation dysfunction (retrograde ejaculation).

Organ Weights.   Organ weight data are commonly analyzed in relationship to body weight and brain weight. In many cases, changes in organ weights are reflective in reductions in body weight rather than direct effects of the test material. Liver, testes, adrenal, and thyroid weight changes are typical with suppression of body weight gain of 20% or more in rodents (8,32). The relative weights of the brain, kidneys, heart, spleen, pituitary, and prostate are not as highly influenced by reductions in body weight in rodents. For dogs, it has been shown that marked weight gain suppression is associated with increased liver weight, variable effects on thyroid and adrenal glands, and reductions in gonad weights. In monkeys, reductions in body weight are associated with lower liver, kidney, and testes weights.

Even in studies where there are marked reductions in body weights, direct test material effects on organ weights cannot be dismissed. For example, testicular weight is very often correlated with testicular toxicity even in anorexic animals. The uterus and ovaries present a particularly difficult interpretive problem because their weights are normally highly variable as a consequence of cyclical reproductive functions.

Increases or decreases in organ weights can be associated with test material induced changes in function and/or morphology of an organ, including disturbances in phospholipid metabolism, induction of enzymes, cellular necrosis, hypo- and hyperplasia, and hypersecretion.

Gross and Microscopic Pathology.   The proper identification of pathologic damage and interpretation of the biological significance in toxicology studies requires extensive training in veterinary pathology. It is not possible in the context of this chapter to delve deeply into this subject or any specific organ pathology. We refer the reader to Chapter 5 or to the many excellent publications for those needing more detailed information (33–36).

There are often numerous descriptions of "nonlesions" in gross necropsy reports that can mask true test material related changes. This can become a particular problem in studies in which many animals died on study. Necropsy reports on found dead animals will contain descriptions of congestion in numerous organs that is simply a reflection of blood settling after death. Similarly, in found dead animals, accumulations of gas in the intestinal tract due to autolysis should not be reported as "dilation of intestine." Thus, many morphologic findings in animals that died on study will not be related to test material treatment.

In general, lesions are evaluated in terms of possible cause. The injury can be spontaneous, related to postmortem events, a direct effect of the test material, or secondary effect to other test material–related changes. The evaluation should utilize comparison to findings in the concurrent control group and, as necessary, historical incidence rates in that strain and species. The incidence of spontaneous lesions increases with the age of the animal and can make interpretation of chronic studies particularly difficult. The functional significance of a pathologic change can be quite different depending on the etiology of the lesion.

Toxicology hazard and risk assessment relies on group and cross-study comparison. Thus, it is important for the pathologist to use standardized classifications. Care must be taken that the same lesions are not described in such different ways so that they cannot be related to one another in the final analysis. This is a particular problem when studies on a test material are conducted in more than one laboratory. In addition, deciding the significance of a particular finding can be difficult in situations where given grades of severity (e.g., mild, moderate, severe) are not predefined and used in a consistent manner by the study pathologist. Subtle lesions are always the most difficult to interpret with regards to significance to human risk assessment.

Hazard and Risk Assessment

One of the most common reactions encountered when presenting toxicology data to "non-experts" is panic. They react to the word "toxic" as if it is a lethal virus that is sure to kill a new project or product. The most important concept that the reader needs to understand is that *everything* is toxic under the right conditions and at high enough concentrations. The primary purpose of conducting animal toxicology studies is not to prove that an agent is nontoxic. Their purpose is to evaluate the particular form of toxicity that a specific compound manifests (i.e., targets of toxicity) and to ascertain the "margin of safety" of a compound (i.e., the difference between the expected exposure level under real life conditions and the exposure levels inducing significant levels of toxicity).

There are four distinct characteristics that go into defining the toxicity of a compound that are important to understand. The toxic *potential* is the actual ability of a chemical to disrupt normal physiology, morphology, and/or function. The toxic *potency* refers to the dosage and frequency of exposure at which the toxicity manifests itself. It has also been used to describe the severity and incidence rate of a particular toxic effect. The toxic *hazard* is a description of the danger (i.e., what are the target organ(s) and adverse effects caused by the agent). The toxic *risk* describes the likelihood of a toxic effect at expected (real-life) exposure levels and conditions (i.e., the steepness of the dose-response curve or, for instance, the distance between a therapeutic and a toxic dosage level). Thus, a compound that has a high or dangerous hazard profile may pose no risk to humans if exposure levels are low and the toxic potency is low.

Key dosage levels identified in toxicology studies include the NOEL or NOAEL, the LOEL or "lowest-observed-adverse-effect-level" (LOAEL), and the MTD. Using the LOEL and/or NOEL, various types of margins can be calculated that estimate expected safe exposure levels. The size of the safety margin can vary according to the route of administration, the toxicokinetics of the test compound, and the biologic activity of the test compound in each species. Extrapolation of animal data to human risk assessment can use a variety of measures of exposure, including the administered dosage (mg/kg/day), dosage corrected for surface area differences (mg/m^2), and actual measured systemic exposure (plasma AUC and C_{max}) (37–40). Irreversible changes are weighted more heavily in any assessment of possible human risk than reversible toxicities.

Most toxicological effects exhibit a normal bell shape (Gaussian) curve for dosage versus effect. The slope of the curve can give an indication of some of the intrinsic characteristics of a test compound. Two test compounds can have the same NOEL but different slopes, indicating quite different characteristics. For example, a steep curve may indicate rapid onset of action or faster absorption. When the slope is relatively flat, a larger margin of safety can be anticipated, because a large increase in dosage would be expected to produce only small increases in adverse effects. The dose-response slope is often used for extrapolation to very low and even no observable effect levels.

The particular calculation method for estimating safety margins, safe exposures, or considering risk is dependent upon whether the test compound is a pharmaceutical, food additive, agricultural chemical, industrial chemical, or environmental pollutant (41–45). Chapters 15, 16, and 17 discuss in more detail the various risk assessment strategies for pharmaceuticals, environmental/occupational exposures, and food/cosmetic products. In general, the acceptable safety margin for pharmaceuticals is highly variable, depending on a risk-benefit analysis (i.e., an acceptable safety margin for a chemotherapeutic agent can be much lower than the safety margin acceptable for a chronic drug used for a nonlethal disease). For chemicals in food, environmental or occupational exposure settings, acceptable exposure limits such as an acceptable daily intake (ADI), reference dose (RfD)-or threshold limit value (TLV) are calculated. Historically, a safety-fold factor approach has been used in such cases, such as 100-fold below the lowest observed effect level, with 10-fold for interspecies differences and 10-fold for intraspecies differences. There is no scientific basis for the use of such factors; rather this is based upon tradition and represents an empirical approach that has generally stood the test of time (46,47).

TARGET ORGANS

The general toxicology of a test agent is usually discussed in terms of identified target organs. Target organs or systems are identified using all of the measured parameters on the study (e.g., clinical chemistry, ECG, ophthalmologic examination, organ weights, and histopathology). The liver and the kidney are the most common targets of chemical toxicity, due to their major metabolic and excretory functions. At the other end of the spectrum, major toxic effects on the various endocrine organs appear to be relatively uncommon. It is unclear whether this reflects the lack of relevant measurements in most studies or the easy dismissal of endocrine gland changes as nonspecific or secondary to other effects.

In a review of published toxicology literature, Heywood estimated that in most cases target organ toxicity was generally seen at 5 to 6 times the NOEL in the rat, dog, and monkey (8). In addition, he found that the NOEL in rodents was usually 3-fold higher than in the dog and monkey. Most target organ toxicity was identified by 13 weeks of treatment. The most likely additional target organ to manifest itself after this duration of exposure was the eye. He also warned that extrapolation of safety data across species should be based on the absence of toxic signs rather than on the demonstrated target organ toxicity because there was less than a 20% correlation in target organs across species. Some correlations between dog and human target organs were established for the gastrointestinal tract, urinary tract, central nervous system, and skin. Correlation between nonhuman primates and humans were found for the gastrointestinal tract, hematopoietic system, liver, central nervous system, and skin.

Effects on a particular organ may be a primary effect of the agent or a secondary effect induced by changes elsewhere in the body. For example, an agent that injured the liver resulting in altered hepatic steroid metabolism may have secondary effects in the reproductive organs, due to subsequent changes in circulating hormones. Various confounding factors must also be considered when evaluating possible target organs. The vehicle used on the study may have adverse effects of its own that need to be separated from effects caused by the test compound. A good example of this is the vehicle cyclodextrin, which can cause renal lesions. This is one reason why it is important to include a vehicle control group in a study. Other method-related effects should also be factored in. If the animal is put under too much stress in the study, this can result in increased cortisol levels leading to acute involution of the thymus and other lymphoid tissues. Lesions can be caused by the method of administration rather than the test agent, especially in repeat dose studies. Species differences in organ morphology and weight are also important to consider. For example, the kidney weight relative to body weight is greater in rodents (0.65% of body weight) than in the dog (0.5%) or monkey (0.42%) and could have an influence on species susceptibility to renal toxins.

Some of the most common target organs are discussed below. The reproductive, nervous, immune, and respiratory system as target organs are not included as they are covered in Chapters 11, 12, 13 and 14, respectively.

Liver

The liver system (including the gallbladder and bile duct) is the most common target organ for chemical toxicity (48,49). This is due to the fact that most chemicals are metabolized in the liver before being eliminated from the body, often through the bile. The centrilobular cells are generally the most susceptible due to the fact that they have higher metabolic rates and fewer detoxification enzymes than periportal cells. Numerous different mechanisms of action have been shown to induce hepatoxicity. The type of liver injury is often dependent upon not only the particular agent and its mechanism of action but also on the length of exposure. Subacute exposures are usually associated with such findings as single cell necrosis, lipid accumulation, or cholestasis. Fibrosis and cirrhotic changes usually require longer-term chronic exposures. In addition to morphological changes, possible early signs of liver injury can be identified by changes in clinical chemistry (50).

Hepatocellular injury is associated with increases in the enzymes ALT, AST, and SDH (Table 8). Hepatobiliary injury is associated with increases in the enzymes GGT and ALP, as well as changes in bilirubin, blood urea nitrogen (BUN), and bile acids (Table 8). Other indicators of possible hepatotoxicity included altered plasma lipids, serum GLDH, and elevated urine taurine levels. GLDH and taurine levels are currently not normally included in standard protocols but have recently been shown to be very specific indicators of hepatic injury (51–53). Indirectly, most coagulation factors are synthesized in the liver and their alteration can be due to hepatic damage.

The incidence of hepatic injury can vary among species and can be reversible in some cases. In addition, the liver often responds to subtoxic and toxic exposures with adaptive responses, including enzyme induction that should be differentiated from toxic responses (54). Some types of hepatic injury are not always apparent from the

Table 8 Chemistry Changes in Blood and Urine Associated with Specific Organ Toxicity

Organ injury	Biochemical markers of injury	Comments
Hepatocellular injury	Increased ALT, AST, SDH, altered coagulation parameters, altered plasma lipids, elevated urine taurine	SDH has greater predictive value than ALT; accuracy increased when both ALT and SHD showed changes Good marker in dog; amount of hepatic ALT $5\times$ that of other tissues The proportion of AST isozymes (cytostolic vs. mitochondrial) may indicate the extent of injury
Hepatobiliary injury	Increased GGT, ALP, total bilirubin, bile acids (urinary bilirubin); decreased amylase	GGT is not a good marker of cholestasis in rats ALP in rat liver is low, limiting its predictability Bile acid and ALP changes confounded by relation to food intake Increased urinary bilirubin may occur in dog before changes in plasma total bilirubin
Renal injury—tubular	Increased serum ALP and glucose (transient) Increased urinary glucose, proteins, GGT, BUN, and creatinine	Increased urinary protein often the first sign of injury Changes in urine pH and volume can also indicate injury
Renal injury—papillary	Increased urinary NAG, proteins	Urine sediments and celluria unreliable indicators
Myocardial cell death	Increased AST, CK, and LDH with no change in ALT	CK not heart specific ECG changes (e.g., S-T elevation) also a marker
Congestive heart failure	Increased AST, ALT, and LDH with no change in CK	CK not heart specific
Muscle necrosis	Increased AST, CK, and LDH with no change in ALT	Some CK changes can also seen with physical stress or injection injury
Pancreatitis	Changes in plasma lipids, increased calcium; increased amylase levels	In severe injury, feces may contain high levels of undigested fat

Abbreviations: ALT, alanine aminotransferase; AST, aspartate aminotransaminase; SDH, sorbital dehydrogenase; GGT, gamma-glutamyltransferase; ALP, alkaline phosphatase; BUN, blood urea nitrogen; NAG, N-acetylglucosamidase; LDH, lactate dehydrogenase; CK, creatine kinase; ECG, electrocardiogram.

dose-response relationship. Standard toxicology study designs are not able to identify agents associated with immunotoxic or idiosyncratic hepatic injury, due the small number of animals. This is a large problem because such injury can occur in man and methods are being developed to help in the identification of such agents.

There are a number of diagnostic functional and clearance assays evaluating hepatic transport, uptake, conjugation, and excretion as well as in vitro test systems that can help in clarifying the extent of injury to the liver or serve as quick screens (49,55,56).

Kidney

The kidney is the second most common target of chemical injury (57,58). This is due to the fact that many chemicals are excreted through the urine. In addition, the kidney has an extensive blood supply and the glomeruli have a large surface area available for exposure.

The kidney's ability to concentrate solutes and substances also enhances its susceptibility to chemical injury. Many chemicals are known to affect renal function, but such adverse effects can vary greatly between species due to the relative morphological differences complicating extrapolation of risk (30,59). As with hepatotoxicity, there are numerous mechanisms of action causing nephrotoxicity. One of the most common sites of chemical injury are the proximal tubules, because most blood flow is delivered to this area of the kidney which functions to concentrate and reabsorb solutes. Tubular necrosis and tubular hyper- or hypoplasia are common findings. Other sites of chemical injury can include the loop of Henle and the glomeruli.

The identification of the potential to cause renal injury in animal studies is of great importance because in humans acute nephrotoxicity usually presents minimal early functional changes and the progression to chronic renal failure is silent. Clinical chemistry changes in the blood and urine can aid in identifying renal injury, although urinalysis is often a more sensitive indicator of renal damage than clinical chemistry changes. Tubular damage is often accompanied by increases in serum ALP, serum glucose, and urinary glucose, proteins, GGT, BUN, and creatinine (Table 8). Injury to renal papillary tissues can be accompanied by increases in urinary NAG and proteins.

Often the earliest sign of renal injury is an increase in urinary protein levels. In some cases tubular injury may be differentiated from glomerular injury by the ratio of high and low molecular weight proteins in the urine. More severe injury may induce reductions in the amount of urine (oliguria). The consistent production of increased volumes of urine (polyuria) may indicate alterations in renal concentrating ability (diuretic effect). Increased urine glucose in the absence of increased plasma glucose may be indicative of damage, to the proximal tubules. Changed in urine pH may also be indicative of tubular damage, but increased urine pH and chloride levels may occur with highly acidic test materials. Urine sediments and celluria is generally an unreliable indicator of nephrotoxicity, except in some incidences of acute proximal tubule damage.

Additional biochemical markers and a combination of qualitative and quantitative screening tests can be used to further define functional changes associated with renal injury (30,60–63).

Some findings in the kidney are not applicable to human risk assessment. For example, alpha 2μ-Globulin nephropathy is an important species-specific toxicologic syndrome that occurs in male rats following exposure to a number of industrial and environmental chemicals (64). In female rats, mineral deposits at the corticomedullary junction are relatively common and attributed to a reduced tubular phosphorus resorption compared to males. This finding is also not considered to predict similar changes in humans.

Cardiovascular System

Histopathologic changes in heart tissue due to chemical exposure in standard toxicology studies are relatively rare. When present, injuries are usually manifested in the myocardium as degenerative lesions and with chronic exposure, fibrosis (65). Prolonged insult can result in cardiac hypertrophy.

The primary markers of cardiotoxicity are changes in serum enzymes. However, the timing and method of sample collection can be particularly important to enable detection of cardiac damage. Serum enzymes that have been associated with injury to cardiac tissues include increases in AST, ALT, LDH, and CK (Table 8). However, it is important to note that none of these enzymes is specific for cardiac tissues. Although increases in hemoglobin and proteins in the urine may occur following cardiac injury, urinalysis is generally not useful in detecting cardiac pathology.

Chemicals can also target the blood vessels producing degenerative and/or inflammatory lesions (66). Identification of vascular toxicity currently relies on histopathological evaluation because there are no unequivocal biochemical markers of arterial injury.

In most cases, cardiotoxicity is manifested as acute, transient, functional responses. If the animal survives, the effect is usually reversible. These functional responses include bradycardia, tachycardia, and various forms of arrhythmia. In pharmacological safety testing, such cardiovascular changes are generally considered to be exaggerated pharmacological effects rather than toxicological effects. Agents that induce such functional changes in the heart are described as having chronotropic effects (act on heart rate), dromotropic effects (act on conductivity), bathmotropic effects (act on excitability), or inotropic effects (act on contractility). Specific changes in ECG waves can indicate possible causation. For example, ischemia conditions are characterized by an inverted T wave, pathological injury to the myocardium is often manifested by elevation of the S-T segment, and altered calcium levels can result in early or late ventricular repolarization characterized by shortened or prolonged Q-T intervals, respectively.

Cardiovascular effects of chemicals can also be manifested as hypotension, hypertension, hemorrhage, thrombosis, and embolism. Nutritional status, electrolyte imbalance, anemia, and thyroid dysfunction can all be secondary factors causing cardiac dysfunction.

Skeletal Muscle

A large number of chemicals and biological agents have been associated with necrosis and degeneration of skeletal muscle in animals and humans (36). Most of these agents can also produce myocardial damage. An increase in CK in the blood is one of the most sensitive and specific enzymes related to muscle injury (Table 8). However, small increases in CK may be indicators of physical stress (i.e., exercise) or injury from intramuscular injection. Furthermore, CK levels are usually not elevated when injury is due to myoneuronal injury. Other enzymes, such as succinate dehydrogenase, aspartate aminotransferase, LDH, and acid phosphatase, may also be associated with muscle injury and repair.

Hematopoietic System

The hematopoietic system is often overlooked as a possible target for chemical injury (67). This complex system includes the bone marrow, circulating blood cells, spleen, lymph nodes, and reticulendothelial tissue in various organs. The bone marrow, which is responsible for the production of all blood components, is particularly vulnerable to cytotoxic agents due to the rapid cell division within the marrow. Many chemicals can injure the system without damaging the marrow by such mechanisms as oxidative hemolysis within the circulation and immunotoxic reactions with blood components. Effects on the hematopoietic system can be manifested as a reduction in the number of all formed elements (pancytopenia), reductions in circulating red or white cells (anemia and granulocytopenia), thrombocytes (thrombocytopenia), or in individual components (e.g., leukopenia, lymphocytopenia). Changes in spleen weight in rodents can be a sensitive indicator of hypo- or hypercellularity of blood cells. However, spleen weight is not generally a reliable indicator of hematopoietic cellularity in the dog.

Gastrointestinal Tract

There are very few agents that specifically target the gastrointestinal tract (68). However, this system, especially the intestines, is particularly vulnerable to cytotoxic agents due to the high rate of cell division. Stomach lesions, such as ulcerations and inflammations, are also relatively common in studies using oral gavage administration with agents that have an irritant effect.

Disturbances of the GI tract are easily observed and usually manifested as vomiting, excessive salivation, or changes in feces (soft stool, diarrhea, absence of stool, bloody stool). These effects will often result in changes in blood and urine electrolytes due to fluid loss. Prolonged or extreme fluid loss will also affect the hematocrit, plasma proteins, and urine osmolality. Severe ulceration and/or necrosis will often result in occult or frank blood in fecal matter. Changes in serum and urine glucose, lipids, and urine ketones are indicative of alterations in carbohydrate metabolism. Testing the functional status of the gastrointestinal tract (e.g., intestinal permeability and stomach motility) usually require a separate study due to potential interference with other general toxicity endpoints.

Eye

The eye contains numerous targets for chemical damage, due to its complexity and wide range of cell types, and is considered a highly sensitive organ system (69). Injury is most often the result of direct irritation due to accidental exposure. However, chemical-induced lesions can also occur in many structures of the eye following systemic exposure. The most common targets include the retina, cornea, and lens. Chemical compounds with a high affinity for melanin are often associated with some levels of retinopathy. Cataracts are also a fairly common, but their significance needs to be considered in relation to the age of the animal. Identification of toxic injury in standard toxicology studies is dependent upon ophthalmoscopic examination and histological evaluation by a veterinary ophthalmologist and pathologist, respectively (70). There are no specific clinical pathology parameters indicative of injury to the eye.

Skin

Toxicity of the skin is usually the result of direct irritation or contact sensitization following dermal or subcutaneous administration (71). Lesions can vary from mild swelling to epidermal necrosis. Systemic toxicants can also result in adverse effects. As mentioned earlier, cytotoxic agents can adversely affect the rapidly dividing skin cells, causing ulceration and inflammation of the epidermis/dermis and can also target the rapid mitotic activity in hair follicles, resulting in alopecia. Some cytostatic agents are known to cause localized damage to the sweat glands resulting in inflammation and necrosis (anhidrosis).

Endocrine Organs

Adrenal

The adrenal cortex is one of the most vulnerable of the endocrine glands to chemical-induced injury (72,73). Its susceptibility is due in part to the lipophilic nature of the organ, which can promote deposition and accumulation of hydrophobic xenobiotics. The gland also has a good blood supply and a relatively high concentration of metabolizing enzymes, making it more likely to be exposed to toxic intermediates.

In addition to androgens and estrogens, the adrenal cortex produces glucocorticoids, which play a role in the metabolism of carbohydrates, lipids, and proteins in the liver, and mineralocorticoids, which play a role in electrolyte transport by regulating renal sodium and potassium reabsorption and excretion. Thus, alterations in adrenal gland function can have numerous secondary effects in the body, including changes in metabolism, electrolyte balance, cardiac function, and steroidogenesis. An important consideration when extrapolating adrenal findings in the rat to risk in man is that such lesions in the rat are usually not hyperfunctional (i.e., do not produce symptoms of hypertension). However, in humans this is usually the case.

Thyroid and Parathyroid

Thyroid hormones regulate the metabolism of virtually every organ. However, the binding and excretion of key thyroid hormones (triiodothyronine, thyroxine, and thyrotropin) can show marked species differences, and findings can often have little relevance to human risk assessment. Most chemicals that interfere with the secretion of thyroid hormones do so through iodine trapping or blockage rather than direct pathological injury to the gland (74). Hyper- or hypothyroidism can be accompanied by changes in serum cholesterol and CK levels.

Pancreas

The pancreas has both exocrine and endocrine functions. Injury to the pancreas is often indicated by increases in plasma glucose, lipid, and calcium levels. Increases in amylase and lipase levels are also associated with pancreatitis but are not usually included in a standard panel of serum enzymes. Species differences in the molecular structure of the pancreatic hormones insulin and glucagons inhibit the use of immunoassays across studies. However, a number of relatively simple assays are available for evaluating pancreatic exocrine function when the pancreas is a suspected target organ (75,76).

Pituitary-Gonadal Axis

Alterations in the mammary gland, ovaries, and testes can be a sensitive indicator of perturbations of the pituitary-gonadal axis. None of the standard clinical pathology parameters included in a standard protocol are specific indicators of alterations in pituitary function. Androgens, estrogens, and other hormones involved in the axis can be added to the clinical chemistry as necessary.

FUTURE TRENDS

The design of multidose toxicology studies has become standardized over the years for both rodent and nonrodents. These studies have an extremely broad responsibility for identifying target organs and NOEL/LOEL values using a small number of study parameters. The regulatory agencies are now asking for mechanistic information on test compounds to aid in risk assessment. In response to this, additional endpoints are often being added to the standard multidose studies. These can include such endpoints as cell division rates within an organ, measurement of hormone concentrations, and functional organ testing. Such endpoints, while added on a case-by-case basis, will continue to grow in popularity.

Investigations still continue into possible in vitro methodologies to replace in vivo animal studies (77–81). Although these methodologies have been used extensively as screening tests and tools to study mechanisms of action, few have been found acceptable as replacement in safety testing to date. One growing area of investigation in toxicology is toxicogenomic and proteomic research. Toxicogenomics can generate gene expression profiles for chemicals that can be compared to the profiles of known toxins. Proteomic analysis of the protein profile at the toxic versus efficacious dose can provide important mechanistic insights. Although not currently part of any regulatory requirements, such methodologies are becoming key tools in mechanistic research and are also being strongly pursued as possible early screening in chemical risk assessment.

REFERENCES

1. Food and Drug Administration. International conference on harmonization: guidance on preclinical safety evaluation of biotechnology-derived pharmaceuticals. Fed Regist 1997; 62:61515.
2. Serabian MA, Pilaro AM. Safety assessment of biotechnology-derived pharmaceuticals: ICH and beyond. Toxicol Pathol 1999; 27:27.
3. Pilaro AM, Serbian MA. Preclinical development strategies for novel gene therapeutic products. Toxicol Pathol 1999; 27:4.
4. Keenan KP. The uncontrolled variable in risk assessment: ad libitum overfed rodents—fat, facts and fiction. Toxicol Pathol 1996; 24:376.
5. Allaben WT, Hart RW. Nutrition and toxicity modulation: the impact of animal body weight on study outcome. Int J Toxicol 1998; 17:1.
6. Kuiper MH, Boeve T, Jansen MW, Roelofs-van J, Thuring JWGM, Wijnands MVW. Ophthalmologic examination in systemic toxicity studies: an overview. Lab Anim 1996; 31:177.
7. Kurata M, Horii I. Blood coagulation test in toxicological studies—review of methods and their significance for drug safety assessment. J Toxicol Sci 2004; 29:13.
8. Heywood R. Target organ toxicity. Toxicol Lett 1981; 8:349.
9. Long GG, Symanowski JT, Roback K. Precision in data acquisition and reporting of organ weights in rats and mice. Toxicol Pathol 1998; 26:316.
10. Carr GJ, Maurer JK. Invited commentary. Precision of organ and body weight data: additional perspective. Toxicol Pathol 1998; 26:321.
11. Roberts R, Cain K, Coyle B, Freathy C, Leonard JF, Gautier JC. Early drug safety evaluation: biomarkers, signatures, and fingerprints. Drug Metab Rev 2003; 35:269.
12. Luft J, Bode G. Integration of safety pharmacology endpoints into toxicology studies. Fundam Clin Pharmacol 2002; 16:91.
13. Marcusson-Stahl M, Cererbrant K. A flow-cytometric NK-cytotoxicity assay adapted for use in rat repeated dose toxicity studies. Toxciology 2003; 193:269.
14. Lewis RW, Billington R, Debryune E, Gamer A, Lang B, Carpanini F. Recognition of adverse and nonadverse effects in toxicity studies. Toxicol Pathol 2002; 30:66.
15. Williams GM, Iatropoulos MJ. Distinguishing adverse from non-adverse effects in drug development. Toxicol Pathol 2002; 30:41.
16. Hamlin R. Extracting "more" from cardio pulmonary studies on beagle dogs. In: Gilman MR, ed. The Canine as a Biomedical Model. Bethesda, MD: American College of Toxicology and LRE, 1985:9.
17. Doherty JD, Cobbe SM. Electrophysiological changes in animal model of chronic cardiac failure. Cardiovas Res 1990; 24:309.
18. Hammond TG, Carlsson L, Davis AS, et al. Methods of collecting and evaluating non-clinical electrophysiology data in the pharmaceutical industry: results of an international survey. Cardiovasc Res 2001; 49:741.
19. Caisey JD, King DJ. Clinical chemistry values for some common laboratory animals. Clin Chem 1980; 26:1877.

20. Loeb WF, Quimby FW. The Clinical Chemistry of Laboratory Animals. New York: Pergamon Press, 1989.
21. Matsuzawa T, Nomura M, Unno T. Clinical pathology reference ranges of laboratory animals. J Vet Med Sci 1993; 55:351.
22. Nachbaur J, Clarke MR, Provost JP, Dancia JL. Variations of sodium, potassium and chloride plasma levels in the rat with age and sex. Lab Anim Sci 1977; 27:972.
23. Uchiyama T, Tokoi K, Deki T. Successive changes in the blood composition of the experimental normal beagle dogs accompanied with age. Exp Anim 1985; 34:367.
24. Matsuzawa T, Sakazume S. Effect of fasting on haematology and clinical chemistry values in the rat and dog. Comp Haematol Int 1994; 4:152.
25. Neptun DA, Smith CN, Irons R. Effect of sampling site and collection method on variations in baseline clinical pathology parameters in fischer 344 rats. Fund Appl Toxicol 1985; 5:1180.
26. Walter GL. Effects of carbon dioxide inhalation on hematology, coagulation, and serum clinical chemistry values in rats. Toxicol Pathol 1999; 27:217.
27. Evans GO. Animal Clinical Chemistry: A Primer for Toxicologists. London: Taylor and Francis, 1996.
28. Beynon AC. Animal models for cholesterol metabolism. In: Beynon AC, Solleveld HA, eds. Biosciences. Dordrecht: Martinus Nijoff, 1988:279.
29. Ramaswamy M, Wallace TL, Cossum PA, Wasan KM. Species differences in the proportion of plasma lipoprotein lipid carried by high-density lipoproteins influence the distribution of free and liposomal nystatin in human, dog, and rat plasma. Antimicrob Agents Chemother 1999; 43:1424.
30. Stonard. Assessment of renal function and damage in animal species. A review of the current approach of the academic, governmental and industrial institutions represented by the animal clinical chemistry association. J Appl Toxicol 1990; 10:267.
31. Jung K, Mattenheimer H, Burchardt U. Urinary Enzymes in Clinical and Experimental Medicine. Berlin: Springer, 1992.
32. Scharer K. The effect of chronic underfeeding on organ weights of rats. Toxicology 1977; 7:45.
33. Farrow MG. Unique aspects of GLP pathology. J Am Coll Toxicol 1987; 6:389.
34. Roe FJC. Toxicity testing: some principles and some pitfalls in histopathologic evaluation. Human Toxicol 1988; 7:405.
35. Ruben Z, Wagner BM. Correlations between morphologic and functional changes induced by xenobiotics: is every induced change a sign of toxicity. Toxicol Appl Pharmacol 1989; 97:4.
36. Haschek WM, Rouseaux CG. Handbook of Toxicologic Pathology. New York: Academic Press, 1991.
37. Davidson IWF, Parker JC, Beliles RP. Biological basis for extrapolating across mammalian species. Reg Toxicol Pharmacol 1986; 6:211.
38. Ruelius HW. Extrapolation from animals to man: predictions, pitfalls and perspectives. Xenobiotic 1987; 17:255.
39. Brown SL, Brent SM, Gough M, et al. Review of interspecies risk comparisons. Reg Toxicol Pharmacol 1988; 8:191.
40. Gephart LA, Salminen WF, Nicolich MJ, Pelekis M. Evaluation of subchronic toxicity data using the benchmark dose approach. Regul Toxicol Pharmacol 2001; 33:37.
41. Kramer HJ, Van Der Ham WA, Slob W, Pieters MN. Conversion factors estimating indicative chronic no-observed-adverse-effect levels from short-term toxicity data. Regul Toxicol Pharmacol 1996; 23:249.
42. Atherley G. A critical review of time-weighted average as an index of exposure and dose of its key elements. Am Ind Hyg Assoc J 1985; 46:481.
43. Sharratt M. Assessing risk from data on other exposure routes. Regul Toxicol Pharmacol 1988; 8:399.
44. Lu FC. A review of the acceptable daily intakes of pesticides assessed by WHO. Regul Toxicol Pharmacol 1995; 21:352.
45. Fairhurst S. Hazard and risk assessment of industrial chemicals in the occupational context in Europe: some current issues. Food Chem Toxicol 2003; 41:1453.

46. Calabrese EJ. Principles of Animal Extrapolation. New York: Wiley-Interscience, 1983:538.
47. Hattis D, Baird S, Goble R. A straw man proposal for a quantitative definition of the RfD. Drug Chem Toxicol 2002; 25:403.
48. Plaa GL, Hewitt WR. Toxicology of the Liver. New York: Raven Press, 1982.
49. Woodman DD. Assessment of hepatic function and damage in animal species. J Appl Toxicol 1988; 8:249.
50. Amacher DE. A toxicologist's guide to biomarkers of hepatic response. Human Exp Toxicol 2002; 21:253.
51. Waterfield CJ, Turton JA, Scales MDC, Timbrell JA. Investigations into the effects of various hepatotoxic compounds on urinary and liver taurine levels in rats. Arch Toxicol 1993; 67:244.
52. Waterfield CJ, Turton JA, Scales MDC, Timbrell JA. Effects of various non-hepatotoxic compounds on urinary and liver taurine levels in rats. Arch Toxicol 1993; 67:538.
53. O'Brien PJ, Slaughter MR, Polley SR, Kramer K. Advantages of glutamate dehydrogenase as a blood biomarker of acute hepatic injury in rats. Lab Anim 2002; 36:313.
54. Willimas GM, Iatropoulos MJ. Alteration of liver cell function and proliferation: differentiation between adaptation and toxicity. Toxicol Pathol 2002; 30:41.
55. Groneberg DA, Grosse-Siestrup C, Fischer A. In vitro models to study hepatotoxicity. Toxicol Pathol 2002; 30:394.
56. Grosse-Siestrup C, Pfeffere J, Unger V, et al. Isolated hemoperfused slaughterhouse livers as a valid model to study hepatotoxicity. Toxicol Pathol 2002; 30:749.
57. Hook JB, Goldstein RS. Toxicology of the Kidney. New York: Raven Press, 1993.
58. Commandeur JNM, Vermeulen NPE. Molecular and biochemical mechanisms of chemically induced nephrotoxicity: a review. Chem Res Toxicol 1990; 3:171.
59. Mudge GH. Comparative pharmacology of the kidney: implications for drug-induced renal failure. In: Bach PH et al. ed. Nephrotoxicity: Assessment and Pathogenesis. Chichester: Wiley, 1982:504.
60. Bovee KC. Renal function and laboratory evaluation. Toxicol Pathol 1986; 14:26.
61. Hottendorf GH. Functional-morphologic correlations in assessing renal toxicity. Toxicol Pathol 1986; 14:123.
62. Fent K, Mayer E, Zbinden G. Nephrotoxicity screening in rats: a validation study. Arch Toxicol 1988; 61:349.
63. Trevisan A, Giralso M, Borella M, Bottegal S, Fabrello A. Tubular segment-specific biomarkers of nephrotoxicity in the rat. Toxicol Lett 2001; 124:113.
64. Swenberg JA. α_{2u}-Globulin nephropathy: review of the cellular and molecular mechanisms involved and their implications for human risk assessment. Environ Health Perspect 1993; 101:39.
65. Acosta D, Jr. Cardiovascular Toxicology. New York: Raven Press, 1992.
66. Louden C, Morgan DG. Pathology and pathophysiology of drug-induced arterial injury in laboratory animals and its implications on the evaluation of novel chemical entities for human clinical trials. Pharmacol Toxicol 2001; 89:158.
67. Irons RD. Toxicology of the Blood and Bone Marrow. New York: Raven Press, 1985.
68. Rosman R, Hanninen O. Gastrointestinal Toxicology. Amsterdam: Elsevier, 1986.
69. Hayes AW. Toxicology of the Eye, Ear, and Other Special Senses. New York: Raven Press, 1985.
70. Balwin HA, McDonald TO, Beasley CH. Slit-lamp examination of experimental animal eyes. Grading scales and photographic evaluation of induced pathological conditions. J Soc Cosmet Chem 1973; 24:181.
71. Hobson DW. Dermal and Ocular Toxicology Fundamentals and Methods. Boca Raton, Florida: CRC Press, 1991.
72. Ribelin ES, Mosley MT. Effects of drugs and chemicals upon the structure of the adrenal gland. Fund Appl Toxicol 1984; 4:105.
73. Colby HD. Adrenal gland toxicity: chemically induced dysfunction. J Am Coll Toxicol 1988; 7:45.
74. Capen CC. Correlation of mechanistic data and histopathology in the evaluation of selected toxic endpoints of the endocrine system. Toxicol Lett 1998; 102-103:405.

75. Boyd EJS, Rinderknecht H, Wormsley KG. Laboratory tests in the diagnosis of the chronic pancreatic diseases. Part 4. Tests involving measurements of pancreatic enzymes in body fluid. Int J Pancreatol 1988; 3:1.
76. Wilmink T, Frick TW. Drug-induced pancreatitis. Drug Saf 1996; 14:406.
77. Nuwaysir EF, Bittner M, Trent J, Barrett JC, Afshari CA. Microarray and toxicology: the advent of toxicogenomics. Mol Carcinogen 1999; 24:153.
78. Cockerell GL, McKim JM, Vonderfetch SL. Strategic importance of research support through pathology. Toxicol Pathol 2002; 30:4.
79. Man WJ, White IR, Bryant D, et al. Protein expression analysis of drug-mediated hepatoxicity in the Sprague-Dawley rat. Proteomics 2002; 2:1577.
80. Thome-Kromer B, Bonk I, Klatt M, et al. Toward the identification of liver toxicity markers: a proteome study in human cell culture and rats. Proteomics 2003; 3:1835.
81. Amin RP, Vickers AE, Sistare F, et al. Identification of putative gene based markers of renal toxicity. Environ Health Perspect 2004; 112:465.

8

Genetic Toxicology

Donald L. Putman†, Jane J. Clarke, Patricia Escobar, Ramadevi Gudi, Ljubica S. Krsmanovic, Kamala Pant, Valentine O. Wagner III, and Richard H. C. San
Genetic Toxicology Department, BioReliance, Invitrogen Bioservices, Rockville, Maryland, U.S.A.

David Jacobson-Kram
Office of New Drugs, U.S. Food and Drug Administration, Silver Spring, Maryland, U.S.A.

INTRODUCTION

Genetic toxicology, unlike other disciplines in toxicology, does not study a specific adverse health effect. Rather, potential genotoxic effects are evaluated because they are considered important prequelae to the development of adverse health effects, such as cancer. Additionally, the induction of mutations in germinal cells can result in increased frequencies of genetic diseases or even the introduction of new genetic diseases into the human gene pool. It has also been suggested, although perhaps not proven, that somatic cell mutation is also important in the initiation of atherosclerotic plaques and may be the basis for the aging process. A number of short-term test systems are available for assessment of genetic hazard. These systems are often categorized by the endpoints that they measure: gene mutation, chromosome damage, or deoxyribonucleic acid (DNA) damage. It is the close association of these well-characterized and easily quantified endpoints with known mechanisms of oncogene activation or loss of tumor suppressor gene function that places such importance on genotoxicity testing. Thus, short-term genetic toxicology tests may be used to identify chemicals that require further testing in long-term animal systems as well as provide support for the evaluation and interpretation of carcinogenicity findings from these animal systems.

Although there is little question that genotoxicity testing should be part of a safety evaluation of all new chemical identities, the appropriate assay systems to be used, as well as the protocol design itself, have often been determined by national regulatory guidelines. Considerable progress has been made in attempts to standardize protocol requirements for genotoxicity testing, particularly through the efforts of the International Conference on Harmonization (ICH) and the Organization for Economic Cooperation and Development (OECD).

---

†In memoriam.

Pharmaceuticals

The ICH process has resulted in the promulgation of guidelines for a "Standard Battery for Genotoxicity Testing of Pharmaceuticals (ICH Harmonised Tripartite Guideline S2B)" (1) and "Guidance on Specific Aspects of Regulatory Genotoxicity Test for Pharmaceuticals (ICH Harmonised Tripartite Guideline S2A)" (2). These guidelines have standardized genotoxicity testing on pharmaceuticals between the United States, Europe, and Japan. The recommended standard battery is: (1) a test for gene mutation in bacteria, (2) an in vitro test with cytogenetic evaluation of chromosomal damage with mammalian cells or an in vitro mouse lymphoma tk assay, and (3) an in vivo test for chromosomal damage using rodent hematopoietic cells. If all results in the standard battery are negative, it will usually provide a sufficient level of safety to demonstrate the absence of genotoxicity activity. However, if one or more positive responses are seen, test materials may have to be evaluated more extensively. Under certain circumstances the standard battery may have to be altered. For example, under certain circumstances, the results of the bacterial assay may not be informative. This could happen when testing materials that are excessively toxic to bacteria, such as certain antibiotics, or materials that are specifically designed to be active in mammalian cells, such as topoisomerase inhibitors or nucleoside analogues. Under these circumstances the guidelines suggest performing the two in vitro mammalian tests (cytogenetics and mouse lymphoma) in addition to the bacterial mutation assay. A second circumstance in which the standard battery may be modified is for compounds that bear structural alerts for genotoxic activity but give negative results in the three standard assays. In such a situation, additional testing may be required. This testing should take into account the nature of the material, its known reactivity, and information on how it is metabolized. The guidelines also note that the standard battery may have to be modified based on limitations in the use of in vivo tests. For example, pharmacokinetic data may suggest that a compound is not systemically absorbed and therefore not available to the target tissues, most often the bone marrow. Cited examples of such materials include radioimaging agents, aluminum-based antacids, and some dermally applied pharmaceuticals. If an in vivo route of exposure cannot be found that will provide target cell exposure, both in vitro mammalian cell tests should be performed. The guidelines also indicate that additional genetic toxicology testing may be required if a material is negative in the three-test battery but gives positive responses in a carcinogenicity bioassay. Examples of additional tests include use of modified conditions for metabolic activation in in vitro tests and in vivo tests that measure DNA damage in tumor target organs. These can include unscheduled DNA synthesis, radioactive phosphorus (^{32}P)-postlabeling, mutation induction in transgenes, or molecular characterization of genetic changes in tumor-related genes. Finally, the guidelines indicate that additional genetic toxicology may be required for compounds with unique chemical structures that have not been tested in carcinogenicity bioassays.

For products of recombinant DNA technology such as vaccines, monoclonal antibodies, blood-derived products, hormones, cytokines, and other regulatory factors, the U.S. Food and Drug Administration (FDA) Center for Biologics Evaluation and Research reviews the requirement for genotoxicity testing on the basis of product application.

Medical Devices

In July, 1995, FDA Center for Devices and Radiological Health (CDRH) announced that it would abandon the Tripartite Guidance Document of 1986 in favor of the 1992 International Organization for Standardization (ISO) guidelines for mutagenicity testing of device materials (3). According to the ISO guideline, a three-test battery is required. The battery must include one test for gene mutation, one test for chromosomal aberrations, and one test for DNA effects; two of the three tests should use mammalian cells as the target. All tests must be conducted according to current OECD testing guidelines. Most recently, CDRH has been requesting the ICH mutagenicity battery in place of the ISO battery. At the present time it is not completely clear which guideline device manufactures should follow.

Industrial Chemicals and Pesticides

United States

U.S. Environmental Protection Administration (EPA) authority for the regulation of chemicals requiring mutagenicity testing is covered under the Toxic Substances Control Act (TSCA) or the Federal Insecticide, Fungicide, and Rodenticide Act (FIFRA). The TSCA regulates both new chemicals (Section 5) and those that were already in commerce at the time the act was passed (Section 4).

Although Section 5 does not require toxicology testing, the Office of Pollution Prevention and Toxics (OPPT) has established testing criteria based on human exposure or release into the environment (4). For certain high-volume chemicals that reach the trigger for occupational or consumer exposure, the requirement includes two genetic toxicology assays, a bacterial gene mutation assay and an in vivo micronucleus test.

Toxicology testing of existing chemicals is determined through test rules or consent orders. Because Section 4 chemicals have wide distribution in the environment or widespread human exposure, the mutagenicity battery includes, in addition to the bacterial mutation assay and in vivo micronucleus test, an in vitro gene mutation assay, preferably the mouse lymphoma mutation assay (4). Submitters have the option of substituting a Chinese hamster ovary (CHO)/hgprt gene mutation assay and an in vitro chromosomal aberration assay in place of a mouse lymphoma test. A positive response in either gene mutation assay triggers a study for interaction with gonadal DNA and may include such endpoints as sister chromatid exchange (SCE), alkaline elution, or unscheduled DNA synthesis (UDS). Positive evidence of interaction with gonadal DNA triggers a specific locus test. A positive response in the in vivo bone marrow micronucleus test triggers a dominant lethal assay, and a positive dominant lethal triggers a heritable translocation assay. Chronic studies for carcinogenicity are triggered by a positive response in all three base sets, or a positive response in either in vitro mutation assay plus the micronucleus assay. Single positive responses or positive responses in the two in vitro assays results in a data review.

The Office of Pesticide Programs (OPP) revised its mutagenicity testing scheme for agricultural chemicals in 1991 (5). Its three-test battery includes a bacterial mutagenicity assay, a mouse lymphoma gene mutation assay, and an in vivo bone marrow cytogenetics assay, either bone marrow metaphase analysis or micronucleus test. The CHO or V79/hgprt gene mutation assay and an in vitro chromosomal aberration assay may be substituted for the mouse lymphoma assay.

Europe

The Seventh Amendment to directive 79/831/EEC stipulates that a bacterial gene mutation assay using both *Salmonella* and *E. coli* and an in vitro cytogenetics assay are required for premanufacturing or preimport notification of new chemicals to be manufactured in quantities between 1 and 10 metric tons per year. Only the bacterial mutation assay is required for chemicals manufactured in quantities between 100 kg and 1 metric ton. For chemicals with more than 10 tonnes per year in commerce or where 50 metric tons in aggregate are in commerce, a mammalian gene mutation assay and in vivo cytogenetics assay are added to the base set.

Japan

Two mutagenicity studies are required for new chemicals and include the bacterial gene mutation assay and chromosomal aberration assay in cultured mammalian cells. The micronucleus test is also recommended as an additional screening test. The guidelines for screening new chemical substances were published in 1986 by the Ministry of Health and Welfare (MHW), the Ministry of International Trade and Industry (MITI), and the Agency of Environment.

The Ministry of Labor also regulates registration of new chemical substances, marketing of chemicals, raw materials, intermediates, by-products, and waste generated in the workplace. Only a single mutagenicity test, the bacterial gene mutation assay using *S. typhimurium* and *E. coli*, is required for these materials. A positive bacterial mutation assay requires performance of an in vitro chromosomal aberration assay.

The Ministry of Agriculture, Forestry, and Fisheries (MAFF) requires a three-test battery including a bacterial gene mutation assay using *S. typhimurium* and *E. coli*, an in vitro chromosomal aberration assay, and a primary DNA damage assay as measured by a bacterial repair test, the Rec-assay (6).

BACTERIAL MUTATION ASSAYS

Introduction

In the early 1970s, several researchers affirmed the use of bacterial mutation assays as a simple and rapid means of detecting mutagens and carcinogens (7–9). Mutations can be detected by either forward or reverse mechanisms. Forward mutation systems detect mutation as a change in the normal phenotype (appearance) of an organism, whereas reverse mutation systems detect mutation as a reversion from a mutant phenotype to a normal phenotype. In forward mutation systems, which theoretically possess a larger genetic target, any one of a number of nucleotides, when altered, can disable the expression or function of a gene. Reverse mutation assays generally focus on one or a few specific sites that, when altered, restore function to a defective gene. However, the advantage of the forward mutation assays is more theoretical than practical. Although other microbial mutation assays have been developed, the two most popular and best validated systems employ, either individually or in combination, *S. typhimurium* and *E. coli*. In their early development, bacterial mutation assays were reported to detect as mutagens 85% to 90% of the carcinogens tested (10,11). More recent validation studies, using 264 chemicals in the U.S. National Toxicology Program database, have found that the *S. typhimurium* assay has a sensitivity to rodent carcinogens of 58% and a specificity for noncarcinogens of 73% (12). Further analysis of such databases has indicated that chemical class and the presence or absence of structural alerts for genotoxicity (13) greatly alter the meaningfulness of the results (14).

Bacteria used in mutation assays are primarily sensitive to three types of mutational events: base-pair substitution mutations, frameshift mutations and DNA crosslinking (15). A frameshift mutation alters the reading frame of the DNA by insertion or deletion of one or more bases. Base-pair substitution mutations retain the correct reading frame but one of the basepairs undergoes a substitution such that the resulting DNA molecule contains an incorrect base. DNA crosslinking agents covalently bind the two strands of the DNA double helix. Because of the importance in maintaining an organism's genetic integrity, nature has invested much energy in minimizing the chance for mutations to occur. All organisms, even the simplest bacteria, have elaborate DNA repair systems. Furthermore, mutations are extremely rare events. For these reasons, mutations are difficult to detect without the use of specialized bacteria that are hypersensitive to specific types of mutations.

Purpose of Study

The purpose of these studies is to evaluate the mutagenic potential of a test article and its metabolites by measuring and quantifying its ability to induce reverse mutations at selected loci of *S. typhimurium* or *E. coli* in the presence and absence of metabolic activation. This test system has been shown to detect a diverse group of chemical mutagens (10,11).

Cell Selection and Justification

The *S. typhimurium* and *E. coli* strains used in this assay each have a defect in one of the genes involved in histidine and tryptophan biosynthesis, respectively. The defect renders the cell dependent (auxotrophic) on exogenous histidine or tryptophan. Unless the cell experiences a mutation that reverts the dysfunctional gene back to the wild type (prototrophic), the cell becomes disabled when the exogenous histidine or tryptophan is exhausted. For this reason, this assay is referred to as a reverse or back mutation assay.

To increase their sensitivity to mutagens, several additional mutations have been incorporated into the strains used in the standard battery. Mutations in the *uvr*A gene of *E. coli* and in the *uvr*B gene of *S. typhimurium* are partial deletions of each respective gene (9,16). The *uvr* genes code for a series of DNA excision repair enzymes involved in removal of T-T dimers induced by ultraviolet (UV) light. Cells with this type of mutation are unable to repair damage induced by UV light and other types of mutagens. The presence of either of these mutations can be detected by demonstrating sensitivity to UV light. The pKM101 plasmid codes for an error prone DNA repair system (17). Because cells with this mutation cannot correctly repair DNA damage, they have increased sensitivity to mutagens. Cells containing this plasmid are resistant to ampicillin. The *rfa* wall mutation prevents the *S. typhimurium* cells from synthesizing an intact polysaccharide cell wall (16). Therefore, large molecules such as benzo[a]pyrene (BaP) that are normally excluded are able to penetrate the cell. Cells containing this mutation are sensitive to crystal violet. The genotypes of some of the more commonly used tester strains are summarized in Table 1.

Because a single strain of bacterium is capable of detecting only a specific type of genetic damage, several strains must be used to effectively screen for mutagenic potential. The *S. typhimurium* strains detect reversion from *his*⁻ to *his*⁺ at a single site in one of the 12 steps of histidine biosynthesis. Strains TA98, TA1537, TA1538, TA97, and TA97a are reverted from histidine auxotrophy to histidine prototrophy by frameshift mutagens, whereas TA100 and TA1535 are reverted by base substitution mutagens (18). Strain TA102 possesses A-T base-pairs at the site of the mutation, unlike other *S. typhimurium* tester strains that possess G-C base-pairs at the mutation sites. In addition, TA102 has been shown to be useful for detecting oxidative mutagens, such as bleomycin, that are not detected by other tester strains. The *uvr*B mutation has not been introduced into this strain; therefore, with an intact excision repair system, it can detect cross-linking agents, such as mitomycin C (19). The *E. coli* strains detect reversion from *trp*⁻ to *trp*⁺ at a site blocking

Table 1 Tester Strain Genotypes

Histidine mutation					Tryptophan mutation	Additional mutations		
hisC3076	hisD3052	hisD6610	hisG46	hisG428 (pAQ1)	trpE	LPS	Repair	R factor
Frame-shift detectors				Base pair detectors				
TA1537	TA1538	–	TA1535	–	–	rfa	ΔuvrB	–
–	TA98	TA97	TA100	–	–	rfa	ΔuvrB	+R
–	–	–	–	TA102	–	rfa	–	+R
–	–	–	–	–	WP2 (pKM101)	–	–	+R
–	–	–	–	–	WP2 uvrA	–	ΔuvrA	–
–	–	–	–	–	WP2 uvrA (pKM101)	–	ΔuvrA	+R

tryptophan biosynthesis prior to the formation of anthranilic acid. These strains have A-T base pairs at the critical mutation site within the trpE gene (20). Tryptophan revertants can arise due to a base change at the originally mutated site or elsewhere in the chromosome causing the original mutation to be suppressed. Thus, the specificity of the reversion mechanism is sensitive to base-pair substitution mutations, rather than frame-shift mutations (21).

To adequately assess the mutagenic potential of a chemical, it is important to select an appropriate battery of tester strains. Although the selection is often guided by the world's regulatory bodies, the nature of the chemical should always be considered prior to making the final selection. If the specific properties of a chemical make one strain particularly sensitive, that strain should most likely be included in the battery. The batteries used by the world's regulatory bodies have been selected to provide sensitivity for a diverse group of chemicals.

The strain battery that was approved under the 1997 harmonization efforts of the OECD and the ICH allow the selection of one strain from each of five categories, as follows: (1) TA98; (2) TA100; (3) TA1535; (4) TA1537, TA97, or TA97a; (5) TA102, WP2 uvrA or WP2 uvrA (pKM101). To detect crosslinking agents it is necessary to select TA102 or to add WP2 (pKM101) (2,22).

Maintenance of Cells

To ensure that the cells are well characterized and traceable, it is best to obtain cultures from a recognized supplier. Dr. Bruce Ames no longer supplies strains. They may be obtained from MolTox (Boone, North Carolina, U.S.A.) and Invitrogen (Rockville, Maryland, U.S.A.). *E. coli* may be obtained from the National Collection of Industrial and Marine Bacteria, Aberdeen, Scotland, and from MolTox. Shortly after receipt of new cultures, both frozen permanent stocks and working stocks should be prepared (18).

Master plates for *S. typhimurium* tester strains are prepared by inoculating onto minimal media supplemented with histidine and biotin. For those strains that contain the pKM101 or pAQ1 plasmid, ampicillin or tetracycline are added as appropriate (18). Master plates for *E. coli* tester strains are prepared by inoculating onto Vogel-Bonner minimal medium E supplemented with 2.5% Oxoid Nutrient Broth No. 2. Master plates are incubated at 37°C for approximately 24 to 48 hours and are stored at 4°C. Master plates can serve as working stocks for up to 6 weeks. On occasion, one can experience the inherent problem of picking a revertant from the master plate for the overnight culture. When this occurs the entire overnight culture contains revertant his^+ or trp^+ cells, resulting in confluent bacterial growth on the plates. By gently placing a replicate plating pad onto the surface of the master plate, a small quantity of each colony can be transferred to a biotin-only plate. After incubation, the revertant colonies are clearly identifiable as isolated areas of bacterial growth on the biotin-only plate. When selecting colonies for inoculating the overnight culture, these his^+ or trp^+ colonies can be avoided. This dramatically reduces the chances of selecting a revertant colony for inoculation of the overnight cultures (23).

Overnight cultures are inoculated from the appropriate master plate or from the appropriate frozen stock. To ensure that cultures are harvested in late log phase, the length of incubation should be controlled and monitored. The shaker-incubator is programmed to begin shaking at approximately 125 rpm at 37°C, approximately 12 hours before the anticipated time of harvest. All cultures should be harvested by spectrophotometric monitoring of culture turbidity rather than by duration of incubation. Cultures should be removed from incubation at a density of approximately 10^9 cells/ml. Because undergrowth or overgrowth of the cultures can cause loss of sensitivity, it is important to monitor the cultures to ensure a sufficient population of viable cells is used. The sensitivity of the bacterial mutation assays is enhanced by the large population of individual cells at risk, approximately 10 to 100 million cells per plate. Wagner and San (24) have reported that cultures with titer values between 10^8 and 10^9 yield comparable sensitivity.

Experimental Design

Bacterial mutation assays are commonly performed in two phases. In the United States and Europe, the first phase has historically been a preliminary toxicity assay or dose range–finding assay. This phase is used to establish the dose range for the definitive assay. The second phase, the mutagenicity assay, which may include both an initial assay and a confirmatory assay, is used to evaluate the mutagenic potential of the test article. If a large number of similar chemicals are being screened, it is often possible to eliminate the preliminary toxicity once an appropriate dose range is established. In Japan, it is customary to conduct the preliminary experiment, termed a toxicity-mutation assay by some laboratories, with all strains and the appropriate concurrent negative and positive controls, using duplicate plates per dose rather than just one or two representative strains and single plate per dose. As part of the harmonization efforts of the ICH, either approach is acceptable as long as two independent trials are included that evaluate the mutagenicity of the test article (2).

Dose Selection

In the preliminary toxicity assay, the maximum dose level tested should be 5 mg per plate, solubility or homogeneity permitting. If the test article cannot be dissolved at a sufficient concentration in a solvent compatible with the test system or if the test article cannot be suspended adequately in a vehicle compatible with the test system, the maximum dose tested should be the highest achievable dose up to 5 mg per plate. A suspension is not ideal because of the difficulty in preparing accurate dosing stocks and in delivering them to the test system. However, unlike mammalian systems where the test article must be removed following a finite exposure period, suspensions will not otherwise interfere with the conduct of the assay. A sufficient number of lower dose levels should be tested in the preliminary toxicity assay to determine the appropriate dose range for the definitive assay.

In the mutagenicity assay, the maximum dose level for each strain and metabolic activation combination should be either 5 mg per plate or should be selected to demonstrate mutagenicity, toxicity or precipitate. The criteria for assessing toxicity, precipitate, and mutagenicity are discussed in following sections. The selection criteria for the maximum dose level in the mutagenicity assay approved by the OECD and ICH are as follows: (1) For a nontoxic, a nonmutagenic, and a nonprecipitating test article, the maximum dose level should be 5 mg per plate; (2) For a toxic or a mutagenic test article, the maximum dose level should demonstrate toxicity or mutagenicity irrespective of the precipitation profile; (3) For a precipitating, a nontoxic and a nonmutagenic test article, the maximum dose level may be the lowest precipitating dose level (2,22).

Although these criteria will most likely meet future regulatory requirements, other criteria may be applied based on the objective of the assay. It has been demonstrated that low-level mutagenic components may not be detected until the test article is tested at a sufficiently high enough concentration for the mutagenic components to be detected. This may necessitate testing at precipitating dose levels. Laboratories in Japan have identified examples of test articles that are clearly mutagenic only at precipitating dose levels (2). For this reason, it is recommended that one select dose levels based on criterion (1) or (2), if the study may be submitted to a Japanese regulatory body. If the testing is being conducted early in the development process, testing at precipitating dose levels may help identify potential low-level mutagenic contaminants in different preparations or analogues of the test material.

Number of Cultures

Because the preliminary toxicity assay is used primarily to determine the appropriate dose range for the definitive assay, it is usually conducted with only a single plate per dose level. A preliminary toxicity-mutation assay, used to evaluate toxicity and mutagenicity, is usually conducted with two replicate plates per dose level. The mutagenicity assay is usually conducted with three plates per dose level. This provides a reliable estimate of the response at each dose level without significantly influencing the mean by divergent plate counts.

Metabolic Activation System

Many mutagens and carcinogens are actually promutagens and procarcinogens that require activation or detoxification to their active forms, e.g., polycyclic aromatic hydrocarbons, aromatic amines, nitrosamines, and azo dyes. The major mammalian activation systems are multicomponent, membrane-bound, nicotinamide adenine dinucleotide phosphate (NADPH)-requiring, molecular oxygen-requiring, cytochrome P450-dependent complexes of mixed-function oxygenases. Because *S. typhimurium* and *E. coli*, as well as many other in vitro test systems, lack these metabolic capabilities, an exogenous activation system must be provided. Ames and others developed an exogenous activation system by centrifuging homogenized mammalian liver at 9000 X g, to recover the microsomal fraction commonly referred to as S9. To effectively detect a wide variety of promutagens and procarcinogens, it is necessary to stimulate production of these enzymes with an inducing agent prior to collecting the liver, most commonly a polychlorinated biphenyl (PCB) (7). Although other tissues, species, and inducing agents may be used, liver microsomes from rats induced with Aroclor 1254 have been found to be a convenient and efficient activating system (25). Because of the carcinogenic properties of Aroclor 1254, the disposal problems associated with PCBs, and the difficulty in working with PCBs in some parts of the world, other inducing agents have been developed. Matsushima et al. (26) and Ong et al. (27) have reported that a combination of phenobarbital and β-naphthoflavone provide an alternative to PCB induction that is similar to Aroclor 1254. Typically, S9 homogenate is prepared from male Sprague-Dawley rats induced with a single, intraperitoneal injection of Aroclor 1254, at 500 mg/kg, five days prior to sacrifice. The S9 is prepared and stored frozen at approximately $-70°C$ for up to 2 year. The OECD 471 guideline (22) requires that 2-aminoanthracene not be the sole chemical for verifying the function of the S9. For this reason each batch of S9 homogenate must be assayed for its ability to metabolize at least two of the following chemicals: 2-aminoanthracene, 7,12-dimethylbenzanthracene, or BAP to forms mutagenic to *S. typhimurium* TA100 (28).

For the S9 homogenate to provide a NADPH-generating system, it must be combined with an appropriate mix of cofactors as follows. Immediately prior to use, the S9 is thawed and mixed with a cofactor pool to contain 10% S9 homogenate, 5 mM glucose-6-phosphate, 4 mM β-nicotinamide adenine dinucleotide phosphate (NADP), 8 mM $MgCl_2$, and 33 mM KCl in a 100 mM phosphate buffer at pH 7.4. This mixture is referred to as S9 mix. Sham mix, containing 100 mM phosphate buffer at pH 7.4, is used in place of S9 mix for the nonactivated portion of the assay. For peak activity, some mutagens may require S9 mixes with between 4% and 30% S9 homogenate (29,30). If specific metabolic requirements (e.g., azo compounds) are known about the test article, this information should be utilized in designing the assay. Furthermore, equivocal results should be clarified using an appropriate modification of the experimental design (e.g., dose levels, activation system or treatment method) (2,22).

Controls

To ascertain that the test system is functioning properly, appropriate controls must be included with each toxicity-mutation or mutagenicity assay. To determine that the tester strains are functioning properly, a set of negative controls must be included for each tester strain–activation combination. If a routine vehicle (e.g., water, dimethyl sulfoxide, ethanol, or acetone) is being used, the negative control only needs to be the vehicle. If an unusual vehicle, with no historical database, is being used, the negative control should include both untreated and vehicle controls. This will allow one to determine any vehicle-induced effects on the test system. To determine that the tester strains are responding to known mutagens, positive controls that are direct-acting and those that require S9 activation must be included for each tester strain–activation combination. It is important to compile the control values and to monitor their performance. These historical values can be used to track performance of the test system over time and to provide a basis for determining outlier values for each experiment. Positive controls that may be used with each tester strain–activation combination are shown in Table 2.

Sterility controls should also be included for the sham and S9 mixes and for the vehicle and test article dosing solutions by plating on selective agar with the same aliquot used in the assay.

Dose Administration

On the day of its use, minimal top agar, containing 0.8% agar and 0.5% NaCl, is melted and supplemented with L-histidine, D-biotin, and L-tryptophan. Supplemented top agar is commonly referred to as selective top agar. Bottom agar is Vogel-Bonner minimal medium

Table 2 Positive Controls

Strain	S9 activation	Positive control	Concentration (µg/plate)
TA98, TA100, TA1535, TA1537, TA1538	+	2-Aminoanthracene	1.0
TA97			2.0
WP2 *uvr*A, WP2 *uvr*A (pKM101)			10
TA102		Sterigmatocystin	10
WP2 (pKM101)			100
TA98, TA1538	−	2-Nitrofluorene	1.0
TA100, TA1535		Sodium azide	1.0
TA1537, TA97		9-Aminoacridine	75
TA102		Mitomycin C	1.0
E. coli		Methyl methanesulfonate	1000

E (31), containing 1.5% agar and 0.2% glucose. The low glucose content enhances the revertant colony formation of tester strain TA97 without affecting the other strains (32).

The test article can be administered to the test system using the plate incorporation method or the preincubation method. The plate incorporation method is the original method developed by Ames (7). In this method, S9 mix or sham mix, tester strain, and test article dosing solution are added to molten selective top agar. The components are mixed and overlaid onto the surface of minimal bottom agar plates. After the overlay has solidified, the plates are inverted and incubated for approximately 48 to 72 hours at 37°C.

Although the plate incorporation method is sensitive to many mutagens, it is not sensitive to all mutagens (e.g., nitrosamines, divalent metals, aldehydes, azo-dyes, pyrrolizidine alkaloids, allyl compounds and nitro compounds) (33). Yahagi et al. (34) developed the preincubation method to overcome this limitation. Although the preincubation method is generally more sensitive than the plate incorporation method because the test article is preincubated with the test system, it is also generally more subject to toxic effects. In the preincubation method, 0.5 ml of S9 mix or sham mix is added to preheated (37°C) glass culture tubes. To these tubes are added tester strain and dosing solution. After mixing it is allowed to incubate for 20 to 60 minutes at 37°C. Selective top agar is added to each tube, and the mixture is overlaid onto the surface of minimal bottom agar plates and incubated as described above. Plates that are not counted immediately following the incubation period are stored at 4°C until counted.

Endpoint Evaluated and Time of Evaluation

Prior to scoring the revertant colonies, the condition of the bacterial background lawn is evaluated for evidence of test article toxicity by using a dissecting microscope. Toxicity and degree of precipitation are scored relative to the concurrent vehicle control plate using the codes shown in Table 3. It is essential that the background lawn is evaluated before scoring the revertants so that grownup, nonrevertant background lawn colonies are not included in the revertant count. This occurs as the level of toxicity increases because histidine or tryptophan available for the surviving population permits the auxotrophic bacteria to form isolated microcolonies that can be misinterpreted as mutant colonies (Fig. 1). True revertant colonies generally appear as isolated colonies about 1 mm to 2 mm in diameter.

Table 3 Background Lawn Evaluation Criteria

Code	Description	Characteristics
1	Normal	Distinguished by a healthy microcolony lawn
2	Slightly reduced	Distinguished by a noticeable thinning of the microcolony lawn and possibly a slight increase in the size of the microcolonies compared to the vehicle control plate
3	Moderately reduced	Distinguished by a marked thinning of the microcolony lawn, resulting in a pronounced increase in the size of the microcolonies compared to the vehicle control plate
4	Severely reduced	Distinguished by an extreme thinning of the microcolony lawn, resulting in an increase in the size of the microcolonies compared to the vehicle control plate such that the microcolony lawn is visible to the unaided eye as isolated colonies
5	Absent	Distinguished by a complete lack of any microcolony lawn exceeding $\geq 90\%$ of the plate
6	Obscured by particulate	The background bacterial lawn cannot be accurately evaluated due to microscopic test article particulate
NP	Noninterfering precipitate	Distinguished by precipitate on the plate that is visible to the naked eye, but any precipitate particles detected by the automated colony counter total less than 10% of the revertant colony count (e.g., ≤ 3 particles on a plate with 30 revertants)
IP	Interfering precipitate	Distinguished by precipitate on the plate that is visible to the naked eye, and any precipitate particles detected by the automated colony counter exceed 10% of the revertant colony count (e.g., >3 particles on a plate with 30 revertants)

Immediately surrounding the revertant colony is a normal to moderately reduced microscopic background lawn. To confirm the genotype of any questionable colonies, each may be replicate plated onto histidine-free or tryptophan-free medium containing trace quantities of biotin. Colonies that grow on the amino acid-free medium are true revertant colonies that should be included in the revertant count. All nonreplicating colonies are excluded from the count. For each plate, all true revertants are tallied and reported as revertants per plate.

A dose level is considered toxic if it causes a $>50\%$ reduction in the mean number of revertants per plate relative to the mean vehicle control value (this reduction must be accompanied by an abrupt dose-dependent drop in the revertant count) or a moderate reduction in the background lawn. In the event that fewer than three nontoxic dose levels are achieved, the affected portion of the assay should be repeated with an appropriate change in dose levels. Because mutagenic activity is inherently toxic, it may be necessary to adjust dose levels to investigate suspect responses.

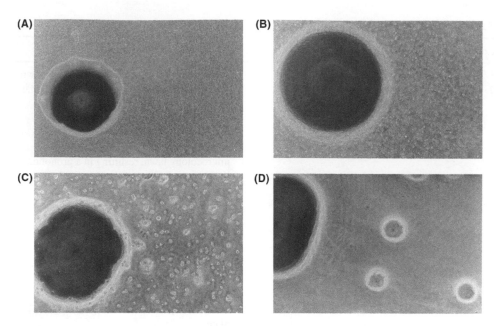

Figure 1 Bacterial background lawn evaluations. In (**A**), a normal, healthy background lawn is shown surrounding a revertant colony to the left. The healthy lawn results from microcolonies that form as the bacteria divide. When the available histidine or tryptophan is exhausted these non-mutated bacteria stop dividing. A slight reduction in the background lawn (**B**) results when a small percentage of the population of bacteria is killed. The resulting survivors become slightly larger and less densely packed. As the toxicity continues to increase, a larger percentage of the bacterial population is killed resulting in more available histidine or tryptophan for the surviving population. At this stage, the background lawn becomes moderately reduced (**C**), with a revertant colony visible to the left and the background lawn appearing as isolated, enlarged microcolonies. As the toxicity approaches near total lethality, a severely reduced background lawn (**D**) results when the microcolony lawn becomes visible to the unaided eye as isolated colonies.

Evaluation Criteria

Data Presentation

For each plate, the background lawn evaluation code and revertant count should be presented along with the mean and standard deviation (SD) of the replicate revertant counts for each dose.

Statistical Analysis

Although several statistical models have been developed, no single, recommended choice has been agreed upon for these assays. Weinstein and Lewinson (35), Bernstein et al. (36) and Stead et al. (37) assume the experimental variation follows a Poisson distribution. Margolin et al. (38) assumed that the random variation follows a negative binomial distribution. Meyers et al. (39) employ an iterative weighted least squares method. Unfortunately, dose-response relationships can vary widely in practice, and all of these methods employ specific models and assumptions that are not always met. Snee and Irr (40) have shown that by using a power transformation, the statistical assumptions of normal distributions and homogeneous variance are more closely met. Therefore, analysis of variance, regression analysis and Student's t-test can be properly used in evaluation of mutagenicity data. This method allows statistical evaluation of the data with regard to reproducibility and linear, quadratic and higher-order responses. Regardless of the statistical model used, if any, sound scientific judgment and biological relevance should be used as the primary criteria, with statistical methods serving as an aid in drawing any conclusions.

Criteria for a Valid Test

To ensure the validity of the test results, certain test system criteria must be met before the data can be properly evaluated. Each tester strain culture must demonstrate the appropriate genotype as listed in Table 1. Ideally, these strain markers should be determined daily for each culture; however, at a minimum, they should be demonstrated following preparation of each new master plate or frozen stock culture. Each culture must demonstrate the characteristic number of spontaneous revertants in the negative control. Each laboratory should establish historical ranges for the performance of the strains in their environment. To ensure that appropriate numbers of bacteria are plated, tester strain culture titers must be greater than or equal to 0.3×10^9 cells/ml. Positive controls must demonstrate the sensitivity of each strain to a known direct-acting mutagen and the capability of the activation system to convert a promutagen to a mutagen.

Positive and Negative Test

The most appropriate criteria for assessment of a positive response are a biologically relevant, reproducible, statistically significant, dose-related increase in revertant colonies per plate. However, in the absence of a clear statistical model and despite the lack of supporting evidence, the following arbitrary guidelines have been commonly used. In a recent survey of laboratories conducting the Ames test, about 80% use some variation of the twofold or threefold rule, and about 20% rely on a statistical model (41).

For a test article to be evaluated positive, it must cause a dose-responsive increase in the mean revertants per plate of at least one tester strain either with or without S9 activation. Data sets are judged positive if the increase in mean revertants at the peak of the dose response is equal to or greater than two or three times the mean vehicle control value. Strains TA1535, TA1537, and TA1538 are judged positive if the peak response is equal to or greater than 3.0 times the vehicle control value. Strains TA98, TA100, TA97, TA102, WP2 *uvr*A, WP2 *uvr*A (pKM101), and WP2 (pKM101) are judged positive if the peak response is equal to or greater than 2.0 times the vehicle control value. An equivocal response is a biologically relevant increase in a revertant count that partially meets the criteria for evaluation as positive. This could be a dose-responsive increase that does not achieve the respective threshold cited above or a nondose responsive increase that is equal to or greater than the respective threshold cited. A response is evaluated as negative, if it is neither positive nor equivocal.

As per the OECD (22) and ICH (2) guidelines, verification of a clear positive response is not required; however, equivocal result should be retested using and appropriate modification of the experimental design (e.g., dose levels, activation system, or treatment method). Per the OECD guideline (22), negative results do not need to be retested when justification can be provided.

Special Considerations

Bacterial mutagenicity assays may be readily modified to accommodate the testing of unusual test articles. These test articles are typically those that are poorly detected by the standard assay or those that cannot be directly delivered to the test system. Several of the more common modifications are briefly discussed below.

Medical Devices

These materials present a unique challenge because of the difficulty in delivering the test article to the test system. This problem is overcome by extracting the test article in an aqueous medium (e.g., saline) and in an organic medium (e.g., dimethyl sulfoxide or ethanol) (3,42). The materials are typically extracted at 37°C or 50°C for three to five days. The extracts are generally prepared at a ratio of 120 cm^2 test article surface area in 20 ml of extraction medium for materials <0.5 mm thick. For test articles ≥0.5 mm thick, the extraction ratio is usually 60 cm^2 of test article surface area in 20 ml of extraction medium. For test articles in which the surface area cannot be readily determined, the extraction ratio is usually 4 g of test article per 20 ml of extraction medium. The extracts are subjected to the normal testing scheme, with 100 μL of each extract being the maximum dose. In light of rare toxicity with such extracts, it is common to only test a single dose of each extract.

Petroleum Extracts

Many complex mixtures of petroleum hydrocarbons that demonstrate dermal carcinogenicity in rodents are undetected or only induce marginal responses in the standard bacterial mutagenicity assay. In 1984, Blackburn et al. (43) described a modified *S. typhimurium* assay with improved sensitivity to complex mixtures of petroleum hydrocarbons with boiling points ≥500°F. The Blackburn method overcame two difficulties in testing petroleum hydrocarbons. First, by extracting the oil sample with dimethyl sulfoxide, aqueous compatible solutions are obtained. Second, the metabolic activation system is enhanced by using an 80% hamster liver S9 mix with a 2X NADP concentration rather than the standard 10% rat liver S9. Blackburn et al. (44) further reported that when using tester strain TA98 in the modified assay, there was excellent correlation between the slope of the initial portion of the mutagenicity curve (termed the mutagenicity index) and the carcinogenic potency of the oil.

Reductive Metabolic Activation

Many dyes used in foods, drugs, cosmetics, and industrial products are azo compounds. These compounds can be reduced, by anaerobic intestinal microflora and mammalian azo reductases in the liver, to free aromatic amines. Because many aromatic amines are carcinogenic and mutagenic, a safety assessment of these compounds is necessary. Prival and Mitchell (45) have developed a modification to the standard assay for optional sensitivity to a wide range of azo dyes. These modifications were adapted from those developed in Sugimura's laboratory and employ use of 30% uninduced hamster S9 under reductive conditions and a 30-minute, 30°C preincubation. The use of reductive metabolic activation should be used in collaboration with the normal activation system.

Vapor and Gas-Phase Test Articles

Vapor or gaseous test articles require an effective containment system to ensure adequate testing. Several exposure systems have been developed. Distlerath et al. (46) developed the taped plate assay to test volatile materials on a small scale. Hughes et al. (47) have used Tedlar® bags for in situ testing of volatiles in small-volume environmental air samples. Wagner et al. (48) reported on the use of the desiccator methodology for the routine testing of vapor-phase and gas-phase test articles. By using 9-liter desiccators to contain the test articles, dose responsive positive increases were observed with methylene chloride as a vapor and with vinyl bromide as a gas.

Biomonitoring

The genotoxicity testing of urine has been used to monitor humans exposed to cigarette smoke, drugs, and to chemicals in the workplace. Chemicals administered to humans can appear in the urine as the free, parent chemical, as one or more metabolites, or as conjugates with glucuronic acid, cysteine, or other substances. Although not all metabolites are excreted in the urine, assays on urine have been used successfully to test the in vivo metabolism and mutagenicity of cigarette smoke, antineoplastic drugs, food mutagens, and other chemicals. To adjust for varying volumes of urine and differences in body weight between individuals, the creatinine content of each urine sample can be used to standardize the quantity and concentration of urine tested in the mutagenicity assay. Due to the presence of histidine in the urine, which can interfere with the assay, and also to concentrate the excreted mutagens, the samples can be extracted with a SEP-PAK® C_{18} column (Millipore Corporation, Bedford, Massachusetts, U.S.A.). The C_{18} column will extract nonpolar components and has been found to be superior to XAD-2 resins in terms of the performance and recovery of nonpolar genotoxic constituents in urine (49). The loss of polar components in both the XAD-2 and C_{18} extraction procedures is anticipated. The extracts are generally tested using an enhanced preincubation procedure developed by Kado et al. (50). In this method, heightened sensitivity (13- to 20-fold) is achieved by using a concentrated preincubation mixture with a 10-fold increase in the number of bacteria per plate and a 90-minute preincubation period.

Screening Assays

Although these assays will not meet regulatory requirements, they can provide a quick, cost effective means of screening a large number of materials. Each method has advantages and disadvantages and can be modified to accommodate the available resources.

Spot Test Assay. Each tester strain is typically tested in duplicate in the presence and absence of S9 activation. Because the test article is applied in the center of a petri dish and a concentration gradient forms as the test article diffuses into the agar, each plate permits evaluation over a limited concentration range (51). Revertant colonies induced by test articles that diffuse poorly tend to be tightly clustered immediately outside the zone of inhibition caused by cytotoxicity of the test article. In these cases it is difficult to accurately count the revertants. On the other hand, some test articles diffuse so readily that the revertants are spread fairly evenly throughout the top agar and can be counted with reasonable accuracy. If the distribution of revertants is skewed toward the area around the test article, the phenomenon is referred to as clustering. For these reasons, the results provide a semiquantitative assessment of the test article's mutagenic activity with all strains in the standard battery and the assay requires about 120 mg of test article.

Abbreviated Standard Assay. This assay generally employs tester strains TA98 and TA100, two strains that are responsive to a diverse group of mutagens. Each strain is tested at multiple dose levels each in the presence and absence of S9 activation. The results provide a quantitative, but limited, assessment of the test article's mutagenic activity, and the assay requires about 90 mg of test article. To test five strains each in the presence and absence of S9 requires about 250 mg of test article.

Microsuspension Assay. This assay is based on the methods of Kado et al. (50) described above. With the enhanced sensitivity achieved with this assay, it provides quantitative data on two strains both with and without S9 using 25 mg.

MAMMALIAN CELL MUTATION ASSAYS

Introduction

The induction of mutations in mammalian cells in vitro was first demonstrated in Chinese hamster V79 cells (52,53). Since that time, investigators have searched for in vitro systems that are sensitive to chemically induced mutations, e.g., in diploid fibroblasts (54), L5178Y mouse lymphoma cells (55,56), Chinese hamster ovary (CHO) cells (57,58), and human lymphoblasts (59,60).

Depending on the specific regulatory requirements, any one of the following three assay systems may be used: the thymidine kinase locus of L5178Y mouse lymphoma cells (TK), the hypoxanthine-guanine phosphoribosyl transferase locus of CHO cells (CHO/HGPRT), and the bacterial xanthine-guanine phosphoribosyl transferase gene that has been inserted into CHO cells (AS52/XPRT). This discussion is focused on the TK and CHO/HGPRT assay systems, which are the more commonly used mammalian cell gene mutation systems.

Purpose of Study

The purpose of the mammalian mutation assay is to evaluate the mutagenic potential of the test article based on quantitation of forward mutations at a selected locus in mammalian cell cultures (specifically, the TK locus of L5178Y mouse lymphoma cells, or the HGPRT locus of CHO cells).

Cell Selection and Justification

The L5178Y mouse lymphoma thymidine kinase assay, first described by Clive et al. (61), has successfully identified a number of mutagenic agents. The assay utilizes L5178Y cells that are heterozygous at the TK Locus. Potential mutagenic agents are tested for the ability to cause the $TK^{+/-} \rightarrow TK^{-/-}$ mutation. $TK^{-/-}$ mutants lack the salvage enzyme TK and can easily be detected by their resistance to lethal thymidine analogues. The selective agent of choice is trifluorothymidine (TFT) (62).

L5178Y mouse lymphoma cells possess several desirable characteristics that facilitate mutagenicity testing. The cells grow in suspension culture, which allows: (1) the cultures to be easily sampled to determine the cell population densities, and (2) the enumeration of mutant colonies in selective soft agar medium. The cell line also exhibits a very high cloning efficiency ($>70\%$ in our hands) and has a generation time of 8 to 10 hours. Within 10 to 14 days after the initial seeding, colonies are large enough to count and size with an automatic colony counter. This cell line is easily cryopreserved, recovers quite readily when reestablished in culture, and is routinely grown in horse serum, which is very cost effective.

The maximum mutagenic response at the TK locus is achieved with a relatively short expression time. A 2- to 3-day expression period is necessary for the L5178Y $TK^{+/-}$ assay (63,64), whereas a range of 6 to 16 days is required for selective systems measuring mutations at the HGPRT locus (56,60,65,66). A short expression period also allows the recovery of slower-growing mutants, which would be overgrown during a longer selection period.

In addition to the detection of point mutation, the use of L5178Y cells, which are heterozygous at the TK locus, also permits the detection of mutants resulting from chromosomal rearrangements. L5178Y $TK^{-/-}$ mutants resulting from point mutations are recoverable because no essential functions are deleted. Mutants resulting from chromosomal deletion or rearrangement may be recovered if the deleted essential function is supplied by the homologous region on the homologous chromosome (67). After treatment with many mutagenic substances, mutant $TK^{-/-}$ colonies exhibit a characteristic frequency distribution of colony sizes. The precise distribution of large and small TFT-resistant mutant colonies appears to be the characteristic mutagenic "finger-print" of carcinogens in the L5178Y $TK^{+/-}$ system (63,67). Clive et al. (63) and Hozier et al. (68) have presented evidence to substantiate the hypothesis that the small-colony variants carry chromosome aberrations associated with chromosome 11, the chromosome on which the TK locus is located in the mouse (69). Large colony $TK^{-/-}$ mutants with normal growth kinetics appeared karyotypically similar within and among clones and with the $TK^{+/-}$ parental cell line. In contrast, most slow-growing, small-colony $TK^{-/-}$ mutants had readily recognizable chromosome rearrangements involving chromosome 11. They suggested that the heritable differences in growth kinetics and resultant colony morphology in large and small mutants were related to the type of chromosome damage sustained. Large-colony mutants received very localized damage, possibly in the form of point mutation or small deletion within the TK locus, whereas small-colony mutants received damage to collateral loci concordant with the loss of TK activity. This view was substantiated by the work of Glover et al. (70). They reported the loss of a 6.2 kb fragment that spans the end of the TK locus and a portion of the collateral loci in small-colony mutants. Therefore, it is possible that a range of genetic lesions (point mutations and chromosomal damage) is detected using the TK locus in mouse lymphoma cells.

The CHO/HGPRT assay was designed to select for mutant cells that have become resistant to such purine analogues as 6-thioguanine (TG) and 8-azaguanine as a result of mutation at the X-chromosome-linked HGPRT locus (57,71–73). This system has been demonstrated to be sensitive to the mutagenic action of a variety of chemicals (57). Unlike the L5178Y cells, which are heterozygous at the TK locus, the CHO cells are functionally hemizygous at the HGPRT locus (the single functional copy of the HGPRT gene being present on only one of the two X chromosomes). Therefore, while mutants resulting from point mutations are detectable in this assay system, mutants resulting from chromosomal mutations are not recoverable because no homologous region is available to supply any deleted essential function and lethality ensues (67).

Maintenance of Cells

L5178Y/$TK^{+/-}$ mouse lymphoma cells, from clone 3.7.2C, should be obtained from American Type Culture Collection (ATCC), Manassas, Virginia, U.S.A. Each freeze lot of cells must be tested and found to be free of mycoplasma contamination. Prior to use in the assay, L5178Y/$TK^{+/-}$ cells are cleansed to reduce the frequency of spontaneously occurring $TK^{-/-}$ cells. Using the procedure described by Clive and Spector (74), L5178Y cells are cultured for 24 hours in the presence of thymidine, hypoxanthine, methotrexate, and glycine to poison the $TK^{-/-}$ cells. L5178Y cells are cultured in Fischer's Media for Leukemic Cells of Mice with 0.1% Pluronics, supplemented with 10% horse serum and 2 mM L-glutamine ($F_{10}P$).

The CHO-K1-BH4 cell line is a proline auxotroph with a modal chromosome number of 20, a population doubling time of 12 to 14 hours, and a cloning efficiency of usually greater than 80% (73). This subclone (D1) was derived by Dr. Abraham Hsie (Oak Ridge National Laboratories, Oak Ridge, Tennessee, U.S.A.). CHO cells should be cleansed in medium supplemented with hypoxanthine, aminopterin, and thymidine (HAT), then frozen. Cells used in the mutation assay should not exceed four subpassages from frozen stock. Each freeze lot of cells must be tested and found to be free of mycoplasma contamination. Exponentially growing CHO-K1-BH4 cells are cultured in F12 medium, with or without hypoxanthine, supplemented with 5% dialyzed fetal bovine serum (F12FBS5 or F12FBS5-Hx).

Experimental Design

With L5178Y/TK$^{+/-}$ cells, the mammalian mutation assay is performed by exposing single or duplicate cultures (depending on protocol) to concentrations of test article as well as positive and negative (solvent) controls. Exposures are for 4 hours in the presence and absence of an S9 activation system. Following a 2-day expression period, with daily cell population adjustments, cultures demonstrating 0 to 90% growth inhibition are cloned, in triplicate, in restrictive medium containing soft agar to select for the mutant phenotype. After a 10- to 14-day selection period, mutant colonies are enumerated. The mutagenic potential of the test article is measured by its ability to induce TK$^{+/-}$ → TK$^{-/-}$ mutations. For those test articles demonstrating a positive response, mutant colonies are sized as an indication of mechanism of action.

In compliance with regulatory guidelines, verification of a clear positive response will not be required (1,2). For equivocal and negative results without activation, an independent repeat assay will be performed in which cultures are continuously exposed to the test article for 24 hours. A preliminary toxicity assay without S9 activation and using 24-hour continuous treatment may be performed (where appropriate) to select doses for the independent repeat assay. For equivocal results with S9 activation, an independent repeat assay will be performed using modified dose levels or study design. For negative results with S9 activation, an independent repeat assay will not be required unless the test article is known to have specific requirements of metabolism.

The CHO/HGPRT mutation assay is performed by exposing CHO cells for 5 hours to concentrations of test article, as well as positive and solvent controls, in the presence and absence of an exogenous source of metabolic activation. After a 7- to 9-day expression period, the treated cells are cultured in the presence of 10 μM TG for selection of mutant colonies. The mutagenic potential of a test article is determined by its ability to induce a dose-related increase in the number of TG-resistant mutant colonies when compared to the solvent control.

Dose Selection

The toxicity profile of a test article is determined in a preliminary toxicity test. For the mouse lymphoma assay system, the preliminary toxicity test is conducted by exposing L5178Y/TK$^{+/-}$ cells to solvent alone and to multiple concentrations of test article, the highest concentration being the lowest insoluble dose in treatment medium but not to exceed 5 mg/ml or 10 mM (whichever is the lower) (2,72). The pH of the treatment medium is adjusted, if necessary, to maintain a neutral pH in the treatment medium. The osmolality of the highest soluble treatment condition is also measured. After a 4-hour treatment in the presence and absence of S9 activation, cells are washed twice with F$_{10}$P and cultured in suspension for 2 days posttreatment, with cell concentration adjustment on the first day.

Selection of dose levels for the mouse lymphoma mutation assay is based on reduction of suspension growth after treatment in the preliminary toxicity test. Typically, the high dose for the mutation assay is that concentration exhibiting approximately 100% growth inhibition. The low dose is selected to exhibit 0% growth inhibition. For freely soluble, nontoxic test articles, the highest concentration is 5 mg/mL or 10 mM (whichever is the lower). For relatively insoluble, nontoxic test articles, the highest concentration is the lowest insoluble dose in treatment medium but not to exceed 5 mg/ml or 10 mM (whichever is the lower). In all cases, precipitation is evaluated at the beginning and at the end of the treatment period using the naked eye (2,77).

For the CHO/HGPRT assay system, the preliminary toxicity test is based upon colony-forming efficiency. Approximately 5×10^5 CHO cells are cultured overnight and then exposed to solvent alone and to multiple concentrations of test article, the highest concentration being the lowest insoluble dose in treatment medium not to exceed 5 mg/mlor 10 mM (whichever is the lower) (72). The pH of the treatment medium should be adjusted, if necessary, to maintain a neutral pH in the treatment medium. The osmolality of the highest soluble treatment condition also should be measured. Exposure is for 5 hours at 37°C in a humidified atmosphere of 5% carbon dioxide (CO_2) in air in the presence and absence of S9 activation. Eighteen to 24 hours after removal of treatment medium, the treated cells are trypsinized and reseeded at a density of 100 cells/60 mm dish. After 7 to 10 days incubation at 37°C in a humidified atmosphere of 5% CO_2 in air, colonies are fixed with 95% methanol, stained with 10% aqueous Giemsa, and counted. The cell survival of the test article–treated groups is expressed relative to the solvent control (relative cloning efficiency). For the mutation assay, whenever possible, the high dose is selected to give a cell survival of 10–30%. Four lower doses are selected, at least one of which will be nontoxic. For nontoxic test articles, the selection of the highest concentration should be based on the same criteria as those described for the mouse lymphoma assay system.

Number of Cultures

For the preliminary toxicity test in the mouse lymphoma assay system, a single culture is exposed to the solvent and each test article dose level. For the mutation assay, typically, duplicate cultures are exposed to the solvent control, positive control, and each of eight test article dose levels; cloning for viability assessment and selection of the mutant phenotype are performed at a minimum of five test article dose levels. The use of single cultures in the mutation assay is also acceptable provided that more test articles doses are used (e.g., ten dose levels) and cloned for viability assessment and mutant selection (e.g., eight dose levels).

For the preliminary toxicity test in the CHO/HGPRT assay system, a single culture is exposed to the solvent and each test article dose level. For the mutation assay, duplicate cultures are exposed to the solvent control, positive control, and each of five test article dose levels; cloning for viability assessment and selection of the mutant phenotype are performed at a minimum of four test article dose levels.

Metabolic Activation System

For the mouse lymphoma assay system, Aroclor 1254-induced rat liver S9 is thawed immediately prior to use and mixed with a cofactor pool to contain 11.25 mg DL-isocitric acid, 6 mg NADP, and 0.025 ml S9 homogenate per ml in F_0P. The S9 mix is adjusted to pH 7.

For the CHO/HGPRT assay system, Aroclor 1254-induced rat liver S9 is thawed immediately prior to use and mixed with a cofactor pool to contain 100 μl S9/ml reaction mixture of approximately 4 mM NADP, 5 mM glucose-6-phosphate, 10 mM $MgCl_2$, 30 mM KCl, 10 mM $CaCl_2$, and 50 mM sodium phosphate buffer, pH 8.0 (72). The S9 reaction mixture must be stored on ice until used.

Controls

The solvent (or vehicle) for the test article is used as the negative control.

For the mouse lymphoma assay system, methyl methanesulfonate (MMS) at two concentrations of 15 and 20 μg/ml for the 4-hour exposure (or 5 and 7.5 μg/ml for the 24-hour exposure) is used as the positive control for the nonactivated test system. For the S9-activated system, 7,12-dimethylbenz[a]anthracene (DMBA) at two concentrations of 0.5 and 0.75 μg/ml is used as the positive control.

For the CHO/HGPRT assay system, EMS is used at a concentration of 0.2 μl/ml as the positive control for the nonactivated study, and BAP will be used at a concentration of 4 μg/ml as the positive control for the S9-activated study.

Dose Administration

For the mouse lymphoma assay system, treatment is carried out in conical tubes by combining test or control article in solvent or solvent alone with medium or S9 activation mixture containing 6×10^6 L5178Y/TK$^{+/-}$ cells in a total volume of 10 ml. All pH adjustments should be performed prior to adding S9 or target cells to the treatment medium. Treatment tubes are gassed with 5% CO_2 in air, capped tightly, and incubated with mechanical mixing for 4 hours at 37°C.

At the end of the exposure period, the cells are washed twice with culture medium and collected by centrifugation. The cells are resuspended in 20 ml $F_{10}P$, gassed with 5% CO_2 in air, and cultured in suspension at 37°C for 2 days following treatment. Cell population adjustments to 0.3×10^6 cells/ml are made at 24 and 48 hours.

For selection of the TFT-resistant phenotype, cells from the appropriate number of cultures demonstrating from 0% to 90% suspension growth inhibition are plated into three replicate dishes at a density of 1×10^6 cells/100 mm plate in cloning medium containing 0.23% agar and 2 to 4 μg TFT/ml. For estimation of cloning efficiency at the time of selection, 200 cells/100 mm plate are plated in triplicate in cloning medium free of TFT (viable cell [VC] plate). Plates are incubated at 37°C in a humidified atmosphere of 5% CO_2 for 10 to 14 days.

For the CHO/HGPRT assay system, the time of initiation of chemical treatment is designated as day 0. Cells are exposed, in duplicate cultures, to five concentrations of test article for 5 hour at 37°C in a humidified atmosphere of 5% CO_2 in air. After the treatment period, all media are aspirated and the cells washed to remove treatment medium and are cultured in F12FBS5 or F12FBS5-Hx at 37°C in a humidified atmosphere of 5% CO_2 in air. After 18 to 24 hours of incubation, the cells are subcultured to assess cytotoxicity and to continue the phenotypic expression period.

For evaluation of cytotoxicity, the replicate cultures from each treatment condition are subcultured independently in F12FBS5 or F12FBS5-Hx, in triplicate, at a density of 100 cells/60 mm dish. After 7 to 10 days incubation at 37°C in 5% CO_2 in air, colonies are fixed with 95% methanol, stained with 10% aqueous Giemsa, and counted. Cytotoxicity is expressed relative to the solvent-treated control cultures.

For expression of the mutant phenotype, the replicate cultures from each treatment condition are subcultured independently at a density of no greater than 10^6 cells/100 mm dish. Subculture, as above at 2- to 3-day intervals, is performed for the 7- to 9-day expression period. At this time, selection for the mutant phenotype is performed.

For selection of the TG-resistant phenotype, cells from each treatment condition are plated into a maximum of five dishes at a density of 2×10^5 cells/100 mm dish in F12FBS5-Hx containing 10 μM TG. For cloning efficiency at the time of selection, 100 cells/60 mm dish are plated in triplicate in medium free of TG. After 7 to 10 days of incubation, the colonies are fixed, stained, and counted for both cloning efficiency at selection and mutant selection.

Endpoint Evaluated and Time of Evaluation

For the mouse lymphoma assay system, the total number of colonies per plate is determined after 10 to 14 days of incubation for the VC plates and the total relative growth calculated. The total number of colonies per TFT plate is then determined for those cultures with $\geq 10\%$ total growth. Colonies are enumerated using an automatic counter; if the automatic counter cannot be used, the colonies are counted manually. The diameters of the TFT colonies from the positive control and solvent control cultures should be determined over a range of approximately 0.2 to 1.1 mm. In the event the test article demonstrates a positive response, the diameters of the TFT colonies for at least one dose level of the test article (the highest positive concentration) is determined over a range of approximately 0.2 to 1.1 mm.

For the CHO/HGPRT assay system, the colonies are fixed with 95% methanol after 7 to 10 days of incubation. This includes the plates for cytotoxicity assessment, mutant selection, and cloning efficiency at time of selection. Once stained, the colonies are counted.

Evaluation Criteria

Data Presentation

For the mouse lymphoma assay system, the cytotoxic effects of each treatment condition is expressed relative to the solvent-treated control for suspension growth over 2 days posttreatment and for total growth (suspension growth corrected for plating efficiency at the time of selection). The mutant frequency (MF) for each treatment condition is calculated by dividing the mean number of colonies on the TFT plates by the mean number of colonies on the VC plates and multiplying by the dilution factor (2×10^{-4}) and is expressed as TFT-resistant mutants per 10^6 surviving cells.

For the CHO/HGPRT assay system, the cytotoxic effect of each treatment condition should be expressed relative to the solvent-treated control (relative cloning efficiency). The mutant frequency for each treatment condition is calculated by dividing the total number of mutant colonies by the number of cells selected, corrected for the cloning efficiency of cells prior to mutant selection, and is expressed as TG-resistant mutants per 10^6 clonable cells. For experimental conditions in which no mutant colonies are observed, mutant frequencies should be expressed as less than the frequency obtained with one mutant colony. Mutant frequencies generated from doses giving $\leq 10\%$ relative survival are not considered as valid data points and are not included in the data analysis.

Criteria for Valid Test

For the mouse lymphoma assay system, the following criteria must be met for a test to be considered valid. These criteria have evolved over the years. Until recently, the criteria were as follows. The spontaneous mutant frequency of the solvent (or vehicle) control cultures must be within 20 to 100 TFT-resistant mutants per 10^6 surviving (i.e., clonable) cells. The cloning efficiency of the solvent (or vehicle) control group must be greater than 50%. At least one concentration of each positive control must exhibit mutant frequencies of ≥ 100 mutants per 10^6 surviving cells over the background level [an induced mutant frequency

(IMF)]. The colony size distribution for the MMS positive control must show an increase in both small and large colonies (75,76). A minimum of four analyzable concentrations with mutant frequency data is required for assays with duplicate cultures [or a minimum of seven analyzable concentrations with mutant frequency data for assays with single cultures (77)].

As a result of the International Workshop on Genotoxicity Testing (IWGT) workgroup meetings about the mouse lymphoma assay, in Plymouth (UK) and Aberdeen (UK), the current criteria are as follows (78,79). The spontaneous mutant frequency of the solvent (or vehicle) control cultures must be within 35 to 140 TFT-resistant mutants per 10^6 surviving cells. The cloning efficiency of the solvent (or vehicle) control group must be between 65% and 120%. The suspension growth (i.e., day-1 fold-increase in cell number multiplied by the day-2 fold-increase in cell number) of the negative controls must be between 8 and 32. There are two acceptable approaches to assuring an adequate positive control response: (1) The laboratory should use a dose of a chemical that yields an absolute increase in total MF (i.e., an increase in IMF) of at least 300 per 10^6 surviving cells. At least 40% of the IMF should be reflected in the small colony MF (2). The laboratory must use a dose of a chemical that increases the small colony IMF by at least 150 per 10^6 surviving cells. A minimum of four analyzable concentrations with mutant frequency data is required for assays with duplicate cultures (or a minimum of seven analyzable concentrations with mutant frequency data for assays with single cultures).

For the CHO/HGPRT assay system, the following criteria must be met for a test to be considered valid. The cloning efficiency of the solvent (or vehicle) control must be greater than 50%. The spontaneous mutant frequency in the solvent (or vehicle) control must fall within the range of 0 to 25 mutants per 10^6 surviving cells. The positive control must induce a mutant frequency at least three times that of the solvent control and must exceed 40 mutants per 10^6 surviving cells. A minimum of four analyzable concentrations with mutant frequency data is required (72).

Positive and Negative Test

In evaluation of the data for the mouse lymphoma assay system, increases in mutant frequencies that occur only at highly toxic concentrations (i.e., less than 10% total growth) are not considered biologically relevant. All conclusions are based on sound scientific judgment; however, the following criteria are presented as a guide to interpretation of the data. As with the criteria for a valid test, the evaluation criteria have evolved. At the inception of the assay, only a 2-fold and dose-related increase in MF over the background were required for a positive response. Until recently, the requirements were as follows (80). The result is considered to induce a positive response if a concentration-related increase in mutant frequency is observed and one or more dose levels with 10% or greater total growth exhibit mutant frequencies of ≥ 100 mutants per 10^6 surviving cells over the background level. A result is considered equivocal if the mutant frequency in treated cultures is between 55 and 99 mutants per 10^6 surviving cells over the background level. Test articles producing fewer than 55 mutants per 10^6 surviving cells over the background level are concluded to be negative.

As a result of the IWGT workgroup meetings about the mouse lymphoma assay, in Plymouth (U.K.) and Aberdeen (U.K.), the current criteria are as follows (78,79). A global evaluation factor (GEF), defined as the mean of the negative/solvent MF distribution plus one SD, of 90 mutants per 10^6 surviving cells over the background and a statistically significant dose response are required for a positive response. If the IMF is <90 mutants per 10^6 surviving cells and there is no dose response, the result is negative. Results that fulfill one criterion but not the other will be evaluated on a case-by-case basis.

For the CHO/HGPRT assay system, spontaneous mutant frequencies in this assay range from 0 to 25 mutants per 10^6 surviving cells. As a result, calculation of mutagenic response in terms of fold increase in mutant frequency above the background rate does not provide a reliable indication of the significance of the observed response. The wide acceptable range in spontaneous mutant frequency also suggests the need to set a minimum mutant frequency for a response to be considered positive. Hsie et al. (57) refer to a level of 50 mutants per 10^6 surviving cells. However, a minimum significant level at >40 mutants per 10^6 surviving cells is commonly used.

Supplemental Information

The full power of the mouse lymphoma assay is not realized without very careful attention to dose selection, culture, and treatment conditions, cloning conditions, colony counting techniques, and mutant colony sizing requirements. To produce a valid assay, it is essential to assure that a sufficient range in toxicity has been induced by the test chemical so that weak positive responses are not missed. Culture condition should provide for rapid, uniform cell proliferation and should be free of exposure to white light or other nonspecific mutagens. Treatment conditions can markedly affect the outcome of genotoxicity tests using cultured mammalian cells. Low pH and high osmolality have been demonstrated to produce false positive responses for mutation, cell transformation, and clastogenicity (81). Perhaps the most sensitive portion of the assay is cloning. Some media and sera that will support suspension growth fail to sustain clonal growth. This is also the part of the assay most susceptible to contamination. Cloning conditions are best judged by the recovery of small-colony mutants (80). If the small colonies do not grow to a detectable size, many mutagens will go undetected. Use of a known small-colony inducer, such as MMS, provides a control for cloning conditions (small colony generation), colony counting, and sizing.

Apart from the conventional mouse lymphoma assay that entails the plating of cells in an agar matrix for viability assessment and mutant selection, a microtiter (or microwell) method has been developed (82,83). In the microtiter method, the procedures for the preparation of cells for assay and the treatment of cells with test article are identical to those used in the conventional assay. For assessment of viability following treatment and mutant selection, cells are transferred into 96-well microtiter plates. Sizing of mutant colonies in the microwells is feasible, and the data are essentially comparable to those generated from the conventional agar method (84,85).

In the AS52/HPRT mammalian cell gene mutation assay system, the CHO cells carry a single copy of the *E. coli gpt* gene stably integrated and express the bacterial gene for the enzyme xanthine-guanine phosphoribosyltransferase (58,86). Mutants deficient in this enzyme can be induced in the AS52 cell line, and both spontaneous and induced mutants can be selected for resistance to 6-TG.

IN VITRO CHROMOSOME ABERRATION ASSAYS

Introduction

For several decades the in vitro cytogenetics assay has proven its worth in assessing chromosomal derangement due to chemicals and radiation and has become an integral element of genetic toxicology testing. The chromosome aberration assay offers the advantage of direct visualization of the damage caused by the test article under investigation and can also be used to screen populations for chromosome anomalies arising as a result of environmental agents. The abnormalities that are detected using this method are structural chromosome aberrations, which involve breaks and rearrangements, and numerical chromosome aberrations, involving variations in the number of chromosomes in the nucleus.

Structural chromosome aberrations, involving one or both chromatids, result in a discontinuity in the chromosomal DNA that may be (1) repaired, restoring the original structure, (2) rejoined inappropriately, forming a rearrangement, or (3) left unrejoined resulting in a break or deletion. The majority of structural aberrations are typically lethal to the cell or to the daughter cells during the first few cell cycles following their appearance. However, these structural anomalies serve as an indicator of the occurrence of transmissible aberrations, such as balanced translocations, duplications, inversions, and small deletions. These transmissible aberrations, can result in fetal and perinatal mortality or defects at birth if they arise in germ cells and may play a role in tumor initiation and progression in somatic cells (87).

Cells with numerical chromosome aberrations feature a chromosome complement different from the number of chromosomes characteristic for the species. A deviation of the chromosome number involving one or a few chromosomes is termed aneuploidy. This condition can be measured in karyotypically stable primary cell cultures (i.e., peripheral lymphocytes). A variation in the complement of chromosomes involving a whole set of chromosomes is called polyploidy or endoreduplication, depending on the underlying mechanism. This anomaly can be measured in primary cell cultures and in established cell lines. Aneuploidy, polyploidy, and endoreduplication are not due to the direct interaction of an environmental agent with the chromosomal DNA. Aneuploidy and polyploidy are usually the result of disruption of some aspect of the spindle apparatus (microtubules, centrioles, kinetochores, and the associated proteins) or due to cell fusion, failure of cytokinesis, or nuclear fusion in binucleate cells (88,89). Endoreduplication appears to be an abnormal variation of cell replication, probably resulting from the action of DNA polymerase β rather than DNA polymerase α, that involves two cycles of chromosome replication in the absence of an intervening nuclear division (90–92).

When aneuploidy appears in germ cells, the result can be spontaneous abortions or defects at birth (93). These numerical aberrations do not seem to play a key role in the initiation of tumors but are indicative of the evolution of karyotypic instability within a population of tumor cells (88). The physiological outcome, and hence the genotoxic impact, of polyploidy and endoreduplication is less than clear. Both phenomena are found in vivo in normal cell populations, and both are caused by a variety of agents some of which do not induce other types of chromosome damage (94–97). The induction of numerical aberrations may be interpreted as cytotoxicity with a concomitant perturbation of DNA replication, and unless it is observed at concentrations that are within a therapeutic (or expected exposure) range it may not reflect a major genotoxic lesion (88).

Purpose of Study

The purpose of an in vitro cytogenetic study is to evaluate the clastogenic or chromosome breakage potential of a test article and its metabolites based upon its ability to induce chromosome aberrations in culture using an established cell line or a primary cell source. The use of cell cultures as a test system has been demonstrated to be an effective method of detection of chemical clastogens (98). Induction of chromosome breakage in vitro is an indicator that the test article is potentially genotoxic.

Cell Selection and Justification

Established cell lines or primary cell cultures can be used as the in vitro test system. The cell types routinely used in these assays are CHO cells, Chinese hamster lung (CHL) cells and human peripheral blood lymphocytes (HPBL). The Chinese hamster cell lines, CHO, and CHL, are established cell lines that are grown as monolayer cultures. Human lymphocytes, HPBL, are a primary cell source and are grown as suspension cultures that must be stimulated with the mitogen phytohemagglutinin (PHA) in order to divide.

Primary cell cultures, such as HPBL, are believed to show some variability between donors in their response to test articles and their sensitivity to test article treatment compared to established cell lines (99,100). However, HPBLs have demonstrated reliability over years of in vitro cytogenetic testing and are sufficiently validated, and their relevancy to human exposure to test articles cannot be overlooked. When obtaining blood cells routine clinical blood handling precautions should be observed, and donor selection should be closely monitored. Blood should be obtained only from healthy volunteers without a recent history of receiving medication, viral infection, or x-ray exposure (101).

Established cell lines from frozen stocks, such as CHO or CHL cells, are genetically more homogeneous than primary cell cultures and tend to show less interexperiment variability within a cell type. Established Chinese hamster cell lines, such as CHO and CHL, are useful in in vitro cytogenetics testing because they are easily cultured in standard medium, have a small number of large chromosomes each with a more or less distinctive morphology, and have a relatively short cell cycle time (102). Several clones of CHO cells are currently available for cytogenetic studies. In comparative studies quantitative differences in responses to test articles between these clones have been demonstrated, and this characteristic makes it imperative that the cell source and type of clone used in any study are well described (100). An inherent property of most established cell lines is that, due to extensive chromosome rearrangements, the chromosome number varies around a modal value (100,101). This property necessitates establishing criteria for defining analyzable cells. The current criteria are that cells with the modal chromosome number plus or minus two chromosomes are acceptable for microscopic analysis.

Maintenance of Cells

Established cell lines can be obtained from laboratories conducting in vitro cytogenetics studies or a supplier, such as the American Type Culture Collection (Manassas, Virginia, U.S.A.). Upon receipt of the cells frozen stocks should be established, and the cells need to be checked for mycoplasma contamination.

Several environmental factors must be monitored closely. Extremes of pH and osmolality under test conditions must be avoided. Low pH and excessively high osmolality can induce chromosome aberrations (103,104). These parameters must be adjusted to physiological levels when necessary. When the test system consists of established cell lines, the monolayers must not reach confluency at any time (i.e., during incubation of seeded cultures prior to test article treatment or during the assay). The target cells in the assay are mitotically active. As the cells approach confluency, the growth rate slows down, thereby diminishing the number of target cells. In addition, with established cell lines, as the monolayers become confluent and the growth rate slows, the cell cultures have a tendency to become karyotypically unstable, and the background levels of chromosome rearrangements (dicentrics, rings, etc.) may increase.

Experimental Design

In vitro chromosome aberration studies are generally conducted in two phases. The first phase, the preliminary toxicity assay, serves as a dose range-finding assay for the definitive portion of the study. In the second phase, the chromosome aberration assay, the clastogenic potential of the test article is evaluated. The second phase may include an initial and an independent repeat or confirmatory assay.

When conducting an in vitro chromosome aberration assay, it is critical to make structural damage assessments in chromosomes that are in the first posttreatment metaphase of the cell cycle. If damaged cells are capable of cycling and allowed to progress through more than one cell cycle, damaged chromosomes (or fragments) may be lost or converted to relatively intricate derivatives (105). Structural damage that appears as chromatid-type in the first posttreatment metaphase can potentially emerge as chromosome-type damage in the second posttreatment metaphase. The loss of damaged chromosomes (or fragments) or the conversion of one type of damage into another during cell cycle progression can be misleading. Ensuring that structural damage is assessed in the first posttreatment metaphase may be accomplished by assessing the cell cycle delay, if any, that results from treatment with the test article in question; or by using multiple harvest times. The harvest times are designed to enrich the proportion of first post-treatment metaphase cells and are described below.

Dose Selection

In the preliminary toxicity assay the maximum concentration tested is either 5 mg/ml or 10 mM (whichever is lower) for freely soluble test articles, or, for poorly soluble test articles, the maximum concentration resulting in a suspension that can deliver a reliable amount of test article to the test system (workable suspension). The preliminary toxicity assay should be conducted in the presence and absence of metabolic activation (S9). A sufficient number of lower concentrations must also be included to determine the appropriate dose range for testing in the definitive assay. A solvent control needs to be included in the preliminary toxicity assay. Toxicity end points are assessed relative to the solvent control and should be such that they give an appropriate indication of the test article impact on cell growth (106). For established cell lines the colony forming efficiency (cloning/plating efficiency), cell monolayer confluency, or a measure of the number of surviving cells, assessed with an automatic cell counter, are reliable indicators of the test article toxicity. Determination of the average generation time using BrdUrd-labeled cells stained for sister chromatid differentiation (107), or mitotic index determination, may be used as supplementary information, but neither is a sufficient indicator of cytotoxicity when used alone. For cells grown in suspension, such as HPBLs, the reduction in mitotic index relative to the solvent control is the most practical method of assessing toxicity. Under test conditions, the pH should be adjusted to physiological values, and the osmolality should be monitored and compared with the solvent control.

In the definitive assay, the maximum concentration to be tested must be selected to demonstrate toxicity (assuming there is measurable toxicity) in the test system. For established cell lines, the highest concentration selected must exhibit a level of toxicity of at least a 50% reduction in cloning efficiency or cell monolayer confluency or a 50% inhibition in cell growth relative to the solvent control. For HPBLs, the highest concentration selected for testing must exhibit a reduction in the mitotic index of at least 50% relative to the solvent. The selection of the maximum dose level for the chromosome aberration assay that is as follows: for a nontoxic, nonprecipitating test article, the maximum dose level should be 5 mg/ml or 10 mM (whichever is lower); for a toxic test article, the maximum dose level should demonstrate toxicity (at least 50%) regardless of the precipitation profile; and for a precipitating, nontoxic test article, the maximum dose level should be the lowest precipitating dose level (2,108).

Number of Cultures

For the preliminary toxicity assay one culture for each dose level and the solvent control is sufficient although more than one culture can be used. Duplicate cultures for each dose level and the solvent control are recommended for the chromosome aberration assay.

Metabolic Activation System

Extended treatment of cells in S9 should be avoided because of the cytotoxic nature of the mixture and the loss of enzymatic activity of the S9 mix over time. Exposures of 3 to 6 hours are sufficient when the concentration of S9 is 10% or less (100). Aroclor 1254-induced S9 may, under some circumstances, induce chromosome breakage, possibly due to the generation of active oxygen radicals (109). Other metabolic activation systems using different rodent species and inducing agents offer an alternative to the use of PCBs (110). The effects of oxygen radicals may therefore be minimized by using S9 induced by agents other than Aroclor 1254, such as β-naphthoflavone plus phenobarbital.

Controls

To determine that the test system is functioning properly and that the test is valid, appropriate positive and negative controls must be included in chromosome aberration assays. A solvent control, in which the cell cultures are treated with the solvent only, is required to assess relative increases in the measured end point (structural or numerical chromosome aberrations). The amount of solvent added to the test system should be the same as in the test article–treated cultures. A solvent control needs to be included in both the S9-activated test system and in the nonactivated test system. If an unusual solvent is being used in the assay and there is little or no historical data to determine its effect on the test system, then an untreated control should also be included as one of the negative controls. The untreated control receives no additional components other than the culture medium for the nonactivated test system or the S9 reaction mixture for the metabolically activated test system. Exposure to S9, in the untreated control cultures, should be for the same length of time as in the test article–treated cultures. Comparison of the solvent control values to the untreated control values allows assessment of any solvent effects. A positive control is required to determine that the test system is capable of detecting clastogenic activity. The positive control articles should be appropriate for the system in which the test is conducted. In the nonactivated test system, the positive control article should be a direct-acting clastogenic compound, such as mitomycin-C (MMC) or N-methyl-N'-nitro-N-nitrosoguanidine (MNNG); in the S9-activated test system the positive control should be an agent requiring metabolic activation, such as BAP or cyclophosphamide (CP). The positive controls should be used at concentrations that adequately demonstrate that the test system is functioning. However, high concentrations and the resulting extreme responses from the positive control articles are to be avoided whenever possible.

Dose Administration, Exposure Time, and Cell Collection Time

Target cells are treated for a defined exposure time that may be continuous up to cell harvest in the absence of S9 but limited (3 to 6 hours) in the presence of S9. Typically the test article is dissolved in solvent at a concentration that will be diluted to the final target concentration when the dosing aliquot is added to test system. Incorporation of the test article–solvent mixture into the treatment medium has been demonstrated to be an effective method of dosing the target cells (98). In the S9-activated test system, the test article-solvent mixture is added to the S9 mixture in the culture flask for the prescribed exposure time (3–6 hours), the test article-solvent/S9 mixture is then aspirated, and the cells are rinsed with a physiological buffer and refed with complete medium. The cultures are then incubated until the cell harvest. It is important to include a concurrent toxicity test (colony forming efficiency, cell monolayer confluency, or cell growth inhibition for CHO cells and mitotic inhibition for HPBLs) along with the chromosome aberration assay.

An attempt to harmonize global regulatory requirements by the ICH and OECD has led to the issuance of guidelines that satisfy global submission (1,107). In this set of guidelines, the conduct of an in vitro cytogenetics or chromosomal aberration assay will be carried out in the absence and presence of S9-activation. The cells are exposed to at least three concentrations of the test article for 3 to 6 hours as well as positive and solvent controls in duplicate cultures. The cells are then harvested for microscopic analysis at a single time point 1.5 times the normal cell cycle from the initiation of treatment. In the event of a negative response in the nonactivated portion of the assay, an independent repeat or confirmatory assay is required. The repeat assay is carried out with a continuous exposure up to cell harvest, which is 1.5 times the normal cell cycle. A negative response in the S9-activated portion of the assay may require a confirmatory assay (to be required on a case by case basis).

The end points measured include structural and numerical aberrations in metaphase chromosomes that are representative of the first cell division after treatment. The harvest times are selected in an attempt to balance the requirement for evaluating first-division metaphase chromosomes with the possibility of test article–induced cell cycle delay. To obtain the metaphase chromosomes, the cells are treated with a spindle apparatus disrupting agent, Colcemid®, two hours prior to cell harvest. The concentration of Colcemid® is typically 0.1 µg/ml treatment medium. This treatment traps the cells in metaphase at the time of cell harvest. The cells are harvested by treatment with trypsin for monolayer cultures or by centrifugation for suspension cultures. The harvested cells are then treated in a hypotonic buffer (0.075 M KCl) for an appropriate time that allows the cells to swell (3 to 20 minutes depending on cell type). The swelling of the cells is necessary to ensure well-separated chromosomes when the cells are dropped onto microscope slides. After hypotonic treatment, the cells are fixed (#:1 methanol and glacial acetic acid), dropped onto slides, and stained with Giemsa.

Metaphase Analysis

To ensure that a sufficient number of metaphase cells are available for analysis on the slides, the percentage of cells in mitosis per 500 cells scored (mitotic index) is determined for each treatment group. In some cases, when test article precipitation has been carried over by centrifugation of suspension cultures, or cannot be adequately rinsed from monolayers, it must be determined that the precipitate will not obscure analysis of the metaphase chromosomes. Slides from the highest scorable dose level and the next two or three dose levels are selected for analysis.

Slides selected for analysis are blind coded. Metaphase cells with the modal number (2n) ± 2 centromeres are examined under oil immersion. Whenever possible, a minimum of 200 metaphase spreads (100 per duplicate flask) are examined and scored for chromatid-type and chromosome-type aberrations (Fig. 2) (101). Chromatid-type aberrations include chromatid and isochromatid breaks and exchange figures, such as quadriradials (symmetrical and asymmetrical interchanges), triradials, and complex rearrangements. Chromosome-type aberrations include chromosome breaks and exchange figures, such as dicentrics and rings. Fragments (chromatid or acentric) observed in the absence of any exchange figure are typically scored as a break (chromatid or chromosome). Fragments observed with an exchange figure are not scored as an aberration but are considered part of the incomplete exchange. Pulverized chromosome(s), pulverized cells, and severely damaged cells (≥ 10 aberrations) are also recorded. Chromatid and isochromatid gaps are recorded but not included in the analysis. The XY coordinates for each cell with chromosomal aberrations are recorded using a calibrated microscope stage. The percent polyploid and endoreduplicated cells are also evaluated per 100 cells. The mitotic index is recorded as the percentage of cells in mitosis per 500 cells counted.

Evaluation Criteria

All conclusions must be based on sound scientific judgment. As a guide to interpretation of the data, the test article is usually considered to induce a positive response if the percent aberrant cells is increased in a dose-responsive manner with one or more concentrations being statistically elevated relative to the solvent control group ($p \leq 0.05$). A reproducible and statistically significant increase at a single dose level may also be considered positive. Test articles not demonstrating a statistically significant increase in aberrations are concluded to be negative. Regardless of results of the statistical analysis, however, the biological relevance of the response must be considered (for example, comparing test results with historical control data), especially when evaluating a borderline response (106).

Data Presentation

The toxic effects of treatment are based upon colony forming efficiency, cell monolayer confluency, cell growth inhibition, or mitotic inhibition relative to the solvent control group. These data are presented for both the preliminary toxicity assay and the definitive assay for all dose levels tested (which may include an initial and an independent repeat or confirmatory assay). The number and types of aberrations, the percentage of structurally aberrant cells (percent aberrant cells), numerically aberrant cells in the total population of cells examined, and the frequency of structural aberrations per cell (mean aberrations per cell) are also reported for each treatment group. Chromatid and isochromatid gaps are presented in the data but are not included in the total percentage of cells with one or more aberrations or in the frequency of structural aberrations per cell.

Statistical Analysis

Numerous statistical methods are available for use in analyzing chromosome aberration data. At the present time, a reliable and commonly used method is the Fisher's Exact Test. The Fisher's test is used to make pairwise comparisons between the percentage of aberrant cells in each test concentration group and the solvent control value. An adjustment of the significance level should be done to take into account that multiple comparisons are made against a single concurrent solvent control. The Cochran-Armitage test is recommended as a trend test for dose responsiveness (111).

Criteria for a Valid Test

The frequency of cells with structural chromosome aberrations in the untreated and solvent control groups should remain within the range of the historical controls. For the positive controls, the percentage of cells with aberrations must be statistically increased ($p \leq 0.05$, Fisher's exact test) relative to the solvent control or to the untreated control.

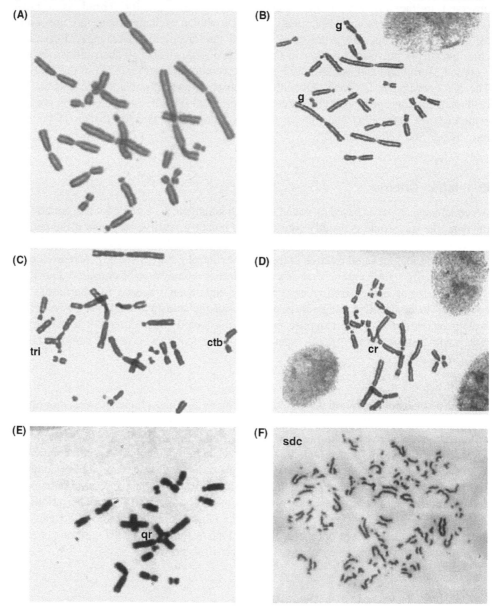

Figure 2 Examples of structural and numerical aberrations in Chinese hamster ovary (CHO) chromosomes. (**A**) Cell in metaphase of mitosis demonstrating the standard modal number (20) of structurally normal chromosomes. (**B**) Gap, g. (**C**) Chromatid break, ctb; chromatid rearrangement (triradial), tri. (**D**) Chromatid rearrangement (complex rearrangement), cr. (**E**) Chromatid rearrangement (quadriradial), qr. (**F**) Severely damaged cell, sdc. (**G**) Numerical aberration, polyploidy. (**H**) Numerical aberration, endoreduplication. Examples of in vivo rat (**I**) and mouse (**J**) bone marrow metaphases showing chromatid type aberrations.

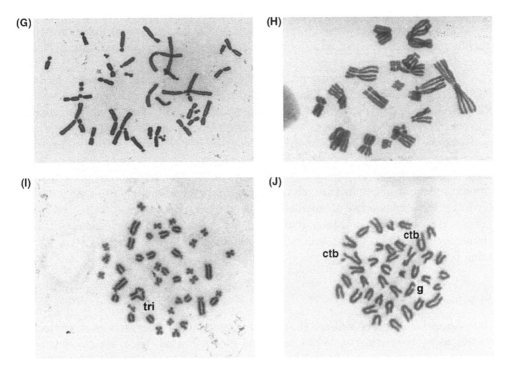

Figure 2 (*Continued from previous page*)

IN VIVO CYTOGENETICS ASSAY SYSTEMS

In vivo cytogenetic assays are used to evaluate the potential of a product to induce structural chromosome aberrations in somatic and germ cells of mammals. There are several advantages to in vivo testing, the most significant being the consideration of metabolic activation and detoxification processes. In vitro assays using S9 or primary hepatocytes to simulate in vivo metabolism may lack critical detoxification enzymes. Additionally, some chemicals are known to be modified by intestinal bacteria (112). In vivo testing also allows for the assessment of chromosome alterations in both somatic and germ cells.

The standard chromosome damage assays include the micronucleus assay in bone marrow or peripheral blood cells and the chromosome aberration assay in bone marrow or spermatogonial cells. Both the micronucleus test and the metaphase analysis assays may be used interchangeably for the demonstration of in vivo clastogenic activity.

Erythrocyte Micronucleus Test

Introduction

The micronucleus test is used for the detection of damage to chromosomes as well as the mitotic apparatus in bone marrow or peripheral blood cells of rodents. The assay system has been well standardized (113–116).

The basic features of the test system are (1) the effect of the test chemical is observed in anucleated polychromatic erythrocytes (PCE); (2) PCE have a relatively short life span, so that any micronuclei they contain must have been generated as a result of recently induced chromosome damage; (3) micronuclei are readily identifiable and their distribution is well defined; and (4) the frequency of induced micronuclei in PCE is dependent upon sampling times.

Erythroblasts in bone marrow undergo a final chromosome replication after which they divide and differentiate into PCE. Chromosomal breaks or interference in the mitotic process that result in the lagging chromosomes during this division lead to the formation of micronuclei that are similar in appearance but much smaller than the nucleus in immature, nucleated erythrocytes. During differentiation, only the nucleus is expelled from the nucleated erythrocyte, leaving behind any micronuclei formed.

The micronucleus assay may be used not only for the detection of acute but also chronic genetic damage. In mice, chromosomal breakage in bone marrow erythroblasts produces an accumulation of micronuclei in normochromatic erythrocytes (NCEs) in peripheral blood and there is little, if any, selective removal of micronucleated cells from circulation. This is not the case with rats, which limits their usefulness in long-term studies using peripheral blood.

Experimental Design

Species.   Mice or rats are the most frequently used mammals in micronucleus studies using bone marrow. When peripheral blood is used, mice are recommended. However, any appropriate mammalian species may be used provided sufficient historical control data are available. At initiation of the study, the weight variation between animals should not exceed $\pm 20\%$ of the sample mean for each sex.

Housing Conditions.   Animals should be obtained from sources that are free of adventitious agents. Animals should be housed in an American Association for the Accreditation of Laboratory Animal Care (AAALAC)–accredited facility with a controlled environment of $23 \pm 3°C$, $50 \pm 20\%$ relative humidity, and a 12-hour light/dark cycle. Animals may be individually or group housed by sex. Animals should have free access to a certified chow that has been analyzed for environmental contaminants and to drinking water. Animals should be identified uniquely and acclimated for no fewer than 5 days prior to study initiation.

Treatment and Sampling Time.   The maximum volume of liquid administered by gavage or injection should not exceed 2 mL/100 g body weight. Except for irritating or corrosive substances that normally reveal aggravated effects with higher concentrations, variability in test volume should be minimized by adjusting the concentration to ensure a constant volume at all dose levels. Dosing may be performed using a single administration, followed by multiple sampling times, or by dose administration on two consecutive days, separated by 24 hours and followed by a single sample time. The choice of treatment protocol is usually made on the basis of any pharmacokinetic data on the test substance. The use of a high dose increases the likelihood that a weak clastogen will be detected. In many cases, a higher total dose can be given in two or more treatments than in a single treatment, and in such cases multiple injections may increase the success rate of the assay. No single sampling time is optimal (117). However, the most frequently used design involves the administration of three concentrations of test article as well as positive and negative (vehicle) controls to male mice after which bone marrow cells are collected at 24 and 48 hours and examined for the presence of micronucleated PCE (mPCEs). In the event that peripheral blood is the target, samples are taken at least twice, starting no earlier than 36 hours after treatment, with appropriate intervals following treatment. The clastogenic potential of the test article is measured by its ability to increase mPCEs in treated animals as compared with vehicle control animals.

Dose Selection. Dose levels to be employed should be selected on the basis of toxicity data but should not exceed 2 g/kg body weight. During the performance of the toxicity study, in addition to the observation of clinical signs and mortality, bone marrow smears may be prepared from all the surviving animals and scored for PCE/total erythrocyte ratio. If both sexes are being tested, the toxicity profile may be different between males and females and will justify dose selection based on sex. Normally, the high dose should be the maximum tolerated dose (MTD) as determined according to mortality, bone marrow cell toxicity, treatment-related clinical signs, or 80% of the lethal dose for 50% of the test animals (LD_{50}) up to a limit of 2 g/kg body weight.

If data are available to demonstrate that there are no substantial differences in toxicity, pharmacokinetics, or metabolism between sexes, testing of a single sex is sufficient (115). Where human exposure to chemicals may be sex-specific, as for example with some pharmaceutical agents, the test should be performed with animals of the appropriate sex. Each treatment group should include at minimum of 5 analyzable animals.

Controls. Concurrent positive and negative (vehicle) controls should be included for each sex tested. Negative controls, consisting of vehicle alone and otherwise treated in the same way as the treatment groups, should be included for every sampling time. The volume of vehicle administered should be equivalent to that given to test animals. In addition, an untreated control group should be included in the absence of historical control data demonstrating no adverse effect of the vehicle alone. If peripheral blood is analyzed, a pretreatment sample should be acceptable as a concurrent negative control but only for short-term studies.

It is advisable to include a concurrent positive control in every experiment to ensure that the assay is performed according to prescribed standards. Convincing positive data may be accepted in the absence of positive control data, but reports of negative assay data unaccompanied by concurrent positive control data are not acceptable. Positive control doses should be chosen so that the effects are clear but do not immediately reveal the identity of the coded slides to the evaluator. The purpose of a positive control is to show that a response can be detected under the conditions of dosing and sample preparation. It is acceptable that the positive control be administered by a route different from the test substance and sampled at only a single time. In addition, chemical class–related positive control chemicals should be considered, when available. Examples of positive controls and concentrations that are used in mice are EMS, 200 mg/kg; ethyl nitrosourea, 25 mg/kg; mitomycin C, 1 mg/kg; and CP, 40 mg/kg. Positive control doses that significantly alter the proportion of PCEs in the bone marrow should be avoided.

Accumulation of historical data for the negative and positive controls is recommended. Comparison of the concurrent negative and positive controls with the historical value provides evidence that the assay is within expected limits.

Route of Administration. The preferred route of administration is the route of human exposure. However, to maximize delivery of the test substance to the target tissue, intraperitoneal injection is the most commonly used method of administration.

Bone Marrow Collection. Bone marrow cells are collected from femurs or tibias into a small amount of fetal calf serum (1 to 2 ml), and smears are prepared and stained using standard methods. The primary consideration in preparation of bone marrow smears is to obtain a single layer of cells sufficiently spread to preserve morphology and to facilitate scoring. A random distribution of the cells is achieved by suspending and mixing the marrow in fetal bovine serum (FBS). The cells are stained to differentiate PCEs from NCEs. Methods include the use of conventional stains, e.g., Giemsa or May-Gruenwald-Giemsa, or

DNA-specific stains, such as acridine orange (116), Hoechst 33258 plus pyronin Y (118), which may eliminate some of the artifacts associated using non-DNA-specific stains.

End Point Evaluation. The minimum number of cells scored per sample should be chosen to minimize the proportion of zero class samples. At a spontaneous frequency of 0 to 2 micronucleated cells per thousand, at least 2000 cells should be scored per sample. Because the frequency of micronucleated cells among NCEs does not increase as markedly as that among PCEs, it is not necessary to score micronucleated NCEs. However, it may be useful to measure this parameter for purposes of quality control, because artifacts in any given slide will produce apparent increases in the frequencies of micronuclei in both NCEs and PCEs and the incidence of artifacts will generally fail to follow the time course through the erythrocyte subpopulations as expected for the true micronuclei.

In addition to the frequency of mPCEs, the ratio of PCEs to total erythrocytes should be determined. This ratio may be obtained by counting the number of PCEs out of 1000 erythrocytes. A reduction in PCE/total erythrocyte ratio is used to indicate bone marrow toxicity and may be used to document bioavailablity of the test chemical to the target tissue. In the absence of bone marrow toxicity, plasma levels may be required to demonstrate bioavailability of the test substance to the target organ (119).

Evaluation Criteria

The criteria for distinguishing positive and negative results should be established in advance. Statistical methods may be used as an aid in evaluating the test results; however, statistics should not be the only criteria for determination of a positive response. Biological relevance of the results should also be considered. Criteria for determining a positive result should include a dose-related increase in mPCEs or a clear increase in mPCEs at the high dose at a single sampling time. A negative result indicates that, under the test conditions, the test substance does not produce mPCEs in the test species.

Data Presentation. Individual animal data are presented in tabular form. The experimental unit should be the animal. The incidence of mPCEs is determined for each animal and treatment group. The number of PCEs scored, the number of mPCEs, and the ratio of PCEs per 1000 erythrocytes should be reported for each animal and summarized for each treatment group by sex and time point.

Statistics. There is little agreement on the distribution of mPCEs, and a variety of tests have been used for statistical analysis, including those based on the binomial, Poisson, and negative binomial distributions (120). Our laboratory uses the statistical tables developed by Kastenbaum and Bowman (121), which are based on the Poisson distribution and which may be used to test pairwise the statistical difference in the mPCE frequencies between test article–treated and vehicle control groups.

Criteria for Valid Test. The mean incidence of mPCEs must not exceed 0.5% (5 mPCEs/1000 PCEs) in the negative (vehicle) control. The incidence of mPCEs in the positive control group must be significantly increased relative to the negative control.

Mammalian Bone Marrow Chromosome Aberration Assay

Introduction

The in vivo chromosome aberration assay is used for the detection of certain structural chromosome changes induced by test compounds in mammals, usually rodents. The gross chromosome damage detected in these assays is frequently lethal to the cell during the first few cell cycles after their induction. The induction of these aberrations indicates a potential to induce more subtle chromosome damage (nonlethal) than may be compatible with cell division and that may lead to heritable cytogenetic abnormalities.

Chromosome aberrations are evaluated in mitotically arrested metaphase cells, following treatment with the test compound. In principle, metaphase analysis can be performed in any tissue containing dividing cells. Whereas the bone marrow is the most appropriate tissue containing rapidly dividing cells for screening purposes, other cells may be examined when tissue-specific effects are of interest. Some aspects that were mentioned in micronucleus study design are common to all in vivo tests, such as the species selection, solubility, route of administration, dose levels, and controls.

Experimental Design

Following the administration of three concentrations of test article as well as positive and negative (vehicle) controls to animals, bone marrow cells are arrested in metaphase using colchicine treatment and are collected for microscopic evaluation. Normally at least two bone marrow collection times are used. The first sampling time is usually 18 hours, which is approximately 1.5 normal cell cycle lengths following treatment. Because cell cycle kinetics can be influenced by the test article, a later sample collection at 42 hours (24 hours after the initial sample time) is also used.

Treatment and Sampling Time. Treatment by a single administration is normally used unless there is a specific reason for doing otherwise. A single injection will, in the majority of cases, provide for maximum sensitivity of the assay. As in the micronucleus test, the volume administered should not exceed 2 ml/100 g body weight.

The efficiency of detection of induced aberrations will depend upon the selected cell sampling time for cytological processing. The aberrations are best observed in contracted metaphase chromosomes at the first mitosis after their induction.

It is necessary to sample cells at their first mitosis (M_1) after treatment to allow for the most accurate measure of the induced aberration frequency. If the cells are scored at M_2 or M_3, the types of aberrations are mixed and lose identity with the cell stage. Because of failure to divide, acentric fragments can be lost from daughter cells, and chromatid-type aberrations can segregate to give normal and aberrant cells. All of these factors lead to a reduced aberration frequency if first-division metaphase cells are not scored.

The selected sample times should be such that cells in different stages of the cells cycle at the time treatment will be analyzed. Also, induced chromatid-type aberrations are converted into derived chromosome-type as a consequence of cell division and subsequent DNA replication. The majority of chemical agents induce chromatid-type aberrations during S phase, irrespective of the cell cycle stage treated. Thus at least one of the populations analyzed should constitute cells that were in the S-phase at the time of treatment (122). This is of particular importance for agents that have a short period of activity in vivo.

For some chemicals, such as benzo[a]-pyrene and 2-acetylaminofluorene, that can cause considerable cell cycle delay, the maximum induction of chromosomal damage occurred between 36 to 44 hours after a single dose administration (123). A cell kinetics study to estimate the cell cycle delay caused by the test article treatment can be performed by implanting BrdUrd tablets subcutaneously at 1 to 2 hours prior to dose administration. Bone marrow is collected at different time points, such as 12 and 24 hour following dosing. Metaphase cells are differentially stained (124) and the proportions of cells in first-division (M_1), second-division (M_2), and third-or-greater-division (M_3) metaphase are determined. The average generation time is estimated based on the proportion of M_1, M_2 and M_3 cells. As long as cells are scored at the first-division metaphase following treatment, the types of aberrations visualized are reflective of the stage of the cell cycle in which they were induced. The types of chromosome aberrations have been extensively described and standardized (125).

Dose Selection. In general, selection of an upper dose level can be based on end points mentioned in the micronucleus assay. In addition to the observation of clinical signs and mortality, bone marrow mitotic index may be considered in dose selection. The high dose should be set at the MTD, based on mortality, bone marrow toxicity, or treatment-related clinical signs. The maximum dose delivered should not exceed 2 gm/kg.

Preparation of Metaphase Cells. At an appropriate time prior to sampling, generally 1 to 3 hours, animals are injected with 2 mg/kg colchicine to arrest cells in metaphase. The bone marrow samples are collected, processed by exposing cells to a hypotonic solution, and then fixed. The fixed cells are spread on slides and stained with Giemsa.

Evaluation Criteria

The criteria for distinguishing positive and negative results should be established in advance. Statistical methods may be used as an aid in evaluating the test results; however, statistics should not be the only criteria for determination of a positive response. Biological relevance of the results should also be considered. Criteria for determining a positive result should include a dose-related increase in percent cells with aberration or a clear increase in percent aberrant cells at the high dose at a single sampling time. A negative result indicates that, under the test condition, the test substance does not produce chromosomal aberration in the test species.

Data Presentation. The mitotic index should be determined as a measure of cytotoxicity in at least 1000 cells per animal. Metaphase cells containing $2n \pm 2$ centromeres should be scored from each animal for chromatid-type and chromosome-type aberrations.

The mitotic index and the total number and types of aberrations found in each animal should be presented. Gaps are presented in the data but are not included in the total percentage of cells with one or more aberrations or in the average number of number of aberrations per cell. The percentage of damaged cells in the total population of cells scored are calculated for each treatment group. The severity of damage within the cell is reported as the average number of aberrations per cell for each treatment group. Male and female animals are analyzed separately. The Fisher's exact test may be used for pairwise comparisons of the percentage of aberrant cells between each treatment group and negative control group. The Cochran-Armitage trend test for the percentage of aberrant cells are performed between test article-treated groups and the negative control to test for evidence of dose response.

Spermatogonial Chromosome Aberration Assay

Introduction

The in vivo mammalian spermatogonial chromosome aberration test is conducted to identify those substances that cause structural chromosome aberrations in mitotically dividing mammalian spermatogonial cells (126–128). Rodent germ cells assays would not normally be conducted for routine screening purposes but may be part of a package of data used in quantitative hazard assessment. In all probability, the clastogenicity of the agents will have been established either in vitro or in vivo using somatic cells prior to germ cell testing.

Requirements for the bone marrow cytogenetic assays apply equally to germ cell studies, but additional technical considerations should be considered.

Experimental Design

Species. Routinely mice and rats are used for the spermatogonial metaphase analysis.

Treatment and Sampling Time. It is advisable to use more than one sampling interval because treatment with the test agent may delay the cell cycle. Differentiating spermatogonia divide at 26 to 38 hour. The majority of mitotic cells in testicular preparations are stage B spermatogonia with an average cell cycle time of 26 hours. Because most clastogens are S-phase dependent, sampling should be performed at 24 and 48 hours after dose administration.

Dose Selection. The MTD is usually selected as the high dose for hazard identification. The MTD is defined as the dose that shows signs of toxicity to the animals or gives an indication for cytotoxicity to differentiating spermatogonia. However, in the spermatogonial metaphase analysis, the number of spermatogonial metaphases from treated animals should not be reduced by more than 50% as compared to the vehicle control. The limit dose for nontoxic chemicals should be 2 g/kg body weight. Two additional doses adequately spaced should be employed to establish a dose response.

Preparation of Spermatogonial Metaphases. Animals are treated with 3 to 4 mg colchicine/kg body weight at 2 to 4 hours prior to sacrifice. The number of spermatogonial cells can be enhanced if the testicular cells are dispersed in 0.1% trypsin prior to hypotonic treatment (128).

Cells to Be Scored. For each animal, at least 100 well-spread mitotic metaphases, with complete number of centromeres, are analyzed for structural aberrations with a minimum of 500 per treatment group. Additionally, the ratio of spermatogonial mitotic cells to I and II meiotic cells may be determined in a total sample of 100 dividing cells per animals to establish possible cytotoxic effects.

Scoring Criteria. Cells with $2n \pm 2$ centromeres are acceptable for scoring. Aberrations should be recorded as described for the bone marrow assay. Numerical abnormalities or polyploids are not scored in this test, which is designed for the assessment of structural chromosome aberrations.

Evaluation Criteria

The statistics, criteria for determination of a valid test and data presentation for the spermatogonial chromosome aberrations assay are same as for the bone marrow assay (see above).

Skin Micronucleus Assays

Introduction

The in vivo rodent micronucleus test is widely used to detect potential of the chemicals, drugs, or other substances to cause chromosome damage, primarily in the haematopoietic cells in the tissues, such as the bone marrow. Other organs that have been used in this test include the liver, gastrointestinal tract, colon, or testis. In recent years, the rodent skin has been used in the micronucleus test because the skin has high probability to be exposed to mutagens or carcinogens (129,130). In addition, the skin is a suitable target organ when the test substance (for topical application) is not absorbed and, therefore, not available to the bone marrow. In such cases, false negative results can be generated and genotoxic substances can be missed.

Experimental Design and Procedures

Mouse or rat skin can be used in this test. The micronucleus induction occurred in the epidermal basal cells (dividing cells) following topical application of the test substance. The test consisted of the following steps:

Dose Administration.   The shaved animal skin is repeatedly exposed to the test substance. Daily treatment for 3 days is recommended.

Separation of Epidermis from Dermis.   The treated skin is dissected, cut into slender pieces, and exposed to cold trypsin (2–8°C) for approximately 15 hours. Following this procedure, the epidermis can be peeled from the dermis layer.

Isolation of Basal Cells.   The epidermal pieces are agitated for approximately 1 hour in minimum essential medium supplemented with calf serum, after which the suspension is filtered. The suspension is then centrifuged to pellet the basal cells.

Hypotonic Treatment and Cell Fixation.   The basal cells are resuspended, treated with 0.075 M KCl, and then fixed with methanol:acetic acid (3:1, v/v). The fixation of cells should be repeated at lest two times.

Smear (Slide) Preparation.   After the last centrifugation, the cell pellet is resuspended in a small amount of the fixative, and a small aliquot of the cell suspension is spread with a Pasteur pipette onto a glass slide.

Staining of Smears.   The air-dried smears are stained with a 40 mg/ml acridine orange solution.

Scoring.   Using a fluorescent microscope, 2000 basal cells are evaluated for the presence of micronuclei.

Definitions.   Basal cells are cells with red cytoplasm and yellow-green (fluorescent) nucleus. A micronucleus is a round, yellow-green structure (fluorescent) with a diameter less than half of that of the main nucleus. A micronucleus is located within the cytoplasm and is always separated from the main nucleus. Some other cells can be seen under the microscope. These cells are epidermal superficial cells that have yellow-green cytoplasm and yellow-green nucleus or yellow green cytoplasm and red nucleus.

Statistical Analysis.   Statistical differences between treated animals and their solvent controls are evaluated using Kastenbaum-Bowman tables (118). The micronuclei frequency is calculated as the number of micronucleated cells per 1000 cells scored.

Evaluation Criteria

The micronucleus test using rodent skin, or the skin of other species, can be used in the assessment of the genotoxicity of different substances. However, further investigational work on study design, sampling time, and dose selection is needed to standardize the test.

PRIMARY DNA DAMAGE ASSAYS

Introduction

The induction of DNA damage by physical or chemical agents in mammalian cells represents the early event(s) that may lead to mutation and/or neoplastic transformation.

Therefore, an assessment of the DNA-damaging capacity of a substance may provide some information on its potential mutagenic and/or carcinogenic activity.

Damage to DNA may be detected directly by the measurement of DNA fragments (e.g., using alkaline elution techniques) or indirectly by the measurement of DNA synthesis that occurs in the process of DNA repair. Several methods are available for the estimation of DNA repair, e.g., (1) by chromatographic detection of the rate of disappearance of altered nucleotides (131), (2) by sedimentation of DNA through alkaline sucrose gradients for detection of DNA fragmentation and rejoining (132), and (3) by monitoring the "re-synthesis" of short sections of the DNA molecule that are eliminated by endo- and exonuclease enzymes following exposure to exogenous DNA damaging agents (133).

Monitoring DNA repair synthesis is the most widely used method for assessing DNA-damaging activity. As opposed to the scheduled DNA synthesis that occurs during the normal phase of semiconservative duplication of DNA in the cell cycle, DNA synthetic activity triggered by DNA damage can occur at any phase of the cell cycle and is commonly referred to as "unscheduled DNA synthesis" or UDS. Measurement of UDS can be achieved by tracking the incorporation of BrdUrd or tritiated thymidine into nuclear DNA of repairing cells, although other purine or pyrimidine precursors can also be used (134). The incorporation of radioactively labeled purine or pyrimidine can be measured by autoradiographic or scintillation counting methods.

Repair of DNA damage in mammalian cells, as evidenced by UDS, was first demonstrated by the autoradiographic detection of the uptake of labeled thymidine into the DNA following UV irradiation (133). A variety of cell types, including fibroblasts and epithelial cells of rodent as well as human origin, have been used as indicator cells for UDS. The use of fibroblasts, which typically have limited metabolic capability for the biotransformation of chemical compounds, usually entails the inclusion of an exogenous enzyme system to provide for metabolic activation. The use of freshly isolated hepatocytes, which are enzymatically proficient, does not require the inclusion of an exogenous metabolic activation system.

Examination of more than 100 chemical compounds representing the major groups of carcinogenic substances revealed a good correlation between the carcinogenic activity and the capacity to elicit DNA repair synthesis in cultured mammalian cells (135–140). A review of the published literature and suggested protocols and evaluation criteria for evaluating UDS were presented in a Working Group Report prepared for the Gene-Tox Program, U.S. Environmental Protection Agency (141). Recommendations for the performance of UDS assays in vitro and in vivo have been presented in subsequent papers (142–144).

This section will focus on the monitoring of UDS by autoradiography because this method is commonly used in the screening of substances for DNA-damaging activity, although some discussion on the use of alkaline elution and scintillation counting techniques will be included.

Purpose of Study

The purpose of the UDS assay is to evaluate the potential of the test article to induce unscheduled DNA synthesis in primary rat hepatocyte cultures following in vitro or in vivo administration of the test article.

Species/Cell Selection and Justification

Primary hepatocytes should be obtained from young adult (6- to 12-week-old) Sprague-Dawley or Fischer rats. This test system has been demonstrated to be sensitive to the

DNA-damaging activity of a variety of chemicals. The response of hepatocytes from either strain of rat to DNA-damaging agents is comparable. The use of male animals only is based on the fact that the in vivo UDS assay was validated in male rodents and the preponderance of data in the literature is from male animals. The use of hepatocytes from male rats is sufficient unless there is evidence of significant male/female differences in toxicokinetics (144).

Monitoring unscheduled DNA synthesis in primary cultures of rat hepatocytes presents several advantages over other cell types used to monitor possible interactions between the test article and DNA. First, the target cells possess the ability to metabolize many promutagens/procarcinogens to their active form. Second, rat hepatocytes in culture are nearly 100% nondividing, so no metabolic blocks are needed to inhibit replicative DNA synthesis. Third, the target cells are epithelial in origin. Because most human cancers are carcinomas, an assay using epithelial cells to monitor genetic damage may be more relevant to the in vivo situation than a similar assay using fibroblasts.

Maintenance of Cells or Animals

Animals should be obtained from a source monitored for evidence of adventitious agents and are quarantined for no fewer than 5 days prior to dose administration. The animals are observed each working day for signs of illness, unusual food and water consumption, and other general conditions of poor health. All animals must be judged to be healthy prior to utilization in the study.

Animals are housed in an AAALAC-accredited facility with a controlled environment of $50 \pm 20\%$ relative humidity and $23 \pm 3°C$ with a 12-hour light/dark cycle. Rats may be individually or group housed by sex in plastic autoclavable cages. Heat-treated hardwood chips are used for bedding. Animals are provided free access to a certified laboratory rodent chow that has been analyzed for environmental contaminants, and to tap water.

Experimental Design

For the in vitro UDS assay, the assay is performed using modifications of the procedures described by Williams (136,145). Primary rat hepatocytes are exposed to concentrations of the test article as well as positive and negative controls in triplicate cultures. For in vivo UDS studies, the experimental design follows that described by Butterworth et al. (143) and OECD Guideline 486 (146). Hepatocytes are isolated from male rats at two time points (2 to 4 hours and 12 to 16 hours) following the administration of three concentrations of test article as well as positive and vehicle controls. The harvests at two time points in the in vivo assay are designed to target the peak UDS response elicited by different test articles (147). Both the in vitro and in vivo UDS assays are evaluated on the basis of incorporation of tritiated thymidine (^{3}H-TdR) into the hepatocyte DNA, presumably as a consequence of DNA repair.

Dose Selection

For in vitro UDS studies, selection of dose levels for the UDS assay is based upon toxicity of the test article. Primary rat hepatocytes, plated 90 to 180 minutes earlier, are exposed to concentrations of test article, the highest concentration not to exceed 5 mg/ml. Approximately 18 to 20 hours after treatment, toxicity is assessed by measuring the amount of lactate dehydrogenase (LDH) that has leaked from the cells into the culture medium relative to the solvent control. Leakage of this enzyme increases with the loss of cell membrane integrity. The treated cultures also are observed microscopically for toxic effects. Whenever possible, the high dose is selected to yield at least 50% toxicity, to a maximum of 5 mg/ml. For freely soluble, nontoxic test articles, the highest concentration is 5 mg/ml. For relatively insoluble, nontoxic test articles, the highest concentration is the lowest insoluble dose in treatment medium but not to exceed 5 mg/ml. If dose-related cytotoxicity is noted, irrespective of solubility, then the top concentration is based on toxicity as described above. In all cases, precipitation is evaluated at the beginning and at the end of the treatment period using the naked eye.

For in vivo UDS studies, selection of dose levels is based on toxicity of the test article but will not exceed 2 g/kg body weight (146). The high dose for the UDS assay should be the MTD, or that which produces some indication of toxicity, such as reduction in body weight gain, clinical signs of pharmacotoxic effect, or mortality. The LD_{50} may be selected for the high dose, provided that a sufficient number of animals are likely to survive to the 16-hour postexposure harvest. Two additional dose levels are tested, approximately one-half and one-fourth of the high dose.

Number of Animals or Cultures

For in vitro UDS studies, hepatocytes from a single rat are sufficient for testing a number of test articles. For in vivo UDS studies, the animals will be assigned to 10 treatment groups of five males each based on equalization of group mean body weights. Only three surviving animals per group are evaluated microscopically for UDS.

For preparation of primary hepatocyte cultures, the rats are anesthetized with isoflurane and a midventral incision is made to expose the liver. The liver is perfused with 0.5 mM ethylene glycol-bis(β-aminoethyl ether) N,N,N′,N′-tetraacetic acid (EGTA) solution followed by collagenase solution (80 to 100 units Type I collagenase/ml culture medium).

The liver is removed, transected, and shaken in a dilute collagenase solution to release the hepatocytes. The cells are pelleted by centrifugation, resuspended in complete Williams' Mimimum Essential Medium (WME buffered with 0.01 M HEPES, supplemented with 2 mM L-glutamine, 50 μg/ml gentamicin and 10% FBS) and approximately 5×10^5 cells are seeded into 35 mm tissue culture dishes containing complete WME. For the preliminary cytotoxicity assay, cells are seeded into two replicate dishes per dose level, without coverslips. For the UDS assay, cells are seeded into three replicate dishes per dose level, containing 25-mm coverslips. In addition, four cultures are seeded without coverslips for determination of total LDH release: two for treatment with the highest dose of test article and two for treatment with the solvent control. The hepatocyte cultures are maintained in a humidified atmosphere of 5% CO_2 and 37°C.

Controls

For in vitro UDS studies, untreated cells are used as the untreated control. The test article solvent (or vehicle) is used as the negative control. For solvents other than water or culture medium, the final concentration in treatment medium should not exceed 1%. For positive control, 7,12-dimethylbenz(a)anthracene (DMBA) at concentrations of 3 and 10 μg/ml is used.

For in vivo UDS studies, the test article vehicle is used as the negative control. Commonly used positive controls, administered via gavage, include MMS and dimethylnitrosamine (DMN) for the 2- to 4-hour time point and 2-acetylaminofluorene (2AAF) for the 12- to 16-hour time point (143). However, the response is greatly influenced by the route of administration and the solubility of the positive control in a vehicle compatible with the route of administration. For example, both MMS and DMN are readily miscible with water, and they can be administered by intraperitoneal or intravenous injection or by gavage. On the other hand, 2AAF, being insoluble in water and with limited solubility in carboxymethylcellulose or corn oil, can be administered only via gavage to elicit a detectable response. When 2AAF is administered via intraperitoneal injection, the response is very marginal in spite of excessive toxicity (148). DMN, administered via intravenous injection or gavage, can be used as the positive control for the 2- to 4-hour and 12- to 16-hour sacrifices (148).

Dose Administration

For in vitro UDS studies, the cells are washed with plating medium at 90 to 180 minutes after plating, refed with serum-free WME (for the UDS assay, the medium will contain 10 μCi/ml ^{3}H-thymidine), and exposed to chemicals for approximately 18 to 20 hour at 37°C.

The test article is dissolved or suspended either directly in serum-free WME at the appropriate concentration or in an appropriate solvent at a 100X concentration. If WME is the solvent, the test article dilutions are prepared directly in the serumfree WME medium. The plating medium is removed from the hepatocyte cultures and replaced with the treatment medium at a rate of 2 ml per dish. If WME is not used as the solvent, the test article dilutions are prepared in the appropriate solvent, and 20 μl of the 100X dosing solutions are added to the treatment medium.

At approximately 18 to 20 hours after treatment, at least one culture from each treatment group is observed microscopically, and a toxicity evaluation of the cultures is made relative to the solvent controls. An aliquot of the medium from two replicate culture dishes per treatment group is removed for measurement of LDH release. In addition, the extra cultures treated with the solvent control and the highest test article dose are lysed with 1% Triton and subsequently sampled for LDH release.

Eighteen to 20 hours after exposure, the coverslips containing cells are washed three times in serum-free WME. The cells are swelled in 1% sodium citrate solution and fixed in three changes of ethanol-glacial acetic acid fixative (3:1, v/v). The coverslips are allowed to dry for at least 1 hour before mounting cell side up on glass slides. The slides are labeled with the study number and a code to identify the dose level.

The slides are dipped in kodak NTB (or equivalent) emulsion (diluted 1:1 in deionized H$_2$O) at 43 to 45°C, allowed to drain and dry for at least 1.5 hours at room temperature and are stored for 5 to 12 days at 2 to 8°C in light tight boxes with a desiccant. Slides are developed in Kodak D-19 developer (diluted 1:1 in deionized H$_2$O), fixed in Kodak fixer, and stained with hematoxylin-eosin stain.

For in vivo UDS studies, the oral route is recommended because the data reported in the published literature are predominantly based on chemicals (including chemicals commonly used as positive controls) administered by gavage (149,150). Other routes of administration (e.g., via intravenous injection) may be used if justified. The intraperitoneal route is not recommended in light of reservations expressed that this route could expose the liver directly to the test article rather than exposure via the circulatory system (144).

The test article–vehicle mixture, the vehicle alone, and the positive control are given as single administrations. The rate of administration for the test article–vehicle mixture and vehicle alone is typically 10 ml/kg unless larger volumes, up to 20 ml/kg body weight, are required to deliver the targeted dose.

The isolation and culturing of hepatocytes are performed as described earlier for in vitro UDS studies. Ninety to 180 minutes after plating, the cells are washed once with complete WME and refed with serum-free WME containing 10 μCi ^{3}H-TdR/ml. Four hours later, the radioactive medium is removed, the cultures washed three times in serum-free WME containing 0.25 mM thymidine, and then refed with serum-free WME containing 0.25 mM thymidine and incubated for 17 to 20 hours. The cultures are then processed for autoradiography as described earlier for in vitro UDS studies.

End Point Evaluation and Time of Evaluation

All coded slides are read without knowledge of treatment group. The slides are viewed microscopically under a 100X oil immersion lens. An automated colony counter is interfaced with the microscope so that silver grains within each nucleus and the surrounding cytoplasm can be counted. First the number of grains in a nucleus are counted. Then the number of grains in three nuclear-sized adjacent cytoplasmic areas are counted. Replicative DNA synthesis is evidenced by nuclei completely blackened with grains and should not be counted. Cells exhibiting toxic effects of treatments, such as irregularly shaped or very darkly stained nuclei, also should not be counted.

For in vitro UDS studies, a total of 150 nuclei should be scored per dose level. If possible, 50 nuclei are scored from each of three replicate cultures.

For in vivo UDS studies, 50 nuclei should be scored from each of three replicate cultures for a total of 150 nuclei from each rat.

Evaluation Criteria

Data Presentation

A net nuclear grain count is calculated for each nucleus scored by subtracting the mean of the cytoplasmic area counts from the nuclear area count. For each treatment group, a mean net nuclear grain count and SD, as well as the proportion of cells in repair (percentage of nuclei showing ≥ 5 net nuclear grain counts), are determined and reported.

Criteria for Valid Test

The following criteria must be met for a test to be considered valid. The proportion of cells in repair in the negative controls must be less than 15%, and the net nuclear grain count must be less than 1. The mean net nuclear grain count of the positive control must be at least 5 counts greater than that of the solvent control.

Positive and Negative Test

All conclusions should be based on sound scientific judgment; however, the following is offered as a guide to interpretation of the data. Any mean net nuclear count that is increased by at least five counts greater than the solvent control is considered significant (136,145). A test article is judged positive if it induces a dose-related increase with no less than one dose significantly elevated above the solvent control. A significant increase in the mean net nuclear grain count in at least two successive doses in the absence of a dose response is also considered positive. A significant increase in the net nuclear grain count at one dose level without a dose response is judged equivocal. The test article is considered negative if no significant increase in the net nuclear grain counts is observed. The percentage of cells in repair (cells with ≥ 5 net nuclear grains) is also reported; this information may also be used in making a final evaluation of the activity of the test article.

Supplemental Information

Apart from the use of autoradiography, UDS can also be monitored by the liquid scintillation counting (LSC) technique for the detection of incorporated radioactivity (139,141,151). The procedures for exposure to test article and labeling with ^{3}HTdR are identical to those for the autoradiographic technique. Following the labeling period, the DNA is extracted. Aliquots of the extracted DNA are used for determination of the DNA content using standard spectrophotometric methods and for the detection of incorporated radioactivity using LSC. The LSC method provides the advantage that the time between exposure and obtaining the results is less than that for the autoradiography approach. However, the LSC method does not provide direct visualization of the cells undergoing UDS. In addition, the LSC method requires more cells, more test article, and more replicate samples than does the autoradiography procedure. The LSC method is potentially prone to interference by the presence of cells undergoing DNA replicative synthesis because of the substantial uptake of ^{3}HTdR by such cells. Therefore, the LSC methodology is less commonly used than the autoradiography approach.

Although hepatocytes are most commonly used in UDS studies, the DNA-damaging effects of chemicals on germinal tissue can also be studied using the in vivo UDS procedure (152). This approach has been used to identify the DNA-damaging effect of chemical mutagens in germ cells (153–157).

Another method of studying the DNA-damaging effect of chemical mutagens is the alkaline elution technique (158–160). This procedure detects DNA damage prior to the onset of UDS. It can be used on both somatic and germinal tissue. Depending on the tissue, the procedure can be used under in vitro and in vivo conditions. Following exposure to the test article, cells are transferred to a filter and lysed under alkaline conditions. Upon passage of an eluting fluid, small DNA fragments will pass through the filter. Larger DNA fragments, depending on their size, may be eluted while intact undamaged DNA will be retained by the filter. The DNA-damaging activity of a test article is assessed by the quantity of DNA eluted and the speed at which DNA from exposed cells elute from the filter. In a survey of selected chemicals that are difficult to detect in conventional in vitro genetic toxicology assays (e.g., bacterial mutagenesis, mammalian cell mutagenesis, UDS), the results of in vitro alkaline elution studies on rat hepatocytes correlated well with in vivo carcinogenicity assay data (161). Using a slight modification of the analytical procedure, the alkaline elution assay can be adapted for the detection of DNA-DNA and DNA-protein crosslinks (158,160,162).

SYRIAN HAMSTER EMBRYO CELL TRANSFORMATION ASSAY

Introduction

Under the strategy for testing carcinogenic potential of a pharmaceutical, the ICH Harmonised Tripartite Guideline S1B indicated that data from in vitro assays, such as a cell transformation assay, can be useful at the compound selection stage (163). This has triggered an interest by regulatory agencies for the Syrian golden hamster embryo (SHE) cell transformation assay for a genotoxic pharmaceutical, especially if the drug is intended to be administered chronically to humans.

The SHE cell transformation assay at pH 6.7 is conducted to determine the ability of a test article to induce morphological transformation in cultured SHE cells. The SHE cell transformation assay is one of the most widely used cell transformation assays. The end points of this assay are related to the conversion of normal cells to preneoplastic or neoplastic cells. The assay provides a valuable tool in the process of assessment and evaluation of the carcinogenic potential of a test article (164–166).

Experimental Design

The SHE cell transformation assay is conducted with cultured Syrian hamster embryonic cells prepared at the gestation period of approximately 13 days. Cells from the embryos are isolated and frozen. A feeder layer of cells is seeded with x-ray irradiated SHE cells prior to seeding the target cells. The SHE transformation assay is performed at pH 6.7. The assay is designed to allow the expression of transformed morphology of clonal SHE cells seeded onto feeder cells, after exposure to at least five concentrations of test article as well as positive and vehicle controls in the absence of a supplemental exogenous mammalian metabolic activation system. For maximum assay sensitivity, two exposure durations can be used, namely a 24-hour exposure assay and a 7-day exposure assay. Following treatment, the cells are cultured for a period of 7 days, and then fixed, stained, and evaluated for the cytotoxic effects of treatment and the induction of phenotypic transformation as measured by morphological transformation of the cells (165,167,168).

Test System

SHE cells have been demonstrated to provide both high sensitivity and high specificity needed to identify rodent carcinogens (168), as measured by morphological transformation of the cells.

Preparation of SHE Cell Stocks

Cells are prepared from approximately 13-day gestational Syrian golden hamster embryos obtained from an approved source. The embryos are removed from the uterus and transferred to a petri dish containing wash solution (calcium- and magnesium-free Hank's balanced salt solution containing 200 U -200 µg/mL Penicillin–Streptomycin). The embryos are aseptically decapitated, delimbed, and eviscerated. The tissue is transferred to another petri dish on ice and cut into smaller pieces (approximately 1 to 3 mm). The pieces are placed in a trypsinization flask containing wash solution and magnetic stir bar placed on a magnetic stirrer. The first supernatant with this wash solution is discarded after approximately five minutes of stirring at low speed to remove as many blood cells as possible. The wash solution is replaced with dissociation solution, and the tissue is stirred gently for 5 minutes. At that time the tissue is allowed to settle for 5 minutes and the supernatant is discarded. More dissociation solution is added to the flask and rinsed gently for 10 minutes. Meanwhile, 2 ml of FBS are added to a series of 50 ml centrifuge tubes (6 to 8 tubes) and kept on ice. The tissue is allowed to settle for 5 minutes, and carefully the supernatant is pipetted off into the prepared 50 ml centrifuge tubes. This step of cell dissociation is repeated 2–4 more times. The cell suspension is centrifuged at 1000 rpm for 10 minutes at 2°C to 8°C. The supernatant from the centrifuge tubes is decanted and discarded, and the cells are resuspended and pooled in 20 to 50 ml of complete Dulbecco's Modified Eagle's Medium—Leboeuf's modification (DMEM-L) containing penicillin/streptomycin at 200 U/ml and 200 µg/ml concentration. The cell number is counted, cell density is calculated, and the cells are seeded in T150, T162 or T225 flasks at a density of 1.333×10^5 viable cells per cm^2 area of the flask in complete DMEM-L containing antibiotics. The flasks are incubated for 1 to 2 hours at $37 \pm 1°C$, $\geq 85\%$ humidity at $10 \pm 0.5\%$ CO_2. After 1 to 2 hours, the culture medium is aspirated off to remove the floating cells and fresh complete DMEM-L containing antibiotics is added to each flask (volumes to add in different size flasks-T150- 30 ml, T162- 32 ml or T225- 45 ml). The flasks are returned to the incubator for approximately 24 hours. After 24 hours of incubation, the flasks should be viewed under the phase contrast microscope and observed for confluence. If the flasks are not 60–80% confluent, they should be placed back in the incubator for another 24 hours. If the cultures have not reached 60–80% confluence at the end of 48 hours from culture initiation, then the cells should not be used in the assay and the cultures should be discarded and a new isolate should be prepared.

Cryopreservation of Cells

When the cells have reached 60–80% confluence, the culture medium is aspirated off and the cells are rinsed twice with 10 ml calcium- and magnesium-free Hanks' balanced salt solution (CMF-HBSS). After the last rinse, 5 ml of detachment solution (trypsin 0.05% and 0.02% Na_2EDTA in CMF-HBSS) are added to each flask and the flasks are returned to the incubator for 4 to 8 minutes. Once the cells are detached, 5 ml of complete DMEM-L are added to the flasks. The cells are triturated, pooled in sterile 50 ml centrifuge tubes, and centrifuged at 1000 rpm at 2 to 8°C for 10 minutes. The supernatant is aspirated off, and the cells are held on ice. Cells from all the flasks are pooled and resuspended in complete DMEM-L. The cell number is counted in a hemacytometer using the trypan blue cell exclusion method, and the cell density is calculated. The volume of additional complete medium needed to dilute the cells to 2.0 or 5.0×10^6 cells/ml is determined and added to the cell suspension, mixed well, and then diluted 1:1 with 2X cryoprotective medium (15% DMSO in complete DMEM-L). One-ml volumes of the cell suspension are distributed into 1 ml cryovials labelled with cell type, freeze date and cell concentration (1.0 or 2.5×10^6 cells/vial). The vials are placed into a −70°C freezer for at least 24 hours and then transferred to liquid nitrogen storage. Prior to using the new isolate in the transformation assay, the isolate is tested for following properties: (1) the number of cells to be seeded as target cells in order to achieve 25 colonies to 45 colonies per plate, (2) the number of transformed colonies in the solvent (negative) control should be within the historical negative control data, and (3) the number of transformed colonies in the positive control should be significantly higher than that in the negative control.

Solubility Determination

A test article solubility determination is conducted to determine the test article vehicle and the maximum soluble concentration up to a maximum of 2500 mg/ml. Vehicles compatible with this test system, in order of preference, include but are not limited to complete growth medium DMEM-L, dimethyl sulfoxide (CAS 67-68-5), ethanol (CAS 64-17-5), and acetone (CAS 67-64-1). The vehicle of choice is the vehicle, selected in order of preference, that permits preparation of the highest stock concentration, up to 2500 mg/ml. The maximum concentration of solvent in the test system is 0.2%, and the maximum test article concentration of test article is 5.0 mg/ml or 10 mM, whichever is lower.

pH and Osmolality Determination

The pH of the culture medium in this assay is critical. It should be measured at the time of media preparation and adjusted to 6.7 ± 0.05 prior to use in the assay. The pH of the test article dosing solutions should be checked after at least four hours of undisturbed incubation at $37 \pm 1°C$ with approximately $10 \pm 0.5\%$ CO_2 in the air. To achieve this, prior to performing the preliminary cytotoxicity assay, the test article should be dissolved in an appropriate solvent and diluted in complete medium at a concentration equal to or greater than the highest concentration to be tested in the cytotoxicity assay. The pH should be determined using a standard pH meter both at the time of media preparation and after at least four hours of incubation. Only test articles of neutral pH can be tested in this assay. The pH of dosing solutions should be adjusted to approximately 7.0 with 1N NaOH or 1N HCl prior to treatment of the cultures.

The osmolality should be determined using a standardized freezing point depression osmometer. The test article concentrations increasing the osmolality considerably (e.g., greater than 20%) above that of the vehicle control should be avoided.

Preliminary Cytotoxicity Assay

Before performing the SHE cell transformation assay, a cytotoxicity assay will be conducted to establish a dose range. This involves exposing SHE target cells in clonal growth for 24 hours and/or 7 days to a range of concentrations of the test article and the solvent control. The highest dose used is 5 mg/ml or 10 mM, whichever is lower (2). Lower doses may be used if the solubility of the test article is limited. At least 5 concentrations of test article should be tested. Following exposure, SHE cell colonies in culture dishes are counted using a stereomicroscope, and then the plating efficiency in each group is calculated (plating efficiency per group = number of colonies obtained per group × 100/ number of target cells seeded). The relative cytotoxicity of each treatment group is measured by the reduction in plating efficiency of the treated SHE cells compared to solvent controls. Selection of dose levels for the transformation assay is based on the following criteria: (1) when there is no toxicity, (no reduction in plating efficiency or colony size as assessed by visual observation) the high dose selected for the transformation assay will be 5 mg/ml or 10 mM, whichever is lower, unless there is precipitation, then the lowest precipitating concentration is used as the high dose; (2) when there is toxicity, a range of doses are selected for evaluation in the transformation assay to ensure at least a 50 ± 5% reduction in plating efficiency is achieved. If it is determined that the treatment results in a reduction in size of the majority of the colonies on the plate that would preclude scoring that dose, then lower concentrations will need to be tested; (3) each assay must include at least five test article treatment groups, a solvent control, and a positive control. The high dose is chosen as described above, and at least four lower doses are tested.

Frequency and Route of Administration

The target cells will be treated for 24 hours and/or 7 days. Treatment is achieved by incorporation of the vehicle and test article vehicle mixture into the medium.

Controls

Vehicle Control. The vehicle for the test article is used as the vehicle control. The final concentration of the vehicle in treatment medium should not exceed 0.2%.

Positive Control. Benzo(a)pyrene (BAP, CAS 50-32-8) is used as the positive control at concentrations between 1.25 µg/ml and 20 µg/ml.

Transformation Assay

Preparation of Feeder Cells. Cryopreserved SHE cells from a tested and approved lot are thawed and grown to 50% to 90% confluency in growth flasks (2 to 4 days). On Day 1 of the assay, feeder cells are detached and suspended in culture medium in a growth flask on wet ice. The cells are x-ray irradiated (with approximately 5000 rad) to a point where they are still viable, yet no longer capable of replication. Confirmation of this is made by preparing five plates containing only feeder cells. Following irradiation, the cells are centrifuged to form a pellet, resuspended in culture medium, and counted using a hemacytometer. The cell concentration is adjusted to 2×10^4 cells/ml in complete medium, and 2 ml of this suspension are placed into each 60 mm culture dish. Each assay should include at least five test article dose groups, at least one vehicle control group, and at least one benzo(a)pyrene positive control group. Each group should include at least 40 culture dishes. Dishes are incubated at $37 \pm 1°C$ in a humidified atmosphere of $10 \pm 0.5\%$ CO_2 for 24 hour prior to addition of the target cells.

Preparation of Target Cells. The day after seeding of the feeder cells, a second vial of SHE cells from the same lot is thawed and seeded in a growth flask for approximately 5 hours. After the 5-hour incubation period, the target cells are detached, counted with a hemacytometer, and diluted with culture medium to a concentration that will yield approximately 25 to 45 colonies/dish. For the target-cell adjusted dose groups, the required number of target cells/dish is determined from the results of the cytotoxicity assay. The number of target cells seeded should achieve approximately 25 to 45 colonies/dish, with an optimum of 35 colonies/dish. Two ml of the target cell suspensions are placed into each culture dish, containing 4×10^4 feeder cells. Dishes are incubated at $37 \pm 1°C$ in a humidified atmosphere of $10 \pm 0.5\%$ CO_2 for 24 hours prior to addition of test article treatment.

Adjusted Target Cell Seeding. In the SHE cell transformation assay, the number of colonies/dish has been observed to affect transformation frequency (167). Therefore, a relatively constant number of colonies/dish across the dose groups should be achieved in the transformation assay. Data obtained from the preliminary cytotoxicity assay are used for adjusting the target cell seeding. Following exposure to the vehicle and test article, SHE cell colonies are counted in all dishes of the vehicle control group and each dose group. The mean number of colonies for the vehicle control group and each dose group is calculated. The mean plating efficiency is calculated for each group (mean plating efficiency = mean number of colonies obtained per group $\times$ 100/number of target cells seeded). The relative plating efficiency (RPE) for each test article dose group is calculated (RPE = PE test article dose $\times$ 100/PE vehicle). Target cell adjustment is performed in test article dose groups with a RPE of <70%. The number of target cells needed = original number of target cells seeded $\times$ 100/relative plating efficiency. In the SHE transformation assay, the adjusted number of target cells for each test article dose group is used. For the control groups (positive and vehicle control), the appropriate number of target cells for this cell lot is used to obtain approximately 25 to 45 colonies/plate, with an optimum of 35 colonies/dish.

Test Article Treatment. Twenty-four hours after seeding of the target cells, the test article stock solution is prepared by dissolving the test article in the chosen solvent at a concentration below maximum solubility. From this stock solution, at least four serial dilutions of test article in solvent should be prepared to achieve 500X the final culture dish concentrations. Each of these test article solutions is diluted 1:250 with culture medium to yield a 2X desired final concentration, such that upon addition to the target cells, final concentrations attained will be 1X in 0.2% solvent. Each test article treatment dish receives 4 ml 2X test article in 0.4% solvent in culture medium. Each culture dish in the solvent control group receives 4 ml of 0.4% solvent in culture medium. Each culture dish in the benzo(a)pyrene positive control group receives 4 ml of 2X BaP:0.4% solvent in culture medium. All culture dishes are incubated (undisturbed) at $37 \pm 1°C$ in a humidified atmosphere of $10 \pm 0.5\%$ CO_2 for 24 hours or for 7 days as required. All dishes with feeder-cells only will receive 6 ml of complete medium on the treatment day.

For the 24-hour dosing regimen, the control and test article treatment medium is removed from the dishes after approximately 24 hours. The cultures are refed with 8 ml of culture medium per dish without test article. Control groups (vehicle and BaP) should also be refed with culture medium at this time. Following refeeding, cultures are incubated for 7 to 9 days (7 to 8 days after initial dosing). The extra 1 to 2 day(s) of incubation may be necessary to compensate for retarded colony growth caused by refeeding.

Scoring of Cloning Efficiency and Transformation Dishes. Following incubation, the culture medium is removed from each dish. The SHE cell colonies in dishes of each dose group are fixed with methanol and stained with Giemsa stain. Using a stereomicroscope, the colonies in each culture dish are counted and recorded. Each colony is evaluated and recorded as either normal or morphologically transformed (MT). Normal colonies contain cells with an organized, often flowing, pattern of growth with minimal cell crisscrossing, particularly where the cells are at a confluent density (Fig. 3). Normal colonies also tend to be in a monolayer. MT colonies contain cells arrayed in an extensive randomly oriented, three dimensional, stacked growth pattern, with crisscrossing of cells at the perimeter and in the interior of the colony. Cells in MT colonies frequently are more basophilic than their normal counterparts and have increased nuclear/cytoplasmic ratios (164). Colonies where the cell growth is too sparse to assess morphology, where the majority of the colony is missing, or where the majority of the colony cannot be adequately assessed because it is growing on the side of the dish should be counted for calculation of the relative plating efficiency but not included in the number of colonies analyzed for morphological transformation. The highest dose to be analyzed for morphological transformation is the lowest dose that causes at least a 50% reduction in RPE.

Evaluation Criteria

Criteria for Determination of a Valid Test

The total number of colonies/group for all groups should be greater than 1000. The transformation frequencies of the BaP positive control group(s) must be statistically greater than the transformation frequency of the vehicle control group ($p < 0.05$), as indicated by the Fisher's Exact Test. The average number of colonies/dish for the negative or solvent control group should be approximately 25 to 45 colonies. The transformation frequency for the solvent control must be within historical solvent control values. The dishes with feeder-cells only should not have any visible colonies. In case colonies are present, the assay should be repeated.

Statistical Analysis

Statistical tests for significant treatment related effects on transformation frequencies should be done, using a one-sided Fisher's Exact Test (169). In this test, the transformation frequency of the vehicle control group is compared pairwise to the transformation frequencies of each test article-treated group including the positive control, BaP group. An unstratified binomial exact permutation trend test for a significant positive dose response trend should also be conducted.

Evaluation of Test Results

Data from identical treatment conditions from multiple trials may be pooled for statistical analysis. The statistical method employed to test for a significant treatment-related effect will be a one-sided Fisher's Exact Test. A test article should be considered positive if it

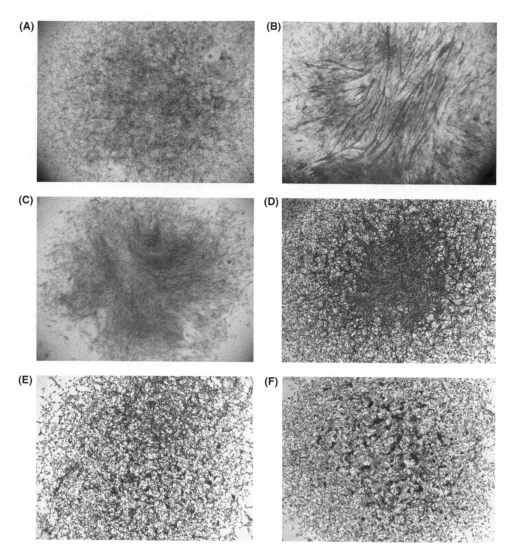

Figure 3 Examples of normal and morphologically transformed (MT) colonies in the Syrian hamster embryo (SHE) cell transformation assay. Normal colonies (**A, B, C**) contain cells with an organized, often flowing pattern of growth with minimal crisscrossing, particularly where the cells are at a confluent density. These colonies tend to be monolayer. The type of colony depicted in (**B**), found frequently among the SHE cell colonies, is called a myclone. MT colonies (**D, E, F**) contain cells arrayed in an extensive randomly oriented, three-dimensional, stacked growth pattern, with crisscrossing of cells at the perimeter and in the interior of the colony. Cells in MT colonies are frequently more basophillic (darker staining) and have increased nuclear/cytoplasmic ratios as compared to cells in a normal colony.

causes a statistically significant increase (i.e., $p < 0.05$) in morphological transformation at a minimum of two doses of test article, compared to concurrent vehicle controls (with pooled data from all trials), or a significant increase at one dose with a statistically significant ($p < 0.05$) positive dose-response trend. If a significant increase occurs at only one dose without a significant positive dose-response trend, or a statistically significant dose-response trend without a statistically significant increase at any dose, additional studies may be warranted.

SINGLE CELL GEL ELECTROPHORESIS (COMET ASSAY)

Introduction

The single cell gel electrophoresis assay, commonly known as the comet assay, is a sensitive technique unique for its ability to measure DNA damage and repair in individual cells. The comet assay is a relatively new technique that is increasingly been used in the testing of new pharmaceutical or chemical compounds for genotoxicity. The comet assay is also widely used for environmental monitoring, human biomonitoring and molecular epidemiology, and fundamental research in DNA damage and repair (170–172).

As previously mentioned in this chapter, the registration of pharmaceuticals or chemical compounds requires a comprehensive assessment of their genotoxic potential in vitro as well as in vivo. In some cases when there is indication of genotoxicity, additional in vitro or in vivo studies are usually performed to further elucidate the mechanism of action and to support the risk assessment. The comet assay has the ability to contribute to this type of investigations relying on its ability to sensitively assess DNA damage in almost any eukaryotic cell, originated from in vitro cultures or animal organ tissues (173,174).

The comet assay in vivo can provide valuable information in organ tissues that were never tested before due to technical limitations. It is used as a supplemental assay for mechanistic and/or target organ specific toxicity (175,176). The comet assay has become popular with new modifications of the technique, such that DNA double strand breaks, DNA oxidative damage, and DNA repair can be easily detected (172).

The comet assay is increasingly being used in genetic toxicology testing even though there are no ICH or OECD guidelines available. However, there is a big movement among scientists from academia, industry, and government to generate guidelines, and an international committee has recently been assembled for this purpose.

Detecting DNA damage in cells is not new; several different techniques have been in use for many years. The comet assay is unique because it can measure DNA damage at the single cell level and it requires only a small amount of cells (170,177).

The innovation with the comet assay was introduced by Ostling and Jonhanson (178) when they embedded cells into agarose gels to immobilize them. Then the cells were put under detergents and high salts to lyse the cellular membrane and break down proteins and RNA, in order to allow the DNA to relax. Subsequently, the cells underwent electrophoresis to enable the relaxed DNA strands to move out of the nucleus. This resulted in the formation of a "tail" on one side of the cell. Because this image resembles a comet, this technique is now universally known as the comet assay.

The comet assay technique in use today is based upon a modification introduced by two independent groups (170,177). They introduced the alkaline versions (pH 13) that measure DNA single strand breaks induced by alkaline labile sites. The main differences are that Singh et al. (170) lysed the cells at pH 10 with 2.5M NaCl, Triton X-100, and Sarkosyl for 1 hour, followed by a treatment and electrophoresis with alkaline buffer (0.3M NaOH) (pH > 13), whereas Olive et al. (177) simply lysed cells in weak alkali (0.03M NaOH) (pH > 13) for 1 hour before electrophoresis. The fact that both buffers are alkaline and have a high pH (> 13), the comet assay has been considered to be in the same category as alkaline unwinding, alkaline elution, or alkaline sucrose sedimentation, where separation of two DNA strands around a break by alkaline denaturation is essential to reveal the break (179).

The protocol from Singh and colleagues is the most widely used (170), and it has been simplified over the years (171).

Since the introduction of the alkaline comet assay, it has become one of the standard methods for measuring DNA damage, as reflected by its exponential use in the last decade, quantified by the increase in the number of publications in peer reviewed journals.

Experimental Design

The comet assay protocols currently used for in vivo and in vitro genetic toxicology testing have been established in publications by Tice et al. (171) and Hartmann et al. (173). The comet assay is a sensitive technique that evaluates the genotoxic potential of a test compound to induce DNA damage in individual cells. DNA damage is measured as DNA strand breaks that can be the results of DNA single strand breaks, double strand breaks, strand breaks induced by alkali labile sites, oxidative damage, and cross-linking.

The comet assay basically consists of mixing cells (isolated/individual cells) with low melting agarose, placing the mixture on microscope slides to allow the gel to solidify and immobilize the cell, submitting the cells to detergents and high salts, and then running the electrophoresis in alkaline buffer (pH 13) (170).

In genetic toxicology testing, the comet assay is conducted both in vitro and in vivo model systems, and the most widely accepted protocols designs are as follows:

The general design of in vitro comet assays includes the following features: standard cell lines (i.e., CHO, CHL or V-79), test article (3 to 9) doses, positive, and solvent control, testing with and without metabolic activation, and exposure times of 4 and 20 hours (171).

In vivo comet assay designs are composed of two phases: (1) dose range finding study to determine the MTD; and (2) definitive study conducted in mice and rats. The design of the definitive assay includes the following features: 5 animals per group, 5 dose groups (negative control, positive control, along with low, medium, and high dose of test article), one route of exposure (i.e., IP, IV or oral gavage); and collection of one or several tissues at 3 and/or 24 hours after treatment (171,173).

Evaluation Criteria

Cells with damaged DNA will show an increase of DNA strand breaks, which are displayed as an increased migration of DNA fragments outside the nucleus (comet shape, Fig. 4). The extension of the migrated DNA and the amount of fragments in the comet tail are quantified to assess the extent of DNA damage. DNA damage quantification can be done manually by classifying the cells into categories of damage (180) or measuring the tail length. Automatic quantification can be done by using specialized software that will determine the comet tail length, tail intensity and Olive tail moment (which combines both tail length and intensity) (177,181).

IMPLICATION OF POSITIVE GENETOX FINDINGS

The implication of a positive genetic toxicology finding can vary tremendously based on the nature of the product and the phase of development. The pharmaceutical industry, for example, screens candidate compounds very early in development. Typically, the earliest safety tests performed include a bacterial mutation assay and an in vitro assay for chromosome damage, often a micronucleus assay in CHO cells. In most instances a positive finding in one of these screening assays is sufficient to eliminate the chemical from further development. In selected instances, further development of a potentially mutagenic drug may be acceptable, for example, if the drug were being developed to

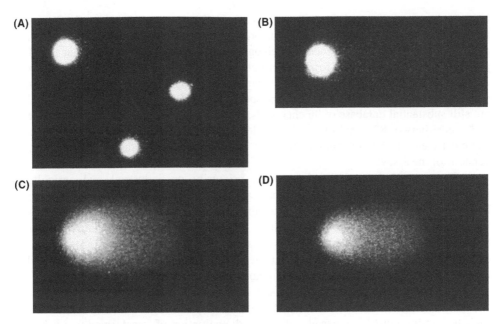

Figure 4 DNA damage levels in skin basal epidermal cells of SKH-1 mice after multiple topical applications of chemicals, measured with the comet assay. Lack of DNA damage following exposure to ethanol (**A**) or vinblastine (**B**). DNA damage following exposure to methyl methanesulfonate (**C**) or N-methyl-N′-nitro-N-nitrosoguanidine (**D**), manifested by an increase in migration of DNA fragments outside the nucleus (comet shape).

treat a life threatening disease, such as cancer. Although this might be an acceptable risk/benefit finding for a drug, the same would not be true for a new agricultural chemical or food additive. In these latter situations, large numbers of individuals would be exposed, and the equation is much more weighted towards safety. For some products, genotoxicity is unavoidable. For example, monomers used in many chemical syntheses must of necessity be reactive to fulfill their function. In these situations, containment is the key to safety.

As stated in the introduction, the ICH guidelines are vague as to how to proceed in the face of a positive genetox result. Data gleaned from the Physicians' Desk Reference (PDR) (182) suggest that positive results in the Ames assay and the in vivo micronucleus test are rare for approved drugs. However, positive responses in the in vitro cytogenetics or the mouse lymphoma assay are not uncommon. As reported by Snyder and Green twenty-nine percent of the drugs in the 1999 PDR had at least one positive finding with a quarter of all in vitro cytogenetics and mouse lymphoma assays being positive (182).

In the recent past a number of Center for Drug Evaluation and Research (CDER) review divisions have requested that sponsors perform either a SHE cell transformation assay or a p53 mouse carcinogenicity study to help clarify positive genetox results. In some cases, the positive results were seen only in the in vitro chromosomal aberration or the mouse lymphoma gene mutation assay. Performing a transgenic mouse carcinogenicity study prior to initiating repeated dose phase 1 clinical trials is problematic. The time required to perform the 28-day range finding study combined with the 6-month in-life for the definitive assay and the postlife phases for the two studies would result in more than a year's delay in the clinical program. The SHE cell transformation assay is shorter in duration but typically would still be expected to take several months. Furthermore, the pharmaceutical industry has not embraced the SHE cell assay. Validation studies, primarily from two laboratories, have demonstrated good concordance between results in the SHE cell assay and the outcome of two-year rodent carcinogenicity studies (183). In particular the "low pH" SHE cell assay is reported to have even better concordance (183). In a database in which 213 chemicals were tested in both a two-year rodent bioassay and in the SHE cell assay, concordance was 80%, sensitivity 82%, and specificity of 69% (183). In a somewhat smaller but still substantial database of 96 chemicals, the low pH SHE assay had concordance of 78%, sensitivity of 82% and specificity of 71% (184). Although the latter is reputed to be technically easier, the concordance with the chronic bioassay seems similar for the two versions of the assay.

These validation studies have been primarily on industrial and agricultural chemicals and pollutants and not on pharmaceuticals. A validation program organized by the International Life Sciences Institute examined the concordance among a series of transgenic mouse carcinogenicity models, the SHE cell transformation assay and traditional two-year rodent bioassays for a series of 19 human drugs (185). Again the data suggested good concordance between the SHE cell assay and the two-year studies, but the correlation with predicted human carcinogens was poor, 37%.

The SHE cell transformation assay also suffers from a number of technical challenges: cells have to be repeatedly isolated and qualified; frozen cells have limited shelf life; serum must be screened and qualified; evaluation of transformed foci is highly subjective; feeder cells must be irradiated; the difference between a positive and negative study can sometimes hinge on one focus; high failure rate with many repeats; and significant overlap in the historical values for the vehicle and positive control transformation frequencies (186). Most drugs that are carcinogenic in two-year bioassays do so by mechanisms unrelated to mutagenesis (182). Modes of action, such as exaggerated pharmacological effects, immune suppression, and hormonal imbalances, are only expected to be operant in whole animal systems. It is unclear how a cell culture-based assay could respond to these mechanisms.

CDER has recently (January, 2006) posted final guidance on its Web site titled "Recommended Approaches to Integration of Genetic Toxicology Study Results." This guidance suggests possible alternatives to the SHE cell and p53 assays for clarifying positive genetic toxicology results. The guidance focuses on three approaches: weight-of-evidence (WOE), mode of action (MOA), and conduct of additional studies to add to the WOE.

Weight of Evidence

In using a WOE evidence approach, the following questions are germane. Was the positive response observed in an in vitro or in vivo assay? Was the positive response reproducible? Was the response dose related? What was the magnitude of the response? Was the response seen only at a highly cytotoxic dose? Was a positive seen in more than one assay? Positive responses that are dose related, seen at doses that induce little or no toxicity, and seen in multiple test systems raise the level of concern. Positive in vitro responses that are not reproducible, are not dose related, and are seen only at highly cytotoxic doses are generally considered to represent little or no human risk. If the WOE suggests a lack of human risk, additional studies may not be required.

Mode of Action

Examination of the MOA of a positive response can help elucidate whether the response represents a human risk. A relevant parameter that should be considered is the possibility of a threshold. Unlike other types of toxicity, risk assessments on carcinogens and mutagens have historically not included consideration of thresholds. This practice was based on the conventional wisdom that a single molecule of an alkylating agent could theoretically cause a mutation and initiate a tumor. However, it is also likely that some agents that induce genotoxic end points may do so by mechanisms that have thresholds. For example, genetic lesions scored as micronuclei can originate through clastogenic events giving rise to acentric chromosome fragments or through damage to the mitotic spindle, which would give rise to whole chromosomes. Because DNA is not the target in the latter situation, this MOA is likely to be associated with a threshold. Other examples of MOA likely to be associated with a threshold include enzyme inhibition, such as induction of chromosomal aberrations by topoisomerase inhibitors, inhibitors of DNA synthesis, and excessively high toxicities (187–189).

Additional Testing to Support the WOE

In instances where results for genetic toxicology studies or other indicators suggest potential risk for carcinogenicity, additional testing may be warranted to either allay concern or confirm the potential risks. Data from a broad spectrum of assays can be used to add to the WOE assessment and help regulators and sponsors determine the existence and magnitude of a cancer risk.

When a positive response is seen in one of the two in vitro mammalian cell assays, it is reasonable to complete the four test battery and perform the other mammalian cell assay. Other end points that can influence the WOE include assessment of DNA adducts, evaluation of DNA damage using the comet assay, mutation in vivo using a transgenic mutagenesis model, in vitro cell transformation assays, including SHE, short-term carcinogenesis studies, and patient monitoring. Although this last option is technically straightforward, the associated ethical and legal issues are not.

REFERENCES

1. International Conference on Harmonisation (ICH) of Technical Requirements for Registration of Pharmaceuticals for Human Use. Genotoxicity: A Standard Battery for Genotoxicity Testing of Pharmaceuticals. S2B document recommended for adoption at step 4 of the ICH process on July 16, 1997. Fed Regist, 1997; 62; November 21: 16026–16030.
2. International Conference on Harmonisation (ICH) of Technical Requirements for Registration of Pharmaceuticals for Human Use. Guidance on Specific Aspects of Regulatory Genotoxicity Tests for Pharmaceuticals. S2A document recommended for adoption at step 4 of the ICH process on July 19, 1995. Fed Regist, 1996; 61; April 24: 18198–18202.
3. ISO 10993. Part 3: tests for genotoxicity, carcinogenicity and reproductive toxicity, AAMI standards and recommended practices, Biological Evalutation of Medical Devices, Association for the Advancement of Medical Instrumentation, Washington, DC, 1994; Vol. 4: p. 31.
4. Auletta A, Dearfield KL, Cimino MC. Mutagenicity test schemes and guidelines: U.S. EPA Office of pollution prevention and toxics and office of pesticide programs, environ. Mutagenesis 1993; 21:38.
5. Dearfield KL, Auletta AE, Cimino MC, Moore MM. Considerations in the U.S. Environmental protection agency's testing approach for mutagenicity. Mutat Res 1991; 258:259.

6. Shirasu Y. The Japanese mutagenicity studies guidelines for pesticide registration. Mutat Res 1988; 205:393.

7. Ames BN, McCann J, Yamasaki E. Methods for detecting carcinogens and mutagens with the *Salmonella*/mammalian-microsome mutagenicity test. Mutat Res 1975; 31:347.

8. Slater EE, Anderson MD, Rosenkranz HS. Rapid detection of mutagens and carcinogens. Cancer Res 1971; 31:970.

9. Bridges BA. Simple bacterial systems for detecting mutagenic agents. Lab Pract 1972; 21:413.

10. McCann J, Ames BN. Detection of carcinogens as mutagens in the *Salmonella*/microsome test: assay of 300 chemicals: discussion. Proc Natl Acad Sci USA 1976; 73:950.

11. McCann J, Choi E, Yamasaki E, Ames BN. Detection of carcinogens as mutagens in the *Salmonella*/microsome test: assay of 300 chemicals. Proc Natl Acad Sci USA 1975; 72:5135.

12. Ashby J, Tennant RW, Zeiger E, Stasiewicz S. Classification according to chemical structure, mutagenicity to *Salmonella* and level of carcinogenicity of a further 42 chemicals tested for carcinogenicity by the U.S. National toxicology program. Mutat Res 1989; 223:73.

13. Tennant RW, Ashby J. Classification according to chemical structure, mutagenicity to *Salmonella* and level of carcinogenicity of a further 39 chemicals tested for carcinogenicity by the U.S. National toxicology program. Mutat Res 1991; 257:209–227.

14. Ashby J, Tennant RW. Definitive relationships among chemical structure, carcinogenicity and mutagenicity for 301 chemicals tested by the U.S. NTP. Mutat Res 1991; 257:229–306.

15. Green MHL. Mechanisms of bacterial mutagenesis and properties of mutagenesis tester strains. Arch Toxicol 1978; 39:241.

16. Ames BN, Lee FD, Durston WE. An improved bacterial test system for the detection and classification of mutagens and carcinogens. Proc Natl Acad Sci USA 1973; 70:782.

17. McCann J, Springarn NE, Kobori J, Ames N. Detection of carcinogens as mutagens: bacterial tester strains with R factor plasmids. Proc Natl Acad Sci USA 1975; 72:979.

18. Maron DM, Ames BN. Revised methods for the *Salmonella* mutagenicity test. Mutat Res 1983; 113:173.

19. Levin DE, Hollstein M, Christman MF, Schwiers EA, Ames BN. A new *Salmonella* tester strain (TA102) with A-T base pairs at the site of mutation detects oxidative mutagens. Proc Natl Acad Sci USA 1982; 79:7445.

20. Wilcox P, Naidoo A, Wedd DJ, Gatehouse DG. Comparison of *Salmonella typhimurium* TA102 with *Escherichia coli* WP2 tester strains. Mutagenesis 1990; 5:285.

21. Green MHL, Muriel WJ. Mutagen testing using trp$^+$ reversion in *Escherichia coli*. Mutat Res 1976; 38:3.

22. OECD Guideline 471 (Genetic Toxicology: Bacterial Reverse Mutation Test), Ninth Addendum to the OECD Guidelines for the Testing of Chemicals, published by OECD, Paris, February, 1998.

23. Wagner VO, III, Sly JE, Klug ML, et al. Practical tips for conducting the *Salmonella* and *E. coli* mutagenicity assays under proposed international guidelines. Environ Mol Mutagen 1994; 23:70.

24. Wagner VO, III, San RHC. The effect of titer on the response of two *Salmonella* strains to positive control mutagens. Environ Mol Mutagen 1993; 21:75.

25. Ames BN, Durston WE, Yamasaki E, Lee FD. Carcinogens are mutagens: a simple test system combining liver homogenates for activation and bacteria for detection. Proc Natl Acad Sci USA 1973; 70:2281.

26. Matsushima T, Sawamura M, Hara K, Sugimura T. A safe substitute for polychlorinated biphenyls as an inducer of metabolic activation systems. In: De Serres FJ, Fouts JR, Bend JR, Philpot RM, eds. In Vitro Metabolic Activation in Mutagenesis Testing. North-Holland, Amsterdam: Elsevier, 1976:85.

27. Ong T, Mukhtar M, Wolf CR, Zeiger E. Differential effects of cytochrome P450-inducers on promutagen activation capabilities and enzymatic activities of S9 from rat liver. J Environ Pathol Toxicol 1980; 4:55.

28. De Serres FJ, Shelby MD. Recommendations on data production and analysis using *Salmonella*/microsome mutagenicity assay. Mutat Res 1979; 64:159.

29. Ashby J. The prospects for a simplified and internationally harmonised approached to the detection of possible human carcinogens and mutagens. Mutagenesis 1986; 1:3.

30. Venitt S, Crofton-Sleigh C, Forster R. Bacterial mutation assays using reverse mutation. In: Venitt S, Parry JM, eds. Mutagenicity Testing: A Practical Approach. Oxford: IRL Press, 1984:45.

31. Vogel HJ, Bonner DM. Acetylornithinase of *E. coli*: partial purification and some properties. J Biol Chem 1956; 218:97.

32. Piper CE, Kuzdas CD. Incorporation of TA97a into a standard Ames test protocol. Environ Mutagen 1987; 9:85.

33. Gatehouse D, Haworth S, Cebula T, et al. Recommendations for the performance of bacterial mutation assays. Mutat Res 1995; 312:217.

34. Yahagi T, Nagao M, Seino Y, Matsushima T, Sugimura T, Okada M. Mutagenicities of N-nitrosamines on *Salmonella*. Mutat Res 1977; 48:121.

35. Weinstein D, Lewinson TM. A statistical treatment of the Ames mutagenicity assay. Mutat Res 1978; 51:433.

36. Bernstein L, Kaldor J, McCann J, Pike MC. An empirical approach to the statistical analysis of mutagenesis data from the *Salmonella* test. Mutat Res 1982; 97:267.

37. Stead AG, Hasselblad V, Creason JP, Claxton L. Modeling the Ames test. Mutat Res 1981; 85:13.

38. Margolin BH, Kaplan N, Zeiger E. Statistical analysis of the Ames *Salmonella*/microsome test. Proc Natl Acad Sci USA 1981; 78:3779.

39. Meyers LE, Sexton NH, Southerland LI, Wolff TJ. Regression analysis of Ames test data. Environ Mutagen 1981; 3:575.

40. Snee RD, Irr JD. A procedure for the statistical evaluation of Ames *Salmonella* assay results: comparison of results among 4 laboratories. Mutat Res 1984; 128:115.

41. Majeska JB, Mayo JK. The Ames *Salmonella* assay—state of the art. Mutat Res 2000; 35:41.

42. U.S. Pharmacopeia, XXVII, 88, Biological Reactivity Test, In Vivo, 2004.

43. Blackburn GR, Deitch RA, Schreiner CA, Mehlman MA, Mackerer CR. Estimation of the dermal carcinogenic activity of petroleum fractions using a modified Ames assay. Cell Biol Toxicol 1984; 1:67.

44. Blackburn GR, Deitch RA, Schreiner CA, Mackerer CR. Predicting carcinogenicity of petroleum distillation fractions using a modified *Salmonella* mutagenicity assay. Cell Biol Toxicol 1986; 2:63.

45. Prival MJ, Mitchell VD. Analysis of a method for testing azo dyes for mutagenic activity in *Salmonella typhimurium* in the presence of flavin mononucleotide and hamster liver S9. Mutat Res 1982; 97:103.

46. Distlerath LM, Loper JC, Dey CR. Aliphatic halogenated hydrocarbons produce volatile *Salmonella* mutagens. Mutat Res 1984; 136:55.

47. Hughes TJ, Simmons DM, Monteith LG, Claxton LD. Vaporization technique to measure activity of volatile organic chemicals in the Ames/*Salmonella* assay. Environ Mutagen 1987; 9:421.

48. Wagner VO, III, San RHC, Zeiger E. Desiccator methodology for *Salmonella* mutagenicity assay of vapor-phase and gas-phase test materials. Environ Mol Mutagen 1992; 19:68.

49. Dunn BP, Curtis JR. Clastogenic agents in the urine of coffee drinkers and cigarette smokers. Mutat Res 1985; 147:179.

50. Kado NY, Langley D, Eisenstadt E. A single modification of the *Salmonella* liquid-incubation assay increased sensitivity for detecting mutagens in human urine. Mutat Res 1983; 21:25.

51. Ames BN. The detection of chemical mutagens with enteric bacteria. In: Hollaender A, ed. In: Chemical Mutagens: Principles and methods for their detection, Vol. 1. New York: Plenum Press, 1971:267.

52. Chu EHY, Malling HV. Mammalian cell genetics II. Chemical induction of specific locus mutations in Chinese hamster cells in vitro. Proc Natl Acad Sci USA 1968; 61:1306.

53. Kao FT, Puck TT. Genetics of somatic mammalian cells, VII. Induction and isolation of nutritional mutants in Chinese hamster cells. Proc Natl Acad Sci USA 1968; 60:1275.

54. Albertini RJ, DeMars R. Somatic cell mutation detection and quantification of x-ray-induced mutation in cultured, diploid fibroblasts. Mutat Res 1973; 18:199.

55. Clive D, Flamm WG, Machesko MR, Bernheim NJ. A mutational assay system using the thymidine kinase locus in mouse lymphoma cells. Mutat Res 1972; 16:77.

56. Knaap AGAC, Simons JWIM. A mutational assay system for L5178Y mouse lymphoma cells, using hypoxanthine-guanine phosphoribosyl transferase (HGPRT) deficiency as marker. The occurrence of a long expression time for mutations induced by x-rays and EMS. Mutat Res 1975; 30:97.

57. Hsie AW, Casciano DA, Couch DB, Krahn DF, O'Neill JP, Whitfield BL. The use of Chinese hamster ovary cells to quantify specific locus mutation and to determine mutagenicity of chemicals. A report of the Gen-Tox program. Mutat Res 1981; 86:193.

58. Tindall KR, Stankowski LF, Jr., Machanoff R, Hsie AW. Detection of deletion mutations in pSV2gpt-transformed cells. Mol Cell Biol 1984; 4:1411.

59. Sato K, Slesinski RS, Littlefield JW. Chemical mutagenesis at the phosphoribosyltransferase locus in cultured human lymphoblasts. Proc Natl Acad Sci USA 1972; 69:1244.

60. Thilly WG. Chemical mutation in human lymphoblasts. J Toxicol Environ Health 1977; 2:1343.

61. Clive D, Flamm WG, Machesko MR. Mutagenicity of hycanthone in mammalian cells. Mutat Res 1972; 14:262.

62. Brown MMM, Clive D. The utilization of trifluorothymidine as a selective agent for TK−/− mutants in L5178Y mouse lymphoma cells. Mutat Res 1978; 53:116.

63. Clive D, Johnson KO, Spector JFS, Batson AG, Brown MMM. Validation and characterization of the L5178Y TK+/− mouse lymphoma mutagen assay system. Mutat Res 1979; 59:61.

64. Brown MMM, Clive D. The effect of expression time on the frequency of carcinogen-induced mutants at the TK and HGPRT loci in L5178Y mouse lymphoma cells. Mutat Res 1978; 3:159.

65. Thilly WG, DeLuca JG, Hoppe H, IV, Penman BW. Phenotypic lag and mutation to 6-thioguanine resistance in diploid human lymphoblasts. Mutat Res 1978; 50:137.

66. Rogers AM, Back KC. Comparative mutagenicity of hydrazine and three methylated derivatives in L5178Y mouse lymphoma cells. Mutat Res 1981; 89:321.

67. DeMarini DM, Brockman HE, de Serres FJ, Evans HE, Stankowski JF, Jr., Hsie AW. Specific-locus mutations induced in eukaryotes (especially mammalian cells) by radiation and chemicals: a prospective. Mutat Res 1989; 220:11.

68. Hozier J, Sawyer J, Moore M, Howard B, Clive D. Cytogenetic analysis of the L5178Y tk+/−, tk−/− mouse lymphoma mutagenesis assay system. Mutat Res 1981; 84:169.

69. Kozak CA, Ruddle FH. Assignment of the genes for thymidine kinase and galactokinase to *Mus musculus* chromosome 11 and the preferential segregation of this chromosome with Chinese hamster/mouse somatic cell hybrids. Somatic Cell Genet 1977; 3:121.

70. Glover R, Clive D. Molecular spectra of L5178Y/TK−/− mutants induced by diverse mutagens. Environ Mutagen 1989; 14:71.

71. O'Neill JP, Brimer PA, Machanoff R, Hirsch JP, Hsie AW. A quantitative assay of mutation induction at the hypoxanthine-guanine phosphoribosyl transferase locus in Chinese hamster ovary cells (CHO/HGPRT system): development and definition of the system. Mutat Res 1977; 45:91.

72. Machanoff R, O'Neill JP, Hsie AW. Quantitative analysis of cytotoxicity and mutagenicity of benzo(a)pyrene in mammalian cells (CHO/HGPRT). Chem Biol Interactions 1981; 34:1.

73. Li AP, Carver JH, Choy WN, et al. A guide for the performance of Chinese hamster ovary cell/hypoxanthine-guanine phosphoribosyl transferase gene mutation assay. Mutat Res 1987; 189:135.

74. Clive D, Spector JFS. Laboratory procedure for assessing specific locus mutations at the TK locus in cultured L5178Y mouse lymphoma cells. Mutat Res 1975; 31:17.

75. Moore MM, Clive D, Howard BE, Batson AG, Turner NT. In situ analysis of trifluorothymidine-resistant (TFT^r) mutants of L5178Y/TK$^{+/-}$ mouse lymphoma cells. Mutat Res 1985; 151:147.

76. Aaron CS, Bolcsfoldi G, Glatt H-R, et al. Mammalian cell gene mutation assays working group report. Mutat Res 1994; 312:235.

77. OECD Guideline for the Testing of Chemicals, Guideline 476 (In Vitro Mammalian Cell Gene Mutation Test), Ninth Addendum to the OECD Guidelines for the Testing of Chemicals, published by OECD, Paris, February, 1998.

78. Moore MM, Honma M, Clements J, et al. Mouse lymphoma thymidine kinase gene mutation assay: international workshop on genotoxicity tests workgroup report—Plymouth, U.K. 2002. Mutat Res 2003; 540:127.

79. Moore MM, Honma M, Clements G, et al. Mouse lymphoma thymidine kinase gene mutation assay: followup meeting of the international workshop on genotoxicity testing, Aberdeen, Scotland, 2003, assay acceptance criteria, positive controls and data evaluation, Environ Mol Mutagen 2005; 46, online.

80. Clive D, Bolcsfoldi G, Clements J, et al. Consensus agreement regarding protocol issues discussed during the mouse lymphoma workshop: portland, oregon, May 7, 1994. Environ Mol Mutagen 1995; 25:165.

81. Scott D, Galloway SM, Marshall RR, et al. Genotoxicity under extreme culture conditions. A report from ICPEMC task group 9. Mutat Res 1991; 257:147.

82. Cole J, Arlett CF, Green MHL, Lowe J, Muriel W. A comparison of the agar cloning and microtitration techniques for assaying cell survival and mutation frequency in L5178Y mouse lymphoma cells. Mutat Res 1983; 111:371.

83. Cole J, Muriel MJ, Bridges BA. The mutagenicity of sodium fluoride to L5178Y [wild-type and TK+/− (3.7.2c)] mouse lymphoma cells. Mutagenesis 1986; 1:157.

84. Clements J, Fellows MD, Oxley PA, Greensitt J, Kirkland DJ. Automation of colony sizing in the microwell TK assay and a comparison of data generated using microwell and agar cloning methods. Environ Mol Mutagen 1994; 23:10.

85. Clements J, Fellows M, Oxley P, Wilkinson J, Armstrong H. The mouse lymphoma assay (MLA) in microtitre plates: mutant colony size distribution for a selection of mutagens and a comparison of methods for determining cytotoxicity (RS vs. RTG). Environ Mol Mutagen 1995; 25:9.

86. Tindall KR, Stankowski LF, Jr., Machanoff R, Hsie AW. Analyses of mutation in pSV2gpt-transformed CHO cells. Mutat Res 1986; 160:121.

87. Tlsty TD, Briot A, Gualberto A, et al. Genomic instability and cancer. Mutat Res 1995; 337:1.

88. de Mitchell I, Lambert TR, Burden M, Sunderland J, Porter RL, Carlton JB. Is polyploidy an important genotoxic lesion? Mutagenesis 1995; 10:79.

89. Schultz N, Önfelt A. Video time-lapse study of mitosis in binucleate V79 cells: chromosome segregation and cleavage. Mutagenesis 1994; 9:117.

90. Schimke RT, Sherwood SW, Hill AB, Johnston RN. Over-replication and recombination of DNA in higher eukaryotes: potential consequences and biological implications. Proc Nat Acad Sci USA 1986; 83:2157.

91. Huang Y, Chang C, Trosko JE. Aphidicolin-induced endoreduplication in Chinese hamster cells. Cancer Res 1983; 43:1361.

92. Aardema MJ, Gibson DP, LeBoeuf RA. Sodium fluoride-induced chromosome aberrations in different stages of the cell cycle: a proposed mechanism. Mutat Res 1989; 223:191.

93. Hook EB. Contributions of chromosome abnormalities to human morbidity and mortality and some comments upon surveillance of chromosome mutation rates. In: Bora KC, Douglas GR, Nestmann ER, eds. Progress in Mutation Research. Amsterdam: Elsevier, 1982:9.

94. Feldman G. Liver ploidy. J Hepatology 1992; 16:7.

95. Siegal RL, Kalf GF. DNA polymerase β involvement in DNA endoreduplication in rat giant trophoblast cells. J Biol Chem 1982; 257:1785.

96. Sutou S, Arai Y. Possible mechanisms of endoreduplication induction. Membrane fixation and/or disruption of the cytoskeleton. Exp Cell Res 1975; 92:15.

97. Thust R, Bach B. Exogenous glutathione induces sister chromatid exchanges, clastogenicity and endoreduplication in V79 Chinese hamster cells. Cell Biol Toxicol 1985; 1:123.

98. Preston RJ, Au W, Bender MA, et al. Mammalian in vivo and in vitro cytogenetic assays: a report of the U.S. EPA's Gene-Tox program. Mutat Res 1981; 87:143.

99. Kirkland D, Garner RC. Testing for genotoxicity—chromosomal aberrations in vitro CHO cells or human lymphocytes. Mutat Res 1987; 189:186.

100. Kirkland D. Chromosomal aberration tests in vitro: problems with protocol design and interpretation of results. Mutagenesis 1992; 7:95.

101. Scott D, Danford ND, Dean BJ, Kirkland DJ. Metaphase chromosome aberration assays in vitro. In: Kirkland DJ, ed. Basic Mutagenicity Tests: UKEMS Recommended Procedures. Cambridge: Cambridge University Press, 1990:62.

102. Ishidate M, Harnois MC, Sofuni T. A comparative analysis of data on the clastogenicity of 951 chemical substances tested in mammalian cultures. Mutat Res 1988; 195:151.

103. Morita T, Nagaki T, Fukuda I, Okumura K. Clastogenicity of low pH to various cultured mammalian cells. Mutat Res 1992; 268:297.

104. Galloway SM, Deasy DA, Bean C, Kraynak AR, Armstrong MJ, Bradley MO. Effects of high osmotic strength on chromosome aberrations, sister-chromatid exchanges and DNA strand breaks, and the relation to toxicity. Mutat Res 1987; 189:15.

105. Galloway SM, Bloom AD, Resnick M, et al. Development of a standard protocol for in vitro cytogenetic testing with Chinese hamster ovary cells: comparison of results for 22 compounds in two laboratories. Environ Mutagen 1985; 7:1.

106. Galloway SM, Aardema MJ, Ishidate M, et al. Report from working group on in vitro tests for chromosomal aberrations. Mutat Res 1994; 312:241.

107. Ivett JL, Tice RR. Average generation time: a new method of analysis and quantitation of cellular repairative kinetics. Environ Mutagen 1982; 4:358.

108. OECD Guideline for the Testing of Chemicals, Guideline 473 (In Vitro Mammalian Chromosome Aberration Test), Ninth Addendum to the OECD Guidelines for the Testing of Chemicals, published by OECD, Paris, February, 1998.

109. Kirkland DJ, Marshall RR, McEnaney S, Bidgood J, Rutter A, Mullineux S. Arochlor-1254-induced rat-liver S9 causes chromosomal aberrations in CHO cells but not human lymphocytes: a role for active oxygen? Mutat Res 1989; 214:115.

110. Hubbard JA, Brooks TM, Gonzalez LP, Bridges JW. Preparation and characterization of S9 fractions. In: Parry JM, Arlett CF, eds. Comparative Genetic Toxicology. Houndmills, Hants: The Macmillan Press Ltd, 1985:413.

111. Margolin BH, Resnick MA, Rimpo JY, et al. Statistical analyses for in vitro cytogenetics assays using Chinese hamster ovary cells. Environ Mutagen 1986; 8:183.

112. Batzinger RP, Bueding E, Reddy BS, Weisburger HJ. Formation of a mutagenic drug metabolite by intestinal microorganisms. Cancer Res 1978; 38:608.

113. Heddle JA. A rapid in vivo test for chromosomal damage. Mutat Res 1973; 18:187.

114. Matter BE, Grauwiler J. Micronuclei in bone marrow cells. A simple in vivo model for the evaluation of drug-induced chromosomal aberrations. Mutat Res 1974; 23:239.

115. Heddle JA, Hite M, Kirkhart B, et al. The induction of micronuclei as a measure of genotoxicity. A report of the U.S. environmental protection agency Gene-Tox program. Mutat Res 1983; 123:61.

116. Hayashi M, Morita T, Kodama Y, Sofuni T, Ishidate M, Jr. The micronucleus assay with peripheral blood reticulocytes using acridine-coated slides. Mutat Res 1990; 245:245.

117. Salamone M, Heddle J, Stuart E, Katz M. Toward a an improved micronucleus test: Studies on 3 model agents, mitomycin C, cyclophosphamide and dimethylbenzanthracene. Mutat Res 1980; 74:347.

118. MacGregor JT, Wehr CM, Langlois RG. A simple fluorescence procedure for Micronuclei and RNA in eyrthrocytes using Hoechst 33258 and Pyronin Y. Mutat Res 1983; 120:269.

119. Probst GS. Validation of target tissue exposure for in vivo tests. In: D'Arcy PF, Harron DWG, eds. Proceedings of the Second International Conference on Harmonisation Orlando 1993. Belfast: The Queen's University, 1994:252.

120. Elder L. Statistical methods for short-term tests in genetic toxicology: the first fifteen years. Mutat Res 1992; 277:11.

121. Kastenbaum MA, Bowman KO. Tables for determining the statistical significance of mutation frequencies. Mutat Res 1970; 9:527.

122. Preston RJ, Dean BJ, Galloway S, Holden H, McFee AF, Shelby M. Mammalian in vivo cytogenetic assays. Analysis of chromosomes aberrations in bone marrow cells. Mutat Res 1987; 189:157.

123. Tice RR, Hayashi M, MacGregor JT, et al. Report from the working group on the in vivo mammalian bone marrow chromosomal aberration test. Mutat Res 1994; 312:305.

124. Perry P, Wolff S. New Giemsa method for differential staining of sister chromatids. Nature 1974; 251:156.

125. Evans HJ. Cytological methods for detecting chemical mutagens. In: Hollaender A, ed. Chemical Mutagens, Principles and Methods for their Detection. In: Cytological Methods for Detecting Chemical Mutagens, Chemical Mutagens, Principles and Methods for their Detection, Vol. 4. New York: Plenum Press, 1976:1.

126. Adler I-D. Clastogenic potential in spermatogonia of chemical mutagens related to their cell-cycle specificities. In: Ramel C, Lambert J, Magnusson J, eds. Genetic Toxicology of Environmental Chemicals: Genetic Effects and applied Mutagenesis. New York: Alan R. Liss, 1986:474.

127. Richold M, Chandly A, Ashby J, Gatehouse DG, Bootman J, Henderson L. In vivo cytogenetic assay: analysis of chromosome aberrations in bone marrow cells. Mutat Res 1990; 189:157.

128. Yamamoto K, Kikuchi Y. A new method for preparation of mammalian spermatogonial chromosomes. Mutat Res 1978; 52:207.

129. Nishikawa T, Haresaku M, Adachi K, Masuda M, Hayashi M. Study of a rat skin in vivo micronucleus test: data generated by mitomycin C and methyl methanesulfonate. Mutat Res 1999; 444:159.

130. Nishikawa T, Haresaku M, Fukushima A, et al. Further evaluation of an in vivo micronucleus test on rat and mouse skin: results with five skin carcinogens. Mutat Res 2002; 513:93.

131. Setlow RB, Carrier WL. The disappearance of thymine dimers from DNA: an error-correcting mechanism. Proc Natl Acad Sci USA 1964; 51:226.

132. McGrath R, Williams RW. Reconstruction in vivo of irradiated *Escherichia coli* deoxyribonucleic acid: the rejoining of broken pieces. Nature 1966; 212:534.

133. Rasmussen RE, Painter RB. Radiation-stimulated DNA synthesis in cultured mammalian cells. J Cell Biol 1966; 29:11.

134. Cleaver JE. DNA repair with purines and pyrimidines in radiation- and carcinogen-damaged normal and *Xeroderma pigmentosum* human cells. Cancer Res 1972; 33:362.

135. San RHC, Stich HF. DNA repair synthesis of cultured human cells as a rapid bioassay for chemical carcinogens. Int J Cancer 1975; 16:284.

136. Williams GM. Carcinogen-induced DNA repair in primary rat liver cell cultures, a possible screen for chemical carcinogens. Cancer Lett 1976; 1:231.

137. Williams GM. Detection of chemical carcinogens by unscheduled DNA synthesis in rat liver primary cell cultures. Cancer Res 1977; 37:1845.

138. Williams GM. Further improvements in the hepatocyte primary culture DNA repair test for carcinogens: detection of carcinogenic biphenyl derivatives. Cancer Lett 1978; 4:69.

139. Martin CN, McDermid AC, Garner RC. Testing of known carcinogens and noncarcinogens for their ability to induce unscheduled DNA synthesis in HeLa cells. Cancer Res 1978; 38:2621.

140. Stich HF, San RHC. Reduced DNA repair synthesis in Xeroderma pigmentosum cells exposed to the oncogenic 4-nitroquinoline 1-oxide and 4-hydroxayminoquinoline 1-oxide. Mutat Res 1971; 13:279.

141. Mitchell AD, Casciano DA, Meltz ML, et al. Unscheduled DNA synthesis tests: a report of the "Gene-Tox" program. Mutat Res 1983; 123:363.

142. Butterworth BE, Ashby J, Bermudez E, et al. A protocol and guide for the in vitro rat hepatocyte DNA-repair assay. Mutat Res 1987; 189:113.

143. Butterworth BE, Ashby J, Bermudez E, et al. A protocol and guide for the in vivo rat hepatocyte DNA-repair assay. Mutat Res 1987; 189:123.

144. Madle S, Dean SW, Andrae U, et al. Recommendations for the performance of UDS tests in vitro and in vivo. Mutat Res 1994; 312:263.

145. Williams GM. The detection of chemical mutagens/carcinogens by DNA repair and mutagenesis in liver cultures. In: de Serres FJ, Hollaender AE, eds. In: Chemical Mutagens, Vol. 6. New York: Plenum Press, 1979:71.

146. OECD Guideline 486, Unscheduled DNA Synthesis (UDS) Test with Mammalian Cells In Vivo, Ninth Addendum to the OECD Guidelines for the Testing of Chemicals, published by OECD, Paris, February, 1998.

147. Mirsalis JC, Tyson KC, Butterworth BE. The detection of genotoxic carcinogens in the in vivo—in vitro hepatocyte DNA repair assay. Environ Mutagen 1982; 4:553.

148. San RHC, Sly JE, Raabe HA. Unscheduled DNA synthesis in rat hepatocytes following in vivo administration of dimethylnitrosamine via different routes. Environ Mol Mutagen 1996; 27:58.

149. Mirsalis J, Butterworth B. Detection of unscheduled DNA synthesis in hepatocytes isolated from rats treated with genotoxic agents: an in vivo—in vitro assay for potential mutagens and carcinogens. Carcinogenesis 1980; 1:621.

150. Ashby J, Lefevre PA, Burlinson B, Penman MG. An assessment of the in vivo rat hepatocyte DNA repair assay. Mutat Res 1985; 156:1.

151. Lieberman MW, Baney RN, Lee RE, Sell S, Farber E. Studies on DNA repair in human lymphocytes treated with proximate carcinogens and alkylating agents. Cancer Res 1971; 31:1297.

152. Sega GA. Unscheduled DNA synthesis in the germ cells of male mice exposed in vivo to the chemical mutagen ethyl methanesulfonate. Proc Natl Acad Sci USA 1974; 71:4955.

153. Sega GA, Ownes JG, Cumming RB. Studies on DNA repair in early spermatid stages of male mice after in vivo treatment with methyl-, ethyl-, propyl-, and isopropyl methanesulfonate. Mutat Res 1976; 36:193.

154. Sega GA, Wolfe KW, Owens JG. A comparison of the molecular action of an S_N1-type methylating agent, methyl nitrosourea, and an S_N2-type methylating agent, methyl methanesulfonate, in the germ cells of male mice. Chem Biol Interact 1981; 33:253.

155. Sotomayor RE, Sega GA, Cumming RB. Unscheduled DNA synthesis in spermatogenic cells of mice treated in vivo with the indirect alkylating agents cyclophosphamide and mitomen. Mutat Res 1978; 50:229.

156. Sotomayor RE, Sega GA, Cumming RB. An autoradiographic study of unscheduled DNA synthesis in the germ cells of male mice treated with X-rays and methyl methanesulfonate. Mutat Res 1979; 62:293.

157. Sotomayor RE, Chauhan PS, Ehling UH. Induction of unscheduled DNA synthesis in the germ cells of male mice after treatment with hydrazine or procarbazine. Toxicology 1982; 25:201.

158. Kohn KW, Ewig RAG, Erickson LC, Zwelling LA. Measurement of strand breaks and cross-links by alkaline elution. In: Friedberg E, Hanawalt PC, eds. Handbook of DNA Repair Techniques. New York: Dekker, 1980:379.

159. Skare JA, Schrotel KR. Alkaline elution of rat testicular DNA: detection of DNA strand breaks after in vivo treatment with chemical mutagens. Mutat Res 1984; 130:283.

160. Skare JA, Schrotel KR. Validation of an in vivo alkaline elution assay to detect DNA damage in rat testicular cells. Environ Mutagen 1985; 7:563.

161. Sina JF, Bean CL, Dysart GR, Taylor VI, Bradley MO. Evaluation of the alkaline elution/rat hepatocyte assay as a predictor of carcinogenic/mutagenic potential. Mutat Res 1983; 113:357.

162. Skare JA, Schrotel KR. Alkaline elution of rat testicular DNA: detection of DNA cross-links after in vivo treatment with chemical mutagens. Mutat Res 1984; 130:295.

163. International Conference on Harmonisation (ICH) of Technical Requirements for Registration of Pharmaceuticals for Human Use. ICH Harmonised Tripartite Guideline. Testing for Carcinogenicity of Pharmaceuticals. S1B document recommended for adoption at step 4 of the ICH process on 16 July 1997. Fed Regist, 1998; 23 February; 63: 8983.

164. Isfort RJ, Cody DB, Doerson C, Kerckaert GA, LeBoeuf RA. Alterations in cellular differentiation, mitogenesis, cytoskeleton and growth characteristics during Syrian hamster embryo cell multistep in vitro transformation. Int J Cancer 1994; 59:114.

165. Kerckaert GA, Isfort RJ, Carr GJ, Aardema MJ, LeBoeuf RA. A comprehensive protocol for conducting the Syrian hamster embryo cell transformation assay at pH 6.70. Mutat Res 1996; 356:65.

166. Engelhardt G, Schwind K-R, Mu B. The testing of chemicals in the Syrian hamster embryo (SHE) cell transformation assay for assessment of carcinogenic potential. Toxicol In Vitro 2004; 8:213.

167. LeBoeuf RA, Kerckaert G. Enhanced morphological transformation of early passage syrian hamster embryo cells cultured in medium with a reduced bicarbonate concentration and pH. Carcinogenesis 1987; 8:680.

168. LeBoeuf RA, Kerckaert GA, Aardema MJ, Gibson DP. Multistage neoplastic transformation of syrian hamster embryo cells cultured at pH 6.70. Cancer Res 1990; 50:3722.

169. Armitage P. Statistical Methods in Medical Research. Oxford: Blackwell Scientific Publications, 1971 p. 135.

170. Singh NP, McCoy MT, Tice RR, Schneider EL. A simple technique for quantitation of low levels of DNA damage in individual cells. Exp Cell Res 1988; 175:184.

171. Tice RR, Agurell E, Anderson D, et al. Single cell gel/comet assay guidelines for in vitro and in vivo genetic toxicology testing. Environ Mol Mutagen 2000; 35:206.

172. Collins AR. The comet assay for DNA damage and repair: principles, applications, and limitations. Mol Biotechnol 2004; 26:249.

173. Hartmann A, Agurell D, Beevers C, et al. Recommendations for conducting the in vivo alkaline comet assay. Mutagenesis 2003; 18:45.

174. Hartmann A, Schumacher M, Plappert-Helbig U, Lowe P, Suter W, Mueller L. Use of the alkaline in vivo comet assay for mechanistic genotoxicity investigation. Mutagenesis 2004; 19:51.

175. Sasaki YF, Kawaguchi S, Kamaya A, et al. The comet assay with 8 mouse organs: results with 39 currently used food additive. Mutat Res 2002; 519:103.

176. Sekihashi K, Yamamoto A, Matsummura Y, et al. Comparative investigation of multiple organs of mice and rats in the comet assay. Mutat Res 2002; 517:53.

177. Olive PL, Banáth JP, Durand RE. Heterogeneity in radiation-induced DNA damage and repair in tumor and normal cells measured using the "comet" assay. Radiat Res 1990; 122:86.

178. Östling O, Johanson KJ. Microelectrophoretic study of radiation-induced DNA damages in individual mammalian cells. Biochem Biophys Res Commun 1984; 123:291.

179. Collins AR, Dobson VL, Dusinská M, Kennedy G, Štetina R. The comet assay: what can it really tell us? Mutat Res 1997; 375:183.

180. Anderson D, Yu T-W, Phillips BJ, Schmezer P. The effect of various antioxidants and other modifying agents on oxygen-radical-generated DNA damage in human lymphocytes in the comet assay. Mutat Res 1994; 307:261.

181. Rojas E, Lopez MC, Valverde M. Single cell gel electrophoresis assay: methodology and applications. J Chromatogr B 1999; 722:225.

182. Snyder RD, Green JW. A review of the genotoxicity of marketed pharmaceuticals. Mutat Res 2001; 488:151.

183. Isfort RJ, Kerckaert GA, LeBoeuf RA. Comparison of the standard and reduced pH syrian hamster embryo (SHE) cell in vitro transformation assays in predicting the carcinogenic potential of chemicals. Mutat Res 1996; 356:11.

184. Zhang H, Myhr BC. High-concordance prediction of rodent carcinogenicity by the short-term in vitro SHE cell transformation assay. Toxicologist 2001; 60:263.

185. Mauthe RJ, Gibson DP, Bunch RT, Custer L. The Syrian hamster embryo (SHE) cell transformation assay: review of methods and results from ILSI/HES program on alternative carcinogenicity testing. Toxicol Path 2001; 29:138.

186. Myhr BC. Unpublished presentation at the Environmetal Mutagen Society meeting, Pittsburgh, PA, 2004; October 2–6.

187. Hilliard CA, Armstrong MJ, Bradt CI, Hill RB, Greenwood SK, Galloway SM. Chromosome aberrations in vitro related to cytotoxicity of nonmutagenic chemicals and metabolic poisons. Environ Mol Mutagen 1998; 31:316.

188. Galloway SM, Miller JE, Armstrong MJ, Bean CL, Skopek TR, Nichols WW. DNA synthesis inhibition as an indirect mechanism of chromosome aberrations: comparison of DNA-reactive and non-DNA-reactive clastogens. Mutat Res 1998; 400:169.

189. Galloway SM. Cytotoxicity and chromosome aberrations in vitro: experience in industry and the case for an upper limit on toxicity in the aberration assay. Environ Mol Mutagen 2000; 35:191.

9
Carcinogenicity Studies[†]

Abigail C. Jacobs
Center for Drug Evaluation and Research/Food and Drug Administration, Silver Spring, Maryland, U.S.A.

INTRODUCTION

The carcinogenic potential of test substances is evaluated so that regulatory agencies can make risk assessments or risk/benefit analyses for exposure of humans to chemicals or drugs, regulate exposure conditions, and label products appropriately. Because of small sample size, difficulties in quantification of exposure, variation in individual susceptibility, the long time to tumor in humans, and other confounding factors, carcinogenicity is generally difficult to establish by epidemiology. Therefore animal studies are relied upon at this time to estimate the risk to humans. The current design of assessing carcinogenicity of chemicals in lifetime studies in rodents was developed by the Weisburgers (1) in the late 1960s and was further refined by the National Cancer Institute/National Toxicology Program (NTP) (2–4), U.S. Interagency staff (5).

Studies are conducted by administering the test materials to two mammalian species, generally rats or mice, and occasionally hamsters, for the majority of their lifetime and evaluating the resulting neoplastic lesions. Although the model has a number of deficiencies, the model has been considered appropriate because chemicals found to be human carcinogens in epidemiologic studies (except for arsenic) have also been found to be carcinogens in rats or mice, and complete replacement models or methods are not yet available.

Regulatory Requirements (United States and Worldwide)

Agencies responsible for the regulation of human pharmaceuticals, veterinary drugs, food additives, consumer products, industrial chemicals, pesticides, and occupational exposure have differing regulatory requirements, guidelines, and evaluation procedures for evaluation of carcinogenicity (Table 1). Some are parts of laws or federal regulations,

---

[†]This review does not represent an official FDA opinion.

Table 1 Regulatory Requirements of Various Agencies

Agency	When tests are needed	Study design	Evaluation of risk
CDER/FDA	ICH S1A (6); when pharmaceuticals are used for a chronic indication	ICH S1B (7), S1C (8), S1CR (9); CFSAN Redbook (10)	No quantitative risk assessment; weight of evidence for risk/benefit is evaluated and mode of actions and multiples of human exposure are considered
CFSAN/FDA	Food and color additives: 21CFR 171 (11)	CFSAN Redbook; OECD 451 (12), 453 (13)	CFSAN Redbook of 1993: food additives: Delaney clause (14) amendment to the FD&C Act; cosmetics: quantitative risk assessment for acceptable levels
CVM/FDA	VICH GL28 (15) for animal drug residues	VICH GL28 (15) CFSAN Redbook (10); OECD 451, 453 (12,13)	Quantitative risk assessment for acceptable levels for food-producing animals
EPA	FIFRA/OPPTS (16); TSCA 40CFR. If chemical is used on food or will result on significant human exposure; for TSCA: priority testing lists (of chemicals) by TSCA's ITC committee; Clean Air Act; Clean Water Act	OECD 451, 453 (12,13); OPPTS 870.4200 (16)	Guidelines for carcinogen risk assessment (Mar 2005); mode of actions considered (http:www.epa.gov) (17)
CPSC	Preliminary screening of substances about which a question of carcinogenicity potential has been raised	OECD 451, 453 (12,13); CPSC hazard assessment and reduction program and regulated products program (http://cpsc.gov); (18) Consumer Products Safe Testing Act;	Classification of chemicals into four categories based on the type of scientific data suggesting cancer-causing potential (http://cpsc.gov) (19)

		animal testing policy 49 FR 22522–22523 (19) (1984); (20) guidelines for determining chronic toxicity according to Federal Hazardous Substance Act and Poison Prevention Pkg. Act
OSHA	Chemical manufacturers or importers assess hazards of chemicals which they produce or import, and all employers provide information to employees about hazardous chemicals to which they are exposed, by means of a hazard communication program, labels, and other forms of warning, material safety data sheets, and information and training	OECD 451, 453; industry evaluating chemicals not required to follow specific methods for determining hazards but must be able to demonstrate they have adequately ascertained hazards of chemicals produced or imported in accordance with criteria set forth in App. B of the hazard communication standard of CFR 29 1910.1200 app. A through E (21)	The hazard communication standard of 29 CFR 1910.1200 App. A through E (21); industry uses agency or other guidelines to evaluate and appropriately label products as to their potential hazards; chemicals is considered to be a carcinogen if: it has been evaluated by the IARC, and found to be a carcinogen or potential carcinogen; or is listed as a carcinogen or potential carcinogen in the Annual Report on Carcinogens published by the NTP or OSHA considers it a carcinogen
Europe/Japan pharmaceutical	ICH S1A; Europe: EMEA	ICH S1B, S1C, S1CR; Europe: EMEA guidance 3Bs7 (22)	Risk/benefit; weight of evidence
Europe chem./pesticide			Dangerous substances directive EEC 99/45/EC/ classification and labeling

Abbreviations: CDER, Center for Drug Evaluation and Research (FDA); CFSAN, Center for Food Safety and Nutrition (FDA); CPSC, Consumer Product Safety Commission; EEC, European Economic Community; EMEA, European Medicines Evaluation Agency. (The European licensing authority that reports to the EU commission); EPA, Environmental Protection Agency; EU, European Union; FDA, Food and Drug Administration; FDC, Food Drug and Cosmetic; FIFRA, Federal Insecticide, Fungicide, and Rodenticide Act (EPA); IARC, International Agency for Research on Cancer; ICH, International Conference on Harmonization; ITC, TSCA, EPA, Interagency Testing Committee of Toxic Substances Control Act (EPA); OECD, Organization for Economic Cooperation and Development; OPPTS, Office of Pollution Prevention and Toxics (EPA); OSHA, Occupational Safety and Health Administration; TSCA, Toxic Substances Control Act (EPA); VICH, Veterinary International Conference on Harmonization.

and others are guidelines or guidances. Some agencies specify very specific protocols, and others accept a variety of protocols. The appropriate agency should always be consulted for current policy and desired protocols.

TRADITIONAL STUDY DESIGN AND PARAMETERS MEASURED

Generally groups of 50–70 animals per group of each sex and species (rats or mice) are used. Three dose groups plus a control group are usually tested. In-life measurements include body weight, feed consumption (for feed studies), and clinical signs. Because hematologic and clinical chemistry analyses in aging animals are affected by diseases and neoplasms, they are not particularly useful after 1 year. Thus these analyses may not be recommended to be included in the 2-year studies unless there is a specific reason and utility for their inclusion. Administration of a drug or chemical is generally for 24 months, after which the rodents are humanely killed at a predetermined time, and gross (naked eye visual) necropsy evaluation followed by histologic examination of a large number of predetermined tissues is conducted. Studies should be conducted according Good Laboratory Practice regulations (23) as outlined in Chapter 1. The animal care, test material preparation, and gross and microscopic pathologic evaluations should be conducted in a manner similar to other toxicology studies. The rodent strains selected should be ones with substantial historical data and experience.

The most difficult aspect of the study design is selection of the highest dose. The highest dose for the 2-year studies should be one that won't shorten survival other than by neoplasms or cause severe clinical signs, severe toxicity, or severe physiologic perturbations. The body weight of the control and highest dose groups should generally not differ by more than 10%, so that the controls are still appropriate for comparison. Doses for males and females and for each species should be independently selected. The same route as used in humans should generally be used in the dose-ranging studies in animals, and not all oral administration routes (gavage vs. feed) are equivalent. Administration in feed may result in much greater or much poorer bioavailability, and palatability problems may lead to scatter of feed.

The International Conference on Harmonization (ICH) Guideline on Dose Selection for Carcinogenicity Studies of Pharmaceuticals (8) discusses both dose-ranging studies and high-dose selection for pharmaceuticals. Rodent species/strains with metabolic profiles as similar as possible to humans should be studied. Dose-ranging studies should be conducted for both males and females for all strains and species to be tested in the carcinogenicity study. The doses are generally determined from 90-day studies using the route and method of administration that will be used in the bioassay. Selection of an appropriate dosing schedule and regimen should be based on proposed clinical use and exposure patterns, pharmacokinetics, and practical considerations. Ideally, both the toxicity profile and any dose-limiting toxicity should be characterized. Consideration should also be given to general toxicity, the occurrence of preneoplastic lesions and/or tissue-specific proliferative effects, and disturbances in endocrine homeostasis. Changes in metabolite profile, or alterations in metabolizing enzyme activities (induction or inhibition) over time, should be understood to allow for appropriate interpretation of studies.

Historically, only a maximum tolerated dose (MTD) was used as the high dose selection. However for pharmaceuticals, alternatives to the MTD for high dose selection were considered acceptable according to an international agreement (8). Per ICH, for pharmaceuticals five generally acceptable criteria for selection of the high dose for pharmaceuticals are: (1) the MTD; (2) a minimum of a 25-fold area under the plasma concentration-time curve (AUC) ratio (rodent:human) of systemic exposure for nongenotoxic drugs; (3) dose-limiting pharmacodynamic effects; (4) saturation of absorption; (5) and maximum feasible dose. Other pharmacodynamic-, pharmacokinetic-, or toxicity-based end points may be considered, as described in the next few paragraphs.

MTD: Factors to consider are alterations in physiologic function that would be predicted to alter the animal's normal life span or interfere with interpretation of the study. Such factors include: no more than 10 percent decrease in body weight gain relative to controls; target organ toxicity; significant alterations in clinical pathological parameters.

Plasma AUC pharmacokinetics end point: a minimum of a 25-fold area AUC ratio (rodent:human) for nongenotoxic drugs with similar metabolic profiles in humans and rodents and low organ toxicity in rodents. For the purposes of the ICH guideline, a pharmaceutical is considered nongenotoxic with respect to the use of pharmacokinetic end points for dose selection if it is negative in the standard battery of assays required for pharmaceutical registration. A 25-fold ratio was arrived at after a retrospective analysis was performed on data from carcinogenicity studies of therapeutics conducted at the MTD, for which there were sufficient human and rodent pharmacokinetic data for comparison of AUC values (24,25). In 35 drug carcinogenicity studies carried out at the MTD for which there were adequate pharmacokinetic data in rats and humans, approximately one-third had a relative systemic exposure ratio less than or equal to 1, another one-third had ratios between 1 and 10. Those pharmaceuticals tested using a 25-fold or greater AUC ratio for the high dose will have exposure ratios greater than 75 percent of pharmaceuticals tested previously in carcinogenicity studies performed at the MTD. For use of a pharmacokinetically defined exposure for high-dose selection, rodent pharmacokinetic data are derived from the strains used for the carcinogenicity studies using the route of compound administration and dose ranges planned for the carcinogenicity study. The rodent AUC values and metabolite profiles may be determined from separate steady state kinetic studies, as part of 90-day toxicity studies or dose-ranging studies. Pharmacokinetic data are derived from studies of sufficient duration to take into account potential time-dependent changes in pharmacokinetic parameters that may occur during the dose-ranging studies. Documentation is provided on the similarity of metabolism between rodents and humans. It is recommended that in vivo metabolism be characterized in humans and rodents, if possible. However, in the absence of appropriate in vivo metabolism data, in vitro metabolism data (e.g., from liver slices, uninduced microsomal preparations) may provide adequate support for the similarity of metabolism across species. In assessing exposure, scientific judgment is used to determine whether the plasma AUC comparison is based on data for the parent, parent and metabolite(s), or metabolite(s). Interspecies differences in protein binding are taken into consideration when estimating relative exposure. Although in vivo determinations of unbound drug may be the best approach, in vitro determinations of protein binding using parent and/or metabolites as appropriate (over the range of concentrations achieved in vivo in rodents and humans) may be used in the estimation of AUC unbound. When protein binding is low in both humans and rodents or when protein binding is high and the unbound fraction of drug is greater in rodents than in humans, the comparison of total plasma concentration of drug is acceptable. When protein binding is high and the unbound fraction is greater in humans than in rodents, the ratio of the unbound concentrations should be used. Human pharmacokinetic data are derived from studies encompassing the maximum recommended human daily dose. Human systemic exposure data may be derived from pharmacokinetic monitoring in normal volunteers and/or patients. The possibility of extensive inter-individual variation in exposure should be taken into consideration. In the absence of knowledge of the maximum recommended human daily dose, at a minimum, doses producing the desired pharmacodynamic effect in humans are used to derive the pharmacokinetic data.

Dose-limiting pharmacodynamic end points for high-dose selection will be highly compound-specific and are considered for individual study designs based on scientific merits. The high dose selected should produce a pharmacodynamic response in dosed animals of such magnitude as would preclude further dose escalation. However, the dose should not produce disturbances of physiology or homeostasis that would compromise the validity of the study. Examples include hypotension and inhibition of blood clotting (because of the risk of spontaneous bleeding).

Currently, the maximum feasible (desirable) dose by dietary administration is considered to be 5 percent of diet per ICH S1C (8). The ICH S1C also discusses the issue of a limit dose. It may not be necessary to exceed a dose of 1500 milligrams (mg)/kilograms (kg)/day in cases where there is no evidence of genotoxicity and where the maximum recommended human dose does not exceed 500 mg/day. When routes other than dietary administration are appropriate, the high dose will be limited based on considerations including practicality and local tolerance.

Regardless of the method used for the selection of the high dose, the selection of the mid and low doses for the carcinogenicity study should provide information to aid in assessing the relevance of study findings to humans. The doses should be selected following integration of rodent and human pharmacokinetic, pharmacodynamic, and toxicity data. The rationale for the selection of these doses should be provided. Although not all encompassing, the following points should be considered in selection of the middle and low doses for rodent carcinogenicity studies:

1. Linearity of pharmacokinetics and saturation of metabolic pathways
2. Human exposure and therapeutic dose
3. The pharmacodynamic response in rodents
4. Alterations in normal rodent physiology
5. Mechanistic information and potential for threshold effects
6. The unpredictability of the progression of toxicity observed in short-term studies.

Pharmacokinetics evaluations could indicate linearity of the plasma AUC values with dose or other discontinuities with dose, suggesting that some threshold has been exceeded. Pharmacokinetics data can indicate saturation of metabolic pathways. Drugs can deplete detoxification reactions as well as those that convert the parent compound to a more toxic species. If the plasma AUC value is not increasing with dose, there is no point in increasing the dose, even if an MTD is not reached. Pharmacokinetics data can indicate accumulation of the drug or when steady state is reached.

DATA REPORTING, ANALYSIS, INTERPRETATION, AND RISK ASSESSMENT

Data reporting for content and format will vary by agency. Studies on pharmaceuticals are reported in an internationally agreed upon format (ICH M2) (26) referred to as the common technical document. After completion of the in-life portions of the studies, the adequacy of the studies and whether there were any chemical or drug-related needs to be determined. Adequacy of dose selection is evaluated, and chemical and chemical/vehicle stability and homogeneity need to be confirmed. That the animals were free of infections and properly cared for and monitored throughout the studies is checked. If there was not at least 50% survival at 18 months, there might not be enough animals at risk to get neoplasms.

Gross pathologic and histologic evaluations are critical elements of the studies (27,28). It is best if tissues of all animals are evaluated microscopically. It is essential that tissues of all animals be evaluated if survival or body weight in the high-dose group is markedly lower than that of the controls. Knowledgeable pathologists disagree about diagnoses even when criteria are agreed upon, and different pathologists may use different nomenclature and criteria for a particular lesion. This confounds comparisons to the use of historical data, especially when secondary and tertiary reviews of the histopathologic data are not conducted, as is done by the National Toxicology Program (NTP) (29) or when the data are not recent and from the same testing laboratory.

Hazard Identification

After the histopathologic evaluations are completed, the statistical analyses for survival and neoplasm incidences are conducted. An important question to be answered is whether the incidence of neoplasms at an organ/system site in dosed groups was significantly statistically increased compared with that in controls. The statistical evaluation for hazard identification in carcinogenicity is more complicated than for general toxicology studies. The evaluation may be confounded by background incidences of neoplasms in aging rodents and survival differences between control and dosed animals. Aging rodents develop neoplasms without having received drugs or chemicals. Sites affected by background incidences vary among species, strains, and sexes. The historical background incidences depend on many factors and vary across time and testing laboratories for a variety of reasons (30–32). These factors include:

1. Genetic differences in inbred animals over time
2. Genetic differences between random bred animals
3. Length of study and age of animals at the end of the study—19–26 months old
4. Differences in nomenclature over time and among pathologists
5. Differences between pathologists with regard to diagnoses
6. Differences in how neoplasms are pooled
7. Group-housed versus individually housed (33)
8. Multiplicity of sections examined may increase the incidences in controls
9. Reevaluation of controls because of an effect in dosed groups
10. Environmental contamination (from feed studies)
11. Different diet (soy, protein, fat, fiber, and nitrosamine contaminant levels)
12. Differences in drinking water, such as chlorinated hydrocarbons
13. Presence of pathogens
14. Genetic drift of animals over time
15. Body weight of the animals; lower weight animals have lower neoplasm incidences, and changes in the composition or quantity of the diet can lower neoplasms incidences after 2 years (32,34–44).

The distribution of neoplasm incidences in studies could have been a chance event resulting from random distribution of background neoplasm incidences. Statistical tests are used to evaluate the role of chance in resulting neoplasm incidences. The lower the P value, the less likely the difference in incidences can be explained by random assignment of animals to groups. The statistical tests involve a comparison of the observed neoplasm incidences with those incidences expected. Statistical analyses are conducted on the number of animals with primary neoplasms, not the number of neoplasms. Each gender of each species is separately evaluated. Males are not pooled with females, and neoplasms at all sites are not routinely combined. Vehicle controls are not pooled with untreated controls. Appropriate pooling of neoplasms for statistical analysis is crucial. Neoplasm types pooled for statistical analysis are generally of the same embryonic origin and morphologic type (45). Statistical analyses are made on both individual neoplasm types and on the appropriate pooling of neoplasm types. Analysis of adenomas might give a P value of 0.01, indicating an effect, but analysis of adenomas or carcinomas at the same site might give a P value of 0.06, indicating no effect. Endocrine neoplasms are not pooled with nonendocrine neoplasms. Epithelial neoplasms are not pooled with non epithelial neoplasms. Pancreatic islet neoplasms are not pooled with pancreatic acinar cell neoplasms. Systemic neoplasms are pooled (e.g., lymphoma or lymphocytic leukemia at all sites; hemangiomas or hemangiosarcomas at all sites; histiocytic sarcomas at all sites).

Different statistical tests may be used by various agencies to evaluate the results of carcinogenicity studies. Tests may include trend tests, pairwise tests, time-adjusted tests (adjusted for survival), and time-unadjusted tests. Trend tests look at incidences in all groups simultaneously as a function of dose (mg/kg). Pairwise tests compare each group individually with the control. For the same neoplasm incidences, the trend test will generally give a lower P value than a pairwise comparison (46–49). Often P values of <0.05 are obtained for a trend test when P values of >0.05 are obtained for pairwise comparisons. The trend tests assume that a linear response with the nominal dose would be achieved if the neoplasms were drug related. This assumption may not be warranted due to change in metabolism with dose, saturation of absorption, saturation of a receptor, markedly lower survival, extensive necrosis or atrophy at a site in the highest dose group, saturation or inhibition of conversion to the carcinogenic chemical species, or antagonism between neoplasm types in the highest dose group, such as a negative association between liver neoplasms and lymphomas in CF-1 mice and between liver neoplasms and leukemia in F344 rats.

Time-unadjusted tests do not take into account the time of appearance of the neoplasms. They are based on the overall proportion of neoplasm-bearing animals. The Cochran-Armitage linear trend test (50) and the Fisher exact test (51) are two unadjusted tests that have been used.

Time-adjusted tests include the life table analyses, Peto incidental tumor test, logistic regression analysis, and the poly 3 test. Such tests are used when there are survival differences (52). Survival differences can be evaluated by various trend tests: the Cox test (53–55); the generalized Wilcoxon or Kruskal-Wallis test (56,57), and the Tarone trend tests (58–61).

Life table analysis (both trend and pairwise comparison) for fatal neoplasms involves summation of comparisons at each point in time that an animal with a neoplasm of interest died (53,60).

The incidental neoplasm or Peto (61) test is for neoplasms that are not considered to have been the cause of death but happened to have been observed when the animal died of an unrelated cause. The Peto analysis uses time intervals (e.g., weeks 0–52, weeks 53–78, weeks 79–92, week 92-week before being killed, and the end of the study). One problem is that we don't always know the cause of death. Distinguishing lethal from incidental neoplasms is often difficult. Except for skin and mammary neoplasms, the time of appearance of neoplasms is not known, only that they were present in an animal that may have died of an unrelated cause. Another problem is that the P value may vary with the time intervals selected.

Logistic regression analyses don't require time intervals and models neoplasm incidences as a logistic function of dose (mg/kg) and time (52,62,63). The poly-3 method of Portier and Bailer (64) adjusts for survival differences but does not use time intervals or require knowledge of whether a neoplasm is fatal or incidental.

Statistical results alone do not prove that neoplasms are drug or chemically related, but they do support conclusions that were made by considering all the evidence. Absence of statistical significance does carry weight. Selection of decision rules for appropriate P values is a policy decision. It depends on the product and what is least desirable, a false positive or a false negative. The lower the P value required for significance, the higher the false-negative rate, and the higher the P value required, the higher the false positive rate. A false negative for pharmaceuticals means that the risk to humans may be underestimated. For a false positive, the risk to humans may be overestimated. In both cases the risk/benefit comparisons between drugs for the same indication will be affected.

The possibility of obtaining a false positive increases as the historical background rate increases (47,65–68), and thus different P values for significance may be indicated for common or uncommon neoplasms, such as $P<0.05$ for uncommon and $P<0.01$ for common neoplasms. The same P value for a common neoplasm carries less weight that that for an uncommon neoplasm. For this reason, sometimes different decision rules for P values are used for trend and pairwise comparisons. Although the most important control group for comparison is the concurrent control group, historical incidences are useful for evaluation of uncommon neoplasms that are never or rarely diagnosed. Use of historical control data is important (31,67,68) and has been considered in a formal statistical sense (69–71). Formal statistical analysis procedures incorporating historical data have not been adopted by regulatory agencies because the historical data are so variable and dependent on the testing laboratory conditions and pathologist and the relevant data set may be small. However, historical incidences are used to supplement statistical analyses in assessing biologic significance of findings.

Risk Assessment and Extrapolation to Humans

The strength of the evidence for a carcinogenic hazard is influenced by neoplastic effects being present in multiple organs, in multiple strains, or in multiple species or in each gender, the magnitude of the increased incidences, dose-related trends, the degree of malignancy, historical control incidences, and rarity of a particular neoplasm in rodents. If a hazard has been identified in rodents, the relevance to humans is then evaluated.

Risk assessment (72) considers the strength of the evidence for the carcinogenic hazard, the frequency, duration, and intensity of the exposure of humans to the material, in addition to data on neoplasm incidences and their dose response, nonneoplastic effects, and mode of action data and other data on relevance to humans (17,73,74).

The EPA conducts formal quantitative risk assessments for estimated lifetime cancer risks for chemicals and pesticides (17,75). In contrast, formal numerical risk assessments from carcinogenicity studies are not conducted for pharmaceuticals. Two extrapolations are necessary to convert the animal data to appropriate human risk estimates: the first extrapolation is from animals to humans, and the second is from the experimental doses (which may be high) in animals to the doses (which may be low with environmental exposure) encountered by humans. The extrapolation to humans from animal data involves comparisons of exposure data and considerations of data on mode of action and biologic relevance to humans. Because pharmacokinetic data in humans are not routinely readily available to the Environmental Protection Agency (EPA), the EPA uses uncertainty factors for interspecies extrapolation or mg/m^2 body surface area comparisons for exposure comparisons, whereas Center for Drug Evaluation and Research (CDER/FDA) generally has pharmacokinetic data available for such comparisons.

The EPA (and much of the literature on cancer risk assessment) usually considers studies in which the rodent dose relative to the human dose is rather large and the human exposure is generally inadvertent with no benefit. A large dose in animals may be extrapolated to a very small dose in humans. Extrapolations may be made from a benchmark dose, a dose or concentration that produces a predetermined change in response rate of an adverse effect compared to background, usually in the range of 5 or 10% (75). Mathematical models for formal extrapolations from high doses in rodents to much lower doses in humans may give widely divergent estimates of the risk to humans, depending on the assumptions made (76,77). Usually there are too few dose groups to characterize the entire dose response. The usefulness of very high dose to low dose extrapolations has been questioned because there may be a nonlinear response between the high dose and the very low doses to which humans may be exposed environmentally; alternate extrapolation procedures for such cases may now be considered (17,73,78,79). Because of limitations of the linearized multistage (LMS) model (17) for low-dose risk assessment, which expresses upper confidence limits on cancer risk as a linear function of dose in the low dose range (80), the revised EPA guidelines have moved away from a routine use of the LMS for low dose risk assessment of environmental exposures (17) to considerations of mode of action and biologic relevance to humans.

Extrapolation of risk (or no risk) to humans is greatly improved by what is known about mode of action (78,81,82). Modes of action of carcinogenesis may include direct DNA interaction, covalent adducts, intercalation, or free radical formation. Indirect modification of DNA may include altered membrane or calcium homeostasis, perturbation or modulation of enzymes or of hormones, altered DNA methylation or chromosomal aberrations, enhancement of DNA replication errors, activation of an oncogene, directly or indirectly, inhibition of apoptosis, and other mechanisms. When the mode of action is understood, relevance to humans is easier to evaluate. Some findings in rodents do not have relevance to humans under conditions of exposure or under any circumstances (74,83–86). For reversible effects considered potentially relevant to humans, there is likely a threshold for an effect (87). If the body can repair modified DNA or compensate for an insult or eliminate a transformed cell, then there is a threshold below which neoplasms will not be formed (88–90). In some cases there may be a biomarker for the threshold. However the threshold level is not often known.

For pharmaceuticals, the human exposure under conditions of use may not exceed or be substantially higher than the highest dose used in the rodent carcinogenicity studies. Qualitative risk assessment by CDER/FDA considers:

1. If the drug is clearly genotoxic by a mechanism relevant to in vivo human use
2. If there any carcinogenicity findings clearly related to the drug in the rodents and how strong the evidence is in rodent
3. If there is multispecies evidence for carcinogenicity; when studies from two species are available, clear findings in two species/genders may be of greater concern than findings in only one species.
4. If there are no drug-related neoplastic findings, whether the rodents express the pharmacologic activity seen in humans and whether the rodents express the main metabolites seen in humans
5. If there are drug-related neoplastic findings, whether the findings are biologically relevant to humans under conditions of use and whether there are biomarkers for the hormonal or exaggerated pharmacologic effects in humans, e.g., if a neoplasm is prolactin related, whether prolactin levels in humans increase after exposure to the drug

6. Whether the effects occur at a high multiple of the human exposure under conditions of use
7. Whether there are other drugs in the same pharmacologic class that gave similar rodent findings but no apparent effects on possible biomarkers (e.g., hyperplasia) in humans.

CDER/FDA considers risk/benefit for humans under the conditions of use and whether there are other drugs for the indication without carcinogenicity findings at relevant exposures. If the medical benefit does not justify the risk, the product may not be approved. If the benefit of the therapy is found to outweigh the risks for the indicated patient populations, the findings in the rodent studies are described in the drug product labeling, and the multiple of the human systemic exposure at which they were found is described. Plasma AUC value comparisons would be used if known and appropriate. Nominal dose per body surface area (mg/m^2) comparisons would be used in the absence of appropriate pharmacokinetic data. In some cases, a postapproval monitoring program may be undertaken.

ONGOING ISSUES AND FUTURE TRENDS

In the future it may not be necessary to conduct traditional 2-year studies for evaluation of carcinogenicity potential. Per ICH S1B (7), for pharmaceuticals, alternative shorter-term carcincogenicity models are already accepted by CDER/FDA in place of traditional 2-year carcinogenicity studies in mice, with prior concurrence of CDER/FDA (91). These mechanistically based models allow the use of fewer animals, and the studies are of much shorter duration (92). Since 1997, about 25% of the carcinogenicity protocols submitted to CDER/FDA have been for alternative transgenic models have included the P53$^{+/-}$ mouse (93–95), the TgAC mouse (96–100), and the rasH2 mouse (101–104). These models were extensively studied by an International Life Sciences (ILSI) consortium, and a standardized protocol was evaluated (105). Other models could be considered if supported by data.

Increasing use of mode of action and other nonneoplastic lesion data in evaluation of relevance of findings to humans (74,106,107) is likely. The future use of various biomarkers, including those from toxicogenomics, proteomics or metabolomics analyses (108), for carcinogenicity to reduce the use of animals is hoped for. However, because not all changes in biomarkers after administration of a chemical will necessarily lead to cancer under conditions of use, it is not a simple matter to establish a valid biomarker, i.e., a biomarker that is measured in an analytical test system with well-established performance characteristics and for which there is an established scientific framework or body of evidence that elucidates the physiologic, toxicologic, pharmacologic, or clinical significance of the test results (109). Many challenges remain to the use such data to predict carcinogenicity potential.

REFERENCES

1. Weisburger JH, Weisburger EK. Tests for chemical carcinogens. In: Busch H, ed. Methods in Cancer Research, vol. 1. New York: Academic Press, 1967:370.
2. Weisburger EK. History of the bioassay program of the national cancer institute. Prog Exp Tumor Res 1983; 26:187–201.

3. Haseman JK. Statistical issues in the design, analysis and interpretation of animal carcinogenicity studies. Environ Health Perspect 1984; 58:385–392.
4. Chhabra RS, Huff JE, Schwetz BS, et al. An overview of prechronic and chronic toxicity/carcinogenicity experimental study designs and criteria used by the national toxicology program. Environ Health Perspect 1990; 86:313–321.
5. U.S. Interagency Staff Group on Carcinogens, Chemical Carcinogens. A review of the science and its associated principles. Environ Health Perspect 1986; 67:201–282.
6. International Conference on Harmonization ICH S1A The Need for Long-term Rodent Carcinogenicity Studies of Pharmaceuticals. 1996, www.fda.gov/cder/guidance/index.htm.
7. International Conference on Harmonization ICH S1B Testing for Carcinogenicity of Pharmaceuticals. 1998, www.fda.gov/cder/guidance/index.htm.
8. International Conference on Harmonization ICH S1C Dose Selection for Carcinogenicity Studies of Pharmaceuticals. 1995, www.fda.gov/cder/guidance/index.htm.
9. International Conference on Harmonization ICH S1C(R). Guidance on Dose Selection for Carcinogenicity Studies of Pharmaceuticals: Addendum on a Limit Dose and Related Notes. 1997, www.fda.gov/cder/guidance/index.htm.
10. CFSAN Redbook of 1993 www.cfsan.fda.gov.
11. U.S. Code of Federal Regulations: Food and Color Additives: 21CFR 171.
12. Organization for Economic Cooperation and Development (OECD) 451 Carcinogenicity Studies (Original Guideline, adopted 12th May 1981) being revised 2006.
13. Organization for Economic Cooperation and Development (OECD) 453 Combined Chronic Toxicity/Carcinogenicity Studies (Original Guideline, adopted 12th May 1981) being revised 2006.
14. Federal Food and Drug Act Delaney clause section 409(c)(3)(A).
15. Veterinary International Conference on Harmonization (VICH) Guidance for Industry VICH Guideline GL 28—Studies to Evaluate the Safety of Residues of Veterinary Drugs in Human Food: Carcinogenicity Testing 2001.
16. U.S. Environmental Protection Agency OPPTS 870.4200 www.epa.gov.
17. U.S. Environmental Protection Agency Guidelines for Carcinogen Risk Assessment (March 2005).
18. U.S. CPSC Hazard Assessment and Reduction Program and Regulated Products Program http://cpsc.gov; Consumer Products Safe Testing Act; Animal testing policy. Fed Regist 49 22522–22523, 1984.
19. www.cpsc.gov.
20. Federal Register Consumer Products Safe Testing Act; Animal testing policy 1984; 49:22522–22523,.
21. U.S. OSHA Hazard Communication Standard of 29 CFR 1910.1200 App. A1. http://www. osha.gov.
22. EMEA European Agency for the Evaluation of Medicinal Products, Note for guidance on carcinogenicity potential 2002 http://www.emea.eu.int/pdfs/human/swp/287700en.pdf.
23. U.S. Code of Federal Regulation: Good Laboratory Practices for Nonclinical Laboratory Studies 21 CFR 58.
24. Contrera JF, Jacobs AC, DeGeorge JJ, et al. Carcinogenicity testing and the evaluation of regulatory requirements for pharmaceuticals. Regul Toxicol Pharmacol 1997; 25:130–145.
25. Contrera JF, Jacobs AC, Prasanna HR, et al. A systemic exposure-based alternative to the maximum tolerated dose for carcinogenicity studies of human therapeutics. J Am Coll Toxicol 1995; 14:1–10.
26. International Conference on Harmonization ICH M2 Guidance for Industry M2 eCTD: Electronic Common Technical Document Specification. 2004 www.fda.gov/cder/guidance/index.htm.
27. Bucci TJ. Evaluation of altered morphology. In: Haschek WA, Rousseaux CG, eds. Handbook of Toxicologic Pathology. New York: Academic Press, Inc, 1991:23–35.
28. Crissman JW, Goodman DG, Hildebrandt PK, et al. Best practices guideline: toxicologic histopathology. Toxicol Pathol 2004; 32:126–131.

29. http:/www.niehs.nih.gov.
30. Chu KC, Cueto C, Jr., Ward JM. Factors in the evaluation of 200 National Cancer Institute carcinogen bioassays. J Toxicol Environ Health 1981; 8:251–280.
31. Everett R. Factors affecting the spontaneous tumor incidence rates in mice: a literature review. CRC Crit Rev Toxicol 1984; 13:235–251.
32. Haseman JK, JE, Huff JE, Rao GN, et al. Sources of variability in rodent carcinogenicity studies. Fundam Appl Toxicol 1989; 12:793–804.
33. National Toxicology Program (NTP). Report of the NTP Ad Hoc Panel on Chemical Carcinogenesis Testing and Evaluation Board of Scientific Counselors, National Toxicology Program, DHHS, August 17, 1984.
34. Ross MH, Bras G. Lasting influence of early caloric restriction on prevalence of neoplasms in the rat. J Natl Cancer Inst 1971; 47:1095–1113.
35. Carroll KK, Khor HT. Dietary fat in relation to tumorigenesis. Prog Biochem Pharmacol 1975; 10:308–353.
36. Conybeare G. Effect of quality and quantity of diet on survival and tumor incidence in outbred swiss mice. Food Cosmet Toxicol 1980; 18:65–75.
37. Turnbull GJ, Lee PN, Roe FJ. Relationship of body-weight gain to longevity and to risk of development of nephropathy and neoplasia in Sprague-Dawley rats. Food Chem Toxicol 1985; 23:355–361.
38. Rao GN, Piegorsch WW, Haseman JK. Influence of body weight on the incidence of spontaneous tumors in rats and mice of long-term studies. Am J Clin Nutr 1987; 45:252–260.
39. Rao GN, Morris RW, Seely JC. Beneficial effects of NTP-2000 diet on growth, survival, and kidney and heart diseases of fischer 344 rats in chronic studies. Toxicol Sci 2001; 63:245–255.
40. Rao GN, Crockett PW. Effect of diet and housing on growth, body weight, survival and tumor incidences of B6C3F1 mice in chronic studies. Toxicol Pathol 2003; 31:243–250.
41. Sheldon WG, Bucci TJ, Hart RW, et al. Age-related neoplasia in a lifetime study of ad libitum-fed and food-restricted B6C3F1 mice. Toxicol Pathol 1995; 23:458–476.
42. Thurman JD, Bucci TJ, Hart RW, et al. Survival, body weight, and spontaneous neoplasms in ad libitum-fed and food-restricted Fischer-344 rats. Toxicol Pathol 1994; 22:1–9.
43. Hart RW, Turturro A. Dietary restrictions and cancer. Environ Health Perspect 1997; 105:989–992.
44. Haseman JK, Ney E, Nyska A, et al. Effect of diet and animal care/housing protocols on body weight, survival, tumor incidences, and nephropathy severity of F344 rats in chronic studies. Toxicol Pathol 2003; 31:674–681.
45. McConnell EE, Solleveld HA, Swenberg JA, et al. Guidees for combining neoplasms for evaluation of rodent carcinogenicity studies. J Natl Cancer Inst 1986; 76:283–289.
46. CDER FDA draft Guidance for Industry Statistical Aspects of the Design, Analysis, and Interpretation of Chronic Rodent Carcinogenicity Studies of Pharmaceuticals http://www.fda.gov/cder/guidance/815dft.pdf.
47. Lin KK, Rahman MA. Overall false positive rates in tests for linear trend in tumor incidence in animal carcinogenicity studies of new drugs. J Biopharm Stat 1998; 8:1–15 discussion 17–22.
48. Chen JJ, Lin KK, Huque M, et al. Weighted p-value adjustments for animal carcinogenicity trend test. Biometrics 2000; 56:586–592.
49. Lin KK. Progress report on the guidance for industry for statistical aspects of the design, analysis, and interpretation of chronic rodent carcinogenicity studies of pharmaceuticals. J Biopharm Stat 2000; 10:481–501.
50. Armitage P. Statistical Methods in Medical Research. New York: Wiley, 1971:362–365.
51. Gart JJ, Chu KC, Tarone RE. Statistical issues in interpretation of chronic bioassay tests for carcinogenicity. J Natl Cancer Inst 1979; 62:957–974.
52. McKnight B, Crowley J. Tests for differences in tumor incidences based on animal carcinogenesis experiments. J Am Stat Assoc 1984; 79:639–648.
53. Cox DR. Regression models and life tables. J R Stat Soc 1972; B34:187–220.

54. Thomas DG, Breslow N, Gart JJ. Trend and homogeneity analyses of proportions and life table data. Comp Biomed Res 1977; 10:373–381.

55. Gart JJ, Krewski D, Lee PN, et al. Statistical Methods in Cancer Research In Volume III—The Design and Analysis of Long-Term Animal Experiments, International Agency for Research on Cancer, World Health Organization, 1986.

56. Gehan EA. A generalized wilcoxon test for comparing K samples subject to unequal patterns of censorship. Biometrika 1965; 52:203–223.

57. Breslow N. A generalized kruskal-wallis test for comparing K samples subject to unequal patterns of censorship. Biometrics 1970; 57:579–594.

58. Cox DR. The analysis of exponentially distributed life-times with two types of failures. J R Stat Soc 1959; 21:4121–4421.

59. Mantel N, Haenszel W. Statistical aspects of the analysis of data from retrospective studies of disease. J Natl Cancer Res 1959; 22:719–748.

60. Tarone RE. Tests for trend in life table analysis. Biometrika 1975; 62:679–682.

61. Peto R, Pike MC, Day NE, et al. Guidelines for Simple, Sensitive Significance Tests for Carcinogenic Effects in Long-term Animal Experiments, in Long-term and Short-term Screening Assays for Carcinogens: an Critical Appraisal, World Health Organization, 1980.

62. Dinse GE, Lagatos SW. Regression analysis of tumor prevalence data. J R Stat Soc C 1983; 32:236–248.

63. Dinse GE, Haseman JK. Logistic regression analysis of incidental tumor data from animal carcinogenicity experiments. Fundam Appl Toxicol 1986; 6:44–52.

64. Portier CJ, Bailer AJ. Testing for increased carcinogenicity using a survival adjusted quantal response test. Fundam Appl Toxicol 1989; 12:731–737.

65. Fears TR, Tarone RE, Chu KC. False-positives and false-negative rates for carcinogenicity screens. Cancer Res 1997; 37:1941–1945.

66. Haseman JK. A reexamination of false-positive rates for carcinogenicity studies. Fundam Appl Toxicol 1983; 3:334–339.

67. Haseman JK, Huff JE, Boorman GA. Use of historical control data in carcinogenicity studies in rodents. Toxicol Pathol 1984; 12:126–135.

68. Haseman JK, Boorman GA, Huff J. Value of historical control data and other issues related to the evaluation of long-term rodent carcinogenicity studies. Toxicol Pathol 1997; 25:524–527.

69. Tarone RE. The use of historical control information in testing for a trend in proportions. Biometrics 1982; 38:215–220.

70. Tamura RN, Young SS. The incorporation of historical information in tests of proportions: simulation study of Tarone's procedure. Biometrics 1986; 42:343–349.

71. Prentice RL, Smythe RT, Krewski D, et al. On the use of historical control data to estimate dose response trends in quantal bioassay. Biometrics 1992; 48:459–478.

72. Van Gelder GA. Risk assessment. In: Haschek WA, Rousseaux CG, eds. Handbook of Toxicologic Pathology. New York: Academic Press, 1991:155–163.

73. Crettaz P, Pennington D, Rhomberg L, et al. Assessing human health response in life cycle assessment using ED10s and DALYs: part 1—cancer effects. Risk Anal 2002; 22:931–946.

74. Cohen SM, Klaunig JE, Meek ME, et al. Evaluating the human relevance of chemically induced animal tumors. Toxicol Sci 2004; 78:181–186.

75. Environmental US. Protection agency. Guidelines for carcinogen risk assessment. Fed Regist 1986; 51:33992–34003.

76. Hoel DG, Kaplan NL, Anderson MW. Implication of nonlinear kinetics on risk assessment in carcinogenesis. Science 1983; 219:1032–1037.

77. Gold LS, Gaylor DW, Slone TH. Comparison of cancer risk estimates based on a variety of risk assessment methodologies. Regul Toxicol Pharmacol 2003; 37:45–53.

78. Gaylor DW. New issues in cancer risk assessment. Drug Metab Rev 2000; 32:187–192.

79. Conolly RB, Lutz WK. Nonmonotonic dose-response relationships: mechanistic basis, kinetic modeling, and implications for risk assessment. Toxicol Sci 2004; 77:151–157.

80. Lovell DP, Thomas G. Quantitative risk assessment and the limitations of the linearized multistage model. Hum Exp Toxicol 1996; 15:87–104.

81. Olin SS, Neumann DA, Foran JA, et al. Topics in cancer risk assessment. Environ Health Perspect 1997; 105:117–126.

82. Meek ME, Bucher JR, Cohen SM, et al. A framework for human relevance analysis of information on carcinogenic modes of action. Crit Rev Toxicol 2003; 33:591–653.

83. Cohen SM, Ellwein LB. Cell proliferation in carcinogenesis. Science 1990; 249:1007–1011.

84. Dietrich D, Swenberg JA. The presence of α2β-globulin is necessary for d-limonene promotion of male rat kidney tumors. Cancer Res 1991; 51:3512–3521.

85. Grasso P, Sharratt M, Cohen AJ. The role of persistent, non-genotoxic tissue damage in rodent cancer and relevance to humans. Annu Rev Pharmacol Toxicol 1991; 31:253–287.

86. Andersen ME, Meek ME, Boorman GA, et al. Lessons learned in applying the U.S. EPA proposed cancer guidelines to specific compounds. Toxicol Sci 2000; 53:159–172.

87. Kroes R, Kozianowski G. Threshold of toxicological concern (TTC) in food safety assessment. Toxicol Lett 2002; 127:43–46.

88. Lima BS, Van der Laan JW. Mechanisms of nongenotoxic carcinogenesis and assessment of the human hazard. Regul Toxicol Pharmacol 2000; 32:135–143.

89. Hengstler JG, Bogdanffy MS, Bolt HM, et al. Challenging dogma: thresholds for genotoxic carcinogens? The case of vinyl acetate. Annu Rev Pharmacol Toxicol 2003; 43:485–520.

90. Bolt HM, Degen GH. Human carcinogenic risk evaluation, part II: contributions of the EUROTOX specialty section for carcinogenesis. Toxicol Sci 2004; 81:3–6.

91. Sistare F, Jacobs AC. Chapter 35 use of transgenic animals in regulatory carcinogenicity evaluations. In: Alternative Toxicology Methods. Boca Raton, FL: CRC Press, 2003:391–411.

92. Tennant RW, French JE, Spalding JW. Identifying chemical carcinogens and assessing potential risk in short-term bioassays using transgenic mouse models. Environ Health Perspect 1995; 103:942–950.

93. Donehower LA, Harvey M, Slagle BL, et al. Mice deficient for p53 are developmentally normal but susceptible to spontaneous tumors. Nature 1992; 356:215–221.

94. French J, Storer RD, Donehower LA. The nature of the heterozygous Trp53 knockout model for identification of mutagenic carcinogens. Toxicol Pathol 2001; 29:24–29.

95. Storer RD, French JE, Haseman J, et al. P53 +/− hemizygous knockout mouse: overview of available data. Toxicol Pathol 2001; 29:30–50.

96. Leder A, Kuo A, Cardiff R, et al. v-Ha-ras transgene abrogates the initiation step in mouse skin tumorigenesis: effects of phorbol esters and retinoic acid. Proc Natl Acad Sci USA 1990; 87:9178–9182.

97. Spalding JW, French JE, Tice RR, et al. Development of a transgenic mouse model for carcinogenesis bioassays: evaluation of chemically induced skin tumors in Tg.AC mice. Toxicol Sci 1999; 49:241–254.

98. Eastin WC, Mennear JH, Tennant RW, et al. The Tg.AC genetically altered mouse: assay working group overview of available data. Toxicol Pathol 2001; 29:60–80.

99. Tennant RW, Stasiewicz S, Eastin WC, et al. The Tg.AC (v-Ha-ras) transgenic mouse: nature of the model. Toxicol Pathol 2001; 29:51–59.

100. Sistare FD, Thompson KL, Honchel Y, et al. Evaluation of the Tg.AC transgenic mouse assay for testing the human carcinogenic potential of pharmaceuticals. practical pointers, mechanistic clues, and new questions. Int J Toxicol 2002; 21:65–79.

101. Yamamoto S, Mitsumori K, Kodama Y, et al. Rapid induction of more malignant tumors by various genotoxic carcinogens in transgenic mice harbouring a human prototype c-ha-ras gene than in control non-transgenic mice. Carcinogenesis 1996; 17:2455–2461.

102. Takaoka M, Sehata S, Maejima T, et al. Interlaboratory comparison of short-term carcinogenicity studies using CB6F1-rasH2 transgenic mice. Toxicol Pathol 2003; 31:191–199.

103. Tamaoki N. The rasH2 transgenic mouse: nature of the model and mechanistic studies on tumorigenesis. Toxicol Pathol 2001; 29:81–89.

104. Suemizu H, Muguruma K, Maruyama C, et al. Transgene stability and features of rasH2 mice as an animal model for short-term carcinogenicity testing. Mol Carcinog 2002; 34:1–9.
105. MacDonald J, French JE, Gerson RJ, et al. The utility of genetically modified mouse assays for identifying human carcinogens: a basic understanding and path forward. Toxicol Sci 2004; 77:188–194.
106. Albertini R, Clewell H, Himmelstein MW, et al. The use of non-tumor data in cancer risk assessment: reflections on butadiene, vinyl chloride, and benzene. Regul Toxicol Pharmacol 2003; 37:105–132.
107. Cohen SM, Meek ME, Klaunig JE, et al. The human relevance of information on carcinogenic modes of action: overview. Crit Rev Toxicol 2003; 33:581–589.
108. Preston RJ. Quantitation of molecular endpoints for the dose-response component of cancer risk assessment. Toxicol Pathol 2002; 30:112–116.
109. Biomarkers Definitions Working Group. Biomarkers and surrogate endpoints: preferred definitions and conceptual framework. Clin Pharmacol Ther 2001; 69:89–95.

10

Juvenile Animal Toxicology Studies[†]

Kok Wah Hew
Non-clinical Safety and Efficacy, Takeda Global Research and Development,
Lincolnshire, Illinois, U.S.A.

INTRODUCTION

This chapter is meant to be a basic guide for scientists who are responsible for contracting juvenile animal toxicology studies to contract research organization (CRO) and need help to understand the subject enough to be able to work with the CRO in designing the study, reviewing study protocol, interpreting study results, and assessing potential risks in children. Juvenile animal toxicology studies are highly specialized studies that require experience and expertise in laboratories conducting these studies. It is very important that juvenile animal toxicology studies should be contracted to a CRO that has considerable experience in performing these studies, preferably one that has a lot of experience in conducting developmental and reproductive toxicity studies. At the minimum, technicians in the CRO should be proficient in handling and caring for young animals, and should have sufficient experience in dosing young animals by the desired route of administration. Ideally, the CRO should have had performed several validation studies in the juvenile animals of interest to demonstrate their scientific and technical capabilities and to provide appropriate historical background data.

Prior to starting the study, the investigator should have a detail discussion with scientists at the CRO so that both parties understand the objectives of the study, review existing data for the compound under investigation, and determine the timing and duration of dosing so that the study can be appropriately designed to assess the potential risks of the compound in children. A poorly designed study and/or a poorly conducted study will make the results difficult to interpret or meaningless. It is critical for the investigator to take the necessary steps to perform a well-designed and properly conducted juvenile animal toxicology study in order to avoid any waste of time and valuable resources. Any technical difficulties involving dose administration and study conduct must be resolved before study initiation.

[†]Juvenile animal is generally defined as a young or immature animal. In this chapter, juvenile animal is defined as animal in the period between birth and attainment of sexual maturation.

In order to ensure that the juvenile animal toxicology study performed for a specific test material is considered acceptable by regulatory agencies, it is preferable to submit the draft protocol for the study to the relevant division of an agency for their review and comment.

Regulatory Background

The current nonclinical safety testing of drugs and chemicals has mostly employed young adult animals at the initiation of dose administration. Similarly, clinical trials with drug candidates have mostly been performed in adults. Although children continue to be exposed to environmental chemicals and take drugs to treat diseases, there is relatively little safety information for these compounds in children. In 1993, the National Academy of Sciences (NAS) indicated that there was a paucity of information on the sensitivity of infants and young children to agricultural and industrial chemicals (1). As a result, the 1996 Food Quality Protection Act mandated the U.S. Environmental Protection Agency (EPA) to assess the risk of pesticide chemicals in infants and children (2). In some cases, the risk of these chemicals may have been assessed in other toxicity studies, such as the two-generation reproduction and/or developmental neurotoxicity studies.

For pharmaceuticals, the International Conference on Harmonisation has indicated that juvenile animal toxicology studies should be considered on an individual basis when previous animal data and human safety data are insufficient (3). In 1998, the U.S. Food and Drug Administration (FDA) published the final Pediatric Rule (effective in April 1999), stating that drug marketing applications for new active ingredients, new indications, new dosage forms, new dosing regimens, or new routes of administration must contain a human pediatric assessment unless the applicant company has obtained a waiver or deferral of pediatric studies (4). In addition, FDA can also require pediatric studies of marketed drugs and biological products that (i) are used in a substantial number of pediatric patients (50,000 or more patients in the U.S.) for the claimed indications, or (ii) would provide a meaningful therapeutic benefit to children over existing treatments. For drugs and biologics not indicated for the pediatric population, pediatric studies are not required.

In 2000 the Pediatric Rule was challenged by the Association of American Physicians and Surgeons in court, arguing that FDA had no statutory authority to promulgate the Rule. The court subsequenly struck down the Rule in 2002 and enjoined FDA from its enforcement . In 2003, Congress passed the Pediatric Research Equity Act (PREA) to provide FDA with the statutory authority to require a drug company to provide pediatric assessment for drugs and biologics unless the applicant has obtained a waiver or deferral (5). In PREA, Congress codified many of the elements of the Pediatric Rule and established the Pediatric Advisory Committee within FDA. PREA indicates that pediatric assessment should contain data adequate to (i) assess the safety and effectiveness of the drug or biological product in the relevant pediatric subpopulation, and (ii) support dosing and administration for each pediatric subpopulation. A study may not be needed in each pediatric age group if data from one age group can be extrapolated to another age group.

Juvenile animal toxicology studies are not automatically required for all drugs and biological products. The need to perform these studies will be dictated by (i) the age group the drug or biological product is indicated for, and (ii) whether the safety of the drugs or biological product can be assessed in clinical trials. If the age group for the intended population has been evaluated in clinical or nonclinical studies, then there is no need to perform juvenile animal toxicology studies for the drug or biological product. Hence before starting any juvenile animal toxicology study, the investigator will need to determine:

1. Whether a juvenile animal toxicology study is required based on available nonclinical and clinical data;
2. If the answer is yes, what juvenile animal toxicology study should be performed, i.e., the study design; and
3. Timing of the juvenile animal toxicology study to support clinical trials in children.

For pharmaceuticals, juvenile animal toxicology studies should be conducted before initiation of long-term pediatric clinical trials. If the trials do not involve long-term exposure, it is not necessary to complete juvenile animal toxicology studies before initiation of pediatric clinical trials, although it may be helpful to use data from juvenile animal toxicology studies to identify potential hazards while designing the short-term pediatric trials. If there are insufficient clinical data or experience because of minimal prior adult and pediatric experience, juvenile animal toxicology studies should be completed before initiation of pediatric clinical trials, regardless of whether the clinical trials involve long-term exposure. Similarly, if there have been reports of adverse effects with off-label use in pediatric patients, and there are no adequate data to evaluate the relationship between the drug and the adverse effects, juvenile animal toxicology studies should be completed before initiation of pediatric clinical trials (6).

STUDY DESIGN AND STUDY PARAMETERS

All definitive juvenile animal toxicology studies conducted for submission to regulatory agencies as part of the Investigational New Drug application, New Drug Application, marketing application, or as requested by the agencies must be conducted in accordance with the Good Laboratory Practices (GLP) guidelines, regulations or standards. The testing facility should have complete Standard Operating Procedures (SOPs) to provide detailed instructions for all procedures necessary for the conduct of the juvenile animal toxicology studies. In addition, all juvenile animal toxicology studies must be performed in accordance with the relevant laws and accepted animal care and use guidelines.

The purpose of conducting a juvenile animal toxicology study is to identify potential adverse effects of the test material in juvenile animals. Therefore, the study can be viewed as a single-dose or repeated-dose toxicity study being performed in developing animals instead of the adult animals. The parameters to be evaluated in the study are mostly similar to those included in single- or repeated-dose toxicity study, with the possible addition of the developmental landmarks, behavioral, learning, and other functional assessments.

However, unlike the adult animal used in routine nonclinical toxicity testing, the juvenile animal undergoes a period of postnatal growth, development, and maturation not seen in the adult. As in the case of humans, different organs within the juvenile animal develop and mature at different rates, and the rate for each organ is different in different species. In addition, postnatal development and maturation of organ systems do not occur at the same chronological age across species. These differences make the design of juvenile animal toxicology studies and the extrapolation of data from these studies to estimate risks in children a challenging task. However, as we learn more about the postnatal development and maturation of the different organ systems in laboratory test animals and in children, this knowledge can help us to better design juvenile animal toxicology studies and interpret data from these studies.

Different organ systems in juvenile animals undergo growth, development, and maturation at different stages of development and at different rates. Some organs, e.g., lungs and kidneys, become fully functional within a short time after birth, whereas other organ systems, e.g., the reproductive and immune systems, only become fully functional following a relatively lengthy development and maturation period. As a result, there is no standard study design for juvenile animal toxicology studies, and each study should be considered individually based on a number of considerations. Since these studies are usually quite costly to perform and can potentially use a significant number of animals, the sponsor company is encouraged to submit draft protocols to regulatory agencies for their comments prior to initiating any juvenile animal toxicology studies.

Prior to starting juvenile animal toxicology studies, one should consider (i) the intended or likely use or exposure of the drug/chemical in pediatric populations, (ii) the timing and duration of dosing/exposure in relation to growth and development in juvenile animals and pediatric populations, (iii) the potential differences in pharmacological and toxicological profiles between mature and immature systems, and (iv) the existing data from nonclinical safety studies and adult clinical trials, where available.

The intended pediatric populations, the stage of postnatal development, and the duration of the clinical trial should be considered when deciding the age of animals at dosing initiation, the route of administration, and the duration of treatment for juvenile animal toxicology studies. Existing data from toxicity studies in adult animals and those from clinical trials may provide useful information with regards to target organs of toxicity as well as toxicokinetic (TK) and pharmacokinetic (PK) profiles in the test species and humans. Many current in vivo toxicity studies use animals that are young adult at dosing initiation. If the intended pediatric population is adolescent and if sufficient toxicity information is available from the young adult animals to assess the potential risk of the drug/chemical in adolescent, juvenile animal toxicology studies may not be necessary. In addition, data from the pre- and postnatal developmental study or from the two-generation reproduction study may have adequately addressed the safety of the drug/chemical for the exposure in the neonatal period, and hence juvenile animal toxicology studies may not be necessary. Therefore, in order to avoid performing unnecessary juvenile animal toxicology studies, the existing safety data for the drug/chemical should be carefully evaluated to determine if there is a need to perform these studies.

In designing juvenile animal toxicology studies, the following should be considered:

1. The timing and chronology of the organ system development in the test species when compared to that in humans. For certain organs, a certain developmental stage may be completed in utero in human but only completed postnatally in the test species. This factor should be considered especially when the organ is a target organ for the compound of interest in adult toxicology studies
2. The test species should be dosed at the appropriate developmental stage of interest
3. A pilot or range-finding study should be performed in order to help select doses for the definitive study, and to determine the exposure or internal dose in the juvenile animals for a particular formulation.

Suggestions have been made to modify the pre- and postnatal development study or the two-generation reproduction study such that a juvenile animal toxicology study can be included as part of these studies. However, these former studies have well defined objectives, dosing regimens as well as evaluation end points, and addition of a juvenile animal toxicology study may complicate study conduct, data presentation and interpretation. Therefore, it is preferable to perform any juvenile animal toxicology study as a stand-alone toxicity study.

Study Basics

Test Material and Vehicle

The test material must be the technical grade with the appropriate purity, and its characteristics should be analyzed and documented according to GLP. This information, documented in the Certificate of Analysis, should be obtained prior to study initiation to ensure that the amount given to the test species is correctly calculated based on the purity information. The Certificate of Analysis and the Material Safety Data Sheet (MSDS) for the test material should be provided to the CRO when the test material is shipped. The protocol should clearly indicate whether (i) any correction factor is used to calculate doses to be administered to the test species, and/or (ii) the doses are expressed in terms of the salt or base. In cases where the drug product is to be delivered to children in a pediatric clinical formulation, the test material should also include any inactive ingredients in the pediatric clinical formulation (6). For studies longer than four weeks in duration, appropriate amounts of archive samples should be taken from the test and control materials used in the study. These samples should be archived together with other specimens/documents from the study. Appropriate documentation should be available to indicate the stability of the test material for the duration of the dosing period under the specified storage conditions. In the absence of this documentation, stability samples should be collected before and after the dosing period and analyzed to demonstrate stability of the test material for the duration of the dosing period under the specified storage conditions.

If a vehicle is needed to deliver the test material to the animals, then the vehicle used should be appropriate for the delivery of the test material, should not affect the chemical and physical properties of the test material, should allow sufficient absorption of the test material in the test species in order to obtain sufficient exposure in the animals, and should not induce toxicity to the animals when given alone. Whenever possible, the vehicle used in the juvenile animal toxicology studies should be the same as that used in the adult toxicity study. This will allow comparison of toxicity in different age groups. Stability of the test material in the vehicle under different storage conditions should be established and documented prior to dosing initiation. This will help the testing facility to determine the frequency of dose formulation preparation and the appropriate storage condition for the dosing formulations.

The actual concentrations of the test material in the dose formulations should be determined prior to administration to the animals. Although it is not necessary to verify the concentrations of dose formulations for each preparation, concentration analysis will need to be performed at regular intervals during the dosing phase of the study. If the dose formulation is in the form of a suspension, then homogeneity of the test material in the formulation will need to be ascertained. Homogeneity analysis should be performed on samples collected from the top, middle, and bottom portions of the dose formulations at the highest and lowest anticipated dosage levels. When the volume of each preparation remains about the same throughout the study, homogeneity analysis is usually performed once during the study, prior to dosing initiation. If the dosing period occurs during a time when the animals are experiencing rapid growth, then the volume of dose formulations required at the end of the dosing period will be much higher than that used at the beginning of the dosing period. When there is a significant change in the volume of a particular preparation from the previous preparations, e.g., the batch size changed by more than 30%, then homogeneity analysis may need to be repeated for that particular preparation.

The acceptable level of recovery for dose formulation analysis, e.g., $\pm 10\%$ of the intended concentration, should be clearly stated in the protocol. Ideally, dose formulations should be analyzed prior to dose administration to the animals, and any formulation that shows unacceptable recovery value should be reprepared and reanalyzed until the desired concentration is achieved. If it is not possible to analyze the dose formulations prior to dose administration and if the results of analysis showed unacceptable recovery values, appropriate action should be taken to document the discrepancies and the doses should be readjusted to reflect the actual amount given to the animals.

In cases where the route of administration is oral or parenteral (e.g., intravenous), it may be useful to verify the concentration of the dose formulations for samples collected from the distal end of the dosing apparatus, e.g., the end of the gavage needle or the end of the intravenous catheter. Occasionally, some test material or dose formulation may adhere to the wall of the gavage needle (especially test material that is micronized prior to dosing) or catheter such that only part of the test material is delivered to the animal. Analysis of the dose formulation collected from the distal end of the delivery device will determine the amount of the test material that will actually be delivered to the animal.

The viscosity and pH of the dosing formulation intended for oral or intravenous administration should be evaluated to ensure that these factors will not result in any undesirable effects in the animals. For studies using the intravenous route as the route of administration, osmolarity of the dosing formulation should also be determined. Studies using inhalation as the route of administration should be performed in a CRO with the appropriate apparatus/setup and with extensive experience with the generation, sampling, and analysis of the test atmospheres.

In cases where the vehicle is different from that used in the adult toxicity study or when the toxicity of the vehicle is unknown in the juvenile animals, a sham control should be considered. Animals in the sham control group are subjected to the dosing procedure but without receiving the vehicle. This group is used to discriminate the effects of the vehicle treatment from the dosing procedure.

In studies using young rodents, the amount of dose formulation that can be administered to the animals may be limited by the size of the young pups. The dose volume should be such that the amount to be administered to the young pups should not affect milk or food consumption. Therefore, the dose volume will need to be adjusted depending on the size of the animal at a particular development stage.

Test System

Species Selection. For pharmaceuticals, a juvenile animal toxicology study conducted in one animal species may be considered sufficient to evaluate toxicity of the drug when existing safety data are available in both adult humans and animals (6). Traditionally, rats and dogs are species of choice due to the extensive experience in the care and handling of the animals and the large amount of historical control data available for these species. The same strain/substrain of animal, obtained from the same supplier and from the same location, as has been used in previous toxicity studies with the same test material should be used in the juvenile animal toxicology study. These animals should be maintained under the same environmental conditions, water and diet as those used in previous toxicity studies with the same test material. This will allow comparison of toxic response to the same test material in a test species across different age groups.

When selecting species to be used in juvenile animal toxicology studies, the following factors should be considered:

1. PK and TK data from previous animal studies should be evaluated in order to select the species whose PK/TK profiles most closely resemble those seen in humans;

2. Comparability of the developmental age and developmental changes for different target organs between the species considered and pediatric populations;
3. The technical feasibility of performing a juvenile animal toxicology study in a particular species.

A pilot or range-finding juvenile animal toxicology study should be performed to identify potential target organs, to evaluate the TK profile of the test material in juvenile animals, and to select doses for the definitive study. If results of the TK analysis show that the TK profile in the juvenile animal tested is very different from that seen in humans, or the current route, vehicle, or dosing regimen only results in exceedingly low exposures in the test animals when compared to the expected exposure in pediatric patients, another route, vehicle, dosing regimen or test species may need to be considered. However, technical feasibility, limited experience, and limited knowledge of the developmental stages of developing organ systems may limit the conduct of juvenile animal toxicology studies to rodents (rats and mice), dogs, rabbits, swine, or nonhuman primates. Therefore, the investigator should understand the limitations of the animal model and the differences between the test species and humans when selecting a particular species to conduct the juvenile animal toxicology study.

Although rabbits and swine may be used in juvenile animal toxicology studies, they have not been as widely used as rodents or dogs. Both rabbit and swine suffer from the scarcity of the developmental data from birth to maturity as well as the dearth of historical control data for juvenile animal toxicology studies.

The use of nonhuman primates in juvenile animal toxicology studies should only be considered when data in the adult animal studies show that it is the only test species whose PK profile resembles that in humans, and other test species are not sensitive to the treatment of the test material. Due to the high cost and the need for judicious use of these animals, only a few animals can be assigned to each group. The small sample size, high interanimal variability, and limited historical control data will make interpretation of the results obtained from juvenile animal toxicology studies using nonhuman primates very difficult. In addition, for studies using preweaning nonhuman primates, there is a high risk of maternal rejection if the young animals are handled excessively.

Animal Source and Age. Study animals should be obtained from reputable suppliers with proper documentation of the health status for the animals. All reputable CROs have procedures in place to have their clinical veterinarian and quality assurance personnel check on the quality of the animals and animal care at their suppliers' facility at regular intervals. The age of the animals to be used in juvenile animal toxicology studies will depend on the study design, and the age can vary from newborns to young adults. The primary consideration in choosing the age of the animals will be the age of the intended pediatric population who will be exposed to the drug or chemical. If the previous adult animal toxicity studies have identified target organs, then the maturation profiles of these target organs, where available, should be considered.

It is useful to order pregnant rats or mice from the supplier so that sufficient numbers of pups are born on the same day to facilitate assignment to the study. Pregnant rats can be ordered to arrive at a specific gestational day, e.g., gestation day 15–16, so that they can be acclimatized to the laboratory conditions prior to scheduled delivery. Pregnant dogs should also be ordered from the supplier to obtain puppies used in juvenile dog study.

Number of Animals. A juvenile animal toxicology study typically contains a vehicle control group and three compound-treated groups. Both males and females should be used in the study. The number of animals to be assigned to each dose group will be determined by the types of evaluations to be performed in the study. The investigator should have thorough discussions with scientists in the CRO to determine the appropriate parameters to be evaluated and the number of animals needed for each evaluation. The number of animals to be used in the study should allow meaningful statistical analysis (in rodent studies) and to allow proper interpretation of results. However, the minimum number of animals should be used in order to achieve this goal. For studies using rodents, range-finding or pilot studies typically use about 5–6 animals/sex/group, whereas the definitive studies with the standard evaluation end points use 10 or more animals/sex/group. For studies using nonrodents, e.g., dogs, range-finding or pilot studies typically use 1–2 animals/sex/group, whereas the definitive studies use 4–6 animals/sex/group. In studies that include interim necropsy, recovery animals or several subsets to perform different evaluations, more animals may be needed.

Recovery animals are usually added to the study group to determine if following an extended period of dose administration, toxicity observed in animals in a compound-treated group is reversible after a treatment-free period. Recovery animals are typically added to at least the control and high-dose groups. For studies using rodents, an additional 5–10 animals/sex/group are usually added to the recovery subset. For studies using non-rodents, an additional 2–6 animals/sex/group are added to the recovery subset.

For studies using rodents, a subset of animals should be assigned to obtain blood for TK evaluation. It is useful to include the same number of groups in the TK subset as that in the main study. Prior knowledge about the sensitivity of the analytical method in order to determine the amount of blood needed at each collection time point is critical. Young pups have limited blood volume, and the number of blood samples that can be obtained may also be limited. The amount of blood needed at each collection time point will determine the number of animals assigned to the TK subset. Again, the minimum number of animals should be used in the TK subset in order to obtain a meaningful TK profile of the test material in the young animals.

For studies using nonrodents, the TK samples are usually obtained from the main study animals. Only the minimum amount of blood should be collected at selected time points to ensure that there is no excessive blood loss in the study animals due to this procedure.

If dosing is to be performed in neonates, it would be prudent to set aside some spare animals for possible replacement during the initial phase of the study when spontaneous neonatal deaths or accidental deaths due to intubation error (in studies using the oral gavage route of administration) are not uncommon.

Assignment to Groups.   In species with relatively large litters, e.g., rats and mice, the pups are usually culled on postnatal day (PND) 4 (the day of birth is defined as PND 0) to reduce the litter size to 4/sex/litter. This is done to standardize the litter size for all dams and to bring the number of pups/litter to a manageable level. The advantages and disadvantages of culling and not culling pups during the early postnatal period are described elsewhere (7,8).

For juvenile animal toxicology studies using young animals, the relationship between litters and dose groups will need to be considered due to the need for the young animals to stay with their mothers prior to weaning. For juvenile studies using animals with relatively large litters, e.g., rodents, animals can be assigned to study groups based on one of the following approaches:

1.   All pups in a litter assign to the same dose group (whole-litter approach)
2.   Pups from different litters can be cross-fostered to a dam, and all pups in each

resultant litter are assigned to one dose group (cross-foster approach)
3. Each litter contains all dose groups (split-litter approach).

If the study requires a large number of animals in each dose group—e.g., main study animals plus animals for recovery, interim necropsy, and TK animals as well as animals to be used for behavioral, learning, fertility, and other functional evaluations—then the method of choice would be the whole-litter approach because many pups in each litter will be needed and it is easy to assign and manage these pups from the same litter. In this case, each litter is considered an experimental unit. If the sample size for each group were 10, using the whole-litter approach would require 10 litters to produce the pups for assignment to each group of the study. In a study using the typical four-dose group design, at least 40 litters will be needed for the study. Table 1 illustrates how, using the whole-litter approach, postculling pups may be assigned to a dose group (10/sex in the main study (M), 10/sex in the recovery (R) subset plus TK animals) in a juvenile animal toxicology study.

The disadvantage of using the whole-litter approach is that there may be interlitter differences (litter effects) so that the experimental units within each group may be different. However, preliminary data based on the analysis of body weights in rat pups using the whole-litter approach and in pups using the cross-foster approach (where the litter effects were eliminated) appear to show that there is little or no difference between the body weights of rat pups at the same age in these two approaches (Personal communication, K. Robinson, 2004). This result suggests that for the body weight, the litter effect in the whole-litter approach, if present, is minimal. However, litter effects under the whole-litter approach may be present for other parameters, e.g., behavioral assessment, etc.

If the study only requires a limited number of animals in each group, e.g., main study and recovery animals only, then the cross-foster approach may be considered. In the cross-foster approach, pups from different litters are cross-fostered to one dam to eliminate litter effects. Each pup is considered an experimental unit, and each pup must be identified individually. As a result, almost all pups in each litter can be used, and fewer litters are needed to obtain sufficient number of animals for the study. For example, if only 20 pups/sex are needed for each dose group, then only 80 pups/sex are needed for the entire study with four dose groups. These pups can be obtained from about 10 litters (preculling) or 20 litters (postculling) instead of the 40 litters needed in the whole-litter approach. The advantage of this approach is that it theoretically removes the litter effects and also results in a decrease in animal usage. For studies using this approach, pups are typically cross-fostered beginning at PND 4.

Table 1 Assignment of Postculled Pups to a Dose Group Using the Whole-Litter Approach

Litter No.	Pup 1 Male	Pup 2 Male	Pup 3 Male	Pup 4 Male	Pup 5 Female	Pup 6 Female	Pup 7 Female	Pup 8 Female
1	M	R	TK	TK	M	R	TK	TK
2	M	R	TK	TK	M	R	TK	TK
.	.	.	.	.	.	.	.	.
.	.	.	.	.	.	.	.	.
.	.	.	.	.	.	.	.	.
9	M	R	TK	TK	M	R	TK	TK
10	M	R	TK	TK	M	R	TK	TK

No. animals = 10/sex/group in the main study (M), 10/sex in the recovery (R) subset, plus TK animals.

In the split-litter approach, all dose groups are represented in each litter. The presence of more than one dose group in a single litter may increase the risk of dosing the wrong pups as well as cross contamination. In addition, competition for the mother's milk would render the weaker pups, i.e., pups that received higher doses of the test material, less able to obtain milk and potentially exacerbate the toxicity of the test material. In rat studies using both the whole-litter and split-litter approaches, results showed that at the same dose level, pups in the split-litter approach have higher mortality and lower preweaning growth (9,10). Therefore the split-litter approach does not have any significant advantage over the whole-litter or cross-foster approach.

For juvenile studies using animals with relatively small litters, e.g., dogs, the whole-litter approach is the preferred method because the cross-foster approach does not provide any advantage with regards to lower animal usage, as many litters are needed to produce the required number of animals in the study. In addition, it is impractical to use the cross-foster approach in nonrodent studies because not all pups are born on the same day, thus making fostering difficult to arrange, and significant efforts may be needed to ensure pups acceptance by their adopted mothers.

When assigning animals to different dose groups, appropriate randomization method should be used in order to allow meaningful comparison of the treatment effects among the different dose groups. The common method used in toxicity studies is randomization using a block design to achieve homogeneity of group means and variances for body weight among all dose groups. Since body weight is an important indicator of growth and development, it is critical to use this randomization method to assign animals in juvenile animal toxicology studies.

Route and Method of Administration.   The route of administration should be the same as the intended route of human exposure. The common routes of exposure for the pediatric populations are oral, intravenous, subcutaneous, and inhalation. All dosing in the juvenile animal toxicology studies should be performed at about the same time on the days of scheduled dose administration.

Rodent pups as well as neonatal dogs can be dosed by the oral route beginning at PND 4 and PND 1, respectively, using an appropriate catheter or a small gavage needle. Although it may be possible to perform oral gavage dosing in the rat on PND 1, the success rate of dose administration at this early age is considerably less than that performed on PND 4, and pup mortality may be high due to excessive handling and the relatively high potential for intubation error. Subcutaneous administrations can be applied to rats and dogs beginning at PND 1. Intravenous (bolus) administrations can be applied to rats and dogs beginning at PND 4–7 and PND 1, respectively. Rats can be dosed by the continuous intravenous infusion route beginning at PND 22 (11). Dogs can be dosed by the continuous intravenous infusion route after weaning (12).

Rodents can be dosed by the inhalation route beginning at PND 1 using the whole body inhalation approach in which litters are placed in the inhalation chamber together with the dams. However, additional exposure for the young pups via the mother's milk, via the skin, and possibly via the oral route will need to be considered when using the whole body inhalation approach. Rats can be dosed by nose-only inhalation beginning at PND 7–10 for up to 4 hours/day (13,14). Dogs can be dosed by nose-only inhalation beginning at PND 10 (15). The inhalation apparatus for dosing the dog pup should be modified to fit the relatively short snout of the dog pup. Depending on the length of the dosing period, the dosing apparatus for the dog pup may need to be modified over time to suit the increasing size of the dog muzzle.

Dosing of the young rodents or dog pups is usually performed in an environment separate from the nursing mothers. Since these animals are at a greater risk of hypothermia after separation from their mother, dose administration and other procedures that require the separation of these animals from their mothers should be performed in an appropriately heated environment, e.g., on a surface with heating pads, etc.

For a more detailed guidance on the direct dosing of preweaning mammals in toxicity studies, the reader is encouraged to consult a booklet published by the International Life Sciences Institute (16).

Dose Selection

In addition to study design, dose selection is the most important component of the study. It is essential to perform a pilot or range-finding study prior to initiating the definitive juvenile animal toxicology study. The purpose of the range-finding study is to obtain data to select doses for the definitive study. Whenever possible, the range-finding study should include limited TK evaluation so that exposure of the test material in the young animals can be estimated. It is especially critical to perform a range-finding study with the appropriate TK evaluation when the dose formulation to be used in the juvenile animal toxicology study is different from that used in the adult animal studies. In addition to being useful in dose selection, the range-finding study may also help to identify potential target organs of toxicity in the young animals. The range-finding study typically contains fewer animals in each dose group, e.g., 5–6 animals/sex/group in rodents and 1–2 animals/sex/group in dogs; and therefore, 4–5 compound-treated groups in addition to controls may be used. A well-designed and well-conducted range-finding study will make the dose selection for the definitive study relatively easy.

Prior to conducting the range-finding study, data from the adult animal studies should be carefully reviewed to evaluate the toxicity of the test material in adult animals, the target organs, and the exposure of the test material at different dose levels. However, due to possible differences in TK and sensitivities between the young and adult animals, it may be risky to assume that the toxicity of the test material in the juvenile animals would be similar to that in the adult animals. Therefore, data from the adult animal studies should only be used as a guide. A sufficient dose range should be used in the range-finding study to allow for the observation of a dose-response effect.

Using data from the range-finding study, the high dose for the definitive study should produce toxic signs in the juvenile animals, without causing excessive mortality or severe toxicity that could affect the survival of the animals. The low dose should produce little or no toxicity in order to identify a no observed adverse effect level (NOAEL) where possible.

An outline of the study designs and draft protocols for the range-finding and definitive studies should be submitted to regulatory agencies for consultation.

Timing and Duration of Dose Administration

Timing and duration of dose administration constitute the core of study design for the juvenile animal toxicology studies. Unlike the adult animal studies, there is no set age when dosing typically starts and no set duration for the juvenile animal toxicology studies. The timing and duration of dose administration will depend on the following factors:

1. Timing and duration of exposure/dosing in relation to growth and development in the intended pediatric populations and juvenile animals;
2. Target organs observed in adult animal studies and the timing of maturation process of these organs in the juvenile animals.

A species comparison of the different age groups in the juvenile laboratory animals and in the pediatric population is presented in Table 2.

This table only provides an estimated age for the test species that corresponds to a particular age group in the pediatric population. It should only be used as a guide in deciding the timing and duration of dose administration in the test species. Other factors, including the potential target organs and their maturation processes, should also be considered. Dose administration should begin at an age that is comparable to the earliest possible exposure in humans and at the same time covering the critical development phase of most if not all target organs identified in adult animal studies. Occasionally, it may be necessary to divide animals in the study into several subsets, and each subset will receive dose administration for a specified interval, e.g., PND 4–7, PND 7–21, PND 21–45, in order to determine effects of the test material when administered to different age groups.

A brief summary of the current knowledge of the PK, postnatal development, and maturation of selected organ systems in the young common laboratory test animals and humans is provided below. In some cases, only information from the juvenile animals or humans is provided due to the lack of information in other species. This summary is not a comprehensive review of the current literature, but rather a short overview of the developmental processes and their timetable that may be important when deciding the timing and duration of dose administration. For more detailed information about these postnatal developmental processes, the reader is referred to selected articles listed in the reference section (17–37).

Pharmacokinetics in Children and Juvenile Animals. PK is defined as how the body handles xenobiotics, i.e., absorption, distribution, metabolism, and excretion of these compounds. Maturation of the different organ systems that control these processes will have an impact on how the test material is being absorbed, distributed, metabolized, and excreted, and hence the potential toxicity of the test material in the body.

Absorption. In humans, gastric secretion is low in the newborn, and gastric pH is relatively high at birth (6–8 compared to 1.5 in adults). The higher pH can result in decreased absorption of weak acids and increased absorption of weak bases. Gastric acidity reaches the adult values at 2 years after birth (38). Gastric emptying is slow and irregular, and reaches adult values at 6–8 months. Intestinal mobility is reduced in the newborn.

The stomach of the newborn rodent is immature at birth and experiences a dramatic change towards maturation beginning at weaning, i.e., around postnatal week 3 (39). The intestines of the rat at birth are not as mature as that in humans at birth (40). As in the case of stomach, the intestines of the rat undergo rapid maturation around weaning or shortly after that. In the beagle dog, the small intestines are functionally immature at birth and most adult functions are attained by PND 63 (41,42).

Table 2 A Species Comparison of the Different Age Groups in Juvenile Laboratory Animals and in the Pediatric Population

	Humans	Rats	Dogs	Mini-swine
Neonates	Birth–1 month	Birth–PND 7	Birth–3 weeks	Birth–2 weeks
Infants	1–24 months	PND 7–21	3–6 weeks	2–4 weeks
Children	2–12 years	PND 21–35	6 weeks–5 months	4 weeks–3.5 months
Adolescents	12–16 years	PND 35–55/60	5–7 or 8 months	3.5–6 months

Abbreviation: PND, postnatal day.

The human infant has a higher ventilation rate per body weight but a lower ventilation volume due to a smaller lung volume. On average, children have a higher respiratory tract exposure per unit surface area as compared to adults. The lung alveoli achieve the adult level at 2 years after birth in humans and at the end of postnatal week 4 in rodents (30).

Distribution. In young infants, there is a greater percentage of body water (80–90% of the body weight compared to 55–60% in the adult) and less body fat (10–15% of the body weight). The additional water is primarily extracellular. This can result in a decrease in the retention of lipid soluble compounds and a larger volume of distribution for water-soluble compounds (20). Body lipid rises steadily after birth for the first 9 months, followed by a steady decrease until about ages 4–7, when a second period of increasing body lipid begins (43,44).

In human newborns and neonates, the blood-brain barrier is immature and more permeable to xenobiotics. This barrier becomes more effective at 3–6 months after birth (45). Neonates have reduced plasma protein binding capacity, resulting in a higher fraction of unbound xenobiotics in this population (46). Decreased plasma protein binding would increase the amount of unbound xenobiotics and possibly cause an exaggerated pharmacologic or toxic response. Also, decreased plasma protein binding and increased extracellular fluid volume in neonates results in a greater volume of distribution for relatively polar compounds.

Metabolism. In humans, the newborns exhibit relatively low levels of cytochrome P450 enzyme levels. The activities of these enzymes increase rapidly and a majority of the P450s achieve the adult levels by about 6 months to 1 year of age (19). However, not all CYP enzymes develop at the same rate. For example, CYP2D6 and 2E1 levels are very low at birth but surge within hours after birth and reach the adult levels by about 1 year of age (47,48); CYP3A4 and CYP2C levels rise during the first week after birth and are fully active after 2 months of age (49,50). By 2–3 years, enzymatic activity of the CYP-dependent metabolism exceeds adult values (45). Therefore, young children have an increased ability to metabolize drugs eliminated by CYP-dependent metabolism. By puberty, CYP enzymatic activity has decreased to adult levels (51).

Human neonates have deficient glucuronidation ability at birth due to low levels of uridine diphosphate glucuronosyltransferase (UDP-GT), which appears to reach adult levels by at least age 3–4 years (21). The UDP-GT activities in the neonatal rat are low at birth but reach the adult levels by 1 month of age (52).

Glutathione S-transferases (GST) represent a family of proteins responsible for the activation and deactivation of electrophilic chemicals. Individual GST enzymes mature at an independent rate in infants (48,53). In the rat, the hepatic GST activities are generally low at birth and gradually increase to reach the adult levels within 2–4 weeks (52).

Excretion. In humans, the renal glomerular filtration rate is low in the newborn (about 40% of the adult level in 1-week old infant) and reaches the adult level at about 3–5 months of age (17,21). The renal tubular secretion capacity reaches the adult level at about 7–8 months of age, and the renal blood flow increased to adult levels by 5–12 months of age (48). Clearance, if normalized for body weight, is lower in the newborn and rapidly increases to reach a maximum at about 6 months, when it is almost twice that of the adult (21). Renal function reaches full maturation by age 2–3 years (51).

Preweaning rats and 3–10 days old dog pups have longer elimination half lives for xenobiotics, and clearance in these animals is lower than that in adults (54,55).

In summary, the metabolic capability of the pediatric population typically reaches the adult levels within 6–12 months after birth. In rodents and rabbits, metabolic capability of these species typically reaches the adult levels by weaning. Therefore, if the intended pediatric population is older than 1 year of age, the metabolic capability of this population can be considered as similar to that in the adult. If the intended pediatric population is younger than 1 year of age, then dose administration in studies using rats or rabbits should begin prior to weaning.

Organ System Maturation.   In the juvenile animals and pediatric populations, the nervous, pulmonary, reproductive, renal, skeletal, and immune systems are the major systems that undergo considerable growth and maturation processes (6). If the test material exerts pharmacological or toxicological effects on one or more of these organ systems, then the postnatal maturation processes of these organs should be considered when deciding the timing and duration of the dose administration.

The following sections provide a brief summary of the cross-species comparison of the maturation process for the nervous, pulmonary, reproductive, renal, skeletal, and immune systems. If the target organ in the adult animal studies or clinical trials is one of these organs, then the developmental age of that organ in humans and the test species as well as the timing of pediatric exposure should be considered such that dose administration in the juvenile animals should begin at the corresponding age of the organ when the pediatric population will be exposed.

Nervous System.   In humans, the brain at birth is more advanced in development compared to rodents. The human brain experiences a period of rapid growth postnatally and achieves its maximum weight before puberty. Myelination of many central tracts begins before birth and continues after birth through the first few years of life (24). In rats, the brain grows at a slower rate and absolute brain weight continues to increase slowly for at least the first full year of life. Myelination in rats typically occurs after birth and is not complete until months after birth (24).

In humans, the sensory and reflex functions are relatively developed at birth, whereas in the common laboratory species the same functions are relatively undeveloped at birth, with the exception of vision and taste (26). Therefore, the investigator should be careful in trying to extrapolate the juvenile animal data to humans.

As in humans, the common laboratory species possess learning capabilities in early life. Therefore, evaluation of cognitive function in juvenile animal toxicology studies can provide information about the effects of the test material on the maturation of this function (26).

Pulmonary System.   The timing of maturation of lungs in humans and the common laboratory species is presented in Table 3 (30).

If the intended pediatric population is for children that are older than 2 years, then juvenile animal toxicology study may not be necessary if adult animal data are available to assess toxicity of the test material on the pulmonary system. This is because the pulmonary system for the pediatric population would have matured at that age and adult animal study data can be used to evaluate the potential toxicity of the test material on this system, assuming that the TK profile for the test material is similar between the juvenile and adult animals. However, if the TK profile for the test material is different between the juvenile and adult animals, juvenile animal toxicology study may be necessary. In this case, rats can begin dose administration at 4 weeks of age or slightly later.

Table 3   Timing of Maturation of Lungs in Humans and the Common Laboratory Species

	Humans	Monkey	Dog	Rabbit	Rat	Mouse
Onset	Prenatal	Prenatal	Prenatal	Prenatal	PND 1–4	PND 1–2
Completion	2 years	1 year	16 weeks	Unknown	4 weeks	4 weeks

Abbreviation: PND, postnatal day.

Reproductive System. The average age at onset of puberty for humans and the common laboratory test species is presented in Table 4 (16).

Some laboratory test species achieve adult reproductive status some time after reaching puberty. For example, the reproductive system in male rats reaches the adult status at 10–14 weeks of age and that in the female rats reaches the adult status at 8–10 weeks of age.

Kidney. In general, the human kidney is more mature than the rat kidney at birth. In humans and mice, nephrogenesis is complete before birth. However, the same process is complete in rat, dog, and pig at 4–6 weeks, 2 weeks, and 3 weeks after birth, respectively. In human kidneys, concentrating ability reaches maturity by the first year of life (33).

Skeletal System. The age of appearance and fusion of the secondary ossification centers in the femur in humans and the common laboratory species is presented in Table 5 (32).

This table shows that although the fusion of epiphysis in the long bone occurs around the time of adolescent in human, dog, and mouse, this process occurs much later in life in rats. Therefore, the investigator should be careful about interpreting changes observed in this process in rats.

Immune System. In humans, the immune system becomes immunocompetent by one year of age, and the immune memory is established between one and 18 years. In rodents, the immune system is relatively immature at birth, and it becomes immuno-competent by PND 30, and the immune memory is established between PND 30 and PND 60. The immune system of dogs and humans are at a similar stage of development at birth (28), and the immunoglobulin levels of the dog reach adult levels at approximately one year of age (28).

Parameters to Be Evaluated

In general, the juvenile animal toxicology studies are similar to single-dose or repeated-dose toxicity studies with the main exception that the age of the animals used in the juvenile animal toxicology studies may vary from one study to another. Therefore, the parameters to be evaluated in the juvenile animal toxicology studies are similar to those used in adult animal studies, with possibly a few additional end points to assess the effects of the test material on the developmental processes and functional maturation of some organ systems. Since the values of many parameters in the juvenile animal toxicology studies are age-dependent, it is critical that comparison of values among different dose groups should be made by using values obtained from animals of the same age. As many of these parameters were discussed in greater detail in other chapters of

Table 4 Average Age at Onset of Puberty for Humans and the Common Laboratory Species

	Human	Rhesus monkey	Swine	Dog	Rabbit	Rat	Mouse
Male	12–15 years	4–5 years	4–6 months	6–8 months	6–7 months	PND 45–48	PND 27–31
Female	12–15 years	4–5 years	4–6 months	6–8 months	5–6 months	PND 32–34	PND 26–32

Abbreviation: PND, postnatal day.
Source: From Ref. 16.

Table 5 Age of Appearance and Fusion of Secondary Ossification Centers in the Femur

	Human	Monkey	Dog	Rabbit	Rat	Mouse
Appearance in proximal epiphysis	1–12 years	Birth—6 months	1 week–4 months	PND 1–5	PND 21–30	PND 14–15
Fusion in proximal epiphysis	11–19 years	2.25–6 years	6–13 months	16 weeks	78–156 weeks	13–15 weeks

Abbreviation: PND, postnatal day.
Source: From Ref. 32.

this book, only a brief description of these parameters is provided in this section. Procedures that are handled differently from the adult animal studies will be highlighted here. The reader who requires additional details is encouraged to refer to chapters containing this information.

Observation of Toxic Signs

As in the case of repeated-dose studies, viability and signs of toxicity in the study animals should be monitored daily following dose administration. If the time of the onset of toxic signs is known, then these signs should be monitored at a scheduled time following dosing, e.g., 1–2 hours postdose. This procedure is important in situations where the toxic signs only appear transiently postdose.

Whenever possible, it is useful to have only one or few technicians to monitor the toxic signs. This arrangement will allow consistency in recording these observations. In addition, in observations where it is necessary to indicate different degrees of severity for particular toxic signs, it is important to have a few technicians agreed on how to grade these signs throughout the study.

Although monitoring of the overt post-dose toxic signs can be performed at the cage-side daily, detailed observations of the general health of the animals should be performed at regular intervals, e.g., weekly. For rodents and rabbits, this task can be performed by technicians. For other nonrodents, this task may be performed by veterinarians or veterinarian aides.

Body Weights

Individual body weights should be recorded at regular intervals beginning at least once prior to the first dose administration. For rodents, body weights should be recorded at least twice a week prior to weaning and weekly thereafter. More frequent recording of body weights may be necessary, especially during the preweaning period when the animals are experiencing significant daily weight gains. The final body weight of each animal, body weight recorded just before or after the animal is euthanized for necropsy, is typically recorded in order to allow for the determination of relative organ weights following necropsy.

Food Consumption

Food consumption is determined in pups following weaning. Although the animals begin to ingest solid food prior to weaning, it is not possible to obtain accurate information about food consumption of individual animals within a litter prior to weaning. Food weights, i.e., the weight of food left and the weight of new food provided, should be recorded at the same time the body weight is recorded. This will allow determination of the amount of food consumed during the last interval. Determination of food consumption at the same interval as that in body weight recording will allow comparisons of body weight gains versus the amount of food consumed during the same interval. Food consumption can be calculated using the individual animal as a unit, i.e., g/animal/day, or using the body weight of the animal as a unit, i.e., g/kg/day.

In studies where the test material is administered in the diet, it is important to record the food consumption value as accurately as possible, i.e., the weight of the spilled feed on the cage pad should be included in the calculation of food consumption where possible. This is because the amount of food consumed by the animal is a reflection of the dose received by that animal. In addition, prior to initiating any studies using diet as a vehicle to deliver the test material to the animals, a pilot study must be performed to ensure that food consumption in the animals is not affected due to the poor palatability of the diet containing the test material.

Ophthalmic Examination

Eye examinations should be performed by a trained ophthalmologist prior to administration of the first dose and at the end of the dosing period. For studies using rats and dogs, if dose administration begins prior to PND 12–14, it is not possible to perform this examination prior to the administration of the first dose because eyes in these animals open after PND 12–14. If findings were observed at the end of the dosing period, eye examination should also be performed at the end of the recovery period to determine if the animals are capable of recovering from the treatment effect. This procedure is performed using the same method employed for the adult animals.

Cardiovascular Assessment

In studies using nonrodents, recording of the blood pressure and electrocardiogram (ECG) is used to assess the potential effects of the test material on the cardiovascular system of the juvenile animals. The changes in blood pressure and heart rate in the young dog pups are qualitatively similar to those observed in young infants and children (56). Therefore, this parameter is considered useful in evaluating potential risk of a test material on the heart function of the pediatric population.

The ECG can be recorded using an electrocardiograph while the animal is sedated or restrained, or by using telecardiography. In telecardiography (or commonly called telemetry), a transmitting device is implanted in the appropriate location on the animal and impulses related to the heart waves are transmitted remotely to a recording devise. The advantage of using telecardiography is that the animal is not sedated or restrained during recording and continuous recording can be performed over an extended period.

Recording of ECG is typically done prior to the first dose administration and at the end of the dosing period. If findings were observed at the end of the dosing period, recording should also be performed at the end of the recovery period to determine if the animals are capable of recovering from the treatment effect. On each day of recording, it is important to perform the recording at about the same time as the previous recording in order to allow a meaningful comparison of these values obtained from different days. In addition, on the scheduled recording day, it may be necessary to record ECG prior to dosing and after dosing.

Clinical Pathology

Evaluations of the hemopoietic status (hematology), serum enzyme and electrolyte concentrations (serum chemistry), and characterization of the urine (urinalysis) will provide useful information about the health status of the animals following dose administration. In juvenile animal toxicology studies where dose administration begins at an early age, it may not be useful to collect data for these parameters prior to the first dose. This is because even in untreated or vehicle-treated animals, these parameters are undergoing changes as the animals continue to grow such that results collected at the end of the dosing period cannot be used to compare with the predose values. Therefore, samples for clinical pathology evaluations are usually collected at the end of the dosing period, and results of the compound-treated groups are compared with the controls. Testing facility that had conducted juvenile animal toxicology studies should have historical control data for clinical pathology in different age groups to provide background data for comparison (see Appendixes A–D). As in the case of adult animal studies, if findings are observed at the end of the dosing period, blood samples should also be collected at the end of the recovery period to determine if the animals are capable of recovering from these changes. For studies using rodents, due to the small blood volume of these animals, only the minimum amount of blood (as approved by the Institutional Animals Care and Use Committee) should be collected from these animals. Blood samples for clinical pathology evaluation are usually not collected from animals found dead or euthanized moribund.

Young rats and dog pups should not be deprived of water overnight for urine collection. To collect urine, these animals should only be deprived of water in the metabolic cages for several hours. The testing facility should obtain historical control data for the parameters in the urine obtained using this method of collection.

Toxicokinetics

Collection of blood samples at specific time points following dosing to determine the plasma concentrations of the test material and its metabolites in the test species is usually performed in safety studies in the development of pharmaceuticals. Results of plasma drug concentration analysis are usually called exposure. Determination of exposure is less common in the development of agricultural or industrial chemicals.

In the pilot or range-finding juvenile animal toxicology study, it is useful to perform limited blood sampling to determine exposure in the juvenile animals. Results of TK analysis in the range-finding study will allow the investigator to determine whether at the same dose level (i) the exposure in the juvenile animals is higher or lower than that seen in the adult animals, and (ii) there is sufficient exposure in the juvenile animals when the dose formulation used in the study is different from that used in the adult animal studies. TK results showing exceedingly low exposure in the range-finding study may necessitate the consideration of a different dose formulation in order to obtain a higher exposure in the juvenile animals. In addition, these data can also aid in the selection of doses for the definitive study.

In studies using rodents, blood samples for TK analysis are usually collected from satellite animals. Satellite animals are additional animals assigned to each dose group specifically for the purpose of collecting blood for TK analysis. This is done in order to avoid the effect of extensive blood loss on the health status of the main study animals. The sparse sampling approach, i.e., using blood samples from different animals to obtain an estimate of the TK profile for a particular dose level, is usually used. Due to the small blood volume of these animals, many satellite animals may need to be assigned to the study in order to obtain sufficient blood for analysis. Care must be taken to only assign the minimum number of satellite animals necessary to obtain the TK profile of the test material.

Although the young rabbit may have higher blood volume than the rodent pup, it is not easy to obtain blood from the auricular vessels (mainly ear veins) or jugular vein of the kit. The ear veins of the kit may be visible at 3 weeks of age, but it is quite difficult to obtain multiple blood samples with consistent volume from these veins at this age. Therefore blood samples needed from the preweaning kit are usually collected from the aorta or vena cava, following euthanasia. In the postweaning kit (4–5 weeks of age or older), multiple blood samples at relatively small volume may be collected from the auricular vessels. As in the case of rodents, the TK blood samples for kits are usually collected from satellite animals.

TK blood samples are typically collected on the first day of dose administration and at the end of the dosing period. This is done to determine if there is accumulation of the test material or its metabolites following repeated dosing. Depending on the age of the animals on the first day of dose administration, the TK profile for the test material or its metabolites on the first day of dose administration may be quite different from that at the end of the dosing period due to differences in metabolic maturity of the animals. Therefore, the investigator needs to be aware of these potential differences and interpret the data accordingly. Due to the limited blood volume in the rodent pups, blood collection in pups prior to weaning is typically terminal bleed, and blood is usually obtained from the aorta or via cardiac puncture. If the first dose administration is to be performed on PND 4, the pups to be culled can be used for TK blood collection. TK blood samples are usually not collected from animals that are found dead or euthanized moribund.

Test material may occasionally be detected in blood samples collected from control animals. This result will complicate data interpretation. Therefore, all necessary precautions must be taken to avoid any potential cross-contamination of the blood samples in different dose groups. These precautions may include having different technicians to collect blood samples from the control animals, using separate tools and instruments to collect and process the control samples, etc.

Evaluation of Developmental Landmarks

As in the case of the pre- and postnatal development study, developmental landmarks are usually evaluated at specific time points during the postnatal period. This is done to determine whether the test material may have an effect on the normal growth and development of the juvenile animals. The parameters to be evaluated in rodent pups typically include physical development such as pinna detachment, eye opening, tooth eruption, acoustic startle, vaginal opening, and preputial separation. In addition, a variety of reflexological and sensory tests, including negative geotaxis, righting reflex, visual placing, and papillary reflex, can also be performed. Since the timing of vaginal opening, preputial separation, and descent of the testes is an indicator of sexual maturation, it is essential to evaluate these parameters for study using test material that may have an effect on the reproductive or endocrine system.

In dog pups, similar tests of physical development, including eye opening, tooth eruption, vaginal opening, and preputial separation, can be performed. Sensory tests for the dog pups are included in a neurological examination.

As another measurement of growth, crown-rump length may be determined in rat pups, and body height and length may be determined in young dogs.

Behavioral, Learning, and Memory Assessments

Behavioral development and development of the learning and memory capabilities can be assessed using various tests. These tests are essential for study using test material that may affect the development of the nervous system. Tests of motor activity and functional observational battery (FOB) are used to evaluate behavioral development, with the FOB also giving an overall assessment of neurological development. Passive avoidance testing and various mazes are typically used to evaluate development of the learning and memory functions.

Physical and Neurological Examinations

In studies using nonrodents, such as dogs and swine, neurological examinations can be performed at specific time points to evaluate the sensory and motor development of the juvenile animals. Physical examinations are performed to determine the general health status of the animals. These examinations should be performed by an experienced veterinarian or veterinarian aide. Physical examinations are usually performed prior to the first dose administration and at the end of the dosing period, and neurological examinations are usually performed at the end of the dosing period. If findings are observed during neurological examination performed at the end of the dosing period, animals should be examined again at the end of the recovery period to determine if the changes have regressed.

Assessment of Pulmonary Functions

In juvenile animal toxicology studies where inhalation is the route of administration or if the lung is the suspected target organ, pulmonary function should be evaluated at the end of the dosing period. If the animals receive the first dose administration after the completion of the lung maturation, e.g., after postnatal week 4 in rodents or after postnatal week 16 in dogs, pulmonary functions should also be evaluated prior to the first dose administration. Assessment of the pulmonary or respiratory function in the juvenile animals is similar to that used in the adult animal studies. The respiratory function of the animals can be recorded using a nose-only plethysmograph to determine the tidal volume and respiratory rate and from these values the calculated respiratory minute volume.

Assessment of Reproductive Function

In juvenile animal toxicology studies where the reproductive or endocrine system is the potential target organ, reproductive function of the study animals should be evaluated. In addition to recording the timing of vaginal opening, preputial separation, and/or descent of the testes, estrous cycles may be evaluated in females following the end of the dosing period. Blood samples can be collected at specific intervals or at necropsy to determine hormone levels, including luteinizing hormone (LH), follicle-stimulating hormone (FSH), estradiol/estrogens, testosterone, and progesterone. Since these hormones are influenced by the circadian rhythm of the animals, blood samples should be collected at about the same time for all animals in the study.

In rodent studies, males and females may be mated to determine the reproductive capability of these animals following dose administrations. Sibling mating should be avoided. Unless it is necessary to produce the offspring for further evaluation, it is a common practice to euthanize the mated female on presumed gestation day 13 and examine the uterine contents of the females. At scheduled necropsy, pituitary, thyroid, adrenals, and the reproductive organs should be preserved and their histology should be examined.

Sperm from the males can be collected from the testis or epididymis for count, morphology, and/or motility assessments. Testes can be preserved, sections prepared and stained, and examined for stages of spermatogenesis. In dogs and rabbits, serial semen samples may be collected for evaluation after the animals have reached sexual maturity.

Necropsy and Pathology

As in the case of the adult animal studies, animals in the juvenile animal toxicology studies are euthanized and necropsied at the end of the dosing and recovery periods. Animals that are euthanized moribund or at scheduled necropsy should be dissected, examined, and tissues preserved as soon as possible in order to avoid autolysis of the tissues/organs. If animals are found dead and cannot be necropsied immediately, they should be placed in an appropriate bag and stored refrigerated (2–4°C) until necropsy can be performed. This is to prevent further autolysis of the tissues/organs.

The method of necropsy and gross tissue examinations is the same as that used in the adult animal studies. All lesions and a full set of tissues/organs as those typically listed in the adult animal studies should be preserved for histopathology examinations.

Organ Weights. The major organs and target organs should be weighed. In the absence of known target organs, brain, lungs, heart, liver, spleen, kidneys, adrenals, and male and female reproductive organs are usually weighed. If target organs are known or suspected, weight of these target organs should be recorded. In addition, other lymphoid organs, such as thymus, may be weighed for assessment of immunological changes.

Histopathology. All lesions and a full set of tissues/organs as those typically listed in the adult animal studies (see Chapter 7 "Multidose General Toxicology Studies") should be processed, stained, and examined under the light microscope. For studies using nonrodents, tissues from all groups should be examined. For studies using rodents, initial examination of all tissues with lesions and all tissues from the control and high-dose animals as well as from animals that were found dead or euthanized moribund may be considered. If treatment-related findings are observed in any tissues, the same tissues from the lower dose groups and from the recovery animals should be examined. If it is important to complete the study report on a specific date for regulatory submission, this approach is not preferable because it requires considerable time to process and examine slides from the lower dose groups. In addition, it may be difficult to schedule the study pathologist in the CRO to examine the additional slides at a short notice. Therefore, in order to ensure that the study report is completed on a specific date, it might be better to examine all tissues from all dose groups. It is not necessary to examined tissues from the recovery animals when the same tissues did not show any treatment-related changes at the end of the dosing period. Special stains may be used to confirm or elucidate specific histopathological findings.

Since the histology of tissues/organs may differ from one age group to another, the testing facility should have historical control data for all tissues from the test species obtained at different ages, at PND 4, 7, 14, 21, etc. In the absence of concurrent control data, this background information will allow the study pathologist to compare the histology of the tissues/organs obtained from animals found dead or euthanized moribund at different time (i.e., age) during the study with that in the untreated animal.

Another qualified pathologist should perform a peer review on a subset of the histology slides in the study. This is to ensure that all histopathological findings are described using the appropriate terminology and that there is agreement between the study pathologist and the peer review pathologist with regards to histopathological observations recorded in the study.

Morphometry may be performed on the target organ or suspected target organ in order to determine any changes in the size of the affected organ or region following dose administrations. Morphometry should be performed by a testing facility that has the expertise and considerable experience in performing the analysis. The availability of historical control data for the parameters of interest in the testing facility would be a plus.

Assessment of Bone Growth.   At necropsy, the length of long bones, such as femur, tibia, or humerus, may be determined. This value can be used as an indicator of growth. Biomarkers of bone formation, e.g., osteocalcin and serum phosphorus, or bone resorption may be analyzed in the blood samples collected for clinical pathology evaluation. Histology of the long bones should be examined to evaluate potential effects on the growth plates, bone, and cartilage. In testing facilities where radiographs can be taken, evaluation of additional bone parameters may be performed (57). Application of radiography allows the investigator to evaluate changes of specific bones in the same animal over time.

Assessment of Immune Function.   Immune functions can be assessed by evaluating hematology parameters at the appropriate intervals as well as histology of lymphoid organs, including bone marrow, lymph nodes, thymus and, spleen. Phenotyping of the lymphocytes, evaluation of the natural killer (NK) cell activity, and T-cell dependent antibody response are additional parameters used to further evaluate effects of the test material on immune functions (58).

DATA REPORTING, ANALYSIS, INTERPRETATION, AND RISK ASSESSMENT

Data Reporting and Analysis

Study report for juvenile animal toxicology studies should, at the minimum, contain the following:

1. Study title, study number, testing facility and sponsor information
2. Regulatory compliance and Quality Assurance Unit statement
3. Key study personnel
4. Study schedules, including dosing initiation and completion dates, necropsy date
5. Study summary or abstract
6. Purpose of the study
7. Materials and methods
8. Results
9. Discussion/Conclusion
10. Summary data
11. Individual data.

The study summary or abstract should be concise and contain all the relevant information about the study, including purpose, summary of materials, methods, and results, as well as conclusion. As a rule, the conclusion should fully address the purpose of the study, and where possible, provide a NOAEL or no observed effect level (NOEL) of the test material in the test species. Any deviations from the protocol, protocol amendments, or the facility SOPs that may impact the results of the study should be stated in the report. Study results may be summarized in specific table for regulatory submission.

Statistical tests are usually used to analyze rodent toxicity study data to aid in the comparison of the results in the control and compound-treated groups. Prior to performing the statistical tests, the experimental unit of the study should be determined. For studies using the whole-litter approach, each litter should be considered the experimental unit. For studies using the cross-fostered or split-litter approach, each individual animal within the litter is considered the experimental unit. Data analysis will be determined by this classification.

Data are typically divided into parametric and nonparametric data. Before these data are analyzed for statistical significance, they should be tested for homogeneity of variance. Parametric data that are not homogeneous can be transformed to stabilize the variance or treated as nonparametric data and analyzed accordingly. Homogeneous parametric data are usually analyzed using one-way analysis of variance. Nonparametric data are usually analyzed using the Kruskal-Wallis method. If results of these analyses show significant differences, then pairwise comparison between the control and individual treatment groups is usually performed. Other statistical methods may be used to analyze study data.

In nonrodent juvenile animal toxicology studies, the small number of animals used in each group may make results of statistical analysis rather meaningless. Therefore, data in these studies are often evaluated based on individual animal data in each group. Data from each animal are either compared with the controls or with predose or previous data from the same animal.

Interpretation of Specific End Points

Results of statistical analyses should only be viewed as a guide in interpreting study data. A significant difference between the control and treatment groups dose not automatically indicate a treatment effect. Occasionally, the mean values of certain parameters in a group may be skewed by extreme values found in 1–2 animals. The test of statistical significance may also be affected by unusually high or low values in the control animals. Historical control data from the testing facility should be consulted to ensure that study data are interpreted appropriately.

Various data within a set of parameters, e.g., developmental landmarks or learning and memory data, may be related and should be evaluated together as a category. Many apparently distinct data are also related and should also be assessed together. For example, changes in clinical pathology may be related to changes in organ histology, severe toxic signs may affect food consumption and hence the body weight of the animals. The presence or absence of a dose-response relationship should be considered before assigning treatment effect. Overall, results of the juvenile animal toxicology studies should be evaluated for their toxicological and biological significance.

Observation of Toxic Signs

Toxic signs observed in the animals should be viewed as a manifestation of toxicity in different organ systems. When viewed together, these toxic signs can often suggest specific target organs. However, at sufficiently high doses, the test material may affect multiple organ systems such that the animals may become moribund, and it may not be possible to pinpoint the affected organs. When dosing is being done in preweaning animals, animals with severe toxicity may be rejected by their mother. Excessive handling of the young animals or animals that bleed due to blood sampling or other procedures may also result in rejection by the mother. Such rejection may be lethal for the young animals. It is important to separate lethality caused by the test material and lethality caused by dam rejection secondary to severe toxicity in the young animals or mishandling of the pups.

Body Weights and Food Consumption

In juvenile animal toxicology studies, body weight is an accurate indicator of growth. Therefore, the body weight, usually related to food consumption, is an important marker for the presence or absence of toxicity in the young animals, and it should be evaluated carefully to determine the presence or absence of treatment effects.

Ophthalmic Examination

Results of eye examinations should be interpreted by a trained veterinary ophthalmologist. Observations recorded at the end of the dosing or recovery period are often compared with the data obtained prior to the first dose administration, if this was possible. If findings are recorded in the eye examinations, these observations should be verified during gross and histology examinations of the eye.

Cardiovascular Assessment

ECG in nonrodents should be evaluated and interpreted by an experienced veterinary cardiologist. Appropriate statistical analysis may be used to analyze the ECG data. The main parameters to be considered are heart rate and QT interval. Various correction formulae are used to calculate the corrected QT interval by including the heart rate as a correction factor. The investigator should discuss with the veterinary cardiologist in deciding the appropriate correction formula to be used for the study. Depending on the age of the animal at the first dose administration and the length of the dosing period, comparing the ECG at the end of the dosing period to that prior to the first dose may not be meaningful because age-related changes in the heart rate during these two periods may result in different ECG profiles. It may be more useful to evaluate the ECG prior to dosing and after dosing on a specific day.

Observation of changes in QT interval may be related to the low level of certain CYP enzymes at an early age and its inability to metabolize drugs, leading to the accumulation of the drugs in the pediatric patients. This is reported in the cisapride-induced QTc prolongation in human neonates. The low content of CYP3A4 in the human neonate liver appears to be responsible for its inability to oxidize cisapride and may have caused its accumulation in the plasma and leading to the QTc prolongation (59).

Clinical Pathology

Since the clinical pathology data contain many parameters that are interrelated, it would be useful to have these data evaluated by an experienced clinical pathologist.

Hematology.   There are age-related changes in hematology parameters in many juvenile animals such that it is not meaningful to compare data obtained prior to the first dose administration to those obtained at the end of the dosing period. Age-related changes of several hematology parameters in rats are shown in Figure 1 (60).

As shown in Figure 1, as the rat continues to grow, the erythrocyte count is increased, whereas the reticulocyte count is decreased. Therefore, it is important to compare hematology data from the compound-treated animals with data obtained from the concurrent controls of the same age.

Hematology data are good indicators of the status of hematopoietic system as well as the immune system. A decrease in erythrocyte count with a corresponding increase in reticulocyte count indicates that the animals are anemic. A low white blood cell count may indicate that the immune system is affected. There are confounding factors, e.g., infections or significant blood loss due to serial or frequent blood collection that may influence the hematology data.

Serum Chemistry. As in the case of hematology data, there are age-related changes in serum chemistry parameters. Age-related changes in total bilirubin in rats are shown in Figure 2 (60).

In rats, the total bilirubin and alkaline phosphatase levels are high among the weanlings while the total protein is relatively low at this age. In dogs, the cholesterol and triglyceride levels decrease with age, whereas aspartate aminotransferase (AST) and alanine aminotransferase (ALT) levels increase with age (61). Therefore, it is important to compare serum chemistry data obtained from animals of the same age.

Although age-related differences exist for the different serum chemistry parameters, interpretation of changes in the individual parameters remains similar except that levels that are lower than adult values should be evaluated in the context of the specific age. The chapter titled "Multidose General Toxicology Studies" (Chapter 7) provides an excellent overview of this information. The reader should refer to this chapter for additional information.

Urinalysis. The chapter titled "Multidose General Toxicology Studies" (Chapter 7) provides an excellent overview of the interpretation of the urinalysis data. The reader should refer to this chapter for this information.

Toxicokinetics

The TK profile in juvenile animals can be characterized by the estimates of the maximum concentration (C_{max}), time to reach the C_{max} (t_{max}) and the area under the plasma concentration curve (AUC_{t1-t2}), representing an estimate of the total amount of the test material or its metabolites in the plasma of the animal during a time period (t1–t2), typically 24 hours. Depending on the age of the animals when the TK profile is

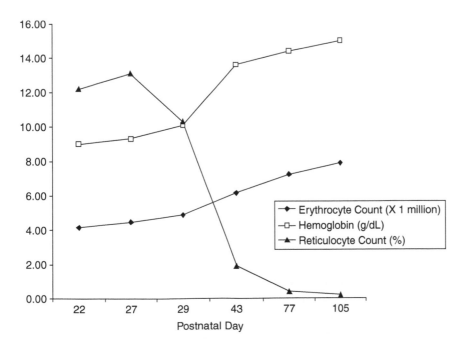

Figure 1 Age-related changes in erythrocyte and reticulocyte counts, and hemoglobin concentration in male Sprague-Dawley rats. *Source*: From Ref. 60.

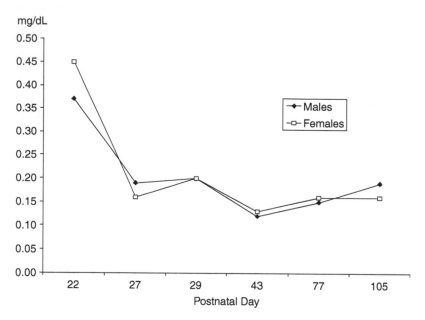

Figure 2   Age-related changes in total bilirubin concentration in male and female Sprague-Dawley rats. *Source*: From Ref. 60.

determined, this profile in juvenile animals may not be the same as that in the adult animals. If the TK profiles between the adult and the juvenile animals are the same or similar, given what is known about the adult clinical trials, it may be easier to estimate the starting dose in the clinical trials in children assuming that the same formulation used in adults will be used in children. If the TK profiles between the adult and the juvenile animals are different, the investigator will need to determine how the TK profile in juvenile animals relates to the intended pediatric population.

Evaluation of Developmental Landmarks

Developmental landmarks should be evaluated together to obtain an overall picture of the potential effects of the test material on the growth and development of the young animals. A delay, or sometimes an acceleration, in achieving the developmental landmarks may suggest a treatment effect. Confounding factors, e.g., overt toxicity affecting suckling and/or food consumption and hence the nutritional status of the animals, should be taken into consideration. Poor nutritional status will impact the maturation of the animals. A delay in vaginal opening or preputial separation is an indication of an effect on sexual maturation, possibly involving the endocrine system. If these effects are observed, both the endocrine and reproductive systems should be closely monitored in clinical trials with children.

Behavioral, Learning, and Memory Assessment

Assessment of behavior, learning and memory parameters is an evaluation of the functional development of the nervous system. Developmental changes in growth, frequently reflected by changes in body weights, may affect the functional development of the nervous system. Changes in these parameters will suggest that the nervous system is a target organ for the test material. These changes may trigger a more extensive evaluation of the histopathology of the nervous system tissues. Monitoring of these parameters should be considered in clinical trials with children.

Physical and Neurological Examinations

For various technical reasons, it may not be possible to perform some developmental landmarks, behavioral, learning, and memory assessments in nonrodents. Therefore, physical and neurological examinations become an important alternative to evaluate potential effects of the test material on maturation and on the functional development of the nervous system. A trained veterinarian should be able to detect abnormal signs in the individual animals to determine whether these signs may be treatment-related. If there is strong evidence that these signs are treatment-related, monitoring of these signs should be included in the protocol for the clinical trials in children.

Assessment of Pulmonary Function

The typical pulmonary function data evaluated in toxicology studies include respiratory rate, tidal volume, and respiratory minute volume (calculated value determined by multiplying respiratory rate with tidal volume). These data are good indicators of the lung function (62). Changes in these values should be evaluated together with results of histopathological evaluation of the lungs. If treatment effects are observed in the pulmonary function of the juvenile animals, these parameters should be closely monitored in clinical trials in children.

Assessment of Reproductive Function

In rodent studies, a change in the cycling or the length of the estrous cycle is an indication of effects on the endocrine system of the females. This can be confirmed by analysis of the hormone levels in the females. Analysis of the hormone levels in the males can also provide information about the function of the endocrine system in the males.

Reproductive function can be evaluated by assessing the ability of the males and females to mate and produce offspring. This is typically done in rodent studies. If the mating failed to produce pregnancy in females, the function can be further assessed by mating compound-treated males with nontreated females, and mating nontreated males with compound-treated females to determine if the effects are present in the males or females. Examination of the uterine contents during midgestation will allow the investigator to determine whether treatment of the test material will affect the female's ability to produce viable fetuses. Absence of implants or presence of early resorptions is an indication that the test material may affect the viability of the embryos or the compound-treated female's reproductive tract cannot maintain the pregnancy. Occasionally, the pregnant females may be allowed to deliver their pups to evaluate the potential effects of the test material on gestation length and the viability of their offspring.

Necropsy and Pathology

Gross and histopathological lesions observed in the study are often good indicators of target organ toxicity. The investigator needs to be cognizant of the presence of background lesions of the common laboratory test species at specific ages. A good CRO should have historical control data that allow the investigator to differentiate between background lesions and possible treatment-related lesions.

Organ Weights.   Organ weights are usually reported as absolute weight, relative to body weight and relative to brain weight. Absolute organ weight may be affected by the nutritional status of the animals. Animals that lose weight may have lower organ weights, a change that may be unrelated to the potential effects of the test material on the organs. Since brain weight in a specific age group usually does not change significantly even in the presence of severe toxicity, the organ weight relative to brain weight provides a good representation of the weight of the organ. Organ weight changes should be evaluated in conjunction with histology of the organ of interest. Changes in liver and kidney weights are good indicators of organ toxicity, whereas heart weight may not be a sensitive indicator of organ toxicity. Lung weight is highly variable and should be evaluated with this variability in mind.

Histopathology.   A study pathologist usually examines the histology slides and prepares a detailed histopathology report for the study. Prior to finalizing the histopathology report, selected slides should be reviewed by a peer review pathologist. All descriptions of the findings in the histopathology report should be agreed upon by the study pathologist and the peer review pathologist. Any disagreement between the study pathologist and the peer review pathologist must be resolved prior to finalization of the histopathology report. This report, signed by the study pathologist, should be included in the study report. A statement, prepared by the peer review pathologist indicating the peer review procedures and the final agreement with the pathology report, is usually included in the study report.

The histopathlogy report should contain a complete description of the treatment-related histological findings in the study. Target organs, when present, should be identified.

Assessment of Bone Growth.   Bone growth can be evaluated using (i) length of long bones, (ii) biomarkers, or (iii) bone histology. If bone is the suspected target organ, all three parameters should be evaluated. In addition, more detailed bone morphometry analyses may be employed to better characterize changes in the affected bones. If bone is not suspected to be the target organ, evaluation of the length of long bones and bone histology may be sufficient. Changes in bone growth should be assessed in conjunction with possible changes in growth hormones in the animals.

Assessment of Immune Function.   Effects on the immune function can be evaluated by assessing (i) hematology parameters, (ii) serum chemistry (immunoglobulin levels), (iii) weights of lymphoid organs, and (iv) histology of lymphoid organs. When necessary, additional parameters, e.g., lymphocyte phenotyping, NK cells activities, etc., may be evaluated. It is critically important to determine the appropriate age when these parameters should be evaluated. Assessment of these parameters before the animals are immunologically competent may result in poor responses. These poor responses are due to the immaturity of the immune system and not due to the treatment of the test material. All parameters in the immune system should be evaluated as a category rather than individually. If treatment-related changes in the immune system are noted at the end of the dosing period, the same system should be evaluated for recovery animals. If there is an absence of recovery in the immune system in the recovery animals, this system should be carefully monitored in clinical trials in children.

Risk Assessment

The purpose of the juvenile animal toxicology study should be clearly stated in the protocol. When evaluating the study data, the study director should integrate all results and provide an overall assessment of the toxicity of the test material in the study animals. In other words, results in individual sections should not be evaluated in isolation and the conclusion of the study should fully address the purpose of the study. All parameters in the study should be evaluated to identify the target organs and toxic dose as well as the NOAEL or NOEL.

The TK profile is a reflection of the internal dose of the test material following dose administration. Although the exposure in the juvenile animal may be similar to that seen in the adult animal, the toxicity observed, including the target organ, and NOAEL or NOEL, may be different from that in the adult animal studies. When comparing the same dose level as in adult animal, higher exposure values in the juvenile animals do not necessarily mean that the test material is more toxic in these animals. Conversely, lower exposure values in the juvenile animals do not necessary mean that the test material is less toxic in these animals. This difference in toxicity may be the result of differences in PK due to the immaturity of the organ systems in the young animals or differences in the sensitivities of the target organs in these animals. Therefore, the TK profile should be evaluated in the context of the age of the testing animals and the intended pediatric population. Any potential differences in PK between the juvenile animals and children should be considered when assessing the potential risks of the test material in the pediatric population.

The juvenile animal toxicology study should identify the target organs, the NOAEL and the plasma exposure value corresponding to the NOAEL. These results should allow an estimation of the possible doses to be used in clinical trials in children, and organ functions to be monitored or biomarkers to be used (if available) based on target organs noted in the juvenile animal toxicology study.

The chapter on Multidose General Toxicology Studies (Chapter 7) provides excellent discussions of the significance of toxicity observed in individual organs. The reader is encouraged to refer to this chapter for detailed discussions of these organs.

In addition, there are several excellent review articles that discuss risk assessment using juvenile animal data. The reader is encouraged to refer to these articles for further discussions of this topic (63–68).

CONCLUSION

The goal of performing juvenile animal toxicology studies is to estimate potential risks of the test material in pediatric populations. Juvenile animals are developing test species and a better understanding of the developing processes of the different organ systems, as well as a knowledge of the kinetics of xenobiotics in juvenile animals compared to adult animals, is critical in the proper evaluation and interpretation of the toxicity data obtained from these studies. Since there is no standard study design for conducting juvenile animal toxicology studies, the materials provided in this chapter only serve as an early guide for the investigators. As more information about the postnatal developmental processes become available and as we continue to gain more experience in conducting these studies, a better guidance document for the design and testing of compounds in juvenile animals may become available in the near future.

ACKNOWLEDGMENTS

The author would like to express his sincere gratitude to Mr. Keith Robinson and Ms. Louise Pouliot of Charles River Laboratories, Preclinical Services Montreal Inc.,

Senneville, Quebec, Canada, for their helpful suggestions and comments for this chapter and for providing the figures and historical control data in this chapter.

REFERENCES

1. National Academy of Sciences (NAS). Pesticides in the Diets of Infants and Children. Washington, DC: National Academy Press, 1993.
2. Food Quality Protection Act (FQPA) of 1996. Pub. L. 104–170.
3. International Conference on Harmonisation. M3 Nonclinical Safety Studies for the Conduct of Human Clinical Trials for Pharmaceuticals. 1997.
4. United States Food and Drug Administration. Regulations requiring manufacturers to assess the safety and effectiveness of new drugs and biological products in pediatric patients, 1998; Fed Reg 63:66632.
5. Pediatric Research Equity Act of 2003. Pub. L. 108–155.
6. United States Food and Drug Administration. Guidance for Industry: Nonclinical Safety Evaluation of Pediatric Drug Products. http://www.fda.gov/cder/guidance/5671fnl.pdf, February, 2006.
7. Agnish ND, Keller KA. The rationale for culling of rodent litters. Fund Appl Toxicol 1997; 38:2–6.
8. Palmer AK, Ulbrich BC. The cult of culling. Fund Appl Toxicol 1997; 38:7–22.
9. Booze RM, Mactutus CF. Experimental design considerations: a determinant of acute neonatal toxicity. Teratology 1985; 31:187–191.
10. Ruppert PH, Dean KF, Reiter LW. Comparative developmental toxicity of triethyltin using split-litter and whole-litter dosing. J Toxicol Environ Health 1983; 12:73–87.
11. Pouliot LS, Groom SN, McCartney J, et al. The effects of continuous intravenous saline infusion upon clinical pathology parameters in the weanling albino rat. Toxicol Sci 2002; 66:235–236.
12. Groom S, Copeman C, Tourigny I, et al. An assessment of the weanling beagle dog as a model for screening pharmaceuticals intended for intravenous infusion to pediatric populations. Toxicol Sci 2003; 72:326.
13. Stoute M, Viau A, Robinson K, et al. Inhalation nose-only exposure of neonatal and juvenile rats. Toxicol Sci 2003; 72:297.
14. Robinson K, Stoute M, Viau A, et al. Inhalation nose-only exposure of neonatal and juvenile rats. Birth Defects Res A Clin Mol Teratol 2003; 67:350.
15. Robinson K, Gordon C, Salame R, et al. Procedures for inhalation treatment of neonatal dogs. Teratology 2002; 65:328.
16. Zoetis T, Walls I, eds. Principles and Practices for Direct Dosing of Pre-Weaning Mammals in Toxicity Testing and Research. Washington DC: ILSI Press, 2003.
17. Benedetti MS, Baltes EL. Drug metabolism and disposition in children. Fund Clin Pharmacol 2003; 17:281–299.
18. Bruckner JV, Weil WB. Biological factors which may influence an older child's or adolescent's responses to toxic chemicals. Regul Toxicol Pharmacol 1999; 29:158–164.
19. Ginsberg G, Hattis D, Sonawane B. Incorporating pharmacokinetic differences between children and adults in assessing children's risks to environmental toxicants. Toxicol Appl Pharmacol 2004; 198:164–183.
20. Ginsberg G, Hattis D, Miller R, et al. Pediatric pharmacokinetic data: implications for environmental risk assessment for children. Pediatrics 2004; 113:973–983.
21. Scheuplein R, Charnley G, Dourson M. Differential sensitivity of children and adults to chemical toxicity. I. Biological basis. Regul Toxicol Pharmacol 2002; 35:429–447.
22. Dourson M, Charnley G, Scheuplein R. Differential sensitivity of children and adults to chemical toxicity. II. Risk and regulation. Regul Toxicol Pharmacol 2002; 35:448–467.

23. Schwenk M, Gundert-Remy U, Heinemeyer G, et al. Children as a sensitive subgroup and their role in regulatory toxicology: DGPT workshop report. Arch Toxicol 2003; 77:2–6.
24. Rice D, Barone S, Jr. Critical periods of vulnerability for the developing nervous system: evidence from humans and animal models. Environ Health Perspect 2000; 108:511–533.
25. Adams J, Barone S, Jr., LaMantia A, et al. Workshop to identify critical windows of exposure for children's health: neurobehavioral work group summary. Environ Health Perspect 2000; 108:535–544.
26. Wood SL, Beyer BK, Cappon GD. Species comparison of postnatal CNS development: functional measures. Birth Defects Res B Dev Reprod Toxicol 2003; 68:391–407.
27. Dietert RR, Etzel RA, Chen D, et al. Workshop to identify critical windows of exposure for children's health: immune and respiratory systems work group summary. Environ Health Perspect 2000; 108:483–490.
28. Holsapple MP, West LJ, Landreth KS. Species comparison of anatomical and functional immune system development. Birth Defects Res B Dev Reprod Toxicol 2003; 68:321–334.
29. Thurlbeck WM. Postnatal growth and development of the lung. Am Rev Respir Dis 1975; 111:803–844.
30. Pinkerton KE, Joad JP. The mammalian respiratory system and critical windows of exposure for children's health. Environ Health Perspect 2000; 108:457–462.
31. Zoetis T, Hurtt ME. Species comparison of lung development. Birth Defects Res B Dev Reprod Toxicol 2003; 68:121–124.
32. Zoetis T, Tassinari MS, Bagi C, et al. Species comparison of postnatal bone growth and development. Birth Defects Res B Dev Reprod Toxicol 2003; 68:86–110.
33. Zoetis T, Hurtt ME. Species comparison of anatomical and functional renal development. Birth Defects Res B Dev Reprod Toxicol 2003; 68:111–120.
34. Pryor JL, Hughes C, Foster W, et al. Critical windows of exposure for children's health: the reproductive system in animals and humans. Environ Health Perspect 2000; 108:491–503.
35. Lemasters GK, Perreault SD, Hales BF, et al. Workshop to identify critical windows of exposure for children's health: reproductive health in children and adolescents work group summary. Environ Health Perspect 2000; 108:505–509.
36. Marty MS, Chapin RE, Parks LG, et al. Development and maturation of the male reproductive system. Birth Defects Res B Dev Reprod Toxicol 2003; 68:125–136.
37. Beckman DA, Feuston M. Landmarks in the development of the female reproductive system. Birth Defects Res B Dev Reprod Toxicol 2003; 68:137–143.
38. Morselli PL. Clinical pharmacology of the perinatal period and early infancy. Clin Pharmacokinet 1989; 17:13–28.
39. Deren JS. Development of structure and function in the fetal and newborn stomach. Am J Clin Nutri 1971; 24:144–159.
40. de Zwart LL, Haenen HE, Versantvoort CH, et al. Role of biokinetics in risk assessment of drugs and chemicals in children. Regul Toxicol Pharmacol 2004; 39:282–309.
41. Paulsen DB, Buddington KK, Buddington RK. Dimensions and histologic characteristics of the small intestine of dogs during postnatal development. Am J Vet Res 2003; 64:618–626.
42. Buddington RK, Elnif J, Malo C, et al. Activities of gastric, pancreatic and intestinal brush-border membrane enzymes during postnatal development of dogs. Am J Vet Res 2003; 64:627–634.
43. Kearns GL, Reed MD. Clinical pharmacokinetics in infants and children. A reappraisal. Clin Pharmacokinet 1989; 17:29–67.
44. Hattis D, Ginsberg G, Sonawane B, et al. Differences in pharmacokinetics between children and adults—II. Children's variability in drug elimination half-lives and in some parameters needed for physiologically-based pharmacokinetic modeling. Risk Anal 2003; 23:117–142.
45. Morselli PL, Franco-Morselli R, Bossi L. Clinical pharmacokinetics in newborns and infants: age-related differences and therapeutic implications. Clin Pharmacokinet 1980; 5:485–527.
46. Notarianni LJ. Plasma protein binding of drugs in pregnancy and in neonates. Clin Pharmacokinet 1990; 18:20–36.
47. Cresteil T. Onset of xenobiotic metabolism in children: toxicological implications. Food Addit Contam 1998; 15:45–51.

48. Alcorn J, McNamara PJ. Ontogeny of hepatic and renal systemic clearance pathways in infants. Part I. Clin Pharmacokinet 2002; 41:959–998.

49. Ginsberg G, Hattis D, Sonawane B, et al. Evaluation of child/adult pharmacokinetic differences from a database derived from the therapeutic drug literature. Toxicol Sci 2002; 66:185–200.

50. Hines RN, McCarver DG. The ontogeny of human drug-metabolizing enzymes: phase I oxidative enzymes. J Pharmacol Exp Therap 2002; 300:355–360.

51. Anderson GD. Children versus adults: pharmacokinetic and adverse-effect differences. Epilepsia 2002; 43:53–59.

52. Gregus Z, Klaassen CD. Hepatic disposition of xenobiotics during prenatal and early postnatal development. In: Polin RA, Fox WF, eds. Fetal and Neonatal Physiology. Philadelphia: W.B. Saunders, 1998:1472–1493.

53. McCarver DG, Hines RN. The ontogeny of human drug-metabolizing enzymes: phase II conjugation enzymes and regulatory mechanisms. J Pharmacol Exp Therap 2002; 300:361–366.

54. Wang L, Edge JH, Ono J, et al. Pharmacokinetics of clonazepam in developing rats. Chinese Med J 1992; 105:726–731.

55. Singh S, Gadgil S, Mirkin BL. Age dependent factors influencing digoxin pharmacokinetics in the postnatal puppy. Res Comm Chem Pathol Pharamcol 1978; 21:87–101.

56. Hew KW, Keller KA. Postnatal anatomical and functional development of the heart: a species comparison. Birth Defects Res B Dev Reprod Toxicol 2003; 68:309–320.

57. Adamo ML, Pinsonneault L, Varela A, et al. Assessing postnatal skeletal development in non-clinical reproductive toxicology and pediatric studies. Birth Defects Res A Clin Mol Teratol 2004; 70:315.

58. Pinsonneault L, Adamo ML, Pouliot L, et al. Techniques for assessing development of the immune system. Birth Defects Res A Clin Mol Teratol 2004; 70:296.

59. Treluyer JM, Rey E, Sonnier M, et al. Evidence of impaired cisapride metabolism in neonates. Br J Clin Pharmacol 2001; 52:419–425.

60. Pouliot L, Robinson K, Beyrouty P. Neonatal toxicology studies: age-related clinical pathology changes in IGS rats. Teratology 2001; 63:277.

61. Pinsonneault L, Gordon C, Robinson K, et al. Gavage dosing in neonatal beagle dogs—growth and clinical pathology. Teratology 2002; 65:327.

62. Anderson BT, McDonald P, Morgan AI. Respiratory volume in young juvenile beagle dogs. Toxicology 2001; 164:116.

63. Baldrick P. Developing drugs for pediatric use: a role for juvenile animal studies? Regul Toxicol Pharmacol 2004; 39:381–389.

64. Bruckner JV. Differences in sensitivity of children and adults to chemical toxicity: the NAS Panel Report. Regul Toxicol Pharmacol 2000; 31:280–285.

65. Ginsberg G, Slikker W, Jr., Bruckner J, et al. Incorporating children's toxicokinetics into a risk framework. Environ Health Perspect 2004; 112:272–283.

66. Miller MD, Marty MA, Arcus A, et al. Differences between children and adults: Implications for risk assessment at California EPA. Int J Toxicol 2002; 21:403–418.

67. Morford LL, Henck JW, Breslin W, et al. Hazard identification and predictability of children's health risk from animal data. Environ Health Perspect 2004; 112:266–271.

68. Renwick AG, Dorne JL, Walton K. An analysis of the need for an additional uncertainty factor for infants and children. Regul Toxicol Pharmacol 2000; 31:286–296.

Appendix A Historical Control Data of Hematology Parameters in Juvenile Charles River Sprague-Dawley Rats [Crl:CD®(SD)IGS BR VAF/Plus®], 1998–2004

Parameter	Days post partum	Male				Female			
		Mean	SD	Min	Max	Mean	SD	Min	Max
WBC (10³/µL)	20 to 29	8.09	3.013	4.50	13.80	7.24	2.848	2.80	14.70
	30 to 39	4.61	1.299	2.27	8.08	3.99	1.126	1.88	6.60
	40 to 49	4.21	1.317	2.82	8.30	4.46	1.940	1.24	9.10
RBC (10⁶/µl)	20 to 29	4.42	0.431	3.81	5.43	4.54	0.506	3.79	5.34
	30 to 39	6.02	0.330	5.39	6.70	6.16	0.322	5.44	6.68
	40 to 49	6.32	0.335	5.77	7.04	6.54	0.384	5.85	7.85
Hb (g/dL)	20 to 29	9.2	1.12	7.4	11.7	9.5	1.25	7.4	11.9
	30 to 39	12.9	0.65	11.5	13.8	13.0	0.64	11.9	14.2
	40 to 49	13.5	0.58	11.8	14.7	13.8	0.75	12.3	15.8
Ht (%)	20 to 29	27.7	3.22	21.8	34.5	28.5	3.61	22.4	36.4
	30 to 39	40.9	2.21	36.2	44.1	40.9	2.19	36.9	45.4
	40 to 49	41.6	2.26	36.8	46.7	41.6	2.65	38.4	51.9
PLT (10³/µL)	20 to 29	921.5	117.55	631	1130	927.8	145.94	770	1509
	30 to 39	1477.9	161.74	1170	1777	1631.4	277.75	1026	2605
	40 to 49	1191.9	135.15	923	1548	1414.1	284.59	1007	2317
RETIC (10⁹/L)	20 to 29	Na	Na	Na	Na	Na	Na	Na	Na
	30 to 39	618.7	42.38	537.4	695.1	504.4	46.67	431.4	598.3
	40 to 49	482.2	40.15	399.4	565.7	375.7	67.26	256.3	496.4
PT (sec)	20 to 29	15.6	0.57	14.7	16.4	15.8	0.54	14.8	16.8
	30 to 39	16.5	1.49	13.5	22.1	16.2	0.79	14.6	18.1
	40 to 49	13.3	1.45	11.9	19.7	13.0	1.34	11.3	15.6
APTT (sec)	20 to 29	13.0	2.11	9.6	16.3	13.3	1.91	10.0	15.4
	30 to 39	20.4	3.59	12.0	33.7	18.1	2.17	13.0	21.1
	40 to 49	18.1	2.58	14.5	31.4	16.5	2.73	13.0	26.1

Abbreviations: SD, standard deviation; Na, not available; WBC, white blood cell; RBC, red blood cell count; Hb, hemoglobin; Ht, hematocrit; PLT, platelet count; RETIC, reticulocyte count; PT, prothrombin time; APTT, activated partical thromboplastin time.
Source: From Charles River Laboratories, Preclinical Services Montreal Inc., Senneville, Quebec, Canada.

Appendix B Historical Control Data of Hematology Parameters in Juvenile Covance Beagle Dog, 2001–2004

Parameter	Age (weeks)	Male				Female			
		Mean	SD	Min	Max	Mean	SD	Min	Max
WBC (10^3/µL)	1 to 3	10.15	2.367	6.90	16.62	9.81	2.364	5.97	13.69
	4 to 6	12.35	3.751	6.88	18.86	13.16	3.604	6.58	19.60
	7 to 9	15.72	3.498	9.91	20.72	13.73	3.752	9.45	20.78
	10 to 12	11.63	3.689	7.23	16.95	11.95	3.689	9.40	17.43
	13 to 15	10.47	3.444	6.30	17.64	9.42	1.857	6.20	12.00
RBC (10^6/µL)	1 to 3	3.79	0.459	2.70	4.67	3.89	0.364	3.19	4.64
	4 to 6	4.11	0.468	3.22	5.02	4.38	0.463	3.57	5.15
	7 to 9	5.06	0.214	4.65	5.34	5.19	0.213	4.96	5.57
	10 to 12	5.62	0.127	5.48	5.85	5.90	0.283	5.68	6.31
	13 to 15	5.93	0.361	5.32	6.68	5.70	0.464	4.68	6.48
Hb (g/dL)	1 to 3	9.8	0.85	8.4	11.5	9.9	0.70	8.9	11.6
	4 to 6	9.2	0.81	7.4	10.9	9.9	0.86	7.8	11.0
	7 to 9	10.6	0.46	9.8	11.5	10.9	0.51	10.0	12.0
	10 to 12	12.0	0.63	11.2	12.7	12.2	0.71	11.6	13.2
	13 to 15	12.9	0.86	11.4	14.9	12.4	0.79	11.1	13.4
Ht (%)	1 to 3	29.7	2.92	23.2	35.4	30.7	2.24	25.7	33.7
	4 to 6	29.4	2.69	23.9	34.8	31.4	2.85	26.4	35.7
	7 to 9	33.6	1.16	31.9	36.0	34.5	2.05	30.8	38.2
	10 to 12	36.7	1.83	34.5	38.7	36.6	1.53	35.1	38.7
	13 to 15	38.9	2.26	34.3	43.5	37.5	2.39	33.1	40.8

PLT (10³/µL)	1 to 3	513.3	143.07	240	767	532.8	134.11	371	782
	4 to 6	422.2	164.39	208	773	421.2	186.49	217	839
	7 to 9	481.1	81.72	333	609	466.8	158.12	235	746
	10 to 12	472.8	108.84	269	556	471.0	135.02	322	650
	13 to 15	415.5	116.73	254	617	415.2	83.58	256	580
RETIC (10⁹/L)	1 to 3	178.4	61.11	115.2	275.1	295.0	55.73	257.6	376.8
	4 to 6	213.7	65.84	130.8	354.9	235.1	34.95	196.9	308.9
	7 to 9	Na	Na	Na	Na	Na	Na	Na	Na
	10 to 12	Na	Na	Na	Na	Na	Na	Na	Na
	13 to 15	74.3	33.28	24.4	119.4	64.2	30.14	33.1	134.9
PT (sec)	1 to 3	8.8	0.89	8.1	10.7	8.5	0.39	7.9	9.2
	4 to 6	9.1	0.80	7.9	11.0	8.8	0.44	8.0	9.5
	7 to 9	8.9	0.59	8.1	10.0	8.6	0.53	8.1	9.6
	10 to 12	10.0	0.68	9.2	11.1	10.1	0.26	9.7	10.3
	13 to 15	8.0	1.38	6.2	10.7	7.4	1.36	5.9	9.7
APTT (sec)	1 to 3	18.9	10.42	12.9	44.4	17.3	2.93	14.0	22.6
	4 to 6	13.0	0.98	11.2	15.3	13.2	1.03	11.9	15.9
	7 to 9	12.2	1.24	10.8	15.3	13.0	1.33	11.0	15.6
	10 to 12	12.0	1.00	11.0	13.4	11.9	0.66	11.1	12.7
	13 to 15	11.1	0.85	10.0	13.8	12.1	1.29	10.5	15.2

Abbreviations: SD, standard deviation; Na, not available; WBC, white blood cell; RBC, red blood cell count; Hb, hemoglobin; Ht, hematocrit; PLT, platelet count; RETIC, reticulocyte count; PT, prothrombin time; APTT, activated partial thromboplastin time.

Source: From Charles River Laboratories, Preclinical Services Montreal Inc., Senneville, Quebec, Canada.

Appendix C　Historical Control Data of Serum Chemistry Parameters in Juvenile Charles River Sprague Dawley Rats [Crl:CD®(SD)IGS BR VAF/Plus®], 1998–2004

Parameter	Days post partum	Male				Female			
		Mean	SD	Min	Max	Mean	SD	Min	Max
AST (U/L)	20 to 29	108.5	14.32	71	144	103.2	17.82	80	146
	30 to 39	118.9	20.15	84	165	108.7	22.22	76	165
	40 to 49	135.6	29.06	82	190	128.5	27.99	71	220
ALT (U/L)	20 to 29	51.0	10.00	33	67	45.9	7.47	35	62
	30 to 39	33.5	5.72	22	43	27.4	5.02	20	40
	40 to 49	35.0	6.27	23	46	28.5	5.11	20	43
ALP (U/L)	20 to 29	402.4	87.41	263	612	377.5	92.81	210	601
	30 to 39	305.2	66.36	174	449	253.5	57.26	169	400
	40 to 49	319.7	87.81	180	556	223.0	60.60	146	388
TBIL (mg/dL)	20 to 29	0.23	0.095	0.10	0.52	0.25	0.159	0.11	0.69
	30 to 39	0.13	0.028	0.06	0.19	0.13	0.042	0.07	0.25
	40 to 49	0.08	0.036	0.02	0.17	0.08	0.036	0.01	0.17
CREAT (mg/dL)	20 to 29	0.5	0.06	0.4	0.6	0.5	0.06	0.4	0.6
	30 to 39	0.4	0.05	0.3	0.5	0.4	0.05	0.3	0.5
	40 to 49	0.3	0.12	0.1	0.5	0.3	0.12	0.2	0.5
GLU (mg/dL)	20 to 29	231.6	53.42	180	370	227.3	53.02	167	368
	30 to 39	120.8	27.79	61	177	120.4	25.67	80	210
	40 to 49	106.8	18.71	78	147	123.4	21.34	61	173

CHOL (mg/dL)	20 to 29	85.5	20.72	55	134	86.9	19.69	62	134
	30 to 39	53.6	11.82	27	79	60.3	13.64	34	95
	40 to 49	63.4	9.67	45	90	67.6	16.65	39	107
TRIG (mg/dL)	20 to 29	115.4	68.21	56	326	113.2	86.18	29	364
	30 to 39	40.9	23.08	13	107	42.8	21.45	19	97
	40 to 49	51.0	26.49	10	141	35.5	17.36	13	88
T PROT (g/dL)	20 to 29	4.8	0.21	4.3	5.1	4.8	0.20	4.4	5.3
	30 to 39	5.1	0.19	4.7	5.6	5.3	0.23	4.9	5.8
	40 to 49	5.2	0.31	4.7	5.9	5.4	0.26	5.0	6.0
ALB (g/dL)	20 to 29	3.1	0.48	2.2	3.7	3.2	0.54	2.3	4.0
	30 to 39	4.0	0.18	3.7	4.4	4.2	0.15	3.8	4.6
	40 to 49	3.8	0.24	3.4	4.3	4.0	0.23	3.7	4.6
PHOS (mg/dL)	20 to 29	10.75	1.277	9.00	15.00	10.56	1.279	8.92	13.33
	30 to 39	11.46	1.557	8.98	14.47	11.43	1.319	8.83	13.93
	40 to 49	10.65	0.803	9.18	12.22	10.73	1.618	8.91	17.47

Abbreviations: SD, standard deviation; AST, aspartate aminotransferase; ALT, alanine aminotransferase; ALP, alkaline phosphatase; TBIL, total bilirubin; CREAT, creatinine; GLU, glucose; CHOL, cholesterol; TRIG, triglycerides; T PROT, total protein; ALB, albumin; PHOS, phosphorous.
Source: From Charles River Laboratories, Preclinical Services Montreal Inc., Senneville, Quebec, Canada.

Appendix D Historical Control Data of Serum Chemistry Parameters in Juvenile Covance Beagle Dog, 2001–2004

Parameter	Age (weeks)	Male				Female			
		Mean	SD	Min	Max	Mean	SD	Min	Max
AST (U/L)	1 to 3	31.0	8.75	16	51	29.3	9.97	18	54
	4 to 6	26.1	4.23	20	33	27.5	4.98	19	37
	7 to 9	29.6	6.60	20	48	33.4	9.13	18	46
	10 to 12	24.5	2.59	22	29	22.8	3.77	18	27
	13 to 15	30.8	5.45	22	41	32.1	5.92	24	47
ALT (U/L)	1 to 3	14.2	7.78	6	37	11.9	6.28	5	36
	4 to 6	17.1	8.49	4	43	22.1	13.20	6	45
	7 to 9	23.8	3.21	18	28	39.0	29.12	20	105
	10 to 12	23.7	5.39	14	28	22.3	6.40	15	29
	13 to 15	38.4	13.16	17	64	45.4	10.83	23	63
ALP (U/L)	1 to 3	229.5	85.95	119	389	237.0	71.84	136	394
	4 to 6	145.6	42.98	89	237	162.4	34.13	100	239
	7 to 9	120.2	29.42	84	173	138.0	30.89	88	183
	10 to 12	113.2	27.14	85	142	134.3	50.06	79	181
	13 to 15	139.6	30.35	95	214	141.8	27.93	91	191
TBIL (mg/dL)	1 to 3	0.60	0.255	0.10	1.08	0.69	0.416	0.12	1.45
	4 to 6	0.44	0.240	0.08	0.90	0.41	0.252	0.14	1.09
	7 to 9	0.24	0.155	0.08	0.57	0.24	0.132	0.08	0.52
	10 to 12	0.09	0.027	0.05	0.12	0.08	0.015	0.07	0.10
	13 to 15	0.09	0.035	0.04	0.14	0.07	0.027	0.03	0.12

Analyte	Week								
CREAT (mg/dL)	1 to 3	0.5	0.06	0.4	0.6	0.4	0.06	0.3	0.5
	4 to 6	0.6	0.30	0.3	1.2	0.6	0.27	0.4	1.1
	7 to 9	0.8	0.26	0.4	1.2	0.8	0.22	0.4	1.2
	10 to 12	0.5	0.04	0.4	0.5	0.5	0.05	0.4	0.5
	13 to 15	0.4	0.13	0.2	0.6	0.4	0.14	0.3	0.6
GLU (mg/dL)	1 to 3	121.2	14.00	87	145	127.8	10.94	109	153
	4 to 6	127.6	12.62	105	149	130.9	8.15	110	147
	7 to 9	120.4	5.84	107	128	121.0	8.02	105	135
	10 to 12	119.7	7.53	113	131	118.8	3.77	114	123
	13 to 15	113.6	7.82	102	129	111.3	5.45	103	122
CHOL (mg/dL)	1 to 3	224.2	37.76	172	301	231.2	41.18	173	338
	4 to 6	242.6	42.06	163	339	228.3	32.38	185	293
	7 to 9	190.6	31.34	136	228	185.8	36.84	127	243
	10 to 12	212.2	32.03	178	264	203.3	42.96	160	257
	13 to 15	187.7	29.81	140	239	175.6	20.93	133	206
TRIG (mg/dL)	1 to 3	146.9	42.47	68	265	155.5	67.34	35	268
	4 to 6	127.2	53.08	47	256	114.1	62.86	49	279
	7 to 9	68.7	36.26	20	137	59.1	19.10	32	100
	10 to 12	41.5	11.84	30	62	40.3	4.99	35	47
	13 to 15	36.5	5.96	27	53	35.1	7.02	20	45
T PROT (g/dL)	1 to 3	3.7	0.31	3.2	4.3	3.8	0.26	3.3	4.4
	4 to 6	4.5	0.31	3.9	4.9	4.6	0.28	4.1	5.2
	7 to 9	4.8	0.22	4.5	5.1	4.7	0.20	4.4	5.0
	10 to 12	5.1	0.24	4.8	5.4	5.1	0.14	5.0	5.3
	13 to 15	5.4	0.25	4.9	5.8	5.3	0.18	4.9	5.6

(Continued)

Appendix D Historical Control Data of Serum Chemistry Parameters in Juvenile Covance Beagle Dog, 2001–2004 (*Continued*)

Parameter	Age (weeks)	Male				Female			
		Mean	SD	Min	Max	Mean	SD	Min	Max
ALB (g/dL)	1 to 3	2.3	0.20	2.0	2.8	2.3	0.22	1.9	2.8
	4 to 6	2.8	0.32	2.3	3.4	2.9	0.31	2.3	3.4
	7 to 9	3.1	0.13	2.9	3.3	3.0	0.14	2.9	3.3
	10 to 12	3.1	0.18	2.8	3.3	3.1	0.15	2.9	3.2
	13 to 15	3.4	0.27	3.0	3.9	3.3	0.13	3.1	3.6
PHOS (mg/dL)	1 to 3	10.18	0.674	9.25	12.36	9.95	0.845	8.50	12.65
	4 to 6	10.25	0.788	8.55	11.48	9.80	0.900	7.88	11.40
	7 to 9	10.05	1.205	8.44	12.18	9.92	1.227	8.17	12.08
	10 to 12	8.83	0.715	7.82	9.53	8.30	0.567	7.45	8.64
	13 to 15	8.59	0.619	7.29	9.65	8.64	0.434	8.10	9.46

Abbreviations: SD, standard deviation; AST, aspartate aminotransferase; ALT, alanine aminotransferase; ALP, alkaline phosphatase; TBIL, total bilirubin; CREAT, creatinine; GLU, glucose; CHOL, cholesterol; TRIG, triglycerides; T PROT, total protein; ALB, albumin; PHOS, phosphorous.
Source: From Charles River Laboratories, Preclinical Services Montreal Inc., Senneville, Quebec, Canada.

11

Developmental and Reproductive Toxicology

Kit A. Keller
Toxicology Consultant, Washington, D.C., U.S.A.

INTRODUCTION

This chapter is meant to be a basic guide for nontoxicologists or nonexperts in developmental and reproductive toxicology (DART) who are responsible for contracting chemical safety studies to outside laboratories and need help in understanding the subject enough to be able to use the appropriate terminology, review protocols, interpret study results, and understand the implications of specific findings to risk assessment. It is not the purpose of this review to discuss specific methodology or specific agents and their mechanisms of toxicity. If the reader is interested, the following books are excellent sources for further inquiries into this area of toxicology (1–5).

The plethora of national guidelines and study designs in DART testing has been replaced in the last decade by harmonized testing guidelines that are generally accepted worldwide. A general outline of the required studies for human drugs, agricultural and industrial chemicals, and food additives can be found in Tables 1–3. However, due to the complexity of study designs in DART testing, it is recommend that the reader let the contract laboratory help in deciding requirements and study design. Any good contract laboratory will have carefully reviewed each guideline and will have prepared protocols to meet the minimum specific requirements for your product type. Testing guidelines for drugs intended for animal use are available but have not been included in this review (8–10).

It is very important that all studies that you are planning to submit to a government agency be run under Good Laboratory Practices (see Chapter 1). The reader should be warned that conducting DART studies require experience and expertise. DART studies should be placed only at contract labs with a good record for conducting these types of studies. If you are not sure about a particular laboratory, ask for a copy of the laboratory's historical control data for fetal, neonatal, and reproductive indices. These data should provide a good indication of how many of these studies are performed each year as well as some insight into the quality and consistency of their data.

One of the most common problems in this field of study is the multiple use and/or misuse of terminology. For this reason, some definitions of common terms used in this chapter have been included as an appendix for the readers benefit. However, it is not

Table 1 International Guidelines for DART Testing of Human Drugs

Study type	Species	No./group	Treatment period	Evaluation
Segment I	Rat	24 male 24 female	F_0 males: 4 weeks premating to sac F_0 females: 2 weeks premating to GD 7	F_0 clinical observations F_0 body wt and food F_0 female estrous cycling F_0 copulatory interval; fertility/fecundity indices F_0 necropsy Corpora lutea count GD 13 uterine exam: viable and inoviable implants
Segment II	Rat	24 female	F_0 female: GD 6–15	Maternal clinical observations Maternal body wt and food Maternal necrospy Corpora lutea count GD 20 cesarean section: early/late resorptions; live and dead fetuses; fetal body wts Fetal external, (1/2) visceral, and (1/2) skeletal exam; high dose and control
Segment II	Rabbit	20 female	F_0 female: GD 6–18	Maternal clinical observations Maternal body wt and food Maternal necrospy Corpora lutea count GD 29 cesarean section: early/late resorptions; live and dead fetuses; fetal body wts Fetal external, visceral, and skeletal exam (high dose and control for skeleton only)
Segment III	Rat	20 female	F_0 female: GD 6–PD 21	Maternal clinical observations Maternal body wt and food Parturition and maternal behavior F_1 litter observations, body wt, and survival indices F_1 developmental and behavioral indices F_1 copulatory interval, fertility/fecundity indices F_1 GD 13 uterine exam: viable and nonviable implants

Guidelines for testing human drugs from International Conference on Harmonization (ICH)—accepted by U.S. FDA, Japan. Ministry of Health and Welfare (MHW), and European EC; no specific requirements, indicated study designs are the author's recommendation. Individual guidelines can be found at www.FDA.gov/CDER.
Abbreviations: PD, postnatal day; FDA, Food and Drug Administration; GD, gestation day; EEC, European Economic Community.

Table 2 International Guidelines for DART Testing of Chemicals and Pesticides

Study type	Species	No./group	Treatment period	Evaluation
Multigen 2G (1–2 litter)	Rat	20 male	F_0 males: 10 weeks prior to mating	F_0 clinical observations, food, and body wt
		20 female	F_0 females: 10 weeks premating to PD 21 F_1 males/females: weaning to sac	F_0 estrous cycle, sperm indices F_0 copulatory interval; fertility/fecundity indices F_0 necropsy with histopathology F_0 parturition and maternal behavior F_1 litter observations, body wts, survival indices, landmarks F_1 copulatory interval; fertility/fecundity indices F_1 necropsy with histopathology and organ wts F_1 parturition and maternal behavior F_2 litter observations, body wts, and survival indices F_2 necropsy
Segment II	Rat	20 female	F_0 female: GD 6–15	Maternal clinical observations, body wt, and food Maternal necropsy, corpora lutea count GD 20 cesarean section: early and late resorptions; live and dead fetuses; fetal body wts Fetal external, (1/2) visceral, and (1/2) skeletal exam
Segment II	Rabbit	20 female	F_0 female: GD 6–18	Maternal clinical observations, body wt, and food Maternal necropsy, corpora lutea count GD 29 cesarean section: early and late resorptions; live and dead fetuses; fetal body wts Fetal external, visceral, and skeletal exam
Neurotoxicity	Rat	20 female	F_0 females: GD 6–PD10	Maternal clinical observations, food, and body wt Maternal parturition and behavior F_1 litter observations, body wts, and survival indices F_1 developmental, reflex, and behavioral indices F_1 neuropathologic examination

Harmonized guidelines accepted by the U.S. Environmental Protection Agency and the Organization for Economic Cooperation and Development. Likely acceptance by Canada MHW and Japan MAFF. Individual guidelines can be found at www.EPA.gov.
Abbreviations: PD, postnatal day; GD, gestation day; MHW, Ministry of Health and Welfare; MAFF, Ministry of Agriculture, Forestry and Fisheries.
Source: From Refs. 6, 7.

Table 3 DART Testing of Food and Color Additives

Study type	Species	No./group	Treatment period	Evaluation
Multigen 2G(2-litter)	Rat	20 male	F_0 males: 10 weeks premating to sac	For each generation
				Clinical observations, food, and body wt
		20 female	F_0 females: 10 weeks premating to PD 21	Copulatory interval; fertility/ fecundity indices
			F_1 males: weaning to sac	Necropsy (histopathology in F_0 and F_1)
			F_1 females: weaning to PD 21	Parturition and maternal behavior
				Litter observations, body wts, and survival indices
				GD 20 cesarean section and fetal evaluation (optional)
				For each generation
Segment II	Rat	20 female	F_0 female: GD 6–15	Maternal clinical observations
				Maternal body wt and food
				Maternal necropsy
				Corpora lutea count
				GD 20 cesarean section: early and late resorptions; live and dead fetuses; fetal body wts
				Fetal external, (1/2) visceral, and (1/2) skeletal exam

U.S. FDA—Redbook 2000. Individual guidelines can be found at www.cfsan.fda.gov/~redbook. Developmental neurotoxicity testing may also be required.
Abbreviations: GD, gestation day; PD, postnatal day.

possible to include a listing of names for even the most common malformations due to space limitations. An internationally developed glossary on abnormalities has been published, and international efforts continue in reaching an accord on the most suitable terminology (11,12).

STUDY DESIGN AND STUDY PARAMETERS

Historically, the entire reproductive cycle has been split into three segments for testing purposes. This aids in data interpretation and helps in identification of specific stages that are targets of a particular toxin. The three segments generally cover the period of premating and mating through implantation (segment I), the period from implantation through major organogenesis (segment II), and finally late pregnancy and postnatal development (segment III). These three segments are: the "reproduction and fertility study," the "teratology study" (or developmental toxicity study), and the perinatal/postnatal study, respectively. For agents anticipated to provide low-level chronic exposure of populations (i.e., environmental pollutants, food additives), complete multigeneration studies over 2 to 3 generations may be required.

Various combinations of these studies may be acceptable as long as all required parameters are included and minimum study requirements met. Examples include combining a Segment I and II study or combining a Segment II and III study. In some cases (for example when test material is in very short supply), it may also be acceptable to conduct a Segment I protocol on the end of a one- or three-month toxicity study by adding in a mating period onto the end of the study.

Other test systems (both in vivo and in vitro) have been developed and used in preliminary, prescreening, or priority selection (13–22). However, these in vivo and in vitro screens and test systems are not considered substitutes for definitive DART testing by any government agency. In addition, these standard studies are not designed to study specific targets or possible mechanism(s) of toxicity. This is quite evident when one compares a list of the standard parameters actually measured in these studies to some of the possible targets in the male or female reproductive system or the developing fetus, which are much more numerous (Table 4). For this reason you will find included a few possible add-on and/or follow-up methods or studies at the end of this chapter that may be useful if further investigation or characterization of a test material is needed.

Study Basics

Test Material and Vehicle

The material to be tested should be the technical grade material or bulk chemical of the active ingredient. The characteristics of the test material (i.e., purity, composition, etc.) must be documented. If a vehicle is necessary for administration of the test material, then the choice of vehicle should be appropriate for the delivery of the test compound, should not interfere with absorption of the test material, and should not induce maternal or developmental toxicity. A vehicle control group should be part of the study design. In addition, a nontreated or sham control may be necessary when using a vehicle of unknown toxicity. Some of the most commonly used vehicles include water, powdered diet, hydroxymethylcellulose, corn oil, and saline. Test material/vehicle mixtures should be analyzed periodically during a study to verify concentration. In the relatively short treatment periods of Segment I, II, and III studies, analysis at the beginning and the end of treatment is sufficient. For longer multigeneration studies, additional analyses should be added. If the dosing preparation is in diet or is a suspension, homogeneity of the test preparation must also be verified at least once.

Test System

Species Selection. There is no "perfect" animal model in DART testing. Indeed, as one can see in Tables 5, 6, and 7, commonly used laboratory species can vary widely in male and female reproductive function as well as in timing and development of offspring. There are many good reviews in the published literature discussing species selection for both developmental and reproductive toxicity studies (23–26). Each species has its benefits and its problems, depending on which particular end points are of importance or what type of agent is being tested. It is very important that an investigator understand the animal model and use this knowledge in interpretation and extrapolation to human risk assessment. You will find that many guidelines suggest that one selects a species whose pharmacokinetics and metabolism most closely resemble that seen in humans. However, in the real world, data of this sort are rarely available at the time that DART studies are initiated. A common assumption that nonhuman primates should be the closest model to humans with regard to pharmacokinetics is simply not true. More often than not pharmacokinetics and toxicokinetics in primates can differ from humans as much as any other species. For all of these reasons, it is highly recommended that the reader avoid

Table 4 Possible Targets in Reproduction and Development Versus End Points Measured

MALE REPRODUCTIVE SYSTEM TARGETS

Production, secretion, and binding of key hormones in the pituitary-hypothalamus-gonadal axis
Production, secretion, and binding of local paracrine and autocrine factors
Production, proliferation, differentiation, and release of sperm in the testes
Transport, maturation, and storage of sperm in the epididymis
Production of seminal fluid/semen
Mating function—libido, mounting behavior, penile erection, ejaculation
Sperm viability, motility, and capacitation in the female reproductive tract

MALE REPRODUCTION PARAMETERS MEASURED

Copulatory interval, sperm in vagina
Resulting pregnancy and litter viability (fertility and fecundity indices)
Testicular, epididymal, seminal vesicle, and prostate histopathology

FEMALE REPRODUCTIVE SYSTEM TARGETS

Production, secretion, and binding of key hormones in the pituitary-hypothalamus-gonadal axis
Production, secretion, and binding of local paracrine and autocrine factors
Estrous cycle, ovarian follicular development, ovulation
Transport of ova in oviduct
Mating behavior—libido and lordosis
Fertilization of ova and blastocyst development
Uterine decidualization and implantation of the blastocyst
Placentation, corpora luteal function, and maintenance of pregnancy
Embryo and fetal nutrition
Parturition triggers and uterine contractility
Maternal behavior, milk production, and ejection

FEMALE REPRODUCTION PARAMETERS MEASURED

Estrous cycling
Copulatory interval, sperm in vagina
Resulting pregnancy and viability (fertility and fecundity indices)
Number of corpora lutea, litter size, early and late resorptions, abortions
Duration of gestation, duration of parturition, stillbirths
General maternal behavior and neonatal survival through weaning
Ovarian and uterine histopathology

TARGETS IN THE DEVELOPING OFFSPRING

Preimplantation development from 1st cleavage to blastocyst
Implantation and developmental of extraembryonic membranes
Organ development and maturation—inductive events, cell proliferation, differentiation, apoptosis, cell migration
Embryo/fetal/neonatal growth—growth factors, activators, and signaling systems
Postnatal physiological adaptation
Suckling behavior
Neonatal development and maturation through puberty

DEVELOPMENTAL PARAMETERS MEASURED

Pre- and postimplantation loss
Gross external, visceral, and skeletal morphology
Fetal and pup body weights
Pup maturational landmarks
Fetal and pup mortality
Pup behavior and reflex tests
Offspring reproductive capacity

Table 5 Species Comparison of Selected Male Reproductive Parameters

	Mouse	Rat	Rabbit	Dog	Monkey	Man
Male breeding age	8–10 weeks	8–12 weeks	6–7 months	10–14 months	3–6 years	Variable
Testis weight (g)	0.15–0.22	1.8–2.6	6.4	11.2–22.4	49	34
Seminiferous cycle (days)	8.9	12.9–13.3	10–10.7	13.6	9.5	16–16.9
Duration of spermatogenesis (days)	35	48–52	39–42	42	38	74
Daily sperm production (10^6)	5	86	160	290–594	110–1000	125–207
Sperm/g testis (10^6/g)	28–63	12–24	24–25	11–24	23	4.4
Epididymal transit time (days)	5–10	7.2–11	9–12.7	11.3	10.5	5.5–12
Cauda sperm reserves (10^6)	49	440	600–1600	2100	5700	182–420
Ejaculate volume (ml)	0.01–0.04	0.03–0.1	0.23–0.64	0.2–2.6	0.09–0.32	1.9–3
Sperm concentration (10^6/mL)	2.5–5	NA	150–263	89–361	419–1154	80
Total sperm (10^6)	0.02	60	NA	84–107	34	350
Motile sperm (mean %)	49–74	50–61	71–83	26–30	54–75	31.7–68

Mean values collected from a wide range of published data and reviews; averages and ranges may vary according to strains within a species.
Abbreviation: NA, not available.

any studies with other than the most commonly used species, the rat and rabbit, for studies that are to be submitted to a government agency unless conferring with an expert. One exception is when testing of a biologics for which rodents may lack the receptor for the test material. Thus, one can expect to use the rat in Segment I, II and III protocols as well as in multigeneration studies. The rabbits are used only in Segment II studies, as the required second, nonrodent species.

Animal Source and Age.   Animals should come from suppliers that can guarantee the health and lineage of the animals. This means animals are often "cesarean-derived," usually from outbred colonies, such as Sprague-Dawley or Wistar rats or New Zealand White or Dutch Belted rabbits. It is beneficial to use the same strain of rat as used in other toxicological studies, if possible, because previous data will help in dosage selection. Animals should be young, but mature adults at the time of mating and the females should be virgin. Age of sexual maturity will be dependent on the strain of the animal selected. Generally, rats should be at least 12 weeks old and rabbits at least five months old at the time of mating. Using animals not fully mature will increase the variability of reproductive parameters, reduce the sensitivity of the study to identify adverse events, and in some cases completely compromise an agency's acceptability of the study. A good study shows a greater than 85–90% pregnancy rate in the controls. Animals to be used in Segment I studies should be acclimated to the study room for at least two weeks prior to initiation of the study. This will allow time for the estrous cycle, which is often irregular following the

Table 6 Species Comparison of Selected Female Reproductive Parameters

	Mouse	Rat	Rabbit	Dog	Monkey	Human
Female breeding age (days)	28–49	46–53	120–240	270–425	1642	4380–4745
Female cycle type	Estrous	Estrous	Estrous	Seasonal	Menstrual	Menstrual
Cycle duration (days)	4–6	4–5	None[a]	150–200	24–38	28–29
Luteotropic hormone(s)	LH/P/E	LH/P/E	E	LH/P	LH	LH
Uterine luteolysis	Yes	Yes	Yes	Yes	No	No
CL dependency[b] (days)	All	All	All	NA	27–28	40
Pituitary dependency[b] (days)	11–12	12	All	NA	32–40	40
Placenta type	Hemotri-chorial	Hemotri-chorial	Hemodi-chorial	Endothelio-chorial	Hemomono-chorial	Hemomono-chorial
Gestation length (days)	18–20	20–22	29–34	53–71	159–174	252–280

Mean values collected from a wide range of published data and reviews; averages and ranges may vary according to strains within a species.
[a]Ovulation induced by coitus.
[b]Number of days that pregnancy is dependent upon the corpus luteum or pituitary. Expressed as days from the time of ovulation.
Abbreviations: LH, luteinizing hormone; P, prolactin; E, estrogen; NA, not available.

stress of shipping, to normalize. Many suppliers will mate or artificially inseminate the animals ("timed pregnant animals") for use in Segment II or III studies. This is especially useful in laboratories that do not want to spend the time or expense of maintaining a colony of breeder males. In these cases, animals will be placed on study as soon as they arrive.

Number of Animals. The numbers of rats and/or rabbits used on a study varies according to study type and expected pregnancy rate. Generally a minimum of 20–30 per

Table 7 Species Comparison of Selected Embryo/Fetal Developmental Parameters

	Mouse	Rat	Rabbit	Dog	Monkey	Man
Blastocyst formation (days)	3–6	3–5	2.6–6	4–5.2	4–9	4–8
Implantation (days)	4–7	5–6	7–8	19–22	9–11	8–13
Major organogenesis (days)	6–16	6–17	6–20	18–35	20–45	21–56
Gestation length (days)	18–20	20–23	29–34	53–71	159–174	252–274
Spontaneous abortion	No	No	Yes	Yes	Yes	Yes
Litter size	4–12	8–12	4–10	1–15	1	1
Birth weight (g)	1.5	5	50	270	500	3300
Spontaneous malfor-mation rate (%)	1–19	0.02–2	0.7–6.3	0.2–2	0.1–0.4	0.14–14

Mean values collected from a wide range of published data and reviews; averages and ranges may vary according to strains within a species.

group for rat and rabbits (3 treated and 1 vehicle control group) are included. Many guidelines give only the required "minimum" number of pregnancies for an acceptable study. It is up to the investigator to decide how many animals they will need to use per group to reach this number at study termination. It is also becoming more common to add additional animals (e.g., 4–5/sex/group) in a study to serve as satellite animals for evaluation of drug blood levels (see Toxicokinetics below). The supplier's and/or laboratory's historical control pregnancy rate for this species should be taken into account when deciding group numbers. The goal is to have sufficient numbers of pregnant animals to make accurate interpretations and maintain consistency studies. The International Conference Harmonization (ICH) Guidelines for testing of human drugs (23) state that: "Below 16 litters per group, study results become inconsistent, above 20 to 24 litters per group, consistency and precision are not greatly enhanced." In multigeneration studies, the starting group size for the first generation (F_0) may need to be larger than in other studies to allow for natural losses and still attain a sufficient number of litters for evaluation of an F_2 or even F_3 generation. In studies with larger animals, such as primates or dogs, smaller group sizes are more common and accepted. Animals used in the study should be individually identified (e.g., tattoo, ear punch, or biochip implant) and should be assigned into dosage groups by some appropriate randomization method based on body weight.

The treated and control groups are always run concurrently. However, it is not unusual in Segment II studies to stagger the day of pregnancy over a few days so that one has, for example, one quarter of each group's animals starting on one day, one quarter more starting on the next day, and so on. This is acceptable to the agencies as long as the stagger evenly distributes animals among each group and each day. It is important not to stagger the animals over too long a period of time. Staggering allows more time on the day of cesarean section for completion of all of the uterine and fetal examinations.

Dosage Selection

Selection of dosages is one of the most critical issues in the design of DART studies and one of the most difficult tasks. In addition, agency expectations with regard to dosage selection and desired outcome can differ between agencies due to their differing approaches to risk assessment (27–31). Dosage selection generally requires quite a bit of experience and is very much test material specific. However, there are a few basic rules that should be kept in mind. One generally wants to see some overt toxicity at the highest dosage level, or in the case of some drugs, a maximally tolerated pharmacological effect. This can be in the form of toxicologically significant reductions in body weight and/or food consumption (i.e., > 10%). Lethality should be kept low (usually stated as below 10%) to ensure adequate numbers for evaluation. If necessary, clinical chemistry parameters, organ weights, and/or histopathology can also be incorporated into the study to document sufficient toxicity. This high dose should also not result in excessive abortion or death of the embryo or fetus, again to ensure adequate numbers for evaluation. However, although excessive toxicity at the high dose can create difficulties in data interpretation, in reality there is more danger of study rejection by the agency if the highest dosage level is too low (i.e., without significant toxicity).

If an agent is simply not very toxic, the maximum dosage level stipulated in the guideline, termed the "limit dose" (i.e., 1 g/kg, 1% or 5% of diet; 5 mg/l; 1000 mg/kg) can be used. In some instances pharmacokinetics can be used for dosage justification when increasing dosages administered do not produce increasing blood or tissue levels of a test substance.

The lowest dosage level should not induce toxicity. For drugs, the lowest dosage level is usually selected based on either the clinically intended pharmacological effect or as a multiple of the anticipated human exposure. The intermediate dose is usually logarithmically placed between the high and low dosage and ideally should induce some minimal observable toxic effect.

Dosage selection for Segment I or multigeneration studies can be based on data collected from previous subchronic toxicity studies in the rat. Using similar dosage levels also has the added benefit of allowing direct comparison of dosage levels producing reproductive toxicity with those producing systemic toxicity. If the guideline requires that maternal treatment be continued through gestation and that offspring be evaluated, then consideration of offspring survival must also be taken into account (see below). In general, dosages used in longer term DART studies are usually lower than those selected for Segment II and Segment III studies.

Dosage selection for the Segment II studies in rat and rabbit are usually based on small non-GLP dosage range-finding (RF) studies in pregnant animals. These RF studies are necessary for identifying dosage levels with sufficient maternal toxicity, but minimal embryonic/fetal loss. They should also flag for possible differences in pharmacokinetics between pregnant and nonpregnant animals. There are no set rules to follow in the design of these studies, but most agencies are now requiring laboratories to report all findings from these studies. Interpretation of RF study results outside of its use as a guide in dosage selection is problematic and full of pitfalls. This is due to the small number of animals per group and the often excessive maternal toxicity. Thus, one needs to be careful that the study is conducted with some forethought. Most often these studies are conducted with 3–5 animals per groups (plus satellite animals for blood level determination) in 4–5 treated groups and one vehicle control group. The highest dosage can be set as high as the LD_{10} (dose lethal to 10% of the animals), as determined in an acute study. The treatment period should be the same as that to be used in the definitive Segment II study. Evaluation of uterine contents can be made at Gestation Day 13 (determining viable and nonviable implants) or near term (Gestation Day 20). Some investigators prefer to sacrifice animals at Gestation Day 20, weigh the gravid uterus, and determine viability of the implants (by fetal movement) without opening the uterus. Estimates of fetal weights are made by dividing the gravid uterine weight by the number of full term fetuses. This allows one to get a general idea about dosages inducing maternal toxicity or embryo or fetal mortality as well as possible effects on fetal growth. Alternatively, fetuses can be removed, individually weighed, and evaluated for gross external, visceral, and/or skeletal morphology. However, many investigators do not feel that it is worth the time and expense of doing this in a RF study.

Dosages selected for the Segment III study are most often the same as those used in the Segment II rat study.

Route and Frequency of Administration

The route of administration should be similar to expected human exposure. Alternative routes may be acceptable if it can be shown that similar systemic exposures are achieved. Oral gavage is the most common method of administration in Segment I, II, and III studies. Addition of test material to the diet or drinking water is the most commonly recommended route in multigeneration tests. Methods have been developed for most routes, from inhalation to sublingual to intravenous infusion. These can vary widely in cost, labor, and accuracy and not all contract laboratories will have the expertise needed, especially on DART studies.

Most DART studies are conducted using single daily dosing. Dosing should be performed at approximately the same time each day. If the test material has a very short half-life in the animal, administration may have to be increased to twice (bid) or even three times a day (tid) to ensure reasonable exposures. In some circumstances where a test material is known to have cumulative effects or is associated with rapid development of tolerance, one may have to dose less frequently or for a shorter treatment period. It is also possible to conduct the DART review using more than three segments (i.e., into 6–8 segments), if necessary. It is not unusual in drug development to have an agent being developed for single use (e.g., diagnostics or surgical medicines, such as anesthetics) where it may not be possible to administer repeated dosages for the required length of time in the guidelines. In such cases, reducing the length of the treatment period but using a higher dosage may be more appropriate than administration over the required treatment period at a much reduced dosage.

The required period of treatment is dependent on the specific guideline (Tables 1–3). In Segment I studies the treatment period begins prior to mating. Historically, a longer period of premating treatment (i.e., up to 80 days) was thought to be necessary in males to extend treatment over at least one full cycle of spermatogenesis. However, recent prospective and retrospective analyses of reproductive data (32,33) reveal that the longer exposure period is not necessary in most standard studies in order to correctly flag male reproductive toxins. For males, current guidelines require premating exposures ranging from 30 to 70 days. Administration to the males is generally continued until they are sacrificed. For females, current guidelines require premating exposures ranging from 14 to 70 days. The end of the treatment period in the female is dependent upon the study design and can range from Gestation Day 6 (when implantation occurs) to the end of the lactation period (Postnatal Day 21).

Historically, in Segment II studies pregnant females are treated during what is commonly referred to as the "major period of organogenesis." This includes the period from implantation to closure of the hard palate (roof of the mouth). This translates into Gestation Day 6–15 in the rat and Gestation Day 6–18 in the rabbit. These are the exposure periods currently required in drug safety testing. Although most of the major organ systems are formed during this period, organogenesis actually extends well into the postnatal period, particularly development of the central nervous system. The new harmonized guidelines for testing of chemicals now required exposures from implantation to the end of gestation.

The treatment period in Segment III studies usually extends at least from closure of the hard palate (Gestation Day 15) until the end of the lactation period (Postnatal Day 21). Some investigators extend this to start treatment as early as Gestation Day 6.

Toxicokinetics

Toxicokinetics simply refers to pharmacokinetic data collected from or to support a toxicology study. It is used primarily to document systemic exposure levels in a study and aids in extrapolation of the study results to other animal studies and to risk assessment in humans. One may also come across the term "pharmacodynamics," which generally refers to the relationship between drug concentration and effect. Such data are usually expressed in terms of the AUC, C_{max} and $t_{1/2}$. AUC or "Area Under the Curve" is an expression of total exposure, i.e., the blood concentration of an agent over a specified time period; ng.hr/ml. The C_{max} refers to the peak concentration measured in the blood. The $t_{1/2}$ refers to the time it takes for half of the test material to clear from the system and is therefore a measure of duration of exposure.

Not all agencies require collection of toxicokinetic data at this time, although there is a growing trend to do so (34). There are no fast rules as to what study day samples should be taken. It is suggested that satellite animals be used for this purpose rather than the main study animals because multiple sampling times result in large amounts of blood withdrawal, which can confound study results and interpretation. Timing of the samples on the selected day is very much dependent on compound and route of administration but usually entails at least four samples anywhere from 5 minutes out to 24 hours postadministration. In the Segment I study, the preferred sampling time for blood collection is just prior to mating from both the F_0 males and females. Selection of the best sampling day for Segment II studies is less clear due to the constantly changing system. Sample collection near the end of the treatment period appears to be the most appropriate time, in most cases.

Most often toxicokinetics data are not collected in Segment III studies. Rather data are collected in a separately run pharmacokinetic study to investigate transfer of test material into milk, often using radiolabeled test material. The data on test material transfer and concentration in milk are very important in the risk assessment of exposure to nursing women and their infants.

Test material concentration may also be measured in fetal blood (or amniotic fluid) to assess levels of placental transfer and possible accumulation. This technique requires quite a bit of expertise and is most easily conducted on term fetuses due to the small blood volumes. If necessary, blood from an entire litter may be pooled.

Parameters to Be Measured

General Observations

There are two basic types of observations. The first is a daily (sometimes twice daily) check for signs of morbidity, mortality, abortion, or early delivery. The second type of observation is a much more detailed assessment in which the animals are removed from their cages and observed for any physical or behavioral abnormalities ("clinical signs of toxicity"). The detailed observation is usually conducted at a selected time after dosage administration. All findings are recorded, including those that may not be considered treatment related. Possible observations are numerous and can range from localized hair loss, excessive salivation, alterations in respiration, and abnormal gaits to tremors or convulsion.

Body Weights and Food Consumption

Body weights are recorded daily, twice weekly, or weekly depending on the guideline and on the reproductive phase (i.e., premating, gestation, lactation). Body weights during the premating and mating period are usually taken weekly or twice weekly. During the gestation period, body weights are recorded either daily or at intervals (i.e., Gestation Day 0, 6, 9, 12, 15, 18, and 20). Maternal and pup body weights in the postnatal period are usually taken weekly (i.e., Postnatal Day 0,7,14, and 21). Food and, in some cases, water consumption are generally measured in the same intervals as body weights.

Vaginal Smears

Vaginal smears can be used for two purposes: to monitor the estrous cycle and to verify mating. Daily vaginal smears allow determination of the cycle stage (proestrus, estrus, metestrus, and diestrus) based on vaginal cytology (35). The estrous cycle in rats normally lasts 4–5 days. Chemicals capable of disrupting the pituitary-hypothalamus-gonadal axis often affect this cycle. For example, chemicals with estrogenic properties will induce the system into prolonged estrus. The method and experience of the technician taking the vaginal smear is important because it is easy to put the female into pseudopregnancy (i.e., prolonged diestrus) with overt vaginal stimulation in rodents. It also takes an experienced technician to interpret the stages properly. Slides can be fixed and stained if a permanent record is needed. Although not required, it is recommended that the estrous cycle be monitored for at least 10 days pretreatment in a Segment I study to ensure that the females placed on study are cycling normally. Females are continued to be monitored during the treatment period until sperm positive during the cohabitation phase. It may be necessary to allow a nontreated recovery period for females who are not cycling before initiating mating. Animal mating is verified by the presence of a vaginal plug or sperm in the vaginal smear (see below).

Cohabitation

The female should always be placed into the male's cage and not vice versa. The rats are usually placed together in the late afternoon and left together overnight. The preferred mating ratio is 1:1 because it is more likely to result in good pregnancy rates and for the ease it allows in compiling and interpreting data. Some guidelines do allow mating two females with one male. Each morning the technician looks for signs of a vaginal plug (coagulated mass of semen), either within the vagina or discharged and found on the bottom of the cage. If a plug is not found, a vaginal smear should be taken to examine for vaginal sperm. The mating period allowed varies from 2 to 3 weeks. Most rats will mate within the first five days of cohabitation (i.e., at the first available estrus) if cycling normally. In some cases females may become pseudopregnant. The longer mating period allows time for these females to restart estrous cycling and hopefully become pregnant. In instances where it appears that fertility problems may be due to a dysfunction of the male system, the mating period usually allows time for an unmated female to be placed with a second proven male from the same test group. The day that mating is verified is usually considered Day 0 of gestation. Records should be made of all cohabitation and matings. The time between initial cohabitation and mating is termed the "copulatory interval."

Female Sacrifice

Gestation Day 13 Uterine Examination. Many investigators prefer to evaluate pregnancy status in an ICH Segment I study at Gestation Day 13. However, other guidelines may require evaluation on Gestation Day 20 or 21 (see below). At Gestation Day 13 the implants should be identified by position within the uterine horns and recorded as simply viable or nonviable. This may be accomplished without opening the uterus. The Gestation Day 13 uterus may be opened and the implants examined for abnormalities, but this requires an expertise that many laboratories do not have. The number of corpora lutea on each ovary is also recorded. The female should be subjected to a gross necropsy, and the reproductive organs, and other tissues as required, should be weighed and saved for possible histopathology.

Term Cesarean Section. In term sacrifices (Gestation Day 20 or 21 in the rat or Gestation Day 29 in the rabbit) the uterus is removed, weighed (termed "gravid uterine weight"), and then opened. The number and uterine positions of any early and late resorptions and viable and dead fetuses are recorded. Early and late resorptions are differentiated by the extent of autolysis (i.e., to what degree fetal features are recognizable). The individual term fetuses are carefully removed from their membranes, the umbilical cord cut, and further examined as described below. The placentas are examined for any abnormalities and saved if required. The number of corpora lutea on each ovary is recorded. Again, the female should be subjected to a gross necropsy and the reproductive organs, and other tissues as required, should be weighed and saved for possible histopathology. For apparently "nonpregnant" rats (but not rabbits), ammonium sulfide staining of the uterus can be used to identify peri-implantation deaths that are otherwise not visible upon gross exam.

Sacrifice at End of Lactation Period.   In Segment III and multigeneration studies, dams are usually sacrificed after weaning of the offspring on Postnatal Day 21. The female should be subjected to a gross necropsy and the reproductive organs, and other tissues as required, should be saved for possible histopathology.

Fetal Evaluations

At Necropsy.   Fetuses should be individually identified so that there is a record of both what litter they are from and in what position they were found in the uterus. Most laboratories do this by means of a stringed tag around the neck. Each fetus is sexed (verified internally at visceral examination) and weighed. The crown-rump length and angiogenital distance may also be recorded; however, this can be time consuming and is usually not required. Each fetus is then externally examined for abnormalities. Only dead fetuses that do not show any significant degree of maceration should be included in the external and subsequent examinations because of the frequent distortions and artifacts encountered in such specimens.

Observed abnormalities are commonly classified into malformations and developmental variations. There is no such thing as a "clean" study; all studies will include at least some incidence of variations. There are no standards for these classifications, and minor differences between laboratories can be expected. Malformations can be defined as "those structural anomalies that alter general body conformity, disrupt or interfere with body function, or are generally thought to be incompatible with life." On the other hand, developmental variations are defined as "those alterations in anatomic structure that are considered to have no significant biological effect on animal health or body conformity, representing slight deviations from normal." Some laboratories include variations in degree of ossification into this category. However, there is a trend to classify variations in ossifications separately as they are generally related to small differences between litters in time of conception and implantation or in many cases related to intrauterine growth. Some guidelines require photographic records of all malformations and representative variations on a study. It is recommended this be done for all studies.

Once the external examination is complete, the fetuses are euthanized. The method of fetal sacrifice can affect the quality of the fetal tissue in subsequent evaluation. For example intraperitoneal injection of drugs may cause a breakdown in abdominal tissues. The most commonly used method of sacrifice is CO_2 asphyxiation or immersion. In rat studies, either one-half or one-third of the fetuses are subjected to visceral examination for anomalies. The remaining fetuses are fixed and processed for subsequent skeletal examination. In rabbit studies, all the fetuses undergo both a visceral and skeletal examination.

Visceral Examination.   Examination of the viscera can be conducted using a variety of methods. Rabbit fetuses are most often evaluated on the day of necropsy as fresh specimens using a necropsy method known as the Staple's method (36–38). This examination includes not only evaluation of abdominal and thoracic organs but also specific cuts into the head to assess eye, brain, nasal passages, palate, and the tongue. Because many laboratories do not have the manpower to conduct all of these evaluations in a single day, the Staple's method has also been used on ethanol and Bouin's fixed specimens. However, fixation can leave the tissues less manageable to manipulate for a proper examination. Historically, Bouin's fixed fetuses are evaluated using a serial slicing method known as the Wilson technique (39) or a combination of both methods. Various modifications and additions to these methods have been published (40–45).

Skeletal Examination. Fetuses selected for skeletal examination are fixed in ethanol, then "cleared" and stained by a KOH-Alizarin Red S technique (46). This method leaves a stained and intact skeleton sheathed within a transparent "body." Some recent guidelines also suggest a preference double staining with alcian blue, which stains cartilage. Examination includes enumeration of the vertebra, ribs, and other bone/cartilage structures, degree of ossification, and any fusions or abnormalities in bone shape or position. Again various modifications and additions to this method have been published (47–51).

Parturition

The pregnant females are placed in "litter" cages with solid floors and nesting material at least two days prior to expected parturition. The start of labor and its progress is noted when possible. In many cases labor will start or finish during off hours, making observations on the entire process difficult. In so far as possible parturition should be observed for any signs of difficulty or unusual duration. The date when all pups are considered delivered is designated as Postpartum, Postnatal, or Lactation Day 0. Usually litters born overnight will be considered to have been delivered on the morning they are found.

Postnatal Observations

As soon as possible after delivery is complete, the pups are counted, sexed, weighed, and externally examined for grossly visible abnormalities. Pups and dams are observed and weighed weekly. Survival checks should be conducted daily. Many laboratories consider any pup found dead on Postnatal Day 0 as stillborn by default. A "lung flotation test" can be used as a more definitive method for differentiating stillborn pups from those dying after birth. In all cases dead pups should be necropsied as soon as possible to evaluate for abnormalities. It is also not uncommon for rodents to cannibalize dead or injured pups. Missing pups are classified with the dead pups when evaluating data.

Reduction of litter size by culling (usually to four males and four females per litter) has been conducted historically, based on the premise that this equalizes or reduces differences in maternal care and nutrition due to litter size. However, some debate still continues with regard to this practice (52). Culling is most commonly conducted on Postnatal Day 4 with pup body weights recorded before and after. All culled pups should be randomly selected.

Pups are weaned from the dams on Postnatal Day 21. A selected number of this F_1 generation can be continued on study for additional behavioral testing and/or to evaluate F_1 reproductive capacity as required. F_1 pups not selected are usually necropsied and tissues saved as outlined for the F_0 generation.

Offspring Developmental, Reflex, and Behavioral Indices

Segment III studies include evaluation of not only offspring growth and survival but also their behavioral development (53,54). At various times throughout the lactation period and early postweaning period, the pups are evaluated using a variety of developmental and behavioral endpoints. Guidelines leave some leeway in the choice of methods, but the testing should include at least some measure of sensory development, activity, and learning/memory function. Developmental indices (Table 8) include such end points as time of pinna detachment, eye opening, tooth eruption, and hair growth and are generally

Table 8 Developmental Landmarks Measured in Rat Offspring

Parameter	Earliest testing start[a] (postnatal day)
Pinna detachment	1
General hair growth	2
Upper incisor eruption	9
Eye opening	13
Testicular descent	22
Vaginal opening	34
Pubertial separation	38

[a]If not present, landmark is looked for daily until acquisition.

coincident with pup growth. Reflex testing (Table 9) should also be part of any standard pup evaluation and can include such reflexes as surface righting as early as Postnatal Day 1 to airdrop righting reflex and startle reflex testing in the late lactation period. It is very important that each parameter be measured at the appropriate time in development. Additional testing can include cliff aversion prior to eye opening, tests of motor development and coordination (negative geotaxis, rotarod, hindlimb support and visual placement), and an open field neuropharmacological evaluation. After weaning on Postnatal Day 21, 1–2 pups/sex/litter are selected to continue behavioral testing and to produce the F_2 litter. Activity level, exploratory and basal, can be quantified in an "activity chamber" using photobeam technology. The most complex testing involves the learning and memory function, which can be measured by various methods, including active or passive avoidance test, maze test, or swimming test.

Offspring Reproductive Capacity

The first end points in the evaluation of offspring reproductive capacity in a Segment III study are two additional developmental indices for sexual maturation: vaginal opening in females and testes descent or preputial separation in males (Table 8). Both of these indices are very sensitive to small changes in hormonal status during gestation and/or lactation. In both Segment III studies and multigeneration studies, offspring reproduction is usually conducted as described for the F_0 generation. Care must be taken so as not to mate siblings. In ICH Segment III studies it is preferable to euthanize and evaluate F_1 pregnancy status using a Gestation Day 13 uterine examination. Guidelines for multigeneration studies may

Table 9 Reflex Indices Measured in Rat Offspring

Parameter	Earliest testing start[a] (postnatal day)
Righting reflex	1
Suckling reflex	1
Cliff aversion	11
Negative geotaxis	12
Corneal reflex	After eye opening
Pupillary reflex	After eye opening
Air-drop righting reflex	16
Pain response (tail pinch)	22
Auditory startle	33

[a]If not present, landmark is looked for daily until acquisition.

require the F_2 litter to be evaluated in a Gestation Day 20 cesarean section with fetal evaluations or to carry out the F_2 or even F_3 generation through weaning. In some instances animals may be required to produce more than one litter. In this case generations will be referred to as the F_{1a} or F_{1b} generation.

Male Sacrifice

It is always advisable to delay the sacrifice of the males until after the outcome of mating is known (via cesarean section or natural parturition). In the event of observed effects on pregnancy, these treated males can be mated again to untreated females to ascertain their role in the adverse effect on fertility. When the males are sacrificed, they too should be subject to a gross necropsy. Evaluations may include organ weights and macroscopic examination of the testes, epididymides, seminal vesicle, and prostate. Tissues are generally saved for possible histopathology. At necropsy one of the testes and/or epididymides may be used to quantify sperm concentration and/or evaluate sperm morphology and motility (55).

Histopathology of Reproductive Tissues

Some guidelines specifically require that microscopic examination be conducted on male and female reproductive organs. It is very important to have histopathology data especially if sufficient histopathology of the reproductive organs is not available or if the quality of the data is dubious from the 1 and/or 3 months general toxicity study. Histopathologic changes in the reproductive organs can be one of the most sensitive end points in DART studies. There has been much debate about adding requirements for labor intensive serial section and cell staging of the testes and ovary. At this time, it is not necessary in DART screening studies to evaluate numerous serial sections of the ovary and testis or to conduct a full staging evaluation. However, the pathologist should have specialized training so as to identify situations in which more complex qualitative and quantitative analysis should be done (56–59).

To correctly evaluate testicular morphology, the tissue must be preserved properly (57,58). The most common tissue preservation method, fixation in formalin and paraffin embedding, are not acceptable for testicular tissue and do not permit adequate assessment of testicular cytoarchitecture or spermatogenic stages. The techniques resulting in the highest quality sections for testicular examination uses Davidson's fixative or perfusion fixation and plastic (i.e., glycol methacrylate) embedding. However, on a routine basis, fixation in Bouin's solution, paraffin embedding and staining with PAS also produces acceptable tissues for proper examination.

DATA COMPILATION, INTERPRETATION, AND RISK ASSESSMENT

The purpose of DART testing is to establish whether a test material has the potential to induce adverse effects on the male and female reproductive system or development of the conceptus and to establish the potency or dosage levels that cause the specific adverse effects. Once this information is established, an assessment can be made of the agent's hazard potential and actual risk it poses to humans by bringing in exposure information as well as data from other toxicology studies, pharmacokinetics, and mechanistic studies (28,30,31,60,61). From a regulatory standpoint, a compound's reproductive and developmental toxicity is of most concern in risk assessment when the dosage level inducing DART effects is below that associated with systemic toxicity in adults. If the dosage level inducing adverse DART effects is above those causing systemic toxicity, then safe exposure levels set to protect against systemic toxicity will usually also protect against adverse reproductive effects. Agents producing DART effects at dosages below those inducing systemic toxicity are generally referred to as "selective" reproductive or developmental toxins.

The minimal acceptability criterion for a DART study is demonstrable toxicity to the F_0 parents or dosing up to the "limit" dose. Although it is advantageous to demonstrate a no-observable-effect level (NOEL), as well as a lowest-observable-effect level (LOEL), for the F_0 generation, as long as a NOEL for developmental toxicity is observed on the study, this is not absolutely necessary. The absence of a parental LOEL and/or a developmental NOEL may require repeating the DART study at either higher or lower dosage levels. In developmental toxicity studies an "inadequate" number of litters for fetal evaluations in a dose group(s), due to excess infertility, resorptions, fetal death, or maternal death, may also lead to the need for an additional dose groups to be tested.

Tools Needed in Interpretation of DART Data

All data needs to be included in the final report. This includes not only summary tables, incorporating group means, but also tables presenting all individual animal data. It is very important in DART studies to include all individual data in such a manner that the reader can associate all maternal and fetal findings with specific animal numbers and times. Not only group means but also individual values should be considered carefully when interpreting results.

Statistical analysis should be used to determine whether results differ significantly from those of the controls. There are no specific types of statistical tests required. The statistical methods applied should be appropriate for the type of end point being evaluated (61–66). There has been a long debate on whether the entire litter or the individual fetus should be treated as the experimental unit in statistical evaluation; most investigators include statistics using both. Some of the tests that have been employed in the statistical analysis of DART data include analysis of variance (ANOVA), analysis of covariance (ANCOVA), Bonferroni inequality test, Bartlett's test for homogeneity, student t-test, chi square test, Fischer's exact test, jackknife procedures, Mann-Whitney U-test, student-Newman-Keuls multiple range test, and rank transformation.

Historical control values for DART parameters are also very important for comparative purposes (67). These are basically data from the control groups of past studies compiled by study date. A lab experienced in conducting DART studies should have historical control records from numerous studies. Because of genetic drift over time in the outbred animal strains used in DART studies, an investigator will usually rely on historical control data that is within $\pm$ 2 years of the initiation of the study being considered. It is best to use historical data from the same laboratory in which the study was conducted. However, published historical control data (68–71) may also be used, when necessary, as long as it is a compilation of data on the same strain and, if possible, the same source (i.e., colony). The vehicle and route of administration used in the control data studies may also be a possible variable and should be considered when deciding what historical control data are appropriate to use for comparison to your study. An example of a typical historical control range of means for cesarean section parameters for rats and rabbits are given in Tables 10 and 11.

For many of the parameters measured in DART studies, the power to discriminate between random variation and true treatment effect (i.e., the statistical sensitivity) is poor

Table 10 Typical Historical Control for Selected Cesarean Section Parameters in Sprague-Dawley Rats

	Range of means
Mean corpora lutea per dam	13.3–18.0
Mean total implantations per dam	11.6–16.0
Mean early resorptions per dam	0.1–1.3
Mean late resorptions per dam	0.0–0.5
Mean dead fetuses per dam	0.0–0.1
Mean viable fetuses per dam	7.4–15.1
Group mean preimplantation loss	0.4–3.4
Group mean postimplantation loss	0.1–1.3
Mean body weight of male fetuses (g)	3.5–4.0
Mean body weight of female fetuses (g)	3.3–3.9
Sex ratio (% males)	41.8–57.3
Mean gravid uterine weight (g)	6.66–94.7

due to the small number of animals, the wide variability of some end points, and the normally low incidence rates of others. For example, with 20 animals per group, it would require an incidence rate 5–12 fold above control levels to detect a statistical increase in malformations compared to a 3–6 fold increase for postimplantation deaths and a 0.15–0.25 fold change in fetal body weight (30). Moreover, the way in which statistical results are used in data interpretation has been under debate (72). The absence of a statistically significant difference from the control value does not necessarily negate the "biologic" significance of an observed change. In this case, the investigator must rely on historical control values, possible dosage-related trend, and experience when deciding whether the "effect" is real or not. On the other hand, the presence of statistical significance also does not make an "effect" biologically or toxicologically significant, especially if the value of the end point in question is within the historical control range for that parameter. The probability of detecting at least one statistical false positive in a study with numerous biological parameters is very high (60).

Table 11 Typical Historical Control for Selected Cesarean Section Parameters in New Zealand White Rabbits

	Range of means
Mean corpora lutea per dam	8.8–17.5
Mean total implantations per dam	2.7–9.9
Mean early resorptions per dam	0.0–2.3
Mean late resorptions per dam	0.0–0.7
Mean dead fetuses per dam	0.0–0.2
Mean viable fetuses per dam	2.7–9.3
Group mean preimplantation loss	1.2–10.3
Group mean postimplantation loss	0.0–2.8
Mean body weight of male fetuses (g)	32.7–49.2
Mean body weight of female fetuses (g)	29.9–45.6
Sex ratio (% males)	36.9–63.3
Mean gravid uterine weight (g)	230.0–596.4

The dose-response can be fundamental in determining if there is, in fact, a true reproductive or developmental effect. The most commonly observed dose-response is characterized by an effect occurring with greater frequency and/or severity as the dosage level is increased. Thus, one would question a possible treatment-related effect if one were to see a higher incidence of an effect in the low- and high-dosage groups compared to controls but not in the mid-dosage group. One must also keep in mind that developmental and reproductive toxicity are assumed to be threshold phenomenon (i.e., they show a threshold dosage level below which adverse effects are not seen). Because of the small number of treated groups and the often steep dose-response curve, it is not uncommon in DART studies to have some apparent effects only at the high-dosage level. This is particularly true under circumstances where developmental toxicity is observed only at levels associated with severe maternal toxicity. There is also the possibility of observing a plateau effect, where no increase in incidence or severity of a particular effect can be induced by increasing the dosage level. This is often due to dose-dependent toxicokinetic limitations. Finally, one needs to consider the impact of "competing" end points on the dose-response patterns (e.g., increase in postimplantation loss covering up any chance of observing a nonlethal effect at high dosage levels).

Effects should be biologically plausible. For example, one may expect to see a test material effect on corpora lutea count in a Segment I study where test material exposure occurred during the time of ovulation and early pregnancy. On the other hand, the number of corpora lutea among test groups in a Segment II or III study should be within the same range as control because compound administration was initiated after implantation. Biologic plausibility would also suggest it unlikely to have an effect, for example, on fetal bone ossification in a Segment I where exposure to the dam did not occur at the time of fetal bone development. Also inherent in plausibility is the stipulation that effects should concur across studies. For example, the validity of a treatment related reduction in offspring weight would be questioned if fetal weights were reduced in the Segment II study, but Day 0 pup weights showed no reduction in the Segment III study at the same dosage level.

Interpretation of Specific Endpoints

Clinical Observation Data

Clinical observations are not always related to toxic effects of the test material. Prior identification of specific findings in previous studies, as well as a dose-response incidence, is an important sign of compound related toxicity. The timing and duration of the observed signs can also help in interpretation. However, confounding factors, including concomitant disease, environmental factors, or technical errors, must also be considered. Hopefully, the use of quality SPF ("specified pathogen free") animals and examination of animals by a veterinarian prior to placement on study should reduce the incidence of spontaneous disease in the test animals. However, there is no procedure that can completely eliminate the possibility. A certain combination of signs and histopathology, as well as a lack of dose-response, can suggest such a confounding factor to the investigator. For example, in rabbits, clinical signs—such as nasal discharge and/or diarrhea, along with histopathological evidence of lung congestion and/or pitted kidneys—have been associated with pasteurellosis and coccidiosis infection. A high enough incidence and severity of such observations indicating questionable health status of the test animals may make a study unacceptable for submission.

Stressful environmental factors, including low humidity, extreme temperatures, or inadequate food and water availability, can also lead to morbidity which can confound study interpretation. Even such factors as suboptimal caging or mishandling of the animals can lead to clinical signs, such as hair loss, abrasions, scabbing, broken teeth, and injured or even broken limbs.

When an animal dies on study, it is very important to try to determine a possible cause of death at necropsy. Findings in oral gavage studies, such as congested or fluid-filled lungs and reddening or puncturing of the trachea, are signs of a gavage error, and the death of the animal would not be considered test material related.

Parental Body Weight and Food Consumption Data

Reduction in body weight gain or actual body weight loss in conjunction with food consumption measurements can be sensitive indicators of systemic toxicity in all types of toxicology studies. In DART studies, body weight, and food consumption data are presented and interpreted separately for each phase of a study (i.e., F_0 premating, F_0 gestation, F_0 lactation, F_1 premating, etc.). Interpretation of premating body weight and food consumption is straightforward. Group mean body weights and/or percent change in body weights are calculated. Reductions in body weights may indicate a direct effect of the test material and/or may reflect reductions in food consumption (anorexia). The role that anorexia may have played in reducing body weights may be assessed by calculating a "food efficiency index." This index is a measure of the efficacy of food utilization (i.e., food consumed/body weight gained). Reduced food intake is not considered a main factor in body weight reductions if the food efficiency index is similar between the treated and control groups. In general, mild to moderate depressions in body weight resulting from reduced food consumption have little or no effect on adult reproductive capacity, and it is not considered appropriate to dismiss reductions in fertility as being secondary to such weight reduction.

For the gestation and lactation periods, mean body weight and food consumption data should be generated for each day it was measured. Most prefer to calculate body weight and food consumption changes as intervals to aid in interpretation. For example, in a rat Segment II study useful intervals to look at would be Gestation Days 0–6, 6–9, 9–12, 12–15, 15–20, 6–15, and 0–20. In this way one can assess the impact of the test material during the early part of the treatment period (6–9), middle of the treatment period (9–12), and during the last part of the treatment period (12–15), and during the entire treatment period (6–15) as well as effects posttreatment (15–20) and over the entire gestation period (0–20). Often included is a "corrected" mean maternal body weight gain that is calculated as the terminal body weight minus the initial body weight minus the gravid uterus weight (or minus the litter weight). It can be difficult to differentiate small reductions in weight gain or weight loss in pregnant and lactating animals due to normally erratic weight gain during pregnancy, as well as such confounding factors as differing litter size and implantation loss. Tables 12 and 13 show a typical mean weight gain in pregnant rats and rabbits based on historical data. Non-pregnant animals as well as does (maternal rabbits) that abort should be excluded from calculation of the means and any statistical evaluations. Also the reader should be aware that food consumption data from the lactation period are of questionable use due to the fact that the pups as well as the dams start to consume the diet during the 2nd week.

Food and body weight effects will most often demonstrate a dose-response pattern. Also it is not uncommon to observe an actual compensatory increase in food consumption, compared to controls after treatment is stopped. However, interpretation of these data is not always simple. For example, when excessive mortality occurs at the high dose there is a possibility of weight reductions appearing larger in the mid-dose group due to the elimination of the most sensitive animals in the higher-dosage group. In these

Table 12 Typical Body Weight Gain in Pregnant Rats

Gestation day	Mean body weight change (g) ± SD
0–6	27 ± 5
6–15	34 ± 9
15–20	64 ± 10

circumstances, the lack of a dose-response would not imply that there were no test material related effects.

Male and Female Reproductive System

Estrous Cycling. Individual daily staging (proestrus, estrus, metestrus, or diestrus) for each female should be presented for the pretreatment period, the treatment period and the posttreatment period, if available. Rat estrous cyclicity can be expressed in a variety of ways. Some laboratories summarize these data as the average duration of cycle in days or number of estruses over a given time period. The normal cycle time in laboratory rats, depending on the strain, is usually 4–5 days. However, this type of compilation will not give you any information on where the changes in cyclicity are occurring or possible mechanisms involved. In toxicology studies, rodents will usually demonstrate some periodic alterations in cycling (e.g., prolonged estrus or prolonged diestrus) prior to becoming completely acyclic, which may aid in interpretation of possible causes (73). Thus, many investigators prefer to summarize estrous cycle data as percent of animals displaying abnormal stages i.e., prolonged estrus (>2 days), abnormal diestrus (<2 or >3 days), prolonged metestrus (>1 day), or prolonged proestrus (>1 day). A summary of the percentage of time spent in each stage would also give similar information about specific stage abnormalities.

Alterations in cyclicity provide some indication that the major endocrine mechanisms controlling normal female reproduction have been affected (74). Prior to ovulation, in the beginning of estrus a marked increase in serum estradiol occurs and the vaginal cytology, consisting of primarily cornified epithelial cells, reflects this influence. Following ovulation, progesterone predominates and becomes the primary controlling factor for vaginal cytology. At diestus, both estradiol and progesterone equally predominate, resulting in vaginal cytology consisting of leukocytes and epithelial cells entangled in mucus.

Mating and Pregnancy. The evidence of mating is expressed as the "copulatory index" and/or "mating index" (Table 14) and as the copulatory interval. A decrease in the copulatory or mating index may be due to physical impairment (e.g., inhibition of penile erection) or to alterations in sexual behavior (e.g., libido, receptivity).

Table 13 Typical Body Weight Gain in Pregnant Rabbits

Gestation day	Mean body weight change (g) ± SD
0–7	93 ± 42
6–13	53 ± 51
12–20	52 ± 63
19–24	37 ± 40
24–29	−16 ± 87

Standard Segment I and multigeneration studies do not directly incorporate end points for assessment of "mating behavior" but rather include only indirect measurement of the end result (i.e., sperm positive smear or vaginal plug). A sperm positive mating does not necessarily indicate that pregnancy will ensue. Rodents actually mount and mate a number of times during a short period of time, and libido and receptivity play an important role. The male must provide a sufficient number of intromissions and ejaculations for the female to respond with sufficient progesterone for the initiation of pregnancy (75,76). For the female, the degree of sexual preparedness strongly influences the site of semen deposition and subsequent transport of sperm in the female genital tract (77). Failure to achieve

Table 14 Calculated Indices Used in DART Studies

Index	Formula
Copulatory index	$\dfrac{\text{\# males mated}}{\text{\# males paired}}$ or $\dfrac{\text{\# females mated}}{\text{\# females paired}}$
Mating index	$\dfrac{\text{\# females mated}}{\text{\# estrus cycles}}$
Fertility index (conception index)	$\dfrac{\text{\# males siring a litter}}{\text{\# males paired}}$ or $\dfrac{\text{\# females pregnant}}{\text{\# females paired}}$
Fecundity index (in females also called pregnancy index)—index of conception rate	$\dfrac{\text{\# males siring a litter}}{\text{\# males mated}}$ or $\dfrac{\text{\# females pregnant}}{\text{\# females mated}}$ or $\dfrac{\text{\# of pregnancies}}{\text{\# of copulations}}$
Implantation index	$\dfrac{\text{\# implantation sites}}{\text{\# corpora lutea}}$
Preimplantation loss	$\dfrac{\text{\# corpora lutea} - \text{\# implantations}}{\text{\# corpora lutea}}$
Postimplantation loss	$\dfrac{\text{\# implantations} - \text{\# viable fetuses}}{\text{\# implantations}}$
Ponderal index	$\dfrac{\text{fetal body weight}}{\text{fetal crown} - \text{rump length}}$
Parturition index	$\dfrac{\text{\# litters delivered}}{\text{\# females mated}}$ or $\dfrac{\text{\# litters delivered}}{\text{\# females pregnant}}$
Live birth index (also called gestation index)	$\dfrac{\text{\# live pups born}}{\text{\# pups delivered}}$ or $\dfrac{\text{\# live litters born}}{\text{\# pregnant}}$
Viability index	$\dfrac{\text{\# pups surviving 4 days}}{\text{\# live pups at birth}}$
Reproduction index	$\dfrac{\text{\# pups surviving 4 days}}{\text{\# females pregnant}}$
Weaning index (also called lactation index)	$\dfrac{\text{\# pups weaned (day 21)}}{\text{\# pups after culling (day 4)}}$
Preweaning loss	$\dfrac{\text{\# pups born per litter} - \text{\# pups weaned per litter}}{\text{\# pups born per litter}}$

Each indices is usually calculated and multiplied by 100 and represented as a percent for each test group.

these conditions will adversely influence these processes and reduce the probability of successful conception.

The actual number of pregnancies resulting from sperm positive matings is calculated as the "fecundity index" (Table 14). The accurate determination of the fecundity index requires careful evaluation of the uterus at necropsy for the presence of implantation sites. All pregnancies should be included here, even those not resulting in viable offspring. A reduction in the fecundity index could be the result of adverse effects on many targets, including effects on sperm motility/viability, follicular rupture and oocyte release, fertilization, oviduct transport, endocrine status, uterine receptivity, or implantation.

The "fertility" (or "conception") index (Table 14) is a much broader reflection of the overall reproductive capacity of the treatment group and takes into account all animals—those that did not mate, those that mated but did not conceive, and those that obtain pregnancy—and thus encompasses both the copulatory index and fecundity index. Unless the study includes mating the treated males and or treated females to untreated rats, it is usually not possible to differentiate whether or not the reduction in fertility is due to dysfunction of the male, the female, or both.

Fertility is not considered a very sensitive indicator of reproductive toxicity. A normal male rodent produces sperm counts well above that required for normal fertility (Table 5). In fact, it has been demonstrated that chemical induced reductions of up to 90% of sperm production can still result in normal fertility rates (78). In contrast, minor reductions in sperm production in human males can have marked effects on reproductive capacity because human males function nearer to the threshold for the number of normal sperm needed to ensure reproductive competence. Female rodents also have a greater reproductive capacity than needed and may require a considerable reduction in oocyte/follicle development before affecting fertility rates. Thus, when "no effects on fertility" is the sole end point available for risk assessment of reproductive competence, not much reliance can be put on this for human risk.

When infertility is observed on a study, especially in association with evidence of histopathological changes in the testes and/or ovary, it is very important to assess whether the effects are reversible. Chemically induced destruction of stem cells (spermatogonia or primordial oocytes) is of great significance because there is no mechanism for repopulation of these germ cells, thus the effect is irreversible.

Gestation Length and Parturition. In rats, the length of the gestation period ranges from 20 to 23 days and averages approximately 21.5 days. Gestation length is most often simply compared using group mean values. However, a graph depicting the percent of the dams undergoing parturition on each possible day of parturition for each dosage group will often give the investigator a better picture of possible dose-related trends. Gestation length is determined by the triggering of parturition, a process that involves numerous endocrine factors and is not completely understood (79–81). Prolonged gestation as well as early delivery of pups are considered dysfunctions of the triggering process and threaten the survival of offspring.

The parturition process itself involves major changes in the contractile potential of the smooth muscle of the uterus to allow for synchronous contractions during labor. Chemically induced dysfunction of parturition (dystocia) often involves interference with uterine contractility. Prolonged parturition (i.e., > 12 hours) is often associated with increased stillbirth.

Calculation of the "parturition index" gives a measure of adult fertility/fecundity through birth (Table 14). However, the index itself provides limited information on actual offspring viability, because litters with only one pup are counted the same as those with more than one pup.

Organ Weights. Organ weight data is usually present as both individual and group mean absolute weights and as relative weights (i.e., organ weight to body or brain weight ratios). In DART studies, absolute organ weights are more important for interpretive purposes because many of the reproductive organs are unaffected by changes in body weight.

In male rats, the reproductive organs to be weighed are the testes, epididymides, prostate, seminal vesicles, and pituitary. Testes weight varies little within a given strain of a test species (82–84). This relatively low intrastrain/intrapecies variability can make testicular weight a sensitive indicator of gonadal injury. Most testicular toxins will reduce testicular weight in rodent studies. However, increases in testicular weight can also be observed with the induction of edema and inflammation, cellular infiltration, or Leydig cell hyperplasia. There is also a chance of observing no change in testicular weight, even with the presence of severe spermatogenic injury upon histopathologic evaluation. Epididymal weight is affected by the number of sperm present in the lumen. Both seminal vesicles and the prostate contain large proportions of luminal fluid, and these fluid levels are easily influenced by changes in androgenic hormone levels.

In female rats, the reproductive organs to be weighed are the ovaries, uterus, and pituitary. The weight of the ovary and uterus do vary during the course of the estrous cycle and obviously during pregnancy. The ovary weight can be closely related to the number of corpora lutea present. Uterine weight can be greatly affected by the presence of estrogen.

Changes in pituitary weight are usually considered as an adverse toxicological effect but are not necessarily reflective of reproductive impairment because gonadotropin producing cells in the pituitary represent only a small portion of the many hormonal cell types.

Unlike changes in the weights of some other organs, testicular, epididymal, and ovarian organ weights are not influenced by small or moderate changes in body weight (83,85–87). Prostate and seminal vesicle weight can vary with body weight changes. Thus, when body weight reductions occur in a study, due to decreased food palatability or consumption, one cannot just assume that changes in the weight of reproductive organs are simply secondary to the presence of general systemic toxicity. In the same vein, reproductive organ weight data should not be used as a lone end point; accompanying histopathology evaluation can be crucial. One cannot assume that a particular agent does not induce adverse effects in the testes or ovary based on the absence of organ weight changes alone. Finally, difficulties in dissection and removal of extraneous tissues from smaller organs, such as the epididymides, seminal vesicles, prostate, and pituitary, can create unwanted variability. Organ weight data should also document whether the specified weight was taken with or without excess fluids. Weights without fluids generally will show less variability.

Histopathology of Reproductive Organs. Properly conducted histopathology is one of the most sensitive indicators of injury to the reproductive system. Not all veterinary pathologists are fully trained to conduct such detailed assessments. Familiarity with the cytoarchitecture of the testis and ovaries, as well as with the kinetics of spermatogenesis and follicle development, are crucial to identifying injury, especially in the identification of less prominent lesions in these organs. Evaluation should include both the germ cells and nongerm supporting tissues. There are a number of excellent reviews that the reader can refer to for more information on identifying pathology in the male and female reproductive organs (56,88–97).

Male Reproductive System. One of the most sensitive end points in the male for determination of reproductive toxicity is histopathology of the testes (98). A thorough histologic evaluation of the testes includes examination of the various cell stages (i.e., spermatogonia, spermatocytes, spermatids), sperm release into the lumen (spermiation), support cells (i.e., Sertoli and Leydig cells), as well as examination of the interstitial area (89,91,93). The most commonly observed finding in the testis is germ cell degeneration and necrosis. Cytotoxic agents will generally target all dividing cell types in the testis. Other male reproductive toxins target very specific germ cell stages or directly target the Sertoli or Leydig cells. However, the majority of testicular toxins, regardless of their site of action, will produce a similar nonspecific degeneration if administered at a high dosage over a prolonged period. Germ cell depletion is often accompanied by Leydig cell hyperplasia or hypertrophy, depending on the hormonal status. It should be remembered that spermatogenesis is a temporally synchronized process, and it is possible to miss an effect by examination of tissues too early or too late posttreatment.

Chemical injury to the epididymis can include necrosis of the epithelium and formation of sperm granuloma and/or spermatocele that can result in obstruction of the lumen. Vacuolization of the epididymal epithelium has been associated with estrogenic stimulation. The pathologist should also take note of any unusual findings in the epididymal spermatozoa.

The accessory sex glands (prostate, seminal vesicles, ampullary glands, bulbourethral glands, and preputial glands) most frequently are targets of chemicals that directly or indirectly alter the balance of reproductive hormones. Histologic changes indicative of toxicity may be degenerative, atrophic, proliferative, or inflammatory. The presence of accessory sex organs varies with species. In many routine toxicology studies, only representative accessory sex organs, such as the prostate, are examined histologically.

Analysis of epididymal sperm can also be conducted at necropsy. Recorded parameters generally include sperm count, viability, morphology, and motility, although additional measured parameters are possible in automated systems (2,83,84).

Female Reproductive System. A thorough histologic evaluation of the ovary includes examination of the epithelial capsule, stroma, and follicular cells. Significant findings in the ovary include a reduction or absence of follicle-enclosed oocytes, unruptured follicles, reductions or absence of corpora lutea, or the presence of ovarian cysts (92,94). Although not required, once an ovarian lesion has been identified, morphometric analysis of follicle subtypes, including primordial oocyte counts, may provide additional information on the extent and possible reversibility of the injury (56,95,96). However, this procedure is labor intensive and requires an advanced level of expertise.

The corpus luteum is a transient ovarian endocrine gland formed by a rapid growth and differentiation of the theca and granulosa cells of the follicle following ovulation (99). The primary function of the corpus luteum in all species is the synthesis of progesterone, which is essential for implantation and subsequent development of the fetoplacental unit. Activation and maintenance of luteal function are species specific and can involve pituitary, placental, and/or ovarian hormones (Table 6). Corpora lutea are found on the surface of the ovary and are counted by macroscopic examination at necropsy. A corpus luteum is formed for every oocyte released. Preimplantation loss (Table 14) can be calculated by the difference between the number of eggs released and the number of implantation sites that develop. The number of implantation sites must be equal to or less than the number of corpora lutea. In some instances not all corpora lutea will be visible on the surface of the ovary, and for statistical purposes the data need to be adjusted in those cases where the number of implants is greater than the number of corpora lutea.

The appearances of the uterus and vagina vary with the stage of the reproductive cycle and with pregnancy. Agents that impair ovarian cycling, alter normal hormonal balance, mimic reproductive hormones, or interfere with autocrine/paracrine regulation may cause significant changes in uterine and vaginal morphology and the ability of the uterus to maintain a fetus to term.

Accessory female sex organs generally are rudimentary and often are not examined unless grossly visible abnormalities lead to histologic observations. However, accessory sex glands, such as the clitoral glands of rodents, may be examined routinely in some studies.

Developmental Data

Adverse developmental effects may be detected at any point in the offspring's life span. In DART studies these effects are manifested as death of the offspring, induction of structural abnormalities (teratogenicity), reduction in growth, and/or functional alterations. All four end points are of toxicological concern if produced at a particular exposure level and in a dose-related manner (28,30,61,100).

A toxicant usually induces more than one type of effect in a dose-dependent manner. In Segment II studies, three general dose-response patterns exist (4,11,101). In the first dose-response pattern, one observes a combination of resorbed, malformed, growth retarded, and "normal" fetuses within the litter. Depending upon the potency of the test material, lower dosages may cause primarily growth retardation or malformation, and higher dosages induce primarily death of the conceptus. This does not necessarily indicate that one type of effect leads to another type of effect but rather indicates that the agent is capable of a full spectrum of effects. This is the type of dose-response pattern that is commonly seen for cytotoxic agents. In the second pattern, the agent is not teratogenic but will induce growth retardation and lethality at sufficiently high dosages. Growth retardation usually precedes significant lethality. In the last pattern, highly potent and target oriented teratogens will generally cause malformations of the entire litter at exposure levels that do not cause embryolethality. Increasing the dosage level will usually result in death of the conceptus but often in conjunction with severe maternal toxicity. In this pattern growth retardation is often associated with the malformed offspring.

Effects on the fetus can be induced by direct effects of the test material on the conceptus or indirectly through toxic effects on the maternal system, placenta, or other tissues. Effects noted after parturition can be the result of previous in utero exposure and exposure to the test material via maternal milk or indirectly through poor maternal care and postnatal nutrition.

Death. Loss of the conceptus anywhere from fertilization to implantation is termed "preimplantation loss." This is calculated from the total number of implants and the total number of corpora lutea (Table 14). Preimplantation loss may be due to a direct effect on the early embryo or indirect interference with such events as movement of the egg/embryo through the fallopian tube, interference with uterine decidualization in preparation for implantation, or adverse effects on corpora lutea function and progesterone synthesis.

Death of the conceptus in the uterus is referred to as "postimplantation loss" (sometimes referred to as "fetal wastage"), which can include early or late resorption of the implanted embryo/fetus and late fetal death. This index is calculated using the number of implants and the number of viable fetuses in a litter (Table 14). Postimplantation loss may be due to a direct lethal effect on the developing conceptus or induction of lethal malformation(s) or indirectly through interference with maternal systems supporting the pregnancy.

Stillborn and neonatal deaths are referred to collectively as "postnatal loss." Postnatal survival is usually expressed in time intervals. Stillborn incidence rate can be expressed as the "live birth index" based on the total number of pups delivered by a dam and the number of live pups delivered (Table 14). An increase in the stillborn rate can be associated with increased late fetal death in the Segment II study. Prolonged gestation and/or problems in parturition (dystocia) are also often associated with increases in stillbirths. Pup adaptation to postnatal life may be affected by treatment induced structural abnormalities or functional alterations. Rodents will often cannibalize stillborn and/or abnormal pups early after delivery making accurate evaluations difficult unless closely observed.

Survival from birth to culling on postnatal day 4, from culling to postnatal week 1, etc. are calculated as "viability indices." Total survival over the entire lactation period can be calculated as the "weaning index" or "preweaning loss" (Table 14). Again, reduced postnatal survival may be due to a direct effect of the test material (via milk and or diet/water administration), induced functional/structural changes affecting survival, or treatment-related effects on maternal nursing behavior, milk production, or milk ejection reflex. The presence or absence of milk visible in the stomach of the pups can help distinguish whether or not lactation played a role in their morbidity/mortality.

In a multigeneration study, an observed reduction in litter size at birth may be associated with a reduced ovulation rate (corpora lutea count), higher rate of preimplantation deaths, higher rate of postimplantation deaths, stillbirths, and/or immediate postnatal deaths. In all types of DART studies, a high incidence of offspring mortality at any point may "mask" the occurrence of other adverse effects, such as growth retardation and/or teratogenicity (102). If a study results in no effects on the conceptus at the mid-dose and very high offspring mortality at the high-dose, an agency may request as additional study to be conducted using dosage groups between the mid- and high-dose levels of the first study.

Growth Retardation. Reductions in offspring body weights are a very sensitive indicator of developmental toxicity due to their relatively small intraspecies variability. Litter size does influence offspring body weight and should be factored into any statistical analyses (i.e., body weight is inversely proportional to litter size; higher weight in small litters and smaller weights in larger litters). There are circumstances where only one or a few of the fetuses/pups in a litter are affected. Therefore, as with other developmental end points, growth should be assessed on both an individual and a litter basis rather than relying solely on group mean values. Pups that are substantially smaller than their litter mates are referred to as runts. In studies where gestation length has been affected, it is recommended that pup body weights be assessed based on the day of conception (Gestation Day 0) rather than from the day of birth (Postnatal Day 0). By doing this, differences between litters in gestation length and age at birth are eliminated.

Male and female body weights should be summarized separately. This, along with data on the sex ratio (males:females) of the litters, can indicate whether or not one gender is preferentially affected by a particular test material. Although there are reports of such gender sensitivity, such occurrences are rare.

Altered growth may be induced at any stage of development and may be permanent or reversible. For example, the mechanism responsible for fetal body weight reductions in a Segment II study may not be carried into the postnatal period, where pup weight may increase parallel to control weights and, in some cases, catch up. Therefore, it is important to examine the data from each day on which body weights were taken to differentiate when actual reductions or losses in body weight actually occurred. Failure to recover from growth retardation is considered permanent stunting. A permanent weight change is usually considered more worrisome than a transitory change, although transitory changes should not be completely dismissed because little is known about the long-term consequences of short-term fetal or neonatal growth inhibition (30).

In utero growth retardation is often accompanied by delays/reductions in skeletal ossification and, in some cases, increases in minor skeletal variations. This is often observed with test agents that exert their effects through maternal toxicity. Agents known to interfere directly with fetal nutrition, growth factors, and other developmental processes may also induce growth retardation by a direct effect on the fetus (103). Postnatally, growth can be affected by alterations in maternal care, milk production, or altered milk ejection reflexes, or it can result from direct effects on pup suckling behavior or continued test-material exposure through milk.

Structural Abnormalities. Highly potent teratogens that consistently induce a large incidence of malformations in offspring are rare (4,11,104). Most agents that are tested have a low potential for causing malformations and/or very specific time and dosage requirements that are not reproduced in a standard study design. Therefore, the chances of observing malformations at a rate high enough to be distinguished against the normal background (i.e., historical control) are small. More often than not it is adverse effects on growth and viability of the conceptus that most often "flags" a compound as a developmental toxin (30,61,104).

When trying to assess whether the presence of malformations in a study represents treatment-induced abnormalities, there are some basic concepts that may help (4). First, almost all types of malformations have been reported to occur spontaneously in rodents and/or rabbits. Secondly, known chemical teratogens produce more or less specific patterns of multiple defects; isolated abnormalities are not the rule. Thus, it is very important to review not only the summary incidence of anomalies but also review individual fetal data for the occurrence of patterns of multiple malformations. A general teratogen, such as a cytotoxic chemotherapeutic agent, usually will produce a whole spectrum of defects, dependent of the time of administration, because all organs are equally susceptible. With all teratogens, some degree of uniformity in induction of malformations is seen. Finally, chemically induced malformations are usually bilateral in the case of paired organs.

A significant change in the incidence may be manifested as an increase in malformed offspring per litter, the number of litters with malformed offspring, or the number of offspring or litters with a specific type or pattern of malformation(s) that appears to increase in a dose-response pattern. The incidence rates should always be compared to the background rate in the historical control data, and statistical significance should not be a limiting factor in deciding whether or not the presence of a particular malformation is test material related.

Developmental variations, because they are not life threatening, occur normally at a much higher incidence rate than major malformations. Developmental variations are not considered true terata. Changes in the incidence of variations are commonly induced at dosages below those causing malformations and can be precursors to teratogenic dosages. It has been suggested that this is because some variations are the result of compensatory mechanisms invoked to halt the progress to malformation and death (105). Variations can also be induced by agents that are not considered teratogenic. However, their presence, with or without increases in malformations, is usually considered indicative of a developmentally toxic effect. Under some circumstances the induction of skeletal variations, such as supernumerary ribs and wavy ribs, are considered the result of maternal toxicity/stress rather than a direct toxic effect on the conceptus (106–109).

Findings related to skeletal ossification can be summarized separately from other developmental variations. Reductions in skeletal ossification rates are usually merely delays in the ossification process and are usually interpreted as being related to growth retardation.

Offspring Function. Investigation into possible functional changes resulting from test-material exposure during gestation and/or lactation is limited in standard DART testing. Currently the guidelines requiring such end points include measurements only for changes in maturational and behavioral indices and reproductive competence. Other systems (e.g., cardiopulmonary, immune, urinary, etc.), are currently not required to be tested for functional competence postnatally. However, some investigators have argued for the inclusion of these additional functions, particularity the immune system (110,111).

Maturational indices (e.g., eye opening, hair growth, pinna detachment) and reflex indices (e.g., righting reflex, startle reflex) are measured as time dependent/growth dependent phenomenon. It is recommended that the development of these parameters be presented as postcoital (from Gestation Day 0) rather than postpartum (from Postnatal Day 0). By doing this, differences between litters in gestation length and pup age are eliminated. Group means, litter means, and individual data should be used when evaluating possible effects. These end points generally display little intraspecies and intralitter variability and are relatively sensitive end points. Delays in the attainment of maturational and reflex parameters are usually associated with reductions in growth of the offspring. The significance of delays in the attainment of these end points is dependent upon how many of the end points are affected, whether both sexes are affected and how long of a delay was observed.

Behavioral testing, including basal and exploratory activity monitoring and learning/memory tests, is conducted over a single or a few days and is generally conducted when the offspring are older. The interpretation of behavioral data is often difficult and limited due to the lack of knowledge about the underlying toxicological mechanisms and their significance (30,112–114). These types of tests also display wide intraspecies variability. However, alterations in behavioral parameters at dosage levels below those causing other developmental injury or maternal toxicity would be of considerable concern particularly if they were permanent. Significant changes in behavioral testing will often warrant follow-up in more sophisticated studies, including brain chemistry and histopathology, to further characterize the test material (115–117).

Evaluation of possible chemically induced effects on offspring reproductive competence can include maturational indices, such as vaginal opening and testes descent or preputial separation as a measure of puberty, initiation and cyclicity of female estrous, and mating procedures, such as those outlined in the parental adults at maturity (118–120). All of these data should be evaluated as described above for similar parameters, including both individual and group mean data. Significant alterations in these parameters can be indicative of in utero and/or postnatal test material effects on sexual differentiation of the brain, altered endocrine status, and possible injury to offspring reproductive tissues and germ cells.

Risk Assessment

Risk assessment and extrapolation of animal data to human risk is a complicated process (2,27–30,60,61). Evaluation methods and safety considerations can be very different, depending on the use, expected human exposure levels and expected exposed population for the agent in question (i.e., drug, occupational chemical, environmental pollutant, etc.). In addition, species vary widely in male and female reproductive function, as well as in timing and development of offspring (Tables 5, 6 and 7), requiring some expertise to accurately extrapolate risk from laboratory animals to humans.

An accurate evaluation must include consideration of all relevant data for the test material, such as acute and chronic toxicity and target organ data, all possible mechanism(s) of action, metabolism and pharmacokinetic data as well as all available DART data. The availability of data in humans can greatly enhance the reliability and accuracy of the risk assessment, but most often risk assessment must rely solely on animal data.

The first step in any risk assessment is a review of the data, including judgment on the quality of the studies available and pertinence to the risk assessment. This judgment is based on a number of factors including, but not limited to, consistency of results, reproducibility of results in the same species, the number of species studied, concordance of effects between species (including humans), demonstrated dose-response relationships, applicability of the various routes of exposure, power of the study to detect a positive result, and the type of end points measured.

Each adverse effect, whether reduced male fertility, embryolethality or pup behavioral changes, may show a slightly different shaped response curve. The LOEL or lowest-observed-adverse-effect level for the study is the lowest dosage inducing at least one type of adverse effect. The no-observed-effect-level or no-observed-adverse-effect-level is the highest dosage showing no adverse effect. As appropriate, an adult systemic, adult reproductive and/or a developmental LOEL/NOEL should be identified.

In the absence of specific data to the contrary, any adverse DART effects seen in the animal studies are presumed to indicate a potential risk to human reproduction. Some end points may be given greater weight in the assessment process than others. An effect perceived to be reversible and non–life threatening would be of less concern than clearly severe life threatening effects. The sensitivity of a particular end point is also considered. The presumption is maintained even if an end point has no counterpart in the human, because concordance of effects are usually an exception rather than the general rule. The lack of uniformity of effects between species is not unexpected if one considers the many critical differences that exist between the conditions of human exposure and those used in animal studies (e.g., the exaggerated dosage levels used in experimental animals; controlled environment and exposure to a single agent; species differences in pharmaco-kinetics, placentation, and pregnancy maintenance).

Many toxicity studies in laboratory animals typically relate the response as a function of the dosage administered without data on actual systemic exposure (i.e., levels of test material in the blood). Yet, it is not uncommon to observe marked species differences in absorption, distribution, and elimination of a chemical. When extrapolating from animals to human, the absence of such comparative pharmacokinetic data increases the uncertainty of the extrapolation. This is especially problematic when extrapolating not just across species but also across differing routes of administration.

Another default assumption, in the absence of pharmacokinetic data, is that treatment of the animal is assumed relevant to human exposure by any route. Also in the absence of adequate pharmacokinetic data, the most sensitive species (i.e., the species with the lowest NOEL) is used in the risk assessment, because humans are generally considered as sensitive as the most sensitive species tested, particularly in developmental toxicity. It can be very beneficial to obtain pharmacokinetic data on a test compound when comparative human data are available. There are many examples of toxicants that require biotransformation before demonstrating any toxic effects. If this biotransformation pathway were shown to be absent in humans, then the toxicity data from the animal studies in that species would be considered irrelevant to human risk assessment. The same holds true for animal data on mechanism(s) of action, which may or may not be relevant to humans.

Actual acceptable levels of exposure for chemicals, other than drugs, vary with the nature of the chemical, the purpose for which it will be used (i.e., food additives, pesticides, and pollutants) and type of benefits expected. There are no mathematical models that are generally accepted for estimating possible DART response below experimental dosage levels. Defining a NOEL in a DART study does not prove or disprove the existence a threshold; it only defines the highest level of exposure under the conditions of the test that are not associated with an adverse effect. Calculating acceptable exposure limits in DART risk assessment is not a precise science but rather an approximation, with allowable exposure concentrations set at a specified fraction of the NOEL based on the available data. The fraction is determined by the use of various "safety factors" as applied using the "uncertainty factor" approach or the "margin of safety" approach

There has been some debate in recent years on the use of the NOEL in setting safe exposure levels, because reliance on the NOEL places substantial importance on the power of a study to detect low-dose effects. Methods for replacing the NOEL with a calculated "benchmark dose" are under consideration (2,121–124).

The margin of safety approach derives a ratio of the NOEL from the most sensitive species to the estimated human exposure level from all potential sources. The adequacy of the margin of safety is then considered based on the weight of evidence, including the nature and quality of the hazard (toxicology data) and exposure data, the number of species tested, dose-response relationships, and other applicable factors.

In the uncertainty factor approach, the size of the applied safety factor varies based on interspecies differences, the nature and extent of human exposure, the slope of the dose-response curve, the types of end points affected, and the relative dose levels for systemic toxicity versus those producing developmental or reproductive toxicity in the most sensitive test species. The safety factor applied can range from 10 to 10,000, depending on the number of adjustments needed. Possibilities include 10 for situations in which the study LOEL must be used because a NOEL was not established, 10 for interspecies extrapolation, and 10 for intraspecies adjustment for variable sensitivity among individuals. Additional adjustments may be applied for length of exposure (acute to subchronic), to correct for inadequacy of the NOEL or LOEL or insensitivity of the end point it is based on. Once the uncertainty factor is selected, this is divided into the NOEL to obtain the acceptable exposure level. Food additives and pesticides generally are given at least 100-fold safety margins. Safety margins for environmental pollutants, on the other hand, are generally 1000-fold.

Acceptable levels of exposure for human drugs are not generally calculated and used in the same way they are used for chemicals. The margin of safety between toxic exposure and therapeutic dosage levels can be as low as 10-fold or even 1-fold for highly beneficial drugs. The Food and Drug Administration (Table 15) and the European Community (Table 16) use "pregnancy categories" and labeling requirements based on available animal and human DART data (125,126), leaving the risk/benefit decision up to the physicians and their patients. Suggestion and discussions on how to improve the information passed on in drug labels and the risk/benefit process for doctors and patients have been published (127).

ADDITIONAL PARAMETERS TO MEASURE AND OTHER FOLLOW-UP STUDIES

This section identifies a few possible add-on and/or follow-up methods or studies that may be useful if further investigation or characterization of a test material is needed. These suggestions are by no means all inclusive. Two methodology books on the male and female reproductive system, edited by Chapin and Heindel (2,3), as well as a book on approaches to mechanistic studies in developmental toxicology (128), are also excellent sources.

Adult Reproduction

Endocrine Status

Measurement of hormone levels can be added to ongoing studies or further evaluated in follow-up studies (129,130). The primary hormones that are measured include luteinizing

Table 15 FDA Pregnancy Categories

A: Controlled human studies show no risk: adequate, well-controlled studies in pregnant women have failed to demonstrate risk to the fetus

B: No evidence of risk in humans: either animal findings show risk, but human findings do not; or, if no adequate human studies have been done, animal findings are negative

C: Risk cannot be ruled out: human studies are lacking, and animal studies are either positive for fetal risk or lacking as well. However, potential benefits may justify the potential risk

D: Positive evidence of risk: investigation or postmarketing data show risk to the fetus. Nevertheless, potential benefits may outweigh the potential risk

X: Contraindicated in pregnancy: studies in animals or human, or investigational or postmarketing reports have shown fetal risk that clearly outweighs any possible benefit to the patient

hormone (LH), gonadotropin releasing hormone (GnRH), follicle stimulating hormone (FSH), estradiol, testosterone, progesterone, and prolactin. However, the reader should be aware that to obtain adequate serum hormone data requires multiple sampling times, due to their pulsatile nature, and must take into consideration the age, reproductive state, and cycle day of the test animal. Also, it is not always possible to differentiate whether endocrine changes are the cause or are secondary to reproductive effects. Endocrine changes that indicate toxicity include multiple values outside the normal physiologic ranges, physiologically plausible changes in direction in hormone levels, or failure of key hormonal events (such as LH surge, preovulatory estradiol rise, maintenance of luteal phase progesterone production, etc.) (131,132). Other strategies for evaluating endocrine status include such hormone challenge assays as measurement of LH following injection of GnRH or measurement of progesterone following injection of chorionic gonadotropin (133).

Sperm Production, Function, and Viability

In addition to standard epididymal sperm evaluations (e.g., sperm count, sperm morphology and molitility) the production and function of the male gamete can be assessed by various additional end points and methods. Most often used methods include

Table 16 European Pregnancy Categories

A: Assessed in pregnant women and no harmful effects are known with respect to the course of pregnancy and the health of the newborn and the neonate

B1: Safety in human pregnancy has not been established; animal studies do not indicate direct or indirect harmful effects with respect to the development of the embryo or fetus, the course of gestation, and peri- and postnatal development

B2: Safety in human pregnancy has not been established; animal studies are insufficient to assess the safety with respect to the development of the embryo or fetus, the course of gestation, and peri- and postnatal development

B3: Safety in human pregnancy has not been established; animal studies have shown reproductive toxicity, e.g., birth defects or other effects on the development of the embryo or fetus, the course of gestation, or peri- and postnatal development

C: Does not increase the spontaneous incidence of birth defects in humans, but it has potential hazardous pharmacologic effects with respect to the course of pregnancy, to the unborn or the neonate

D: Is known or suspected to cause birth defects and/or other irreversible adverse effects on pregnancy outcome. It may also have potential hazardous pharmacologic effects with respect to the course of pregnancy, to the unborn, or the neonate morphometric or flow cytometric evaluation of spermatogenic stages in the testes, in vitro Sertoli and Leydig cell function assays, and assays measuring capacitation, sperm-egg binding, and fertilization (2,32,59,78,93,134–138).

Ovarian Function

Follow-up studies on possible roles of the ovary in fertility reduction include morphometric or flow cytometric evaluation, investigations on ovarian steroidogenesis and corpora lutea function, in vivo time-response studies to assess oocyte maturation, follicular rupture and oocyte release, in vivo oocyte toxicity assay in juvenile mice, and in vitro cultures of growing follicles (3,139–144).

Copulatory Behavior

Possible follow-up studies on sexual behavior could include female receptivity and lordosis response and copulatory measures, such as latency of male to mount, number of intromissions prior to ejaculation, number of mounts without intromission, and lordosis to mount ratios (145–148). However, a more detailed evaluation of sexual behavior is not warranted for all toxicants associated with reductions in fertility. The most likely candidates include agents associated with neurotoxic effect or those with possible androgenic or estrogenic properties.

Fertilization, Transportation, and Implantation

Increases in preimplantation loss can be further investigated using in vivo time-response studies and in vitro assays to assess fertilization, oviduct transport, uterine receptivity and decidualization, and implantation (3,140,149,150).

Parturition

Follow-up studies on parturition effects have utilized in vitro uterine strips to study contractility, uterine smooth muscle cell cultures, endocrine assays, and prostaglandin challenge (151–154).

Lactation and Maternal Behavior

Increases in pup morbidity or death can be further investigated using measurements of maternal milk production and ejection functions as well as pup suckling reflexes (155,156). Maternal behavior can also be scored for measures of anxiety and aggression, nest building, pup retrieval, and other markers (157,158).

Fetal Development

The approaches to evaluating possible mechanisms responsible for developmental toxicity, including teratogenicity, are as numerous as the differing types of effects that are possible, ranging from investigations on possible effects on uterine blood flow to receptor specific targeting in fetal organs (128,159,160). One of the most useful tools in distinguishing whether a test material is acting in utero via toxicity to the mother or directly acting on the fetus are in vitro embryo/fetal culture (161–163). In the postnatal period this can be differentiated using cross-fostering with untreated animals (164).

CONCLUSION

Reproduction and development of offspring are the primary goal of genetics and involve a complicated and not fully known interplay of physiology, endocrinology, and biology. Much of these reproductive and developmental processes are measured indirectly in standard DART studies by the ultimate production of viable and reproductively competent offspring. The large number of chemicals needing to be screened each year make more detailed investigations into each impossible. Government requirements for testing of possible chemically induced effects on reproduction are dependent on the end use, exposure potential, target population, and perceived benefit of the chemical. The laboratory animals used in these studies are not perfect models. However, daily research is increasing our understanding of these animal models, aiding in the extrapolation of potential risk to human populations. Ultimately, a clear understanding of the mechanism(s) inducing chemically related reproductive and developmental toxicity will provide the most accurate extrapolation of potential risk to humans.

APPENDIX: COMMONLY USED TERMS IN REPRODUCTIVE AND DEVELOPMENTAL TOXICITY

Abortifacient

An agent which causes abortion.

Abortion

Premature expulsion from the uterus of products of conception (embryo or a nonviable fetus). Rodents cannot abort. Rabbits do, beginning at approximately 20 days; by day 28 are considered an early delivery (see premature birth) due to the survivability of the fetus. [EMBRYOTOCIA].

Agalactia

Absence or failure of the secretion of milk.

Amenorrhea

Absence or abnormal cessation of the menses or estrous cycles.

Amnion

The inner of the fetal membranes; a thin, transparent sac which holds the fetus suspended in the amniotic fluid.

Androgen

A class of steroid hormones produced in the gonads and adrenal cortex that regulate masculine sexual characteristics; a generic term for agents that encourage the development of or prevent changes in male sex characteristics; a precursor of estrogens.

Anovulation

Suspension or cessation of the release of ova from the follicles.

Blastocyst

Mammalian conceptus in the post-morula stage; spherical structure produced by cleavage of the fertilized ovum, consisting of a single layer of cells (blastoderm) surrounding a fluid filled cavity (blastocele) [BLASTULA; BLASTOSPHERE].

Cannibalism

The consumption of one by the other; in reproduction context, the eating of offspring by the mother.

Cesarean Section

Laparotomy to deliver fetus(es); usually performed on day 18 (mouse), day 20 (rat), day 29 (rabbit).

Chorion

The outermost of the fetal membranes, consisting of on outer trophoblastic epithelium lined internally by extraembryonic mesoderm; its villous portion, vascularized by allantoic blood vessels, forms the placenta.

Conceptus

The sum of derivatives of the fertilized ovum at any stage of development from fertilization until birth including the embryo/fetus and the extra-embryonic membranes.

Copulation

Mating [COITUS].

Copulatory Interval

Time (mean days) animals cohabit until mating occurs [PRECOITAL TIME].

Corpora Lutea (Corpus Luteum, SI)

Endocrine body formed in the ovary at the site of the ruptured Graafian follicle; appear as small raised translucent, creamy or yellowish colored bumps which appear like small grapes on the surface of the ovary (see also Luteinization); secrete an estrogenic and progestagenic hormone.

Culling

In reproductive context, the selective removal of young in a litter, usually to eight (in rat), in order to reduce intralitter competition in nursing.

Decidualization

Changes in uterine tissues in preparation for embryo implantation; characterized by extensive proliferation and differentiation of endometrial stromal cells.

Developmental Variations

For practical purposes, variations are defined as those alterations in anatomic structure that are considered to have no significant biological effect on animal health or body conformity, representing slight deviations from normal. Most examples placed in this category are minor variations in size and form of normally present ossification centers. While these are evaluated on a precise day of development, some variation is expected due to when conception and implantation actually occurred. Thus differences in the pattern of ossification, manifested either as retardation or as acceleration of apparent osteogenesis, are common findings. Also included in this category are slight misshapening or misalignment of structures, processes involving continued development (bilateral skeletal centers not yet fused, incomplete maturation of renal papillae, presence of vestigial structures, etc.), and development of extra ossification sites. Slight malpositioning and hypoplasia are also considered variations in development. The presence of multiple variations in many instances are observed concomitant with maternal and/or developmental toxicity.

Dystocia

Prolonged, abnormal or difficult delivery [PARODYNIA].

Early Delivery

Expulsion of a survivable conceptus prior to normal term parturition. In rodents and rabbits expulsion 2 days prior to term is considered an early delivery.

Embryo

The early or developing stage of an organism, especially the developing product of fertilization of an egg. Its development is termed EMBRYOGENESIS. The embryonic period is as follows:

> *Rat*: 9–14 days postconception
> *Mouse*: 6–13
> *Rabbit*: 10–15
> *Human*: 21–55

Epididymis

A secondary sex organ through which spermatozoa pass and in which spermatozoa acquire ability to become motile and to fertilize; the distal segment (cauda) is also a site for storage of spermatozoa.

Estradiol

An estrogenic hormone produced by follicle cells of the vertebrate ovary; provokes estrus and proliferation of the human endometrium.

Estrogen

Estrogenic hormone; generic term for various natural or synthetic substances that produce estrus.

Estrous Cycle

The recurring periods of estrous in the adult female of most mammals and the correlated changes in the reproductive tract from one period to the next. (stages are PROESTRUS, ESTRUS, DIESTRUS, and METESTRUS).

Fecundity

The physiological ability to reproduce (as opposed to fertility); the biologic competence of the reproductive system.

Fertility

Capacity to conceive or induce conception following mating.

Fertilization

The act of rendering gametes fertile or capable of further development. Begins with contact between spermatozoa and ovum, leading to their fusion, which stimulates the completion of ovum maturation with release of a second polar body. Male and female pronuclei then form and perhaps merge; synapsis follows, which restores the diploid number of chromosomes and results in biparental inheritance and the determination of sex. The process leads to the formation of a zygote and ends with the initiation of its cleavage.

Fetus

The unborn offspring; the developing conceptus following embryogenesis. The fetal period is as follows:

> *Rat*: 15–22 days postconception
> *Mouse*: 14–20
> *Rabbit*: 16–32
> *Mouse*: 14–20
> *Human*: 56–238

Follicle

Small excretory or secretory sac or gland; one of the vascular bodies in the ovary, containing the oocytes.

Atretic Follicle
A Graafian follicle which has involuted.

Graafian Follicle

Mature mammalian ovum with its surrounding epithelial cells.

Ovarian Follicle

The egg and its encasing cells at any stage of development.

Primordial Follicle

Ovarian follicle consisting of an undeveloped egg enclosed by a single layer of cells.

Follicle-Stimulating Hormone

A glycoprotein hormone secreted by the anterior pituitary that promotes spermatogenesis and stimulates growth and secretion of the Graafian follicle.

Gamete

One of two cells produced by a gametocyte, male (spermatozoon) and female (ovum), whose union is necessary in sexual reproduction; a 1N (haploid) cell in sexual fusion.

Gastrula

Early embryonic stage which follows the blastula. The simplest type consists of two layers, the ectoderm and mesectoderm, and two cavities, one lying between the ectoderm and the entoderm; the other (the archenteron) formed by invagination so as to lie within the entoderm and having an opening (the blastopore).

Gastrulation

The process by which a blastula becomes a gastrula or, in forms without a true blastula, the process by which three germ cell layers are acquired.

Gestation

The period of intrauterine development from conception to birth.

Gonadotropin

A substance that acts to stimulate the gonads.

Gravid

Pregnant.

Hydramnios

Altered volume of amniotic fluid.

Oligohydramnios
Reduced quantity at term.

Polyhydramnios
Increased quantity at term.

Hydrometra

Excess fluid (clear, colorless) in the uterus [UTERINE DROPSY].

Implantation

Attachment of the blastocyst to the epithelial lining of the uterus, its penetration through the epithelium, and its embedding in the compact layer of the endometrium [NIDATION].

Infertility

Absence of the ability to conceive, or to induce conception.

Lactation

The secretion of milk; the period following birth during which milk is formed.

Luteinization

The process taking place in the ovarian follicle cells which have matured and discharged their ova; the cells become hypertrophied and assume a yellow or cream color, the follicles becoming corpora lutea.

Luteinizing Hormone

Glycoprotein hormone secreted by the adenohypophysis that stimulates hormone production by interstitial cells of gonads.

Malformation

Defective or abnormal function; anatomic or morphologic abnormality; deformity [BIRTH DEFECT; CONGENITAL ANOMALY; DYSMORPHOSIS; CACOMORPHO-SIS]; defined by the EPA as "a permanent deviation which generally is incompatible with or severely detrimental to normal postnatal survival or development (Fed. Regist. 51(185); 34028–34040, 1986);" For practical purposes: Malformations are those structural anomalies that alter general body conformity, disrupt or interfere with body function, or are generally thought to be incompatible with life. Specific examples of processes that result in maldevelopment include marked or severe mishapening, asymmetry or irregularity of structure brought about by fusion, splitting, disarticulation, malalignment, hiatus, enlargement, lengthening, thickening, thinning, or branching. Absence (agenesis) of parts or whole structures is also considered a malformative process.

Multigravida

A female pregnant for the second (or more) time.

Multipara

A female that has had two or more pregnancies which resulted in birth of viable offspring.

Multiparous

Giving birth to several offspring at one time [POLYTOCOUS].

Morula

The solid mass of blastomeres (embryonic cells) formed by cleavage of a fertilized ovum.

Neonate

Newly born; the neonatal period in humans pertains to the first 4 weeks after delivery.

Nilliparous

A female that never had borne viable offspring [NULLIPAROUS].

Oligomenorrhea

Prolongation of menstrual cycle beyond average limits.

Oocyte

Female ovarian germ cell.

Organogenesis

The period of major organ development in the embryo/fetus; entire period of organogenesis actually continues into the postnatal period, including development of the CNS.

Osteogenesis

Formation or development of the bone (skeleton);

Ovulation

Discharge of an ovum or ovule from a Graafian follicle in the ovary.

Parity

Condition of a female with respect to the number of pregnancy(ies) which resulted in viable born offspring.

Parturition

The act or process of giving birth (delivery; labor).

Perinatal

Occurring shortly before, during or shortly after birth.

Postpartum

After birth or delivery; postnatally (postparturition).

Premature Birth

Birth prior to expected time but capable of surviving ex utero;

Rabbit
After Gest Day 28-up to expected parturition (Day 30).

Mouse
Prior to expected parturition (Day 19).

Rat
Prior to expected parturition (Day 21).

Primigravida

A female pregnant for the first time [UNIGRAVIDA].

Primipara

A female who has born but one offspring [UNIPARA].

Primiparous

Producing only one ovum or offspring at one time [UNIPAROUS].

Progesterone

A steroid hormone produced in corpus luteum, placenta, testes, and adrenals that plays a physiological role in the luteal phase of menstrual cycles and maintenance of pregnancy; also an intermediate in biosynthesis of androgens and estrogens.

Prolactin

A protein hormone produced by the adenohypophysis that stimulates secretion of milk and promotes functional activity of the corpus luteum.

Pseudopregnancy

False pregnancy; the condition mimics those of pregnancy; in rats, accompanied by prolonged diestrus.

Puberty

Period at which the generative organs become capable of reproduction.

Resorption

A conceptus which, having implanted in the uterus, subsequently died and is being, or has been, resorbed.

Early Resorption

Evidence of implantation without recognizable embryonic characteristics evident.

Late Resorption

Recognizable fetal features but undergoing evident autolysis.

Runt

Normally developed fetus or newborn significantly smaller than the rest of the litter.

Semen

A mixture of sperm and fluids from the excurrent ducts and accessory sex glands.

Seminiferous Epithelium

The normal cellular components within the seminiferous tubule consisting of Sertoli cells, spermatogonia, primary spermatocytes, secondary spermatocytes, and spermatids.

Seminiferous Tubules

The structures within the testes in which spermatozoa are produced and begin transport toward the excurrent ducts.

Sertoli Cells

Cells in the testicular tubules providing support, protection and nutrition for the spermatids.

Spermatogenesis

The process of formation of spermatozoa, including spermatogenesis and spermiogenesis; more specifically, the process by which type A spermatogonia germ cells periodically differentiate at a given point within a seminiferous tubule of the testis and divide to give rise to more differentiated spermatogonia and ultimately, primary spermatocytes. The duration of spermatogenesis is the interval from this point until release of the resulting spermatozoa at spermiation.

Spermiation

Complex series of events during which sperm are separated from the seminiferous epithelium and released into the seminiferous tubule lumen.

Spermatogenic Cycle [Cycle of Seminiferous Epithelium]

The interval required for one complete series of cellular associations (spermatogenic stage) to appear at a fixed point within a tubule.

Spontaneous Malformations

The normal background incidence of maldevelopment unrelated to known causes.

Steroidogenesis

Enzymatic steps converting acetate and cholesterol to sex steroids, glucosteroids, or mineralocorticoids.

Stillbirth

Birth of a dead fetus.

Teratogen

An agent or factor that causes the production of physical defects in the developing embryo; the production of defects is termed TERATOGENESIS.

Term

The earliest time at which a fetus can survive outside the mother; fetus at the end of the gestation period (i.e. term fetus).

Testis

The male gonad which contains the seminiferous tubules wherein spermatozoa are produced and the interstitial cells, including Leydig cells, produce androgenic hormones.

Testosterone

A biologically potent androgenic steroid released from the gonads and adrenal glands.

Vaginal plug

A mass of coagulated semen which forms in the vagina of some mammals after coitus [BOUCHON VAGINAL; COPULATION PLUG].

Weaning

The day on which an animal is separated from its mother; usually on postnatal day 21 in the rat.

Yolk sac

An extraembryonic membrane composed of endoderm and splanchnic mesoderm; it is the organ in which the first red blood cells are formed ("blood islands"); In rodents, it is the primary absorptive surface prior to formation of the placenta.

REFERENCES

1. Taylor P. Practical Teratology. New York: Academic Press, 1986.
2. Chapin RE, Heindel JJ. Methods in toxicology. Male Reproductive Toxicology. Vol. 3A. New York: Academic Press, 1993.
3. Chapin RE, Heindel JJ. Methods in toxicology. Female Reproductive Toxicology. Vol. 3B. New York: Academic Press, 1993.
4. Kimmel CA, Buelke-Sam J. Developmental Toxicology. New York: Raven Press, 1981.
5. Witorsch RJ. 2nd ed. Reproductive Toxicology. New York: Raven Press, 1995.
6. Kimmel CA, Makris SL. Recent developments in regulatory requirements for developmental toxicology. Toxicol Lett 2001; 120:73.
7. Reuter U, Heintich-Hirsch B, Hellwig J, et al. Evaluation of OECD screening tests 421 (reproduction/developmental toxicity screening test) and 422 (combined repeated dose toxicity study with the reproduction/developmental toxicity screening test). Regul Toxicol Pharmacol 2003; 38:17.
8. U.S. FDA, Target Animal Safety Guidelines for New Animal Drugs, Office of Scientific Evaluation, Bureau of Veterinary Medicine, Food and Drug Administration, November, 1983.
9. U.S. FDA, General Principles for Evaluating the Safety of Compounds used in Food-Producing Animals, Office of Scientific Evaluation, Bureau of Veterinary Medicine, Food and Drug Administration, November, 1986.
10. Japanese Ministry of Agriculture, Forestry and Fisheries, Guidelines for Toxicity Studies of New Animal Drugs, Notification No. 63–44 of the Pharmacuetical Affairs Office, Tokyo, Japan, 1988.
11. Wise LD, Beck SL, Beltrame D, et al. Terminology of developmental abnormalities in common laboratory mammals (version 1). Teratology 1997; 55:249.
12. Solecki R, Bergmann B, Burgin H, et al. Harmonization of rat fetal external and visceral terminology and classification. Report of the fourth workshop on the terminology in developmental toxicology, Berlin, 18–20 April 2002. Reprod Toxicol 2003; 17:625.
13. Harris MW, Chapin RE, Lockhart AC, et al. Assessment of a short-term reproductive and developmental toxicity screen. Fundam Appl Toxicol 1992; 19:186.
14. Scala RA, Bevan C, Beyer BK. An abbreviated repeat dose and reproductive/ developmental toxicity test for high production volume chemicals. Regul Toxicol Pharmacol 1992; 16:73.
15. Neubert D. Benefits and limits of model systems in developmental biology and toxicology (in vitro techniques). In: Marois M, ed. Prevention of Physical and Mental Congenital Defects. New York: Alan R Liss, 1985:91.
16. Neubert D, Blankenburg G, Lewandowski C, Klug S. Misinterpretations of results and creation of "artifacts" in studies on developmental toxicity using systems simpler than in vivo systems. Developmental Mechanisms: Normal and Abnormal. New York: Alan R Liss Inc., 1985:241.
17. Piersma AH, Verhoef A, Dortant PM. Evaluation of the OECD 421 reproductive toxicity screening test protocol using butyl benzyl phthalate. Toxicology 1995; 99:191.
18. Gray LE, Jr., Kavlock RJ. An extended evaluation of an in vivo teratology screen utilizing postnatal growth and viability in the mouse. Terat Carcin Mutagen 1984; 4:403.
19. Homburger F, Goldberg GN. In Vitro Embryotoxicity and Teratogenicity Tests. Basal: S. Karger, 1985.
20. U.S. EPA, OPPTS 870.3550 Reproduction/Develpmental Toxicity Screening Test. July 2000.
21. U.S. EPA, OPPTS 870.3650 Combined Repeated Dose Toxicity Study with the Reproduction/ Develpmental Toxicity Screening Test. July 2000.

22. O'Connor JC, Cook JC, Slone TW, et al. An ongoing validation of a tier I screening battery for detecting endocrine-active compounds (EACs). Toxicol Sci 1998; 46:45.
23. International Conference on Harmonization: Guideline on Detection of Toxicity to Reproduction. Fed Regist 59: 48746, issued September 22, 1994.
24. Tuchmann-Duplessis J. Selection of animal species for teratogenic drug testing. In: Neubert D, Merker HJ, Kwashigrouch TE, eds. Methods in Prenatal Toxicity. Stuttgart: Georg Thieme Publisher, 1977:25.
25. Stanton HC. Factors to consider when selecting animal models for postnatal teratology studies. J Environ Pathol Toxicol 1978; 2:201.
26. Amann RP. Use of animal models for detecting specific alterations in reproduction. Fundam Appl Toxicol 1982; 2:13.
27. Frankos VH. FDA perspective on the use of teratology data for human risk assessment. Fundam Appl Toxicol 1985; 5:615.
28. Tanimura T. Japanese perspectives on the reproductive and developmental toxicity evaluation of pharmaceuticals. J Am Coll Toxicol 1990; 9:27.
29. European Chemical Industry Ecology and Toxicology Centre, Technical Report No. 21, A Guide to the Classification of Carcinogens, Mutagens and Teratogens Under the Sixth Amendment. Brussels, Belgium, 1986.
30. U.S. EPA. Guidelines for the health assessment of suspected developmental toxicants. Fed Regist 1986; 51:34028. U.S. EPA. Guidelines for the health assessment of suspected developmental toxicants proposed amendments. Fed Regist 1989; 54:9386.
31. Moore JA, Daston GP, Faustman E, et al. An evaluation process for assessing human reproductive and developmental toxicity of agents. Reprod Toxicol 1995; 9:61.
32. Ulbrich B, Palmer AK. Detection of effects on male reproduction—a literature survey. J Am Coll Toxicol 1995; 14:293.
33. Takayama S, Akaike M, Kawashima K, Takahashi M, Kurokawa Y. A collaborative study in Japan on optimal treatment period and parameters for detection of male fertility disorders induced by drugs in rats. J Am Coll Toxicol 1995; 14:266.
34. Schwartz S. Providing toxicokinetic support for reproductive toxicology studies in pharmaceutical development. Arch Toxicol 2001; 75:381.
35. Fox RR, Laird CW. Sexual cycles. In: Hafez ESE, ed. Reproduction and Breeding Techniques for Laboratory Animals. Philadelphia, PA: Lea & Febiger, 1970:107.
36. Staples RE. Detection of visceral alterations in mammalian fetuses. Teratology 1974; 9:A37.
37. Barrow MV, Taylor WJ. A rapid method for detecting malformations in rat fetuses. J Morphology 1969; 127:291.
38. Stuckhardt JL, Poppe SM. Fresh visceral examination of rat and rabbit fetuses used in teratogenicity testing. Teratog Carcinog Mutagen 1984; 4:181.
39. Wilson JG. Methods for administering agents and detecting malformations in experimental animals. In: Wilson JG, Warkany J, eds. Teratology: principles and technigues. Chicago: University of Chicago Press, 1965:263.
40. Sterz H. Routine examination of rat and rabbit fetuses for malformation of internal organ combination of Barrow's and Wilson's methods. In: Neubert D, Merker HJ, Kwashigrouch TE, eds. Methods in Prenatal Toxicology. Stuttgart: Georg Thieme Publisher, 1977:113.
41. Sterz H, Lehmann H. A critical comparison of the freehand razor-blade dissection method according to Wilson with an in situ sectioning method for rat fetuses. Teratog Carcinog Mutagen 1985; 5:347.
42. Machemer L, Stenger EG. Examination of fetuses in teratological experiments. Modification of "Wilson Technique". Arzneimittel Forschung 1971; 21:144.
43. Faherty JF, Jackson BA, Greene MF. Surface staining of 1 mm (Wilson) slices of fetuses for internal visceral examination. Stain Technol 1972; 47:53.
44. van Julsingha EB, Bennett CG. A dissecting procedure for detection of anomalies in the rabbit fetal head. In: Neubert D, Merker HJ, Kwashigrouch TE, eds. Methods in Prenatal Toxicology. Stuttgart: Georg Thieme Publisher, 1977:126.
45. Igarashi E. New method for the detection of cardiovascular malformations in rat fetuses: gelatin-embedding-slice method. Teratology 1983; 48:329.

46. Dawson AB. A note on the staining of the skeleton of cleared specimens with Alizarin red S. Stain Technol 1926; 1:123.

47. Jensh RP, Brent RL. Rapid schedules for KOH-clearing and Alizarin red S staining of fetal rat bone. Stain Technol 1966; 41:179.

48. Staples RE, Schnell VL. Refinements in rapid clearing technique in the KOH-Alizarin red S method for fetal bone. Stain Technol 1964; 39:61.

49. Fritz H, Hess R. Ossification of the rat and mouse skeleton in the perinatal period. Teratology 1970; 3:331.

50. Marr MC, Meyers CB, George JD, Price CP. Comparison of single and double staining for evaluation of skeletal development: the effects of ethylene glycol (EG) in CD rats. Teratology 1988; 33:476.

51. Kawamura S, Hirohashi A, Kato T, Yasuda M. Bone-staining technique for fetal rat specimens without skinning and removing adipose tissue. Congenit Anom 1990; 30:93.

52. Agnish ND, Keller KA. The scientific rationale for culling of rodent litters. Fundam Appl Toxicol 1997; 38:2.

53. Claudio L, Kwa WC, Russell AL, et al. Testing methods for developmental neurotoxicity of environmental chemicals. Toxicol Appl Pharmacol 2000; 164:1.

54. Kaufmann W. Current status of developmental neurotoxicity: an industry perspective. Toxicol Lett 2003; 161:140–141.

55. Perreault SD, Cancel AM. Significance of incorporating measures of sperm production and function into rat toxicology studies. Reproduction 2001; 121:207.

56. Hirschfield AN. Histological assessment of follicular development and its applicability to risk assessment. Reprod Toxicol 1987; 1:71.

57. Russell LD, Ettlin RA, Hikim APS, Clegg ED. Histological and Histopathological Evaluation of the Testis. Clearwater, Florida: Cache River Press, 1990.

58. Lamb JC, IV, Chapin RE. Experimental models of male reproductive toxicology. In: Thomas JA, Korach KS, McLachlan JA, eds. Endocrine Toxicology. New York: Raven Press, 1985:85.

59. Creasy DM. Evaluation of testicular toxicology: a symposium and discussion of the recommendations proposed by the society of toxicologic pathology. Birth Defects Res B Dev Reprod Toxicol 2003; 68:408.

60. Rao KS, Schwetz BA, Park CN. Reproductive toxicity risk assessment of chemicals. Vet Hum Toxicol 1981; 23:167.

61. Interagency regulatory liaison group workshop on reproductive toxicity risk assessment. Environ Health Perspect, 1986; 66: 193.

62. Gad SC, Weil CS. Statistics for toxicologists. In: Hayes AW, ed. Principles and Methods of Toxicology. New York: Raven Press, 1982:273.

63. Shirley EAC, Hickling R. An evaluation of some statistical methods for analysing numbers of abnormalities found amongst litters in teratology studies. Biometrics 1981; 37:819.

64. Ten Have TR, Hartzel T. Comparison of two approaches to analyzing correlated binary data in developmental toxicity studies. Teratology 1995; 52:267.

65. Dunson DB. Assessing overall risk in reproductive experiments. Risk Anal 2000; 20:429.

66. Allen AS, Barnhart HX. Joint models for toxicology studies with dose-dependent number of implantations. Risk Anal 2002; 22:1165.

67. Fritz H, Giese K. Evaluation of the teratogenic potential of chemicals in the rat. Pharmacology 1990; 40:1.

68. Feussner EL, Lightkep GE, Hennesy RA, Hoberman AM, Christian MS. A decade of rabbit fertility data: study of historical control animals. Teratology 1992; 46:349.

69. Morita H, Matsumoto A, Nagato I. Spontaneous malformations in laboratory animals: frequency of external, internal and skeletal malformations in rats, rabbits and mice. Congenit Anom 1987; 27:147.

70. Spence S. The Dutch-belted rabbit: an alternative breed for developmental toxicity testing. Birth Defects Res B Dev Reprod Toxicol 2003; 68:439.

71. Aoyama H, Kikuta M, Shirasaka N, et al. Historical control data on reproductive abilities and incidences of spontaneous fetal malformations in Wistar Hannover GALAS rats. Congenit Anom (Kyoto) 2002; 42:194.

72. Savitz DA. Is statistical significance testing useful in interpreting data? Reprod Toxicol 1993; 7:95.
73. May PC, Finch CE. Aging and responses to toxins in female reproductive functions. Reprod Toxicol 1988; 1:223.
74. Hansel W, Convey EM. Physiology of the estrous cycle. J Anim Sci 1983; 57:404.
75. Adler NT, Resko JA, Goy RW. The effect of copulatory behavior on hormonal change in the female rat prior to implantation. Physiol Behav 1970; 5:1003.
76. Chester RV, Zucker L. Influence of male copulatory behavior on sperm transport, pregnancy and pseudopregnancy in female rats. Physiol Behav 1970; 5:35.
77. Adler NT, Toner JP. The effect of copulatory behavior on sperm transport and fertility in rats. Ann NY Acad Sci 1986; 474:21.
78. Meistrich ML. Quantitative correlation between testicular stem cell survival, sperm production and fertility in the mouse after treatment with different cytotoxic agents. J Androl 1982; 3:58.
79. Fuchs AR, Fuchs R. Endocrinology of human parturition: a review. Br J Obstet Gynecol 1984; 91:948.
80. Neulen J, Breckwoldt M. Placental progesterone, prostaglandins and mechansims leading to initiation of parturition in the human, Exp Clin Endocrinol 1994; 102:195.
81. Chan WY, Chen DL. Myometrial oxytocin receptors and prostaglandin in the parturition process in the rat. Biol Reprod 1992; 46:58.
82. Schwetz BA, Rao KS, Park CN. Insensitivity of tests for reproductive problems. J Environ Pathol Toxicol 1980; 3:81.
83. Heywood R, James RW. Assessment of testicular toxicity in laboratory animals. Environ Health Perspect 1978; 24:73.
84. Blazak WF, Ernst TL, Stewart BE. Potential indicators of reproductive toxicity: testicular sperm production and epididymal sperm number, transit time, and motility in Fischer 344 rats. Fundam Appl Toxicol 1985; 5:1097.
85. Ribelin WE. Atrophy of rat testis as index of chemical toxicity. Arch Pathol 1963; 75:229.
86. Chapin RE, Gulati DK, Barnes LH, Teague JL. The efffects of feed restriction on reproductive function in Sprague-Dawley rats. Fundam Appl Toxicol 1993; 20:23.
87. Parshad RK. Effect of restricted feeding of prepubertal and adult male rats on fertility and sex ratio. Indian J Exp Biol 1993; 31:991.
88. Jones TC, Mohr U, Hunt RD. Genital System. Berlin: Springer Verlag, 1987.
89. Creasy PMD. Foster, male reproductive system. In: Haschek WM, Rousseaux CG, eds. Handbook of Toxicologic Pathology. New York: Academic Press, Inc., 1991:829.
90. Mori H, Christensen AK. Morphometric analysis of Leydig cells in the normal rat testis. J Cell Biol 1980; 84:340.
91. Creasy DM. Evaluation of testicular toxicity in safety evaluation studies: the appropriate use of spermatogenic staging. Toxicol Pathol 1997; 25:119.
92. Yuan. Female reproductive system. In: Haschek WM, Rousseaux CG, eds. Handbook of Toxicologic Pathology. New York: Academic Press, Inc., 1991:891.
93. Russell, Ettlin RA, Sinha Hikim AP, Clegg ED. Histological and Histopathological Evaluation of the Testis. Clearwater, FLA: Cache River Press, 1990.
94. Mattison DR. How xenobiotic compounds can destroy oocytes. Contemp Obstet Gynecol 1980; 15:157.
95. Pederson T, Peters H. Proposal for a classification of oocytes and follicles in the mouse ovary. J Reprod Fertil 1968; 17:555.
96. Smith BJ, Plowchalk DR, Snipes IG, Mattison DR. Comparison of random and serial sections in assessment of ovarian toxicity. Reprod Toxicol 1991; 5:379.
97. Miller RT, Davis BJ. Toxicologic pathology of the reproductive and endocrine systems. Toxicol Pathol 2001; 29:1.
98. Mangelsdorf I, Buschmann J, Orthen B. Some aspects relating to the evaluation of the effects of chemicals on male fertility. Regul Toxicol Pharmacol 2003; 37:356.
99. Keyes PL. The corpus luteum. Int Rev Physiol 1983; 27:57.

100. Johnson EM, Christian MS. When is a teratology study not an evaluation of teratogenicity? J Am Coll Toxicol 1984; 3:431.
101. Manson JM. Teratogens. In: Klaassen CD, Amdur MO, Doull J, eds. Casarett and Doull's Toxicology: The Basic Science of Poisons. 3rd ed. New York: Macmillian Publisher Co., 1986:195.
102. Beck F, Lloyd JB. An investigation of the relationship between foetal death and foetal malformation. J Anat 1963; 97:555.
103. Holson R, Webb PJ, Grafton TF, Hansen DK. Prenatal neuroleptic exposure and growth stunting in the rat: an in vivo and in vitro examination of sensitive periods and possible mechanisms. Teratology 1994; 50:125.
104. Schardein JL, Keller KA. Potential human developmental toxicants and the role of animal testing in their identification and charaterization. CRC Crit Rev Toxicol 1989; 10:251.
105. Palmer AK. Assessment of current test procedures. Environ Health Perspect 1976; 18:97.
106. Yasuda M, Maeda H. Significance of the lumbar rib as an indicator in teratogenicity tests. Teratology 1972; 6:124.
107. Beyer PE, Chernoff N. The induction of supernumerary ribs in rodents: role of maternal stress. Teratog Carcinog Mutagen 1986; 6:419.
108. Joosten HFP, Yih TD, Waarlkens DH, Hoekstra A. The relevance of wavy rib in teratological evaluation. Toxicol Lett Spec Issue Abstr 1980; 188:109.
109. Khera KS. Pathogenesis of undulated ribs: a congenital malformation. Fundam Appl Toxicol 1981; 1:13.
110. Van Loveren H, Vos J, Putman E, Piersma A. Immunotoxicological consequences of perinatal chemical exposures: a plea for inclusion of immune parameters in reproduction studies. Toxicology 2003; 185:185.
111. Chapin RE. The use of the rat in developmental immunotoxicology studies. Hum Exp Toxicol 2002; 21:521.
112. Kimmel CA. The evaluation of behavioral teratogenic effects. Congenit Anom 1987; 27:139.
113. Stanton ME, Spear LP. Workshop on the qualitative and quantitative comparability of human and animal developmental neurotoxicity, work group I report: comparability of measures of developmental neurotoxicity in humans and laboratory animals. Neurotoxicol Teratol 1990; 12:261.
114. Kimmel C, Rees DC, Francis EZ. Qualitative and quantitative comparability of human and animal developmental neurotoxicity. Neurotoxicol Teratol 1990; 12:173.
115. Claudio L, Kwa WC, Russell AL, et al. Testing methods for developmental neurotoxicity of environmental chemicals. Toxicol Appl Pharmacol 2000; 164:1.
116. Hass U. Current status of developmental neurotoxicity: regulatory view. Toxicol Lett 2003; 155:140–141.
117. Altman J. Morphological and behavioral markers of environmentally induced retardation of brain development: an animal model. Environ Health Perspect 1987; 74:153.
118. MacLusky NJ, Naftolin F. Sexual differentiation of the central nervous system. Science 1981; 211:1294.
119. Urbanski HF, Ojeda SR. Neuroendocrine mechanisms controlling the onset of female puberty. Reprod Toxicol 1987; 1:129.
120. Rajfer J, Walsh PC. Hormonal regulation of testicular descent: experimental and clinical observations. J Urol 1977; 118:985.
121. Allen BC, Kavlock RJ, Kimmel CA, Faustman EM. Dose-response assessment for developmental toxicity II. Comparison of generic benchmark dose estimates with no observed adverse effect levels. Fundam Appl Toxicol 1994; 23:487.
122. Kimmel CA, Kavlock RJ, Allen BC, Faustman EM. The application of benchmark dose methodology to data from prenatal developmental toxicity studies. Toxicol Lett 1995; 549:82–83.
123. Foster PMD, Auton TR. Application of benchmark dose risk assessment methodology to developmental toxicity: an industrial view. Toxicol Lett 1995; 555:82–83.
124. Krump KS. Calculation of benchmark doses from continuous data. Risk Anal 1995; 15:79.

125. U.S. FDA. Pregnancy labelling. FDA Drug Bull 1979; 9:23.

126. U.S. FDA. Pregnancy Categories. Fed Regist 1979; 44:37464.

127. Teratology Society Public Affairs Committee. FDA classification of drugs for teratogenic risk. Teratology 1994; 49:446.

128. Welsch F. Approaches to Elucidate Mechanisms in Teratogenesis. Washington: Hemisphere Publisher Co., 1987.

129. Hess DL. Neuroendocrinology of female reproduction: review, models, and potential approaches for risk assessment. Reprod Toxicol 1988; 1:139.

130. Desjardins C. Endocrine regulation of reproductive development and function in the male. J Anim Sci 1978; 47:56.

131. U.S. EPA. Proposed guidelines for assessing male reproductive risk. Fedl Regist 1988; 53:24850.

132. U.S. FDA. Proposed guidelines for assessing female reproductive risk. Fed Regist 1988; 53:24834.

133. Hughes CL. Effects of phytoestrogens on GnRH-induced luteinizing hormone secretion in ovariectomized rats. Reprod Toxicol 1988; 1:179.

134. Amann RP. Detection of alterations in testicular and epididymal function in laboratory animals. Environ Health Perspect 1986; 70:149.

135. Janca FC, Jost LK, Evenson DP. Mouse testicular and sperm development characterized by dual parameter flow cytometry. Biol Reprod 1986; 34:613.

136. Kangasniemi M, Veromaa T, Kulmala J, et al. DNAflow cytometry of defined stages of rat seminiferous epithelium: effects of 3 Gy of highenergy Xirradiation. J Androl 1990; 11:312.

137. Cross NL, Meizel S. Methods for evaluating the acrosomal status of mammalian sperm. Biol Reprod 1989; 41:635.

138. Barbato GF, Cramer PG, Hammerstedt RH. A practical in vitro sperm-egg binding assay that detects subfertile males. Biol Reprod 1998; 58:686.

139. Laskey J, Berman E, Carter H, Ferrell J. Identification of toxicant induced alterations in steroid profiles using whole ovary culture. Toxicologist 1991; 11:111.

140. Perreault SD, Jeffay S, Poss P, Laskey JW. Use of the fungicide carbendazim as a model compound to determine the impact of acute chemical exposure during oocyte maturation and fertilization on pregnancy outcome in the hamster. Toxicol Appl Pharmacol 1992; 114:225.

141. Felton JS, Dobson RL. The mouse oocyte toxicity assay. In: Waters MD, ed. Application of Short-Term Bioassays in the Analysis of Complex Environmental Mixtures. New York: Plenum Press, 1982.

142. Nayudu PL, Kiesel PS, Nowshari MA, Hodges JK. Abnormal in vitro development of ovarian follicles explanted from mice exposed to tetrachlorovinphos. Reprod Toxicol 1994; 8:261.

143. Blondin P, Dufour M, Sirard MA. Analysis of atresia in bovine follicles using different methods: flow cytometry, enzyme-linked immunosorbent assay, and classic histology. Biol Reprod 1996; 54:631.

144. Rao MC, Gibori G. Corpus luteum: animal models of possible relevance to reproductive toxicology. Reprod Toxicol 1987; 1:61.

145. Gerall AA, McCrady RE. Receptivity scores of female rats stimulated either manually or by males. J Endocrinol 1970; 46:55.

146. Etgen AM. 1-(o-Chlorophyenyl)-1-(p-chlorophenyl)2,2,2-trichloroethane: A probe for studiying estrogen and progestin receptor mediation of female sexual behavior and neuroendocrine responses. Endocrinology 1982; 111:1498.

147. McClintock MK, Adler NT, Suer SF. Postejaculatory quiescence in female and male rats: consequences for sperm transport during group mating. J Comp Physiol Psychol 1982; 36:542.

148. Madlafousek J, Hlinak Z. Sexual behavior of the female laboratory rat: inventory, patterning, and measurement. Behavior 1977; 63:129.

149. Cummings AM. Toxicological mechanisms of implantation failure. Fundam Appl Toxicol 1990; 15:571.

150. Toyoda Y, Chang MC. Fertilization of rat eggs in vitro by epidiymal spermatozoa and the development of eggs following transfer. J Reprod Fertil 1974; 36:9.

151. Juberg DR, Webb RC, Loch-Caruso R. Characterization of o,p'-DDT-stimulated contraction frequency in rat uterus in vitro. Fundam Appl Toxicol 1991; 17:543.

152. Criswell K, Loch-Caruso R, Stuenkel E. Lindane inhibits gap junctional communication (GJC) in rat myometrial cells via a calcium-independent process. Toxicologist 1993; 13:354.

153. Latrille F, Perrand J, Stadler J, Monroe AM, Sutter BC. Effects of tioconazole on parturition and serum levels of 17b-oestradiol, progesterone, LH and PRL in the rat. Biochem Pharmacol 1987; 36:1119.

154. Powell JG, Jr., Cochrane RL. The effects of a number of non steroidal anti inflammatory compounds on parturition in the rat. Prostaglandins 1982; 23:469.

155. Sampson DA, Jansen GR. Measurement of milk yield in the lactating rat from pup weight and weight gain. J Pediatr Gastroenterol Nutr 1984; 3:613.

156. Russel JA. Milk yield, suckling behavior and milk ejection in the lactating rat nursing litters of different sizes. J Physiol 1980; 303:403.

157. Maestripieri D, Badiani A, Puglisi-Allegra S. Prepartal chronic stress increases anxiety and decreases aggression in lactating female mice. Behav Neurosci 1991; 105:663.

158. Giordano AL, Johnson AE, Rosenblatt JS. Haloperidol-induced disruption of retrieval behavior and reversal with apomorphine in lactating rats. Physiol Behav 1990; 48:211.

159. Beckman DA, Brent RL. Mechanisms of teratogenesis. Ann Rev Pharmacol Toxicol 1984; 24:485.

160. Wilmut I, Sales DI, Ashworth CJ. Maternal and embryonic factors associated with prenatal loss in mammals. J Reprod Fertil 1986; 76:851.

161. Homburger F, Goldberg AN. In Vitro Embryotoxicity and Teratogenicity Tests. Basal: S. Karger, 1985.

162. Brinster RL. Teratogen testing using preimplantation mammalian embryos. In: Shepard TH, Miller JR, Marios M, eds. Methods for Detection of Environmental Agents that Produce Congenital Defects. New York: American Elsevier Publisher Co. Inc., 1975:113.

163. Dushnik-Levinson M, Benvenisty N. Embryogenesis in vitro: study of differentiation of embryonic stem cells. Biol Neonate 1995; 67:77.

164. McClain RM, Hoar RM. The effect of flunitrazepam on reproduction in the rat. The use of cross-fostering in the evaluation of postnatal parameters in rat reproduction studies. Toxicol Appl Pharmacol 1980; 53:92.

150.

151.

152.

153.

154.

12

Neurotoxicology Testing[†]

Kathleen C. Raffaele
Health Effects Division, Office of Pesticide Programs, U.S. Environmental Protection Agency, Washington, D.C., U.S.A.

Walter P. Weisenburger
Advanced Neuro Health LLC, Kalispell, Montana, U.S.A.

INTRODUCTION: WHAT IS NEUROTOXICITY?

The last several decades have seen a great increase in concern regarding possible effects of exposure to environmental chemicals (including drugs, pesticides, and other commercial products) on the nervous system. Increases, perceived or real, in the incidence of such developmental defects as autism or attention deficit disorder, as well as possible associations between environmental exposure and neurodegenerative diseases, such as Alzheimer's disease and Parkinson's disease, have focused public attention on the brain as a target for adverse effects of such chemicals (1–4). At the same time, there have been major advances in neuroscience over the past several decades (recognized by the U.S. Congress in declaring the 1990s the "Decade of the Brain"), expanding our ability to understand the function of the nervous system and how a variety of chemical classes may impact the normal functioning of that system. Impetus for improving our evaluation of the developing nervous system was further provided by a report from the National Academy of Sciences (5) issued in 1993, which suggested that in many cases the immature organism may be more sensitive to adverse effects of environmental chemicals. Subsequent passage of the Food Quality Protection Act [FQPA] by the U.S. Congress mandated more thorough assessment by the U.S. Environmental Protection Agency (EPA) of toxicity to the developing organism for pesticides in food (6), stimulating additional focus on evaluating neurotoxicity in the young. The U.S. Food and Drug Administration (FDA) also has had an increased interest in testing in juveniles drugs that have previously been tested in adults only, in order to provide better data for evaluating safety of these drugs for use in children.

Although other countries have recognized that nervous system disease might sometimes be a consequence of exposure to manmade chemicals and drugs, the EPA was the first regulatory agency to systematically propose, develop, and promulgate detailed and specific guidelines for the testing of compounds for neurotoxic potential. The 1982 Pesticide

---

[†]This chapter does not necessarily reflect the policy of the U.S. Environmental Protection Agency.

Assessment Guidelines (7) were revised and expanded in scope in 1991 to include a set of neurotoxicity guidelines originally developed for testing industrial chemicals under the Toxic Substances Control Act (TSCA) (8). A revised set of neurotoxicity guidelines, harmonized between these two EPA programs, was published in 1998 (9). In addition to a Neurotoxicity Screening Battery, the harmonized guidelines added limited assessments of neurotoxicity-related parameters into most subchronic and chronic toxicity studies. A similar strategy is seen in the current Organization for Economic Cooperation and Development (OECD) test guideline series, and the OECD Neurotoxicity Guideline (10) is very similar to the current EPA Neurotoxicity Screening Battery test guideline. In addition to the Neurotoxicity Screening Battery, EPA has developed guidelines for more detailed assessments of several aspects of nervous system function, including Schedule-controlled operant behavior (SCOB) (870.6500), Peripheral nerve function (870.6850), and Neurophysiology: Sensory evoked potentials (870.6855) (9). These guidelines were intended for use as follow-up studies to develop more detailed information regarding impacts of compounds on nervous system functioning than can be achieved by use of the screening battery alone.

The EPA neurotoxicity guidelines were developed to test pesticides and chemicals used in industry, when available evidence suggests that there could be a potential for neurotoxicity. Neurotoxicity testing has long been recommended for the registration of new pesticides and the reregistration of old pesticides; these recommendations have been made more formal with the inclusion of both the acute and subchronic neurotoxicity screening battery as part of the required toxicology database in the recently proposed revisions to the Part 158 pesticide toxicity testing requirements (11). Neurotoxicity testing is also required by EPA on a case-by-case basis for chemicals used in industry, when a specific concern has been raised or when other members of the chemical class have been shown to be neurotoxic.

Neurotoxicity is an obvious concern in the development of new pharmaceutical entities. The risk-benefit analysis for drugs is quite different from that for most other chemical uses in that pharmaceuticals are developed specifically to assist in the amelioration or prevention of disease. Although no pharmaceutical regulatory agency in any country to date has specific requirements for the routine testing of new drugs for neurotoxicity, a general requirement to evaluate effects on the central nervous system (CNS) (including motor activity, behavioral changes, coordination, and other end points) is included in the International Conference on Harmonization (ICH) Harmonized Tripartite Guideline for Safety Pharmacology Studies for Human Pharmaceuticals (12), and the FDA and comparable agencies around the world sometimes ask for additional studies. In the U.S., the FDA also regulates food additives; current guidelines used in developing safety data for food additives also do not include a separate guideline for evaluation of neurotoxicity (13). Current recommendations for safety evaluation of food additives are that neurotoxicity be routinely assessed in the form of more detailed clinical observations but that additional data may be requested in specific instances. Many of the studies requested by FDA are performed according to the tests specified in the EPA neurotoxicity guidelines and use criteria published in the guidelines to aid in test selection. For these reasons, the EPA guidelines will be used to develop the protocols to be presented in this chapter.

The definition of neurotoxicity accepted here is as it appears in the EPA neurotoxicity guidelines: "Neurotoxicity is any adverse effect on the structure or function of the nervous system related to exposure to a chemical substance" (14). Similar definitions are used by the EPA Neurotoxicity Risk Assessment Guidelines (15), and by the OECD (16) and International Programme on Chemical Safety (IPCS) (17) in their guidance documents. This broad definition includes effects on function as observed and/or inferred from the behavior of the animal or person, neurochemical or neurophysiological changes, as well as lesions and other effects on the underlying structures of the central and peripheral nervous systems as observed macroscopically and microscopically with the various techniques of histopathology and neuropathology. One type of end point cannot fully substitute one for the other, as behavior can be altered without any observable or detectable structural pathology, and some nervous system lesions, particularly during the early stages of intoxication, do not have obvious functional correlates. Similarly, neurochemical or neurophysiological changes may often be detected in the absence of obvious behavioral changes. The absence of functional correlates should not be taken to indicate a lack of adverse effect, because our behavioral assessments are often quite limited, especially when considered in the context of the behavioral repertoire of most animal species.

As mentioned previously, concern for neurotoxicity includes effects on both adult and developing organisms. In some instances, it has been shown that developing animals and people can be considerably more affected than adults by exposure to harmful chemicals. Disruption or delay of development either during gestation, infancy, or childhood can cause irreversible changes in the nervous system. Although toxic effects on the adult system result most often from interference with communication among nerve cells or direct damage to cellular structures, the developing nervous system presents additional targets, including interference with cellular proliferation and migration, or with intercellular signaling necessary for proper organization of the nervous system. Thus, although the developing nervous system displays more plasticity than the adult, raising the possibility of some functional compensation, developmental exposure may result in permanent change (either structural or functional) that would not be seen following a similar exposure in an adult. Well-known examples of this type of effect in humans include fetal alcohol syndrome (18) and the sequelae of exposure to methyl mercury (19).

As a result of concern for this type of developmental effect, regulatory agencies in Japan and the United Kingdom began in the 1970s to require studies for new pharmaceutical agents that examine effects on the offspring of treated pregnant rats. Those regulatory agencies identified the types of functions that were of interest in terms of "auditory, visual, and behavioral function" for the United Kingdom (20) and "motor and sensory activity, emotion, learning…." etc. for Japan (21). Those guidelines did not dictate specific tests to be performed, allowing for and encouraging greater use of judgment on the part of each investigator and more flexibility in designing studies appropriate for the specific drug under investigation. At least that was the intent. The reality was that a battery was rarely modified for individual compounds once that battery was adopted by a company or contract testing facility. A major problem for the pharmaceutical companies was that this kind of testing was expensive, and differences in the two guidelines often resulted in many behavioral and functional measures being incorporated into all three of the reproductive segment studies (see Chapter 11 for descriptions of the segment studies) if the drug was intended for global marketing. After many years of efforts at "harmonization," the ICH Guidelines on Detection of Toxicity to Reproduction for Medicinal Products were adopted by the European Union and Japan prior to being published in the United States in 1994 (22). Although behavioral testing is incorporated into the ICH Guideline for reproductive toxicity testing, the requirements remain nonspecific, including examination of sensory functions and reflexes and behavior (with suggested assessment of sensory functions, motor activity, and learning and memory), but without specifying any particular procedures or timepoints for assessment. The FDA never required such functional testing and currently "accepts" such testing without actually requiring it. This kind of testing is often referred to as developmental neurotoxicity (DNT) testing, although pharmaceutical companies rarely use that term; usually referring to the study as the perinatal study or the segment III reproductive study.

Studies conducted by the pharmaceutical industry to satisfy the various regulatory mandates from the mid-1970s until the present provided a very good foundation for the testing of chemicals currently required on a case-by-case basis by the EPA for pesticides and chemicals acknowledged to be toxic to adults, and guidelines for DNT testing were included in the 1991 version of the Pesticide Assessment Guidelines cited above (7). As mentioned previously, passage of the FQPA in 1996 (6) led to an increased emphasis on evaluation of toxicity to the developing organism following exposure to pesticides. This in turn led to an increase in the requirement that pesticide chemicals be tested for DNT, and criteria for invoking that requirement have been developed by the Office of Pesticide Programs in EPA (see below). Protocols for studies to be done according to the EPA DNT guidelines will be discussed further below (see section "Developmental neurotoxicity testing: study design" in this chapter).

ADULT NEUROTOXICITY TESTING: STUDY DESIGN

The basic study design dicussed here is from the EPA 860.6200 Adult Neurotoxicity Screening Battery, as described in the harmonized toxicity testing guidelines published in 1998 (23). This study is designed to evaluate possible effects on the human nervous system resulting from exposure to environmental chemicals and can be conducted using either single or multiple exposures, depending on the exposure scenario of concern. The OECD Guideline for a Neurotoxicity Study in Rodents (Guideline Number 424) includes similar end points to those in the EPA guideline, with only small differences in recommended timing of the assessments (8). Elements from the EPA Neurotoxicity test guideline are also currently included in other types of toxicity studies, for example, the EPA 870 series test guidelines recommend inclusion of a weekly detailed clinical examination similar to the functional observational battery (FOB) discussed below, as well as an assessment of motor activity, grip strength, and sensory reactivity to visual, auditory, and proprioceptive stimuli, toward the end of most subchronic and chronic toxicity studies. Similar assessments are also included in the OECD guidelines for subchronic toxicity studies (e.g., 407 and 408) (24,25).

The neurotoxicity screening battery includes a FOB, assessment of spontaneous motor activity using an automated device, and a detailed neuropathological evaluation (Table 1). The battery is intended for use in conjunction with general toxicity study data, and the resulting data should be interpreted in light of other toxicologically relevant information. The battery is a first-tier screen and will not provide a complete evaluation of neurotoxic potential, nor will it provide sufficient information to determine mechanisms. The need for additional, more specific neurotoxicity data could result in the conduct of studies using more focused guidelines (e.g., detailed evaluation of peripheral nerve function or evoked potentials) or in the conduct of studies assessing neurochemical changes that may be related to the mechanism of action for the compound being evaluated (e.g., cholinesterase inhibition for organophosphate or carbamate pesticides).

Study Basics

The EPA guidelines specify that the test material should be well characterized and in a stable form. The vehicle should provide for homogeneous dispersion of the test material as

Table 1 U.S. Environmental Protection Agency Neurotoxicity Screening Battery for Adult Rats: Measured Parameters and Evaluation Timepoints

Functional observational battery	Autonomic signs (lacrimation, salivation, piloerection, exophthalmus, urination, defecation, pupillary function, palpebral closure): convulsions, tremors, abnormal movements; reactivity to handling, arousal; grip strength, landing foot splay; pain perception; posture and gait, unusual/abnormal behaviors; stereotypies, altered appearance; body temperature
Motor activity	Automated apparatus, animals tested individually, session long enough to approach asymptotic levels for last 20% of session
Timing of testing for FOB and motor activity:	
Acute studies	Before dosing, estimated time of peak effect within 8 hours of dosing, 7 days and 14 days after dosing
Subchronic studies	Before first dose; 4th, 8th, and 13th week of exposure[a]
Chronic studies	Before first dose and every 3 months thereafter[b]
Neuropathology	End of study, at least 5/sex/group, in situ perfusion with aldehyde fixative, paraffin, and/or plastic embedding for central nervous system tissues, plastic embedding for peripheral nervous system tissues, special stains as necessary (GFAP encouraged)
Qualitative analysis	Nervous system regions affected, types of neuropathology due to test substance, range of severity of alterations
Subjective analysis	Done if alterations found, determine dose response, evaluations without knowledge of treatment (blind)

[a]OECD Test guideline 424 includes testing prior to exposure, during the first or second week of exposure, and monthly thereafter.
[b]OECD Test guideline 424 includes testing prior to first exposure, at the end of the first month of exposure, and every 3 months thereafter.
Abbreviations: FOB, functional observational battery; GFAP, glial fibrillary acidic protein.

either a solution or a suspension and should not in itself be toxic at the levels administered. If the test material is administered in the diet, homogeneous dispersion and stability in that medium should be verified.

In general, a standard strain of laboratory rat should be used. It is usually recommended that the same strain and supplier of rats used, or intended to be used, for other types of toxicity studies be utilized. This will facilitate the integration of results of the various studies. Occasionally another species may be more appropriate. If, for example, the dog or mouse is known to metabolize the compound of interest in a manner more similar to humans than the rat, that species would be more appropriate for testing. Certain parts of the battery must be modified to accommodate a change in species, and this can be difficult. For purposes of the discussion here, use of the rat will be assumed.

The guidelines specify that young adults at least 42 days of age be used. A concurrent vehicle control group is required, and all aspects of housing and handling should be the same as for the treated groups. If the vehicle is known to be toxic at the levels administered, then an untreated or saline control group should be added to the design. Animals must be randomly assigned to treatment and control groups. A minimum of 10 males and 10 females is required for each dose and control group for behavioral testing. At least five of each sex for each dose and control group are required for terminal neuropathology assessment, although additional animals will be needed if interim evaluations are planned.

Although the guideline specifies that neuropathology evaluations be performed only on five animals per sex, evaluation of larger group sizes (up to 10 animals/sex) for neuropathology should be considered, as lesions in small numbers of treated animals [e.g., axonal degeneration seen in 2/5 high dose animals (40% incidence), and 0/5 control animals (0% incidence)] can be difficult to interpret when a very small sample size is used.

The guidelines emphasize the need for positive control data to be generated by the testing laboratory. Positive control data can either be collected concurrently with the test study or in separate studies. There are several reasons to conduct positive control studies. The most important reason is for the testing laboratory to demonstrate that the FOB methods and motor activity measuring devices are capable of detecting differences in the relevant end points that are associated with neurotoxicity; positive control studies can also be useful in comparing the magnitude of effects caused by test chemicals to those of known neurotoxicants. For the FOB, major neurotoxic end points include limb weakness or paralysis, tremor, and autonomic signs. For motor activity assessments, the equipment and procedure must be capable of detecting both increases and decreases in activity. Pharmacologically induced changes, as opposed to frank neurotoxicity, are usually acceptable to demonstrate testing competence. Positive control data for groups exhibiting central and peripheral nervous system neuropathology are also required.

Another important reason for conducting positive control studies is for the training of technical staff so that they can recognize and competently describe abnormal behavior when it occurs. Observing normal rat behavior is useful, but only the observation of abnormal behavior will prepare technicians for the assessment of behavioral toxicity. Recent publications include additional information about conduct and reporting of positive control studies (26). Training information is also available regarding typical responses to certain types of positive control chemicals (27).

The specialized techniques used in the histopathology examinations for the neurotoxicity studies also require considerable practice and skill beyond typical histopathology assessments. Untreated control group data from training studies may then be submitted to the agency as part of the laboratory's historical control data. Historical control data can be useful in evaluating the significance of effects observed in studies with test compounds and can also provide information regarding the reliability of the measured parameter (e.g., does the baseline shift across studies, how variable are normal control animals, etc.). Positive control data should be generated within a few years of the data in the submitted study (generally not more than five years), assuming that laboratory conditions and personnel are constant, and more often if they are not (28).

In addition to the vehicle control group and any other control groups deemed necessary, the guidelines specify that at least three dose levels of the test compound should be used. Equally spaced dose levels are recommended, and a rationale for selection of the dose levels is required. A primary goal in dose level selection is the ability of the study to determine dose-effect relationships. The highest dose for neurotoxicity testing should be the highest dose tolerated by the animal that does not preclude behavioral testing. For acute, single-dose studies, the results of preliminary lethality studies may be used to select the highest nonlethal dose. When such a dose level is determined, the other dose levels for the acute study can be successive fractions, e.g., one-half and one-quarter of the high dose. If no toxicity is found during preliminary lethality testing, a limit dose may be used for the high-dose level. Limit doses have been set as 2 g/kg body weight for acute studies and 1 g/kg for subchronic and chronic studies. High-dose levels for all of the study lengths should not be so high that the incidence of fatalities would interfere with evaluation of the data from that group. Otherwise, the high-dose level should ideally produce significant neurotoxicity or other toxic effects. The low-dose level should ideally produce minimal or no toxic effects.

As specified in the guideline, criteria for selecting the route of administration for neurotoxicity studies can include the most likely route of human exposure, bioavailability, practical considerations, the likelihood of observing effects, and the likelihood of producing nonspecific effects, such as systemic toxicity. More than one route of exposure may be important. When this is the case, the route that best satisfies the criteria should be selected and a clear rationale should be included with the report. Exposures are usually daily for repeated-dose studies, and administration in the diet is generally acceptable. Exposures for single-dose studies are usually administered by oral gavage. Other regimens should be discussed with the relevant agency prior to the study start. Administration by inhalation is sometimes appropriate, and weekday exposures (5 days/week) are reasonable for practical logisitic reasons.

The neurotoxicity screening battery may be combined with any other toxicity study, provided that neither of the goals of the combined studies is compromised; combining studies can lead to significant savings in terms of time and resources. The revised OECD Guidelines for the Testing of Chemicals advocate this approach for the 28-day repeated-dose toxicity study (guideline #407) and the 90-day repeated-dose toxicity study (guideline #408), both in rodents. As mentioned previously, elements of the neurotoxicity screening battery are also routinely included in most subchronic and chronic toxicity studies in the revised EPA testing guidelines (870 series).

Parameters to Be Measured

Standard measures used in general toxicity studies, such as body weight and food consumption, should be collected in neurotoxicity studies. Although the guidelines do not specify if and when food consumption should be measured, periodic assessment of food consumption is often useful in interpreting the results of the study and is necessary to verify dosing of the compound in studies where administration is in the diet. The guidelines do specify that the animals should be weighed on each day of testing and at least once per week during the exposure period.

In acute studies, the guideline specifies that FOB and motor activity testing should be conducted before dosing (preferably not on the same day as dosing), at the estimated time of peak effect within 8 hours after dosing, and at 7 and 14 days after dosing. The guideline recommends that an estimation of the time of peak effect be made by dosing small numbers of rats with a range of doses and making regular observations of gait and arousal. It is important to note that the time of peak behavioral effect may not coincide with the time of peak plasma levels and should not be chosen based on kinetic studies alone, but in the absence of clinical signs, peak plasma levels may be a good choice.

In subchronic studies, the EPA guideline specifies that FOB and motor activity testing should be conducted before the first dose is administered and during weeks 4, 8, and 13 of exposure. In chronic studies, FOB and motor activity testing should be conducted before the first dose is administered and every 3 months. The OECD guidelines recommend an additional evaluation at 2 weeks in subchronic and one month in chronic studies. If short term effects are anticipated based on acute studies, or for other reasons, early testing may be advisable. If there is concern for different exposure durations, behavioral assessments can also be conducted at additional intervals. If behavioral testing is scheduled on a day when there is dosing, behavioral testing conducted prior to dosing will minimize detection of short-term (acute) effects from the dose; depending on the exposure scenario of concern, pre- or postdosing testing may be most appropriate.

It is important to control for time of day when conducting FOB and motor activity testing, because normal performance on many behavioral tasks varies with the animal's circadian rhythm. This can be accomplished by restricting testing to specific hours during the day or by balancing testing of groups so that all groups are represented throughout the day of testing. The best procedure is to implement both strategies, although the numbers of animals to be tested can place practical constraints on that approach. Because the guidelines do not state that all animals in a study need to be tested concurrently, a balanced replicate design, where two or more cohorts (replicates) that have each treatment and control group equally represented begin the study on different days (or weeks), can reduce otherwise long test days and will distribute the workload into a more sustainable schedule.

Functional Observational Battery

The FOB is a series of noninvasive observational and interactive measures that assess the neurobehavioral and functional integrity of rodents or other species (29,30). Testing in the FOB generally proceeds from the least interactive to more interactive measures. The animal is first observed in its home cage for posture, involuntary motor movements, vocalization, and palpebral closure. The animal is then removed from its cage and rated for ease of removal and reactivity to being handled. While holding the animal, the observer carefully examines it for palpebral closure, lacrimation, eye abnormalities, salivation, and piloerection.

The animal is then placed into an open field (the top of a cart or a standard arena) for a defined period of one to several minutes, during which time the animal is allowed to move about freely. During this period, observations are made of involuntary movements, such as tremors and convulsions, gait, mobility, arousal, respiration, and stereotypical and bizarre behaviors. The number of times the animal rears, defined as any time both front paws leave contact with the floor, is often counted for the defined period selected. The number of fecal boli and urine pools are also counted, and diarrhea and polyuria are noted, if present. Following the defined period during which the animal is allowed to move about freely, several standard stimuli are presented to assess reactivity. The animal is approached from the front with a blunt object, such as a pencil, touched lightly on the rump, presented with a click sound of moderate intensity, and finally has its tail pinched with forceps. The animal's responses to these stimuli are rated and recorded, using a defined rating scale.

A variety of reflexes are then elicited and evaluated. Pupil response to light is assessed with a penlight, and the corneal reflex may be elicited by gentle stroking of the eye with a stiff hair while holding the animal. Extensor thrust, a reflex elicited by applying pressure to the hindfeet, may also be assessed. Air righting is scored after the animal is dropped from a height of approximately 30 cm from a supine position to evaluate the functioning of the vestibular system and the motor components of the righting reflex as the animal turns over in midair to land on all four feet. The animals may be evaluated for their responses to a "hot plate" (typically about 52° C) or in a tailflick apparatus. Both use heat stimuli to assess the degree of analgesia induced by the test compound. Hindfoot splay, a measure of coordination and muscular strength that is sensitive to peripheral nerve damage, may be assessed by dropping the animal one or more times from a height of approximately 30 cm from the prone position and recording the distance between spots made when the animal lands after dabbing the outside digits on the rear limbs with nontoxic ink or paint. Quantitative grip strength is measured two or three times for both fore- and hindlimbs, using wire mesh screens or bars that the animal reflexively grabs and holds while being lifted across the apparatus. The maximum force that the animal exerts before letting go is recorded by strain gauges, and averages for the trials are calculated later. Body temperature measured by rectal probe is often recorded. If body temperature is measured, it should be done near the end of the test session, as the animals often struggle during the 15 to 30 seconds of restraint required for the procedure. The entire FOB battery usually requires approximately 8 to 10 minutes per animal, unless there are unusual behaviors to assess and record.

Observers should be carefully trained and should be unaware of (i.e., blind to) the animals' treatment to avoid potential experimenter bias. There are many variables that can affect the behavior of an animal during FOB testing. Every effort should be made to minimize the effects of such extraneous variables and to maintain a consistent testing environment, including the behavior of the observer(s). Scoring criteria, or explicitly defined scales, should be developed for those measures that involve subjective ranking. Scales for variables such as "arousal" or "reactivity to handling" should be designed such that there will be some range of response in normally behaving animals; scales in which all normal animals consistently achieve identical scores may not be sensitive enough to detect compound-related changes in behavior. If more than one observer will be used during the course of the study, it is important to demonstrate interobserver reliability. Otherwise, results for different animals and/or different time points may not be comparable.

Spontaneous Motor Activity

Motor activity evaluations in animals and people have been found to be useful indicators of nervous system function that are obvious and directly quantifiable by many methods. An additional advantage of these types of procedures for animal testing is that they can be easily automated and, therefore, divorced from potential experimenter bias. Motor activity is considered to be "apical" in that it represents the integration of sensory, motor, and higher-level processes of the CNS (31).

The EPA neurotoxicity testing guidelines specify that motor activity be monitored by an automated apparatus that is capable of detecting both increases and decreases in activity. If more than one device is used for testing, steps must be taken to ensure reliability across devices, and treatment groups must be balanced across devices to minimize the possibility of introducing experimental bias. Animals should be tested individually and all sessions should be the same length. The literature contains numerous examples of session lengths from 1 minute to continuous recording for 24-hr periods and longer. The guidelines do not specify or suggest any particular session length. They do provide the criterion for session length of being long enough for motor activity to approach asymptotic levels by the last 20% of the session for untreated control animals. This criterion allows each laboratory to determine empirically an adequate session length and allows for assessment of habituation by the animal to the test environment. Most laboratories have found the range of times that satisfies this criterion to be 20 to 60 minutes, depending on the apparatus and test environment. As is the case for the FOB, a number of variables are known to affect motor activity and care must be exercised to control for the effects of such variables.

Neuropathology

Neuropathological analysis of tissues from the central and peripheral nervous systems is the third pillar of the neurotoxicity screen. The first step in the preparation of nervous system tissues for histological analysis is in situ perfusion with an aldehye fixative. This procedure pumps the fixative through the blood vessels and allows diffusion of the fixative into the tissues of the brain from the inside; providing faster and more complete preservation of that organ than is possible with standard immersion fixation. The peripheral nerves are more delicate as they project more distally, and perfusion makes them much easier to dissect and more resistant to damage that can result from handling and slicing.

The guideline states that paraffin embedding is acceptable for CNS tissues, although plastic embedding is encouraged. Plastic embedding is required for peripheral nervous system tissues. Histological sections should be stained using hematoxylin and eosin (H&E) or a comparable stain and additional special stains, such as a silver-based method, are recommended. The application of glial fibrillary acidic protein (GFAP) immunohistochemistry and radioimmunoassay is recommended for use in conjunction with standard stains to determine the lowest dose at which cellular alterations are detected (32,33).

Increases in GFAP are sensitive to cytopathology at lower dosages of many neurotoxins than are the stains used in routine histopathology. Detailed descriptions of the vascular perfusion and dissection techniques, as well as other details of appropriate fixation, staining, and processing of nervous system tissues for histological examination, may be found in standard histology texts, including Spencer and Schaumburg (34), and standardized histological protocols, such as those published by the World Health Organization in 1986 (35). Representative tissue samples should be obtained from all of the major regions of the nervous system.

During the qualitative examination phase of the neuropathology examination, the guideline specifies that the regions known to be sensitive to neurotoxic insult and those regions suspected to be affected based on the results of the behavioral tests should receive particular attention. A "stepwise" examination of tissue samples is recommended. With this approach, the sections from the high-dose group are examined first and compared with those from the control group. If no alterations are found in the samples from the high-dose group, additional examinations are not required. If alterations indicative of neuropathology are found in the high-dose samples, samples from the low-dose group must be examined.

When neuropathological alterations are found in the qualitative examination, the guideline specifies that a subjective diagnosis (i.e., semiquantitative analysis) should be performed to further characterize dose-response relationships. All regions of the nervous system with any evidence of pathology must be included in this analysis. Sections from all of the dose groups from each region should be coded so that the pathologist examining the slides will not know to which dose or control group a sample belongs. The sections are randomized, and in the course of the examination the frequency and severity of each lesion are rated and recorded. Photomicrographs of treatment-related lesions are recommended for inclusion in the report to accompany the textual descriptions and to illustrate the rating scale used to quantify the degree of severity of the lesions from very slight to very extensive.

DEVELOPMENTAL NEUROTOXICITY TESTING: STUDY DESIGN

The DNT study was developed in order to evaluate toxic effects on the nervous system of offspring following exposure of the mother to a potentially neurotoxic chemical during development. The discussion below is based on Guidelines first published by the EPA in 1991 (14) and the slightly revised (harmonized) version published in 1998 (36). Although no additional revisions to the EPA guideline have been published, current recommendations from the EPA Office of Pesticide Programs include slight modifications to the guideline; several of these modifications were included in a requirement for DNT studies on organophosphate pesticides (37). These recommendations, as well as differences between the EPA guideline and the current OECD draft test guideline 426 (38), will be also be discussed. Studies using some or all of the elements of the DNT study design are also conducted for some pharmaceutical chemicals, when exposure to offspring during pregnancy may be of concern.

The DNT battery includes exposure to the mother starting during early gestation (gestation day six in the EPA guideline) and continuing through some portion of lactation [postnatal day (PND) 10 in the EPA guideline, PND 21 in the current OECD draft]. The study includes some minimal assessments in the maternal animals, including clinical observations, but focuses largely on assessment of the offspring. A variety of behavioral and neuropathological assessments are performed in the pups, at multiple time points. The specific parameters assessed in the EPA guideline study are listed in Table 2. Table 3 describes differences between the EPA guideline, recommended modifications to the EPA guideline, and the current OECD draft. Table 4 presents a DNT battery that has been used for pharmaceutical testing.

The DNT study is not currently included in the initial toxicity data set required by EPA for pesticides or other environmental chemicals but may be requested on a chemical-by-chemical

Table 2 Parameters Evaluated in the EPA Developmental Neurotoxicity Screening Battery

Parameter	Minimum number per group	Assessment time points
Dams		
Body weight/food consumption	20 dams per dose group	Approximately weekly
Reproductive parameters (e.g., fertility, litter size, pup survival)	20 (litters) per dose group	At birth and during lactation
Functional observations	10 per dose group	$2\times$ during gestation, $2\times$ during lactation
Offspring		
Body weight/food consumption	All pups	At birth, postnatal days 4, 11, 17, 21, and weekly thereafter
Developmental landmarks	All pups	
Vaginal opening		Approximately PND 32–38
Preputial separation		Approximately PND 36–45
Functional observations	10/sex/dose	Postnatal days 4, 11, 21, 35, 45, and 60
Motor activity	10/sex/dose	Postnatal days 13, 17, 21 and 60 (±2)
Auditory startle habituation	10/sex/dose	Around the time of weaning and around day 60
Learning and memory	10/sex/dose	Around the time of weaning and around day 60
Brain weight	10/sex/dose (current recommendation)	PND 11–22[a] and at study termination
Qualitative neuropathology	10/sex/dose (current recommendation)	PND 11–22[a] and at study termination
Quantitative neuropathology (morphometric evaluation)	10/sex/dose (current recommendation)	PND 11–22[a] and at study termination

[a]Current EPA Guideline specifies assessments to be done at PND 11, but EPA accepts assessments done at PND 22 if exposure has been extended. Immersion fixation is acceptable for PND 11 tissue, but perfusion fixation should be used at PND 22 and at study termination.
Abbreviation: PND, postnatal day.

Table 3 Major Differences Between Required Assessments for EPA 870.6300 Developmental Neurotoxicity Study and OECD 426 Guideline (2005 Draft)

Element	EPA	OECD
Dosing period	Gestation day 6 through postnatal day 11 (PND 21 recommended)	Gestation day 6 through lactation (PND 21)
Functional observations	Specific days recommended	Recommended to be weekly preweaning and biweekly postweaning
Minimum group size for pup behavioral assessments	10/sex/dose for most tests	20/sex/dose for most tests
Early neuropathology assessment	Postnatal day 11, with immersion fixation (postnatal day 21 usually accepted, with perfusion fixation)	Between PND 11 and 22, either perfusion or immersion fixation
Behavioral ontogeny[a]	Not discussed	At least two measures required
Motor activity	Specific days recommended (PND 13, 17, 21, and around 60)	1–3 times preweaning, once during adolescence (around PND 35) and once for young adults (PND 60–70)
Motor and sensory function	Auditory startle habituation specified	Quantitative sampling of sensory modalities and motor functions specified, auditory startle habituation listed as example
Neuropathology— number of animals	6/sex/dose specified (10/sex/dose recommended)	10/sex/dose
Direct dosing to pups	Not discussed (recommended in some situations)	Should be considered for some situations

[a]Behavioral ontogeny is not specifically required in the EPA guideline, but two measures are required in the OECD guideline, one of which can be assessment of preweaning motor activity. Other examples provided in the guideline include righting reflex and negative geotaxis.
Abbreviations: EPA, Environmental Protection Agency; OECD, Organization for Economic Cooperation and Development; PND, postnatal day.

basis. Although DNT testing was rarely required by EPA in the past, the recent legal requirements included in the FQPA, as discussed previously, have focused increased attention on assessment of toxicity to young animals. Specific criteria for requesting DNT studies were developed and are currently included in the proposed revisions to part 158 (9). Specifically, the agency proposes to require a DNT for pesticide chemicals when:

1. Treatment-related neurological effects are seen in studies using adult animals (e.g., clinical signs, neuropathology, or changes in functional/behavioral tests)
2. When treatment-related neurological effects are seen in available studies on developing animals (e.g., nervous system malformations, neuropathy, brain weight changes, functional/behavioral changes); when neurological effects in humans have been causally related to the pesticide
3. When there are mechanistic data supporting a possible adverse effect on the developing nervous system
4. When the chemical structure of the pesticide is similar to the structure of chemicals known to act on the developing nervous system.

Table 4 A Developmental Neurobehavioral Test Battery for a Perinatal Reproduction Study for Pharmaceutical Safety Evaluation

Measures	Postnatal day(s) of testing	Mean day of appearance or pass
All in litter		
Surface righting	1 until pass	3.0
4/sex/litter		
Incisor eruption	7 until pass	10.7
Eye opening	10 until pass	14.9
Air righting	14 until pass	18.3
2/sex/litter		
FOB for weanling	21	–
Ophthalmoscope exam	Between 21–28	–
Motor activity (20 minutes)	23	–
Auditory function	30	–
Vaginal opening	28 until pass	32.5
Preputial separation	35 until pass	44.7
1/sex/litter		
Auditory startle habituation	Once as adults	–
Cincinnati water maze (learning)	Between 55–75	–
Passive avoidance (memory)	Between 55–75	–

Abbreviation: FOB, functional observational battery.

Study Basics

The test material should be well characterized and in a stable form. One or more concurrent control groups are required. If a vehicle is used for delivery of the test compound, then a vehicle control group is necessary. The vehicle should be neither developmentally toxic (e.g., teratogenic) nor have effects on reproduction. If a vehicle is not used, a sham-treated group is required. All details of handling and maintaining mothers (maternal rats are referred to as dams) and offspring should be the same for the control group(s) as for the treated animals.

Testing should be performed in rats. Use of the same strain as used in other toxicity studies, and especially reproductive and developmental toxicity studies if they have been done, is preferable but not required. The only limitation placed on strain selection in the guidelines is the admonition to not use the Fischer 344 strain because of differences in the timing of developmental events compared to other strains. A detailed justification is necessary if the Fischer 344 or other mammalian species is used. Communication with the relevant regulatory agency prior to the start of the study in such a case would be advised.

At least 20 young adult pregnant females that have not been pregnant previously (i.e., nulliparous females) should be used for each treated and control group. It is important for these studies to keep in mind that it is the dam that is randomized and administered test compound. Therefore, any measurements made on the offspring should be analyzed with the litter as the experimental unit and not individual offspring.

After the litters are born, on PND 4, each litter should be culled by random selection so that each litter has, as nearly as possible, four males and four females remaining. The issue of culling is the topic of an ongoing debate by researchers in the U.S. and Europe, and a number of references are available discussing the advantages and disadvantages of this procedure (39–41). Some opponents consider the practice of culling to have the potential to mask developmental toxicity, whereas proponents consider the practice necessary to control for differences in litter size. The EPA guideline has not changed, and culling is currently recommended in the draft OECD 426 guideline as well. The OECD guideline, however, does not recommend a specific final litter size, but only that it should include equal numbers of males and females (to the extent possible) and should not exceed average litter size for the strain being tested. Both guidelines emphasize that the culling should be done randomly, and elimination based on body weight is not acceptable. If a litter does not have enough pups of either sex, partial adjustment (e.g., five males and three females) is acceptable. Litters having fewer than seven pups are not acceptable, and those litters should be removed from the study.

After standardization of litters, each pup should be uniquely identified, and one male and one female from each litter (e.g., a total of 20 males and 20 females) should be randomly assigned to one of the following behavioral tests: detailed functional observations, motor activity, auditory startle habituation (motor and sensory function in the OECD draft guideline), or learning and memory. Each of these tests is performed multiple times, as detailed in Table 2. The exact number of animals required varies among tests and by test guideline: the current EPA guideline requires a minimum of 10/sex/group (representing as many litters as possible, e.g., males from 10 litters and females from the other 10) for most behavioral tests, but 20/sex/group (1 pup/sex/litter) are recommended for most parameters evaluated in the OECD guideline [the exception being learning and memory assessments, for which the current draft requires a minimum of 10/sex but recommends a higher number be considered, depending on the specific test being used (38)]. For behavioral testing, the same individual may be evaluated for multiple parameters, as long as the testing is conducted in such a way that results from one parameter are not confounded by carry-over effects from other assessments [e.g., tests should be performed in the same order for all individuals, and (as one example) motor activity should not be evaluated immediately following auditory startle testing, as that experience could change activity levels in the motor activity test]. Neuropathological evaluations are conducted at two time points, currently listed as PND 11 and at study termination in the EPA guideline, and as between PND 11 and 22 and at study termination in the OECD draft guideline (EPA is currently accepting studies in which these evaluations were conducted on PND 21, when dosing is also extended through that period). Although the EPA guideline requires these assessments be conducted in only 6 animals/sex/ group, assessment of 10/sex/group is strongly recommended (based on difficulties with interpretation of data involving such a small sample size) and has been sometimes been required. The OECD draft guideline specifies assessments in 10/sex/group.

In addition to the vehicle and/or any other control groups deemed necessary, the guideline specifies that at least three equally spaced dose levels of the test compound should be used. If the test compound has been previously shown to be developmentally toxic, the high-dose level should be the highest dose that did not cause malformations or death to the fetuses or neonates in developmental or reproductive toxicity studies. The high-dose level should induce some overt maternal toxicity, but should not result in a reduction in body weight gain exceeding 20% during gestation and lactation. The low dose should, ideally, not induce maternal toxicity or DNT.

Administration of the test compound should be daily by the oral route from gestation day six through PND 10–21, with day zero of gestation as the day of presumed mating. Other routes of administration must be justified, and the reasons for the route selected explained clearly. Test compounds and vehicle should be given at the same time each day. If test compound is administered by gavage, dosing should not occur on the day of parturition for animals that are in the process of delivering pups. The day of delivery of a litter is considered PND 0 for that litter.

Although in most DNT studies, test substance is administered to the dams, either via gavage or inclusion in the diet, recent concerns regarding possible increased susceptibility of young animals, including the requirement under FQPA to assess relative sensitivity of young and adult animals, have led to recommendations for direct administration of test substance to the pups in some cases. This possibility should be considered in situations where there will be direct exposure to infants or children but where there is no (or minimal) exposure to pups via lactation in the DNT study. The EPA has in some cases required that pesticide registrants document the adequacy of pup exposure in DNT studies and consider direct dosing in cases where exposure cannot be documented (e.g., in the case of DNT studies recently required for all organophosphate pesticides). The draft OECD 426 guideline also includes language regarding the need for administration of test compound directly to the pup in some cases. Guidance regarding the use of direct dosing in young animals has recently been developed by ILSI (42); in cases where direct dosing of pups is being considered, it is advisable to consult with the relevant agency regarding the age at which dosing should be started, timing of dose with relation to testing, etc.

Parameters to Be Measured

Observations in Dams

In addition to the routine daily clinical observations, more detailed observations should be conducted for dams during gestation and lactation (listed as twice during gestation and twice during lactation in the EPA guideline, and at least twice weekly in the draft OECD guideline). Time of observation with respect to dosing (i.e., before or after dosing) is not specified and should be determined based on compound-specific issues, as discussed previously. The observer(s) should be unaware of the animals' treatment group and standardized procedures, such as those used in the FOB, should be used. As in the adult test battery discussed above, if the same observer cannot be used to evaluate all of the animals in a study, some demonstration of interobserver reliability is required. The guidelines are rather specific about the types of observations that should be conducted, which are similar to those used in the adult neurotoxicity FOB but slightly less extensive. Observations of the dams should include assessment and, for some measures, ranking of signs of autonomic function, such as lacrimination, salivation, piloerection, exophthalmus, urination, defecation, pupillary function, and palpebral closure. Convulsions, tremors, abnormal movements and behaviors, posture, gait abnormalities, stereotypical behaviors, emaciation, dehydration, hypo- or hypertonia, altered fur appearance, the appearance of the eyes, nose, and mouth, and any other signs of toxicity that might aid in the interpretation of the data should be recorded when they are observed. The time of onset, degree, and duration of all observations should be included. The guidelines specify that body weight be recorded for the dams at least weekly, on the day of delivery, and on postpartum days 11 and 21 (weaning). More frequent measurement of dam body weight is often useful in overall interpretation of the study results. Although food consumption is not required for the dams, periodic assessment is also useful in understanding maternal body weight changes and fetal weight differences in some cases. In addition, if the test compound is administered via the diet, measurement of food consumption is essential for determination of dose to the dam.

Observations in Offspring

According to the guidelines, offspring should be examined in their cages at least once each day for signs of morbidity and mortality. All offspring should be observed outside of their cages for gross signs of toxicity whenever they are removed from their cages for weighing or for behavioral testing. The technician(s) trained to conduct these observations should be unaware of the animals' treatment group, and standardized procedures should be used to maximize interobserver reliability if the same observer cannot evaluate all of the animals in a given study. The observations outlined above for the dams represent the minimum for the offspring and the monitored end points should be appropriate for the developmental stage of the animal (examples of appropriate modifications for pups could include evaluation of surface righting, use of a smaller arena size, etc.). Any signs of toxicity in the offspring should be recorded when they are observed and should include the time of onset, degree, and duration, as for the dams.

Live pups should be weighed individually as soon as practically possible after birth, on PNDs 4, 11, 17, and 21 and at least every 2 weeks thereafter. Food consumption is not required for offspring and is not generally recognized as being useful in these studies, as compound administration usually does not extend past weaning. The only developmental indices that are required in the EPA guideline are the age of vaginal opening in females (usually occurs between PNDs 32 and 38) and the age of preputial separation of the penis in males (usually occurs between PNDs 36 and 45). For observation details, see Adams et al. (43) and Korenbrot et al. (44), for females and males, respectively. Although the guidelines do not mention it, measuring the body weight of each offspring on the day of attainment of vaginal opening or preputial separation can be quite useful in interpreting positive findings for delay, or acceleration, of these developmental landmarks.

The behavioral tests required or recommended in the DNT test guideline (motor activity, auditory startle, and learning and memory tests) are apical in nature, i.e., they do not test discrete CNS functions but require integration of various processes. These processes may include sensation, motivation, neuromuscular function, and other aspects of nervous system functioning. The actual behavior measured is the culmination and integration of the function of several underlying processes. According to one pioneering researcher in this area (45), the point of apical testing is to grossly analyze the integrated response of the organism. The value of testing apical performance lies in its potential sensitivity to detect a deficit in any of several subsystems. This sensitivity, due to the involvement of many CNS subsystems, allows many factors to influence behavioral output. An argument against the use of apical tests is that it is often difficult to identify specifically which subsystems are affected. This problem can be overcome by careful examination of the results and correlation with results of several tests that tap similar subsystems, but this may be far from easily or quickly accomplished. In a screening approach, such as the one under discussion, it is less important to define a mechanism of action than it is to determine impairment of function resulting in potential increased risk. Apical tests compromise specificity in favor of sensitivity and are, therefore, useful in detecting impairment. Specificity can be recouped in additional follow-up tests that can be applied on a case-by-case basis to further characterize the nature of the impairment and the site of the lesion, if one can be found.

Spontaneous Motor Activity.   Motor activity should be monitored by an automated device on PNDs 13, 17, 21, and 60 (± 2 days). The same criteria and recommendations listed in the section on adult neurotoxicity assessment pertain to evaluating motor activity in offspring in the DNT study. Unlike the adult guidelines, the DNT guidelines specify that the recording intervals within a monitoring session should not be more than 10 minutes in duration. The same criterion for empirical determination of the length of the monitoring session that appears in the adult guidelines applies to the DNT study, although it should be noted that habituation may not be achieved in very young animals, depending on the type of device being used (46). When testing preweanling animals, it is important to ensure that sensors are at the appropriate height and distance to detect movements of smaller animals; adjustments may be needed, depending on the type of device used.

Auditory Startle Habituation. An auditory startle habituation test should be performed on the offspring around the time of weaning (e.g., PND 22) and around day 60. The mean response amplitude must be determined for each block of 10 trials, with a daily session consisting of five blocks of 10 trials, for a total of 50 trials on each test day. Habituation is assessed by comparison of the degree that the startle amplitude decreases with successive presentations of the startle stimulus. The slope of the recorded data for each treatment group can be compared with the control group to determine whether the slopes differ from one another. Details of the procedure for this test can be found in Adams et al. (43). The auditory startle test can be made more powerful by the addition of prepulse inhibition. Prepulse inhibition contributes information regarding sensory processing to the auditory startle test and can also be used to detect changes in auditory thresholds after exposure to toxicants. Although the guidelines do not require prepulse inhibition, its addition is highly recommended. Details of the conduct of this test may be found in an article by Ison (47). Assessment of auditory startle habituation is specifically required in the EPA guideline. Although its use is not specified in the OECD draft guideline, assessment of auditory startle habituation can serve as a quantitative assessment of motor and sensory function, which is required in the OECD draft guideline.

Learning and Memory. The guideline specifies that one or more tests of learning and memory be administered around the time of weaning (PNDs 21 to 24) and again in adulthood (PND 60 ± 2). Although the guideline indicates that the same or different procedures may be used at these two stages of development, it is important to note that memory of previous testing may confound assessment of learning at the later time point, if the same animals are used for both assessments. If the same procedure is used at both ages, use of different animals at the second time point will ensure that learning can be similarly assessed at both ages.

Considerable flexibility in test selection is allowed. However, two criteria for test selection must be fulfilled. First, learning must be assessed either as a change in behavior across several learning trials or sessions, or, in tests involving a single trial (e.g., one-trial learning passive avoidance), with a condition that controls for nonassociative factors in the training experience that can provide assurance that extraneous factors are not influencing the measure of learning. Second, some measure of memory, either short-term or long-term, must be included in the test in addition to the original measure of learning (i.e., acquisition). Whichever measure of memory is selected, the measure of acquisition should also be obtained from the same test.

Testing for learning and memory and interpreting the resulting data can be quite complex because it is impossible to demonstrate learning without invoking memory and it is impossible to demonstrate memory without invoking learning to establish that which is remembered. When treatment-related effects are found in the test or tests of learning and memory, additional tests may be needed to discover whether the impairment is caused by a change in cognition or due to some confounding factor. Depending on the test and the pattern of results obtained, alterations in sensory functioning and/or processing, motivation to complete the test, motor capabilities, and general activity levels could contribute to the observed effects. Use of appropriate control procedures (e.g., evaluation of straight channel swim speed prior to evaluation of learning, in a water maze) can minimize these interpretive difficulties.

A recommendation in the guideline that is often overlooked is to select a test or tests for learning and memory that has been shown to be sensitive to compounds in the same structural or functional class as the compound under investigation. There are a great many tests of learning and memory in the literature, but it is beyond the scope of this chapter to review them. A few tests that fulfill the criteria in the guidelines for these types of studies in adult rats are delayed-matching-to-position (48), olfactory conditioning (49), and acquisition and retention of schedule-controlled behavior (49,50). Additional tests for weanling rats are described by Spear and Campbell (51) and Krasnegor et al. (52), for adult rats by Miller and Eckerman (53), and for both young and adult rats in Riley and Vorhees (54). Water mazes, especially the Morris water spatial task, often called the Morris maze (55,56), have become popular for assessment of rodent learning and memory in many contexts. Another test that has a relatively large compound effect base after prenatal exposures is the Cincinnati water maze (57,58). Only a few formal comparisons of tests of learning and memory are published. Examples of such comparisons after prenatal exposures include Akaike et al. (59), Tsutsumi et al. (60), and Weisenburger et al. (61).

Neuropathology. A thorough neuropathological analysis of the offspring must be conducted to satisfy this guideline. Both EPA and the draft OECD guidelines specify that evaluations be performed at two time points. For the early time point, the current EPA guideline specifies that one male and one female pup should be removed from each litter on PND 11, such that equal numbers of male and female offspring are removed from all litters combined. Neuropathological examination should be performed on a minimum of ten male and ten female pups per treatment group (as noted previously, although the EPA guidelines require only 6/sex, both EPA and OECD currently recommend use of 10 offspring/sex at each evaluation time). After euthanasia (e.g., by carbon dioxide inhalation), the brains should be removed, weighed, and fixed by immersion in an aldehyde fixative. The remaining offspring in the subset should be sacrificed in the same manner, and their brains removed and weighed. Alternatively, both EPA and OECD recommendations currently allow the early assessment to be performed as late as PND 21; if this later time point is used, perfusion fixation, as described below for adult brains, should be conducted for those brains to be used for histopathological assessment.

In addition to the animals above, both EPA and OECD recommend that ten animals of each sex in each dose group (one male or female per litter) should be sacrificed at the end of the study for neuropathological evaluation, with the same procedures used for the adult neurotoxicity study. Neuropathological evaluation of the animals sacrificed on PND 11–21 and at the termination of the study must include a qualitative analysis and simple morphometric evaluation. As described for adult assessments, findings in the qualitative analysis may trigger the need for an additional semiquantitative analysis. Samples from the PND 11 pups should be immersion-fixed in an aldehyde fixative and then postfixed and processed according to standardized histological protocols, such as the Armed Forces Institute of Pathology (AFIP) (62), Spencer and Schaumberg (34), or Pender (63). Paraffin embedding is acceptable, but plastic embedding is recommended. Although histopathological evaluation of the tissue is conducted in a stepwise manner, starting with high dose and control groups, it is advisable to process tissue from all groups, at least through embedding, in order to prevent shrinkage of tissue; this is particularly important for DNT studies, as tissue shrinkage can invalidate morphometric assessments performed in tissues that have remained in fixative for prolonged periods (e.g., in situations where later evaluation of intermediate dose groups is required). The guidelines recommend that histological sections should be stained using H&E or a similar stain according to such standard protocols as AFIP (62) or Bennet et al. (64).

The brains of pups sacrificed on PND 11–22 should be examined for any evidence of neuropathological alterations. The guidelines specify that samples should be collected from all major brain regions to include the olfactory bulbs, cerebral cortex, hippocampus, basal ganglia, thalamus, hypothalamus, midbrain (i.e., tectum, tegmentum, and cerebral peduncles), brain stem, and cerebellum. Further guidance for examination of the nervous system for indications of developmental insult can be found in Friede (65), Suzuki (66), and Garmen et al. (67). In addition to the typical kinds of cellular alterations that can be assessed in neuropathological studies (e.g., astrocytic proliferation, leukocytic infiltration, and cystic formation), there should be special emphasis placed on structural changes that are indicative of developmental insult. Examples of such changes include gross changes in the size or shape of brain regions, such as the pattern of foliation of the cerebellum, death of neuronal precursors, abnormal proliferation or migration, alterations in transient developmental structures such as the external germinal zone of the cerebellum, evidence of hydrocephalus, particularly enlargement of the ventricles, stenosis of the cerebral aqueduct, and thinning of the cerebral hemispheres.

There are three purposes for the qualitative histological examination in the DNT screen. The first is to identify regions within the nervous system with evidence of neuropathological alterations. The second is to identify the types of alterations resulting from exposure to the test substance. The third purpose is to determine the severity of the lesions. As in the neuropathological examination in the screen for adult animals, the developmental neuropathological examination is conducted using a stepwise approach wherein the high-dose group tissue sections are compared first to the control group samples. If no alterations are found in the high-dose group animals, no further analysis is required. If alterations indicative of neuropathology are found in the high-dose sections, samples of the same tissue(s) from the intermediate-dose group are examined, and so on, until a dose level is encountered that does not exhibit the alterations or there are no more dose groups to examine. The recommendations for the use of additional stains and methods to determine the lowest dose level at which neuropathology is detected in the adult neurotoxicity screen also apply to the DNT screen.

If any evidence of neuropathology is found in the qualitative examination, guidelines indicate that a subjective (i.e., semiquantitative) analysis must be performed to further characterize dose-response relationships. All regions of the brain exhibiting any evidence of neuropathology should be included in this analysis. Sections of each region from all dose groups should be coded as to treatment and randomized prior to examination. After all sections from all dose groups have been rated for severity using a scale, such as $1+$, $2+$, and $3+$, to indicate the degree of severity ranging from very slight to very extensive, the code should be broken and statistical analyses performed to evaluate dose-response relationships. This approach was designed to minimize the potential effects of observer bias in determining the presence or absence of treatment-related neuropathological findings.

Simple morphometric analysis is useful in evaluating disruption of developmental processes that are often reflected in changes in the rate or extent of growth of particular brain regions. Such an analysis is required for some of the pups that are sacrificed on PND 11 (or 22) and at the end of the study. At a minimum, the guidelines specify that this analysis should include an estimate of the thickness of the major layers within the neocortex, hippocampus, and cerebellum. In addition to the regions noted in the guideline, evaluation of other brain regions is often useful, especially in cases where information about the mechanism of action indicates likely involvement of specific brain regions (e.g., dopaminergic toxins impact on the basal ganglia). Details of the procedures for conducting these measurements can be found in Rodier and Gramann (68) and Duffel (69). Evaluations of morphometric data submitted with DNT studies to the EPA have indicated that these evaluations detect changes in brain structure not found using qualitative neuropathological evaluations (70).

DATA COLLECTION, REPORTING, EVALUATION, AND INTERPRETATION

Appropriate data evaluation and reporting are equal in importance to generation of the original data. In order for the data to be useful in evaluating potential health consequences of exposure to a particular chemical, the data must be analyzed and presented in a way that is transparent and easily understood. In addition, various aspects of the results should be integrated and interpreted in the context of other available data (including positive and historical control data from the performing laboratory). The discussion below is relevant for both adult and DNT testing.

Data Organization and Analysis

The final test report must include all of the information and data necessary to properly interpret the results. More specifically, detailed information should be provided regarding study design, equipment used, and the methods used for each included procedure. Any deviations from the guidelines or decisions involving professional judgment should be explained and justified. Examples of what is expected in the report are, for the FOB, the dimensions of the arena, the scoring criteria, and description of the procedures used to standardize the observations, as well as operational definitions for scoring observations. For motor activity, the procedures for calibrating the devices and the balancing of treatment group across the relevant parameters, such as time of day, should be included. The amount of time allowed for the animal to acclimate to the test room is relevant for all types of behavioral procedures. Information regarding stimulus strength (e.g., shock intensity in a passive avoidance task or loudness of tone in an auditory startle habituation task) and intertrial intervals, as well as criteria used to define errors or correct responses in learning tasks, can be very important in interpreting test results and should always be included in the study report. A good "rule of thumb" is that if one is not sure whether or not to include specific information on the conduct of the experiment, include it!

Obviously, the test system (i.e., the animals used) should be well described in terms of species, strain, age, sex, supplier, and any other available information. Many of the end points in neurotoxicity studies are known to vary with strain of rat tested.

Positive control data generated by the laboratory performing the test should be included in the report to demonstrate the sensitivity of the procedures being used and the competence of the personnel performing the tests. These data are vital in documenting the ability of the laboratory to detect effects on evaluated parameters. Use of positive control chemicals should result in statistically significant changes in measured performance, using the same procedures used in the submitted study. The changes in performance should be in the direction expected for the positive control chemical being used (e.g., impairment of memory following scopolamine treatment, increased motor activity following amphetamine treatment). Detailed procedural information for the positive control studies should be included in the study report, in order to facilitate the comparison between study data and positive control data. Results of positive control studies should be presented both in summary tables and as tables of individual animal data, and statistical evaluations should be the same as those used in the submitted study. Failure to submit adequate positive control data has been cited as a major source of difficulty in interpretation of the results of DNT studies (26). Historical, nonconcurrent, positive control data may be used if the essential aspects of the protocol are the same (in order to assure their relevance, these data should normally be from studies conducted within five or fewer years of the submitted study). In DNT studies, positive control data do not need to be from prenatal exposures but do need to use animals of the same age as those tested in the guideline study. Testing of age-relevant animals is of key importance, as performance varies with the age of the animal, and devices or procedures appropriate for adult animals may not be similarly sensitive in younger animals, and vice versa.

In addition to positive control data, historical control data are often useful in the interpretation of study findings, as these kinds of data expand the basis of comparison for possible treatment effects beyond the single study. Care must be taken, however, in comparing data across studies, as performance baselines can shift over time, even within the same laboratory. Thus, comparisons involving historical controls must include relevant procedural information for the available studies, including date of performance (studies conducted outside a 5-year time frame may not be useful); the more comparable the control data is across a number of studies, the more useful it may be in aiding interpretation of data from treatment groups in any given individual study. The submission of positive and historical control data along with the test report is encouraged to facilitate and expedite the review of the study results and interpretation.

Presentation of results of a study should be arranged by test group and dose level, using tabular formats. Data for each individual animal should include its unique identification number, body weights, scores on each sign at each observation time, values for each replicate evaluation of grip strength and hindlimb splay, total session and intra-session (i.e., interval) subtotals for each day of motor activity measurement, and the time and cause of death if the animal died on study or was sacrificed as moribund. For developmental studies, the following measures also need to be presented: the litter from which each offspring came; body weight and score on each developmental landmark (i.e., preputial separation or vaginal opening) at each observation time; auditory startle mean response amplitude per session and by block (i.e., mean for each subset of 10 consecutive trials), and latency to maximum response on each day measured; and appropriate data for each repeated trial (or session) showing acquisition and retention scores on the test(s) of learning and memory on each day tested. Data presented for the learning and memory test should include all trials conducted and should include sufficient detail to permit evaluation of both learning and memory components of the task at each assessment age.

Summary data for each dose and control group must include the number of animals at the start of the test, the number of animals with each observation score at each observation time, the mean and standard deviation for each continuous end point at each observation time, and the results of statistical analyses for each measure, where appropriate. For developmental studies, the following should be added: body weight of the dams during gestation and lactation, maternal clinical and functional observations, litter size, and mean weight of the offspring at birth. As noted above, it is important to remember that the unit of analysis for developmental studies, when compound is administered to the dams, is the litter, as it was the dam that was randomized to treatment group.

All neuropathological observations should be included in the report, arranged by test group. The recommended format for presentation includes descriptions of the lesions for each animal showing the unique identification number, sex, treatment, dose, duration of dosing, a list of structures examined, as well as the location, nature, frequency, and severity of lesion(s). The EPA strongly recommends the inclusion of photomicrographs that illustrate examples of the type and severity of the neuropathological alterations observed. Any diagnoses derived from neurological signs and lesions, including naturally occurring diseases or conditions, should be included. The neuropathology data should be tabulated to show the number of animals examined in each group, the number of animals in which any lesion was found, the number of animals affected by each different type of lesion, and the location, frequency, and severity of each type of lesion. Additional data to be reported for developmental studies include whole brain weights (both absolute and relative), regional brain weights (if determined), and the values for the morphometric measurements made for each animal, listed by treatment group (when similar measurements are taken in both sides of the brain, data should be reported for each side separately).

The findings from the screening battery should be evaluated in the context of other toxicity studies and any other pertinent information that exists for the compound of interest.

The evaluation should include the relationship between the doses of test substance and the presence or absence, incidence, and severity of any toxic effects. Appropriate statistical analyses are crucial to evaluation of the data. Parametric statistical tests are usually appropriate for such continuous data as body weights, motor activity counts, auditory startle data, and body temperature. Nonparametric tests are usually appropriate for the remainder of the measures. It is beyond the scope of this chapter to attempt a discussion of the application of various statistical techniques to each of the measures in a neurotoxicity study. Choice of analyses should consider tests appropriate to the experimental design, including repeated measures when appropriate. Data sets for which parametric statistics are appropriate are analyzed routinely by most laboratories with either analysis of variance (ANOVA) in its several forms or one of several trend tests that assess the relationship of the measure to dose (71). Nonparametric tests (e.g., chi-square, Mann-Whitney U) are often used for data that are not normally distributed. Adjustments for multiple comparisons are not explicitly discussed in the guideline, but significant results should be discussed in the context of the number of analyses performed.

Interpretation of Specific Measures

The tests that comprise the adult and DNT screening batteries cover a wide range of behavioral and pathologic measures that increase the likelihood of detecting neurotoxic effects. The behavioral tests generally lack specificity for distinct neural systems but were selected to survey the integrated functional output. The pattern of effects seen on the parameters measured in the adult or DNT screening batteries can vary from effects on a single measure (e.g., increased startle amplitude during several blocks on the auditory startle habituation test, at a single time point) to effects on multiple measures (e.g., increased reactivity to handling, increased motor activity, increased startle amplitude, and impaired retention in a passive avoidance task). Ideally, one would see a pattern of effects that support each other, along with histopathological changes in the brain region that mediates such functions. However, results are often not so clear. Although it is not possible to discuss all possible outcomes, or even provide a detailed survey, in the context of the current chapter, some general discussion of particular types of findings is provided below.

Given the apical nature of most tests used in both the adult and DNT screening batteries, along with the limited evaluation of other types of toxicity included in these studies, it is often not possible to determine whether effects measured in these studies result from direct effects of the test compound on the nervous system or whether they may be occurring secondary to toxic effects on other organ systems. For example, direct effects on the digestive tract or liver may result in the animal feeling "sick" and thus e.g., less active in an automated motor activity test. In the absence of frank lesions of the nervous system (central or peripheral), it may not be possible to determine the "mechanism" by which the decrease in motor activity occurred, and thus a determination of whether or not the compound causes direct toxic effects on the nervous system may not be possible. Information available from other toxicity studies with the same compound may provide information regarding effects on other organ systems but will not be able to rule out the possibility that there are direct effects on the nervous system at doses similar to those causing other types of toxicity. In cases where it is necessary to clearly distinguish the ultimate origin of behavioral changes seen in the neurotoxicity screening batteries, it may be necessary to perform additional follow-up studies to further refine the interpretation of any effects seen.

Clinical Observation Data

Unusual clinical signs are frequently the first clue that a compound is neurotoxic. More often than not, standard toxicity studies will have been conducted with the compound of interest before a formal evaluation of neurotoxicity is performed. Clinical signs, as well as other findings from such studies, should be reviewed and the likelihood of nervous system damage considered. The most important point to be made from the assessment of clinical signs and the more formal FOB is to "look at your animals!" There is no substitute nor more important source of information than this simple directive. Direct observation and careful recording of clinical signs is critical to well-conducted neurotoxicity assessments.

Obviously, the nature of the clinical signs observed is crucial as they can range from general findings, such as "unkempt appearance," to truly bizarre behaviors, such as repetitive circling, straub tail, and ragelike behaviors. Many of these specific behaviors and syndromes are well documented, and a literature search with appropriate key words will often lead to diagnosis, clarification of mechanism, or at least some ideas on how to proceed.

Clinical observations may also be useful in distinguishing between short-term and long-term actions of a compound. Signs seen directly after dosing, which may resolve prior to subsequent observations, may be due to direct interaction of the compound with the nervous system (e.g., enzyme inhibition or receptor activation) and may reverse when the compound has been cleared from the system. Alternatively, signs that appear only following repeated dosing, or that persist after the compound is no longer present, may indicate a different type of toxic mechanism, with damage persisting and possibly increasing with time after exposure. Either type of effect may be of concern, depending on the proposed uses of the test compound.

Body Weights and Food Consumption

Body weight effects are sometimes the first indication of treatment-related toxicity, but their interpretation is not always clear. It is obvious that reduced food consumption can lead to decreased body weight and/or decreased body weight gain. However, decreased food consumption can have multiple causes. One common cause, decreased palatability of a treated diet, should result in body weight changes directly correlated with the magnitude of decrease in food consumption. When the degree of reduced food consumption does not adequately explain the body weight data, a metabolic difference might be responsible and might lead to unusual behaviors as well, such as increased water intake or altered eliminative processes. The main point to keep in mind for these measures is that both are sensitive to many different kinds of physiological perturbations and can be sensitive to psychological factors as well. A hypothetical example for the latter point is that of an animal that is hallucinating or is experiencing negative emotions, such as fear or disorientation. Under such conditions, the animal may not eat normal amounts, which would lead to decreased body weight if that mental state persisted for more than a day.

Functional Observational Battery

A FOB typically consists of 25 to 35 end points that are measured at several time points before, during, and/or after compound administration. One method of analysis is to group these measures into functional domains (29). One type of grouping includes six domains: autonomic, neuromuscular, convulsions, activity, excitability, and sensorimotor. Statistical analyses have shown measures within these groupings to be correlated, but correlations between groupings in different domains have also been found (30,72). Grouping end points in this manner may simplify analysis and interpretation of this type of data but is not a required part of the data evaluation and does not substitute for evaluation of individual endpoints.

Some toxicologists have expressed concern that with so many measures in the FOB to statistically analyze, one or more statistically significant differences will be found by chance but might not be related to neurotoxicity. However, it is important to remember that multiple correlated measures are evaluated for many types of toxicological end points. For example, the situation with clinical chemistry and hematological data is directly analogous to what is often found with FOB data. As with clinical chemistry, hematology, and any other sets of data that require many statistical comparisons, statistical significance will be found for approximately 1 in 20 comparisons, independent of effect of the treatment. The magnitude, direction, additional findings that do or do not form a logical pattern, and, of course, professional judgment should be used to determine whether or not a particular finding that is statistically significant is biologically significant.

In addition to the concern regarding spurious statistically significant findings (i.e., false positives), the possibility of biologically but not statistically significant findings must also be considered. Certain rare findings, such as convulsions or tremors, may be treatment-related even if statistical significance is not achieved. An example of such a situation would be an incidence of convulsions in 3/10 high-dose animals, when convulsions were never seen in the control group. In such cases, comparison to historical control data may be helpful in determining normal background incidence of such behaviors.

Some measures in the FOB can be viewed as complementary, although they do not measure the same function. An example of this complementarity is the relationship of landing foot splay to grip strength. Landing foot splay involves a reflex to the stimulus of falling that coordinates input from the vestibular, visual, and motor response systems. Grip strength is mainly a measure of the strength of the limbs that relies on a reflex of the toes and claws to touch stimuli. Peripheral nerve damage, such as that induced by acrylamide, is clearly manifested by decreased grip strength with accompanying increased landing foot splay distance. Administration of CNS depressants, such as codeine and pentobarbital, will also result in decreased grip strength when the drugs are present at pharmacologically active levels, but landing foot splay is not affected. The effects of acrylamide become more severe with time after dosing has ceased. The effects of codeine and pentobarbital disappear after the drugs have cleared from the animal. The recommended practice of conducting FOB studies with positive effect compounds allows the researcher to explore the relationships of the various measures comprising the FOB and adds experience to the "tool box" to be used later for interpreting test data.

Motor Activity

Assessment of locomotor activity has been a mainstay of behavioral investigations almost as long as animal studies have been considered as models for human response. In our everyday lives we all realize that activity levels differ among people and increased or decreased levels are often associated with psychological states, such as anxiety or depression, respectively, in the same person at different times. A simple mental review of one's own activity levels that occurred concurrently with changes in psychological state over the past day or week will clarify this point.

An example will serve to illustrate a common pharmacological effect. The didactic scenario is as follows: A person goes to an establishment where alcoholic beverages are served, music is played, and dancing is encouraged with the goal of increasing pleasant stimulation and social behavior. Initially the activity level is low to moderate. After one or two measured doses of alcoholic beverage, the activity level increases as dancing commences and social behavior increases. One or two additional doses are self-administered over a period of time (minutes to hours), and the frequency and intensity increases for dancing and social behavior, there is more frequent and louder verbal behavior and body movements become more exaggerated and less coordinated. If self-administration continues, a point will likely be reached where activities decrease and may eventually be restricted to simple maintenance of necessary physiological functions with little or no apparent activity.

This example from everyday life not only illustrates how we all use observable behaviors, including motor activity, to draw conclusions about the psychological and pharmacological states of ourselves and others, but is also a good example of an "inverted U" dose-response function for a commonly used drug, alcohol. The "inverted U" function refers to the observation in our example that increasing dose administration results in increased response (i.e., more dancing, talking, and exaggerated body language), but that at some point, further increasing the dose results in decreased response (i.e., slower, and then no dancing, less, and then no talking, and little or no active body language). Such nonlinear dose-response relationships occur often in behavioral pharmacology and are also seen in behavioral toxicology and neurotoxicology. Because a basic tenet of toxicology is that there should be a dose-response relationship for a toxicant, the assumption is often made that the dose-response curve should reflect either more or less response with increasing dose. A complex dose response relationship in a three dose study may be erroneously interpreted as inconsistent and considered a spurious finding.

In animal studies, motor activity is assessed over a specified period of time, usually for periods of 30 to 90 minutes up to the assessment of circadian cycles over 24 hours. In versions of this type of assessment where the animal is allowed to move about a standardized test environment that is not the animal's home cage, such as an open field or a figure-eight apparatus, the rat will initially exhibit relatively high levels of activity as it explores the novel or different environment and will move about less over time as it "gets used to" or habituates to the new setting. The rate of habituation can be a sensitive index of the animal's ability to adapt to its environment and is altered by many pharmacological (e.g., amphetamine) and neurotoxic (e.g., trimethyltin) agents.

When evaluating motor activity data from DNT studies, it is important to be aware of the expected developmental pattern for this behavior. In addition to the possible failure of very young animals (e.g., postnatal day 13) to display habituation, there is a normal developmental pattern for the expected level of activity; activity should be lowest on day 13, increase on day 17, and decrease (compared to day 17) on day 21 (46). Although the exact magnitude of the developmental changes may vary from device to device, if the same general pattern is not seen, some problem with task performance may be indicated. If the expected pattern is seen in control animals, but not in treatment groups, a treatment-related change in brain development may have occurred.

As is true for all of the measures in the neurotoxicity battery, observed differences in motor activity levels must be interpreted in the context provided by other measures in the neurotoxicity and general toxicity studies as well as what is known about the pharmacology of the compound. An animal that has been administered a peripheral neurotoxicant, such as acrylamide, that induces a "dying-back" axonopathy resulting in loss of neural control of the limbs, will likely exhibit decreased motor activity, regardless of how one measures it. Habituation will be difficult to demonstrate, as the initial level of activity within a session will probably be very low to begin with. Obviously, this example would not be interpreted as the compound being active only in the CNS because we know that the peripheral effects of acrylamide confound the motor activity assessment. But what if we were dealing with a compound with unknown toxic potential? The point here is that all of the data generated on the compound's effects in our target species must be reviewed before a proper interpretation can be rendered. In the example above, FOB data and the neuropathology data collected would lead us to a more accurate interpretation than an examination of motor activity alone could.

Auditory Startle

The startle response consists of a characteristic sequence of muscular responses elicited by a sudden intense stimulus. Loud sounds and air puffs elicit startle responses in all mammals studied, including humans, whereas visual stimuli are generally ineffective. Only stimuli with very rapid onset times elicit startle. A sound that slowly increases in intensity (i.e., loudness) will not elicit the startle response.

Startle represents a short-latency reflex that is mediated by a simple neural circuit (73). The auditory startle response (also referred to as the acoustic startle response or reflex) can be differentiated from motor behaviors and other movements due to its very short latency and dependence on the onset of the tone. Auditory startle can be measured electromyographically in cats with latencies of approximately 5 msec when measured in the neck muscles and approximately 8 to 10 msec when measured in the hindlimbs. Measurement and testing of auditory startle falls midway between most observational behavioral tests and electrophysiological measurements. The data are quantified as units of force (e.g., newtons) or voltage (for accelerometers) and are quite reproducible for the same animal over different test sessions on different days.

Much of the neural circuitry for the auditory startle response resides in the brain stem and includes the ventral cochlear nucleus, ventral nucleus of the lateral lemniscus, nucleus reticularis points caudalis, and motor neurons in the spinal cord (74). Obviously, the cochlea and other structures involved in hearing must be intact and functioning correctly for the auditory stimulus to be effective in eliciting startle. In toxicity experiments, when the amplitude of the auditory startle response is reduced, the possibility that the treatment has affected the organs of hearing should be investigated. One simple approach is to test the same animals with air puff startle (tactile modality) to assess whether or not the reduced response amplitude is specific to one of the sensory modalities or represents an effect on other components of the neural circuit. Some testing laboratories routinely include air puff startle for this and other reasons.

There are three main parameters that are measured when auditory startle is tested in neurotoxicity assessments: latency, amplitude, and habituation. Latency refers to the time that elapses measured from the onset of the tone to either the beginning of the whole-body startle or that point in time when the maximum force of the startle response is recorded. This measure is related to the speed of the nerve impulse as it travels through the neural circuit. Changes in latency are often indicative of compound-related changes in nerve conduction speed. Amplitude refers to the force with which the rat reflexively responds to the sound stimulus. Changes in amplitude can be due to alterations in the CNS, in the peripheral nervous system, at the neuromuscular junction, or in the muscles involved in the response. Habituation refers to the decrease in the amplitude of response over repeated stimulus presentations and is considered to be a simple form of nonassociative learning. Changes in habituation that are related to exposure to a compound usually indicate a difference in the way the animal adapts to aspects of its environment. Rats, like people, are programmed to dampen responses to repetitive stimuli that do not have consequences for them. In assessing habituation, one should keep in mind that if the mean amplitude of the auditory startle response is dramatically decreased compared to controls, adequate evaluation of habituation may not be possible.

Additional useful information may be obtained through the application of prepulse techniques. The introduction of a low-intensity stimulus shortly before the intense, startle-eliciting stimulus will result in modification of startle amplitude and latency. Those modifications of amplitude and latency are robust and predictable and can lead to assessment of the processing capability of the subject (47). Because prepulse inhibition occurs with tones that are near the threshold of audibility, this technique is used by a few laboratories to assess auditory thresholds in animals (75) and represents a relatively efficient method for the rapid determination of compound effects upon hearing. This is a promising technology for incorporation into toxicity studies in the future to determine the functional status of the auditory system in animals noninvasively. An efficient test of animal hearing would be very helpful as there is currently no efficient and sensitive procedure in general use for the evaluation of hearing in animals, although many drugs and neurotoxicants have been found to affect hearing in animals and people.

Learning and Memory

Tests of learning and memory are often referred to as "cognitive tests" because they are assumed to require considerable processing and integration by the brain. There are many tests of learning and memory in use in animal studies, and they vary greatly in their complexity, as well as in the exact types of learning or memory they evaluate. Although the specific type of learning and/or memory affected will vary depending on the compound being tested (and thus the sensitivity of any given task will vary accordingly), in general, the greater the complexity of the test, the greater the power of that test to detect compound-related deficits in learning and memory. Although the current concept of "learning and memory" is very broad, encompassing many elements of brain function, most tests currently used in rats for DNT studies are very simple, assessing a single type of learning and memory, often in a fairly limited way [see (76) for a discussion of learning and memory evaluations in DNT studies that have been submitted to EPA]. Thus, our assessment of the impact of a particular test compound on these functions (as specified in current guidelines) may not be sufficient to detect all types of treatment-related effects. This may be of particular concern, given that we know mental retardation in children is a real consequence of prenatal exposures to some compounds. Examples of these types of effects include the mental retardation often seen in the fetal alcohol syndrome (77) or in utero exposure to isotretinoin (78,79). Given the limitations of our current assessments, it is particularly important to evaluate these data with care, and not disregard potential effects based on spurious reasoning.

In evaluating results from a learning and memory task, it is important to look separately at the "learning" and "memory" portions. First learning, measured as an improvement in performance over repeated trials, should be evaluated to make sure that the animal actually learned the task. When performance (either as number of errors, time to goal, or other appropriate measure) is plotted over several trials, there should be a gradual improvement, possibly reaching asymptote if training is continued for a sufficient number of trials (the acquisition curve). If no or limited improvement is seen, the animal has not learned the task, and it will not be possible to evaluate memory (if control animals have not learned the task, some procedural problem is indicated). Once it has been determined that learning has occurred, an evaluation of memory can be made. Memory is evaluated as the change in performance following a delay period (the appropriate length of delay depending on the type of task). If performance is maintained at the same or similar level following the delay, then memory is intact. If not, there may be some impairment. The degree of impairment can be compared across treatment groups. Again, if the controls show no memory, the procedure used was probably not appropriate and it would be impossible to detect any treatment-related impairment. As with any other type of task, a comparison of the performance of control and treated groups will indicate whether a treatment-related impairment has been detected on either the learning or memory component of the task.

What weight should be given to positive findings on a learning and memory task, in relation to other findings in a neurotoxicity experiment? Findings on many types of behavioral tests may be accompanied by decreases in body weight (or, indeed, changes in a variety of other measured parameters), but such a correlation provides no information about the cause of either effect. Growth and development are related, but different, aspects of what occurs during the period prior to adulthood. Some would dismiss decreased performance on a learning and memory task associated with transient decreases in body weight. This is not a cogent response, unless it can be shown that size or weight actually affected the performance in the test.

Results of tests of learning and memory must be considered in the context of the other pharmacological and toxicological information available for the compound of interest. For example, if the animals were severely hypoactive and lethargic at the time of testing, a valid assessment of learning and memory was probably not possible. In animal experiments, as in human learning and memory, the factor of motivation should be considered. If the animal was not motivated sufficiently by the reward or adverse consequence, normal performance is not likely. If performance is sustained by electric shock, as in most passive and active avoidance procedures, the equivalence of the effects of the shock should be assessed for the different exposure groups. Similarly, if animals in the treatment group take longer to reach the goal than untreated animals, an assessment of speed in a straight alley would answer the question as to whether or not a motor deficit may contribute to the poorer performance. Depending on the type of task, a comparison of performance as evaluated by number of errors versus that evaluated as latency to reach a goal may provide information regarding the contribution of motor versus cognitive deficits to poor task performance.

Sometimes a clear-cut or borderline decrement cannot be explained by other factors. If one has selected and conducted the test using appropriate criteria and procedures, the findings should be considered treatment-related. More sophisticated and sensitive tests, such as SCOB tests, will likely provide additional information and characterization of the effects on motivation and cognition. The effects should be considered a real effect on learning and memory unless a confounding factor is identified.

Neuropathology

Integration of neuropathological findings with the other findings in a neurotoxicity study is crucial. Neuropathology can identify specific lesions that will elucidate the other findings or can stand alone to indict a compound as a neurotoxicant. However, as has been previously emphasized, the absence of behavioral correlates is not sufficient reason to discount neuropathological lesions, nor is the absence of neuropathological lesions sufficient reason to discount behavioral findings.

There are examples in which a good correlation is seen between behavioral changes and histopathological changes in the nervous system. A good example that has been cited already is acrylamide, which causes a "dying back" axonopathy. Abnormalities detected in the behavioral screening battery on such measures as gait in the FOB, hypoactivity in the motor activity assessment, or poor performance in a test of learning and memory requiring coordinated movement (most of those tests do) might all be due to peripheral neuropathy for which the lesions can be identified. In such a case, interpretation of findings is straightforward and should proceed without difficulty.

More often than not, however, a behavioral or functional change is observed, and no lesion is found. As has been emphasized throughout this chapter, behavior is the result of the combined functioning and integration of many different regions and systems in the brain and spinal cord. Lesions may occur at levels that standard neuropathological techniques cannot detect. Alteration in regional levels of neurotransmitters can affect behavior dramatically but cannot be detected with routine histopathology. The same can be said for changes in the manner that neuronal synapses function. Naturally, one can currently focus on the molecular level and find effects that ultimately may or may not be detectable with the technology of neuropathology.

Conversely, serious lesions are sometimes found in the central or peripheral nervous system without any behavioral correlates. There may be several reasons why this can occur. Possibly the behaviors or reactions that could be affected were not tested. Perhaps the time course of the study was too short and behavioral effects would become manifest if the study continued. It might be that the dose response on other measures interfered with detecting functional effects.

Neuropathology in the offspring of exposed animals may be less dramatic and more elusive than that observed in adults exposed directly to the compound. Crude measures, such as the brain weight assessments and morphometric analysis of the layers of the neocortex, hippocampus, and cerebellum, can, theoretically, show the consequences of interference with developmental processes by the compound of interest. Although conclusions regarding compound-related effects on neuropathology may be strengthened by concordance of these measures (e.g., seeing brain weight changes, nerve cell loss in the hippocampus, and differences in hippocampal thickness), recent data indicate that these measures are often not correlated and each contributes independently to the evaluation of neuropathological effects in the developing brain (70). The comprehensive examinations of the nervous system detailed in the EPA neurotoxicity guidelines make the detection of more subtle lesions and errors in development more likely than behavioral tests alone.

CONCLUSION

A general approach for the examination and detection of neurotoxicity in adult and developing animals, usually rats, has been reviewed. This area is constantly evolving and is expected to become more complex and powerful to detect neurotoxicants in the future. The field of neuropathology will provide greater sensitivity with the application of refined techniques, such as the quantification of GFAP, increased use of peripheral nerve conduction velocity assessments, and more sophisticated staining and tissue preparation, including the increased use of electron microscopy. Techniques involving stereology (including ways to more accurately evaluate changes in cell number or volume of particular brain regions), and the development of such noninvasive imaging techniques as MRI also hold great potential for refining our evaluation of compound-related effects on the nervous system (80,81).

Behavioral techniques are also being improved. Tests of learning and memory, in particular, will provide greater sensitivity to potential effects on cognitive functioning. There has been considerable work on development of screening batteries that use comparable tests in experimental animals and humans, allowing comparable evaluations to be done across species and increasing our confidence that animal testing will provide good prediction of effects in exposed humans (82,83,84). There have also been proposals for the addition of tests for other types of behavior, including attention, anxiety, and social interaction (85). Animal tests are available or being developed to assess these functions, which are obviously very important to humans in our day-to-day life. Research in these areas will continue in the next several years, and it is possible these types of functional tests may become important for neurotoxicological assessments in the future.

Improved techniques for evaluating pharmacokinetics will also play a larger role in future neurotoxicity testing, aiding in the design of more relevant exposure scenarios and in our interpretation of experimental results (86). For example, a flat dose-response curve might make more sense if we knew that oral absorption of the compound was rate-limiting. Similarly, knowledge about lactational transfer might aid in deciding the appropriate route of exposure for a DNT study.

Research on improved approaches to assess neurotoxicity is ongoing in many scientific disciplines, especially the neurosciences broadly defined. The improvement in our understanding of how the nervous system functions in its healthy, normal state, and in various disease states, has been enormous. For example, our understanding of neurochemistry, and the specific mechanisms of some types of neurotoxicants, has been greatly expanded in recent years. In cases where mechanistic information is available (e.g., inhibition of a specific enzyme or interaction with a specific type of neural receptor or channel), it may be appropriate to include some of these types of tests into our neurotoxicity screening studies for those chemicals. In the absence of such information, however, most of these basic research methods (as powerful as they are) are not currently amenable to incorporation into screening approaches.

Although most current neurotoxicity screening approaches use various types of in vivo exposures and evaluate the resulting effects in animals, new screening approaches are under development in an attempt to decrease our reliance on these types of studies. In particular, new "omics" techniques can be used to evaluate changes in nerve cell function following exposure to test chemicals. As we improve our understanding of how changes in cell function relate to nervous system toxicity, "omics" techniques could be used to screen for potentially neurotoxic chemicals. Another, related, approach using high throughput screening techniques, including a variety of cell culture and other in vitro methods, may allow us to directly evaluate compound effects on synaptogenesis or other neurodevelopmental processes. Use of these types of methods, along with new methods in computational toxicology, would allow us to screen larger number of compounds than is possible using current methods and to improve our ability to identify neurotoxic compounds. Although it will likely be some time before these methods are developed sufficiently for routine use, their development will add to our knowledge of neurotoxicity and our ability to use this knowledge in protection of the public health.

REFERENCES

1. London E, Etzel RA. The environment as an etiologic factor in autism: a new direction for research. Environ Health Perspect 2000; 108:401–404.
2. Rice DC. Parallels between attention deficit hyperactivity disorder and behavioral deficits produced by neurotoxic exposure in monkeys. Environ Health Perspect 2000; 108:405–408.
3. Olney JW. New insights and new issues in developmental neurotoxicology. Neurotoxicology 2002; 23:659–668.
4. Weiss B. Vulnerability to pesticide neurotoxicity is a lifetime issue. Neurotoxicology 2000; 21:67–74.
5. National Research Council. Pesticides in the diets of infants and children. Committee on Pesticides in the Diets of Infants and Children. Washington, DC: National Academy Press, 1993.
6. U.S. Congress. Food Quality Protection Act. Public Law 104-170. Washington, DC: Government Printing Office, 1996.
7. U.S. Environmental Protection Agency, Office of Pesticide Programs, Pesticide Assessment Guidelines, Subdivision F—Hazard Evaluation; Human and Domestic Animals. EPA Pub. No. 540/9-82-025, Washington, DC, 1982.
8. U.S. Environmental Protection Agency. Toxic Substances Control Act Test Guidelines: Final Rules. 40 CFR Parts 796-798. September 27 (1985). 39252–39516. Part 798 Subpart G. Neurotoxicity, pp. 39458–39470, 1985.
9. U.S. Environmental Protection Agency. Health Effects Test Guidelines, OPPTS 870-100-870.7800. EPA Document 712-C-98-189 through 712-C-98-351. Washington, DC: U.S. Environmental Protection Agency, 1998.
10. Organization for Economic Cooperation and Development. Test Guideline 424. OECD Guideline for Testing of Chemicals. Neurotoxicity Study in Rodents 1997.

11. U.S. Environmental Protection Agency. Pesticides; data requirement for conventional chemicals. Fed Regist 2005; 70:12276–12353.
12. International Conference on Harmonisation of Technical Requirements for Registration of Pharmaceuticals for Human Use. ICH Harmonised Tripartite Guideline, Safety Pharmacology Studies for Human Pharmaceuticals, S7A, 2000.
13. Sobotka TJ, Ekelman KB, Slikker W, et al. Food and drug administration proposed guidelines for neurotoxicological testing of food chemicals. Neurotoxicology 1996; 17:825–836.
14. U.S. Environmental Protection Agency, Pesticide Assessment Guidelines, Subdivision F—Hazard Evaluation; Human and Domestic Animals, Addendum 10—Neurotoxicity Series 81, 82, and 83; PB 91-154617. Springfield, VA: National Technical Information Service, 1991.
15. U.S. Environmental Protection Agency. Guidelines for neurotoxicity risk assessment. Fed Regist 1998; 63:26926–26954.
16. Organization for Economic Cooperation and Development. Guidance Document for Neurotoxicity Testing. OECD Environment, Health and Safety Publications, Series on Testing and Assessment No. 20, OECD: Paris, 2004.
17. Harry J, Kulig B, Lotti M, et al. Environmental Health Criteria 223: Neurotoxicity risk assessment for human health: Principles and approaches. International Programme on Chemical Safety, World Health Organization, Geneva, 2001.
18. Clarren SK, Smith DW. The fetal alcohol syndrome. N Engl J Med 1978; 298:1063–1067.
19. Chang LW, Guo GL. Fetal minamata disease: congenital methylmercury poisoning. In: Slikker W, Chang LW, eds. Handbook of Developmental Neurotoxicology. San Diego, California: Academic Press, 1998:507–515.
20. Committee on the Safety of Medicines. Notes for guidance on reproduction studies. Committee on the Safety of Medicines. London, Great Britain: Department of Health and Social Security, 1974.
21. Ministry of Health and Welfare. On studies of the effects of drugs on reproduction, Notification No. 529 of the Pharmaceutical Affairs Bureau. Japan: Ministry of Health and Welfare, 1975.
22. U.S. Food Drug Administration, International Conference on Harmonization: Guideline on Detection of Toxicity to Reproduction for Medicinal Products: Availability Notice. Federal Register, September 22, 1994, Part IX, 48746–48752.
23. U.S. Environmental Protection Agency. Health Effects Test Guidelines, OPPTS 870-100 through 870.7800. EPA Document 712-C-98-238. Washington, DC: U.S. Environmental Protection Agency, 1998.
24. Organization for Economic Cooperation and Development, Guideline 407 on repeated dose 28-day oral toxicity study in rodents, OECD: Paris, 1995.
25. Organization for Economic Cooperation and Development, Guideline 408 on repeated dose 90-day oral toxicity study in rodents. OECD: Paris, 1998.
26. Crofton KM, Makris SL, Sette WF, et al. A qualitative retrospective analysis of positive control data in developmental neurotoxicity studies. Neurotoxicol Teratol 2004; 26:345–352.
27. Moser VC, Ross JF, eds. Training video and reference manual for a functional observational battery. U.S. Environmental Protection Agency and American Industrial Health Council, 1996.
28. U.S. Environmental Protection Agency, Generic Non-OP Protocol Review Format (10/21/02). Unpublished document used as template for DNT Study Reviews. Health Effects Division, Office of Pesticide Programs, 2002, p. 7.
29. Moser VC, McCormick SP, Cresson JP, et al. Comparison of chlordimeform and carbaryl using a functional observational battery. Fund Appl Toxicol 1988; 11:139–206.
30. Tilson HA, Moser VC. Comparison of screening approaches. Neurotoxicology 1992; 13:1–14.
31. Crofton KM, Howard JL, Moser VC, et al. Interlaboratory comparisons of motor activity experiments: implications for neurotoxicological measurements. Neurotoxicol Teratol 1991; 13:599–609.
32. Brock TO, O'Callaghan JP. Quantitative changes in the synaptic vesicle proteins, synapsin I and p38 and the astrocyte specific protein, glial fibrillary acidic protein, are associated with chemical induced injury to the rat central nervous system. J Neurosci 1987; 7:931–942.

33. O'Callaghan JP. Neurotypic and gliotypic proteins as biochemical markers of neurotoxicity. Neurotoxicol Teratol 1988; 10:445–452.

34. Spencer PS, Schaumberg HH, eds. Experimental and Clinical Neurotoxicology. Baltimore: Williams and Wilkins, 1980.

35. World Health Organization (WHO), Principles and Methods for the Assessment of Neurotoxicity Associated with Exposure to Chemicals (Environmental Health Criteria 60). World Health Organization Publication Center U.S.A., Albany, New York, 1986.

36. U.S. Environmental Protection Agency, Office of Prevention, Pesticides, and Toxic Substances. Developmental Neurotoxicity Guideline OPPTS 870.6300, EPA Document 712-C-98-239. Washington, DC, 1998.

37. U.S. Environmental Protection Agency, Office of Prevention, Pesticides and Toxic Substances, Office of Pesticide Programs. Data Call-in Notice, Attachment F. U.S. Environmental Protection Agency, Washington, DC: Sept. 10, 1999.

38. Organization for Economic Cooperation and Development. OECD Guideline for the Testing of Chemicals, Draft Proposal for a New Guideline 426, Developmental Neurotoxicity Study. Environment Directorate, OECD: Paris, May 2005.

39. Agnish ND, Keller KA. The rationale for culling of rodent litters. Fund Appl Toxicol 1997; 38:2–6.

40. Lore R, Avis H. Effects of auditory stimulation and litter size upon subsequent emotional behavior in the rat. Dev Psychobiol 1970; 2:212–215.

41. Palmer AK. A simpler multi-generation study. International Congress of Pesticide Chemistry, 1986:1–20.

42. Zoetis T, Walls I. Principles and Practices for Direct Dosing of Pre-Weaning Mammals in Toxicity Testing and Research. Washington, DC: ILSI Press, 2003.

43. Adams J, Buelke-Sam J, Kimmel CA, et al. Collaborative behavioral teratology study: protocol design and testing procedure. Neurobehav Toxicol Teratol 1985; 7:579–586.

44. Korenbrot CC, Huhtaniemi IT, Weiner RW. Preputial separation as an external sign of pubertal development in the male rat. Biol Reprod 1977; 17:298–303.

45. Butcher RE. Behavioral testing as a method for assessing risk. Environ Health Perspect 1976; 18:75–78.

46. Ruppert PH, Dean KF, Reiter LW. Development of locomotor activity of rat pups in figure-eight mazes. Dev Psychobiol 1984; 18:247–260.

47. Ison JR. Reflex modification as an objective test for sensory processing following toxicant exposure. Neurobehav Toxicol Teratol 1984; 6:437–445.

48. Green RJ, Stanton ME. Differential ontogeny of working memory and reference memory in the rat. Behav Neurosci 1989; 103:98–105.

49. Kucharski D, Spear NE. Conditioning of aversion to an odor paired with peripheral shock in the developing rat. Dev Psychobiol 1984; 17:465–479.

50. Cory-Slechta DA, Weiss B, Cox C. Delayed behavioral toxicity of lead with increasing exposure concentration. Toxicol Appl Pharmacol 1983; 71:342–352.

51. Spear NE, Campbell BA, eds. Ontogeny of Learning and Memory. New Jersey: Erlbaum, 1979.

52. Krasnegor NA, Blass EM, Hoffer MA, et al. Perinatal Development: A Psychobiological Perspective. Orlando, FL: Academic Press, 1987.

53. Miller DB, Eckerman DA. Learning and memory measures. In: Annau Z, ed. Neurobehavioral Toxicology. Baltimore: Johns Hopkins University Press, 1986:94–149.

54. Riley EP, Vorhees CV, eds. Handbook of Behavioral Teratology. New York: Plenum Press, 1986.

55. Morris RGM. Spatial localization does not require the presence of local cues. Learn Motiv 1981; 12:239–260.

56. DeQuervain DJF, Roozendaal B, McGaugh JL. Stress and glucocorticoids impair retrieval of long term spatial memory. Nature 1998; 394:787–790.

57. Vorhees CV, Weisenburger WP, Acuff-Smith KD, et al. An analysis of factors influencing complex water maze learning in rats: effects of task complexity, path order, and escape assistance on performance following prenatal exposure to phenytoin. Neurotoxicol Teratol 1991; 13:213–222.

58. Weisenburger WP, Minck DR, Acuff KD, et al. Dose-response effects of prenatal phenytoin exposure in rats: effects on early locomotion, maze learning, and memory as a function of phenytoin-induced circling behavior. Neurotoxicol Teratol 1990; 12:145–152.

59. Akaike M, Ohno H, Tsutsumi S, et al. Comparison of four spatial maze learning tests with methylnitrosourea-induced microcephaly rats. Teratol 1994; 49:83–89.

60. Tsutsumi S, Akaike M, Ohno H, et al. Learning/memory impairments in rat offspring prenatally exposed to phenytoin. Neurotoxicol Teratol 1998; 20:123–137.

61. Weisenburger WP, Kozsk CL, Hagler AR, et al. Perinatal phenytoin and methimazole in rats to compare five tests of learning and memory: factors relevant to the selection of tests for pharmaceutical safety evaluation. Neurotoxicol Teratol 1997; 19:257–258.

62. Armed Forces Institute of Pathology (AFIP). Manual of Histologic Staining Methods. New York: McGraw-Hill, 1968.

63. Pender MP. A simple method for high resolution light microscopy of nervous tissue. J Neurosci Methods 1985; 15:213–218.

64. Bennet HS, Wyrick AD, Lee SW, et al. Science and art in the preparation of tissues embedded in plastic for light microscopy, with special reference to glycol methacrylate, glass knives, and simple stains. Stain Technol 1976; 51:71–97.

65. Friede RL. Developmental Neuropathology. New York: Springer-Verlag, 1975.

66. Suzuki K. Special vulnerabilities of the developing nervous system to toxic substances. In: Spencer PS, Schaumberg HH, eds. Experimental and Clinical Neurotoxicology. Baltimore: Williams and Wilkins, 1980:48–61.

67. Garmen RH, Fix AS, Jortner BS, et al. Methods to identify and characterize developmental neurotoxicity for human health risk assessment. II: neuropathology. Environ Health Perspect 2001; 109:93–100.

68. Rodier PM, Gramann WJ. Morphologic effects of interference with cell proliferation in the early fetal period. Neurobehav Toxicol 1979; 1:129–135.

69. Duffel SJ, Soames AR, Gunby S. Morphometric analysis of the developing rat brain. Toxicol Pathol 2000; 28:157–163.

70. Raffaele K, Sette W, Doherty J, et al. Neuropathological findings in developmental neurotoxicity testing: comparison of qualitative and quantitative evaluations. Society of Toxicology, New Orleans, LA, March 2005. Also in The Toxicologist, 2005; 84:200.

71. Tukey JW, Ciminera JL, Heyes JF. Testing the statistical certainty of a response to increasing doses of a drug. Biometrics 1985; 41:295–301.

72. Baird JS, Catalano PJ, Ryan LM, Evans JS. Evaluation of effect profiles: functional observational battery outcomes. Fund Appl Pharmacol 1997; 40:37–51.

73. Koch M. The neurobiology of startle. Prog Neurobiol 1999; 59:107–128.

74. Davis M. The mammalian startle response. Neural Mechanisms of Startle Behavior In: Evans R, ed. New York: Plenum, 1984.

75. Crofton KM, Janssen R, Prazma J, et al. The ototoxicity of 3,3′iminopropionitrile: functional and morphological evidence of cochlear damage. Hear Res 1994; 80:129–140.

76. Raffaele K, Gilbert M, Crofton K, et al. Learning and memory tests in developmental neurotoxicity testing: a cross-laboratory comparison of control data. Society of Toxicology, Baltimore, MD, March 2004. Also in The Toxicologist, 2004; 78:276.

77. Streissguth AP, Barr HM, Martin DC. Alcohol exposure in utero and functional deficits in children during the first four years of life. In: Porter R, O'Connor M, Whalen J, eds. Mechanisms of Alcohol Damage in Utero. London: Pitman (Ciba Foundation Symposium 105), 1984.

78. Adams J, Lammer EJ. Relationship between dysmorphology and neuro-psychological function in children exposed to isotretinoin "in utero." Clin Neuropharm 1991; 13:159–168.

79. Adams J, Holson RR. The neurobehavioral teratology of vitamin A analogs. In: Slikker W, Chang LW, eds. Handbook of Developmental Neurotoxicology. San Diego, California: Academic Press, 1998:631–642.

80. Hyman BT, Gomez-Isla T, Irizarry MC. Stereology: a practical primer for neuropathology. J Neuropathol Exp Neurol 1998; 57:305–310.

81. West MJ. Stereological methods for estimating the total number of neurons and synapses: issues of precision and bias. Trends Neurosci 1999; 22:51–61.

82. Stanton ME, Spear LP. Workshop on the Qualitative and Quantitative Comparability of Human and Animal Developmental Neurotoxicity, Work Group I Report: Comparability of Measures of Developmental Neurotoxicity in Humans and Laboratory Animals. Neurotoxicol Teratol 1990; 12:261–267.

83. Paule MG. Using identical behavioral tasks in children, monkeys, and rats to study the effects of drugs. Curr Ther Res 2001; 62:820–833.

84. Chalonis JJ, Daniels-Shaw JL, Blake DJ, et al. Developmental aspects of delayed matching-to-sample task performance in children. Neurotox Teratol 2000; 22:684–694.

85. Cory-Slechta DA, Crofton KM, Foran JA, et al. Methods to identify and characterize developmental neurotoxicity for human health risk assessment. I. Behavioral effects. Environ Health Perspect 2001; 109:79–91.

86. Dorman DC, Allen SL, Byczkowski JZ, et al. Methods to identify and characterize developmental neurotoxicity for human health risk assessment. III. Pharmacokinetic and pharmacodynamic considerations. Environ Health Perspect 2001; 109:101–111.

13

Toxicological Assessment of the Immune System

Dori R. Germolec
National Institutes of Environmental Health Sciences, National Toxicology Program, National Institutes of Health, Research Triangle Park, North Carolina, U.S.A.

Robert W. Luebke
Immunotoxicology Branch, U.S. Environmental Protection Agency, Research Triangle Park, North Carolina, U.S.A.

Robert V. House
Science and Technical Operations, DynPort Vaccine Company LLC, Frederick, Maryland, U.S.A.

Gary J. Rosenthal
Drug Development, RxKinetix, Inc., Boulder, Colorado, U.S.A.

INTRODUCTION—OVERVIEW OF THE IMMUNE SYSTEM

The immune system is a complex set of cellular and soluble mediators that protects the body against foreign substances, including infectious agents and certain tumor cells. Immune cells are located throughout the body, either in discrete organs, such as the spleen, thymus, and lymph nodes, or in diffuse accumulations of lymphoid and myeloid cells, as are found in association with the skin, lung, and gastrointestinal tract—strategic locations for detection of entering pathogens and exogenous proteins. Protection may rely on responses to proteins or carbohydrates that are unique to a particular pathogen or cell (antigens) or to components of organisms that are widely shared (e.g., viral double stranded RNA, components of bacterial cell walls). Antigen-driven responses are referred to as antigen-specific or adaptive, whereas responses to shared components are referred to as nonspecific or innate. Adaptive responses require recognition of foreign antigens via complex interaction of cell surface molecules, production of growth factors, lymphocyte proliferation (clonal expansion), and implementation of effector mechanisms that ultimately mediate destruction of the foreign threat. The response is very specific but is rather slow (generally 3–7 days to the peak response). In contrast, innate responses do not require antigen recognition or clonal expansion and thus provide a rapid response (<24 hours) to infection. Innate responses are well conserved phylogenetically; the same or very similar responses that mediate resistance to infection in invertebrates act as a first line of defense in mammals to destroy similar classifications of pathogens. In mammals, nonspecific effector cells include macrophages (production of proinflammatory mediators, phagocytosis of pathogens and dead cells), natural killer (NK) cells (contact-dependent killing of certain tumor cells and certain pathogens), and neutrophilic leukocytes (phagocytosis of bacteria). A variety of soluble mediators are important to innate responses as well, including complement (through lysis of cells and augmented phagocytosis of bacteria) and cytokines (through modulation of the inflammatory response).

Macrophages originate in the bone marrow as promonocytes and are then released and carried into the circulation as monocytes in a relatively immature state, prior to further differentiation at various organ sites. In addition to lymphoid organs, macrophages and functionally related cells (e.g., dendritic cells) are found in most every other organ/tissue, including the liver (Kupffer cells), lung (alveolar macrophages), and skin (Langerhans cells). These cells participate in immune responses at a variety of levels including: (1) bi-directional interactions with lymphocytes (i.e., antigen processing and presentation); (2) production of soluble mediators that control other cellular as well as acute and chronic inflammatory responses; (3) scavenger function for the removal of debris and damaged cells; and (4) host defense against intracellular or extracellular microorganisms or neoplastic cells.

The NK cell is a unique lymphocyte population, which, unlike the cytotoxic T lymphocytes (CTL) described below, can target and lyse virally transformed or neoplastic cells independent of the major histocompatibility complex (MHC) antigens on the target cell surface. NK cells are normally present in measurable levels in healthy individuals and are frequently considered to be the first line of protection against certain kinds of malignancies, particularly those of the hematopoietic system. Recent work has shown that NK cells may also be important in the early defense against certain infectious agents as well, as demonstrated by the ability of NK cells to lyse virus-infected fibroblasts or epithelial cells and target intracellular bacteria residing in monocytes. Mechanistically, certain soluble mediators, including IFN-α, -β and -γ and IL-2, can augment the tumoricidal and anti-infective activity of NK cells. In addition to being activated by cytokines, the NK cell itself is a potent source of certain soluble mediators including IFN-γ and granulocyte/monocyte-colony stimulating factor (GM-CSF).

The granulocytic series of leukocytes includes neutrophils, eosinophils, and basophils, so named because of the staining reactions of their cytoplasmic granules. These cells are also collectively referred to as polymorphonuclear leukocytes (PMN), based on the multilobular shape of the cell nucleus in all three cell types. From a practical, if inexact, standpoint, the term "PMN" is often used interchangeably with "neutrophil." Neutrophils account for 50–70% of circulating white blood cells (WBC) in humans and roughly 20% of circulating WBC in rats and mice. They provide critical protection against extracellular bacteria, particularly during the first few days of infection. Unlike lymphocytes, which depend on specific recognition of antigens and subsequent clonal expansion before affording protection to the host, neutrophils respond to microorganisms immediately via surface receptors for components and products of bacteria. Cells are rapidly recruited from the circulation by products of the inflammatory response (chemokines), a process referred to as chemotaxis. Binding of ligands to surface receptors mediates phagocytosis of pathogens and cellular activation. Internalized organisms are destroyed by products of the respiratory burst (e.g., superoxide anion, H_2O_2 hydroxyl-radicals and singlet oxygen). During the later, antigen-specific portion of the host response to infection, antibodies produced by the adaptive immune response adhere to bacteria;

specialized receptors for the constant region of antibody molecules provide an additional binding site for neutrophils, enhancing phagocytosis of the invaders.

Lymphocytes are the prime cellular effectors of adaptive responses, are classified by their tissue of origin or equivalent, and can be subdivided based on function or maturity. Bone marrow–derived lymphocyte progenitor cells that migrate to and mature in the thymus are referred to as T lymphocytes or T cells; B lymphocytes or B cells are also derived from the common lymphocyte progenitor population and take their name from the Bursa of Fabricius, the site of B cell maturation present only in avians. In other vertebrates, B cells migrate to bursal equivalents (the spleen and lymph nodes in mammals). T cell subpopulations include cells that assist in and amplify other immune responses (T helper cells: T_H), downregulate other immune responses (T suppressor cells; T_S) or act as effectors to destroy infected or neoplastic cells (T cytotoxic cells; T_C) as part of the cell-mediated immune (CMI) response. The T_H cells produce cytokines that regulate immune function and can be further subdivided into subpopulations that assist other T cells (T_H1) or that stimulate and perpetuate antibody responses (T_H2). T_H cytokine production predominates in newborns and is also associated with increased allergy and asthma. Soon after birth there is a switch to the T_H1-dominated adult phenotype—important in eliminating certain bacteria and viruses.

Generally, induction of immune responses follows a process where small naïve lymphocytes differentiate into large "blast-transformed" cells and ultimately divide or clonally expand, giving rise to cells responsible for immunologic memory and effector cell function. Naïve circulating B cells encounter antigen in lymph nodes or tissue-associated lymphoid tissues and become activated. B cells recognize antigen via membrane-bound antibody/immunoglobulin (Ig) molecules that act as antigen receptors. Cross-linking of Ig molecules on the cell surface initiates a signal transduction cascade and, with the appropriate stimulus from T_H2 cytokines, leads to activation and proliferation. These activated B cells clonally expand by repeated division, followed by differentiation into plasma cells that secrete Ig, the soluble mediator of humoral immunity. Ig molecules possess two identical heavy chain and two identical light chain polypeptides that form both an antigen binding site (Fab portion) and a primary effector segment (Fc portion). The Fab portion is a variable region at the N-terminals of both chains that constitutes the antigen-binding site and shows considerable heterogeneity in the composition and arrangement of the amino acids that make up the region, allowing for the recognition of a large number of widely diverse antigens. Five classes of antibodies—IgM, IgG, IgE, IgA, and IgD— have been described based on the characteristics of their heavy chain polypeptides, and each of these antibody classes have distinct expression patterns and functional properties during the immune response. IgM, the first antibody to be produced in the humoral immune response, is generally of low affinity; however, its pentameric conformation allows it to bind effectively to multivalent antigens, such as bacterial cell wall polysaccharides, and it plays a significant role in the activation of the complement system. IgG is the most abundant isotype in serum, is important in the neutralization of bacterial toxins and opsonization of pathogens for phagocytosis, and complement mediated cell lysis. IgA is important in immunity at the mucosal surfaces of the body and protects via binding and cross-linking of pathogens. IgE binds with high affinity to mast cells, leading to the release of inflammatory mediators involved in the clearance of parasites and allergic hypersensitivity responses. Although IgD is present on the surface of all naïve B cells, it is generally lost during maturation, and its function is not well defined.

The majority of T CMI functions depend on maturation of precursor cells in the thymus. Prior to release into the circulation, T cells go through a selection process in the thymus that is critical in establishing and maintaining tolerance to constitutively expressed "self" proteins (antigens) present on somatic cells and certain cell products. Most ($>95\%$) immature T cells that initially migrate to the thymus are eliminated, either because of inefficient or overzealous recognition of host antigens. Failure to remove these autoreactive clones is one cause of autoimmune disease.

IMMUNOSUPPRESSION, HYPERSENSITIVITY, AND AUTOIMMUNITY

Within the field of toxicology, investigation of the immune system is concerned with adverse effects of physical or chemical agents on the function of the complex interactions of specific tissues and soluble mediators referred to as immunity. Host protective events at the cellular and molecular level of this diffuse system are the province of lymphocytes, macrophages, neutrophils, complement components, and such soluble mediators as cytokines and antibodies. The methodologies employed in immunotoxicology use the central principles of toxicology in combination with advances in basic and applied immunology to better understand the actions of xenobiotics on the immune system. Immunotoxic agents identified to date include environmental and industrial chemicals, pharmaceuticals, consumer products, food and food additives, as well as such natural entities as mycotoxins and such physical agents as radiation. From the perspective of pathophysiology, the biological manifestations of altered immune homeostasis can generally be divided into three diverse forms of disease: immunosuppression, hypersensitivity, and autoimmunity. Examples of xenobiotics capable of inducing adverse immune responses are shown in Table 1.

The consequences of xenobiotic-induced immunosuppression can be devastating, as evidenced by the high incidence of secondary cancer in transplant patients following therapeutic immunosuppression, and by the increase in susceptibility to pulmonary infections characteristic of Yusho disease seen in China and Japan following consumption of immunosuppressive polychlorinated biphenyls and furans from contaminated rice oil (1). Even moderate alteration of immune function, as occurs in the case of chronic stress, alters the response to vaccination and the ability to resist new infections or the reactivation of latent viral infections (2). In addition to these and many other clinical cases, a large body of experimental data also exists showing that xenobiotic exposure can produce marked changes in immune competence and significantly decrease resistance to infectious or neoplastic challenge (3).

From an industrial toxicology perspective, hypersensitivity diseases are probably the most common manifestation of immunotoxicity. Although hypersensitivity diseases afflict millions of Americans (3), the incidence associated with environmental or occupational exposure is unclear, although it is likely to be significant in light of the numerous chemicals shown to produce a hypersensitivity response after occupational exposure. Well-known examples include the diisocyanates, trimellitic anhydrides, and platinum dusts. The characteristic that distinguishes the allergic responses from immune mechanisms involved in host defense is the inappropriate nature of the response to specific antigens, which often leads to tissue damage. Almost any organ can be targeted by hypersensitivity reactions, including the gastrointestinal tract, blood elements and vessels, joints, kidneys, central nervous system, and thyroid. However, the skin and lung, which demonstrate urticaria and asthma, respectively, are the most commonly affected.

Although the immune system can adequately defend against infectious agents and prevent adverse reactions to self because of the exquisitely organized network of interacting, discriminatory components, self-tolerance is not always preserved, and disregulated recognition of autoantigens may lead to autoimmune disease. The well-documented

Table 1   Agents Associated with Adverse Immune Responses

Immunosuppression
  Pharmaceuticals
    Cytoreductive agents
    Opiates/opioids
    Transplantation drugs (cyclosporine)
    AIDS therapeutics
  Environmental chemicals
    Air pollutants
    Heavy metals
    Pesticides
    Dusts (silica; asbestos)
  Recreation adjuncts
    Cannabinoids
    Cocaine
    Ethanol
    Tobacco smoke
Hypersensitivity
  Pharmaceuticals
    Phenylglycine acid chloride
    Piperazine amprolium hydrochloride
    Antihistamines
    Anesthetics
    Antibiotic dusts
  Food-associated materials
    Grain and flour dust
    Molds
    Pancreatic extracts
    Papain
Autoimmunity
  Pharmaceuticals
    Chlorpromazine
    Interferons
    Hydralazine
    Methyldopa
    Penicillamine
    Procainimide
  Food-associated materials
    Alfalfa sprouts
    L-tryptophan

  Industrial chemicals
    Polycyclic aromatic hydrocarbons
    Halogenated aromatic hydrocarbons
    Glycol ethers
    Organic solvents
  Physical agents
    Ultraviolet radiation
    Gamma radiation
    Physical stress
    Electromagnetic radiation

  Industrial chemicals
    Anhydrides
    Detergents
    Diisocyanates (TMI, HDI, MDI)
    Ethylenediamine
    Metallic salts (nickel, platinum)
  Organics
    Animal dander
    Cotton dust
    Fragrance components
    Wood dusts

  Industrial chemicals
    Organic solvents (vinyl chloride, TCE)
    Heavy metals
    Pesticides
  Environmental factors
    Infectious agents
    Silica

examples of drug-induced autoimmune syndromes (i.e., procainamide, isoniazid, sulfa drugs, penicillamine) suggest that exposure to other xenobiotics could contribute to the incidence of these diseases through disruption of normal immune processes (4). For example, a number of drugs or their metabolites conjugate to self-proteins, inducing changes in their antigenic determinants such that the molecules are no longer recognized as self. Autoimmune disorders are manifestations of immunologic disregulation in which many predisposing factors (e.g., infection, genetic predisposition) can play an etiologic role. The pathogenesis of autoimmune disease is diverse and includes the production of autoantibodies, damaging inflammatory cell infiltrates into target tissues, and immune complex formation and deposition in numerous tissues.

CONSIDERATIONS AND APPROACHES FOR DETECTING IMMUNOSUPPRESSION

Chemical modulation of the immune system by exogenous agents is due as much to the physicochemical properties of the agent as to the complex nature of immunity. Because of this inherent complexity, the initial strategies devised by immunologists working in toxicology and safety assessment have been to select and apply a broad and often tiered panel of assays to identify immunomodulatory agents in laboratory animals or via focused epidemiological studies.

Although the configurations of these tiered testing panels vary depending on what the data are to be used for, the regulatory requirements to be met, and the animal species employed, they usually include assessment of one or more of the following: (1) lymphoid organ weights and histopathology; (2) quantitative assessment of lymphoid tissue cellularity, hematology, and bone marrow differential; (3) immune cell function at the effector or regulatory level; and/or (4) host resistance studies involving infectious or neoplastic challenge. Table 2 lists some of the more commonly used functional methods in experimental testing of immune status.

A number of test panels have been proposed for evaluating immune suppression in experimental animals [(5–9) section Regulatory Issues In Immunotoxicology below]. The tier testing approaches employed by these regulatory agencies are similar in design in that the first tier is a screen for immunotoxicity, with the second tier consisting of more specific or confirmatory studies, host resistance studies, or in-depth mechanistic studies. At present, most information regarding these models comes from the U.S. National Institute of Environmental Health Sciences, National Toxicology Program (NIEHS/NTP) followed

Table 2 Methods Used to Assess Immunotoxicity

Method	Immune parameter evaluated
Nonspecific markers immunotoxicity	Complete blood count and differential
	Immunopathology
	Acute phase proteins
	Complement (CH50)
Cell mediated immunity	Surface marker phenotypic analysis
	Mixed lymphocyte response
	Mitogen induced proliferation
	Delayed-type hypersensitivity/skin testing
	Cytotoxic T-lymphocyte mediated cytolysis
Humoral immunity	Antibody plaque forming cell assay
	Basal or antigen specific serum antibody titers
	Mitogen induced proliferation
Nonspecific immunity	Natural killer cell cytotoxicity
	Macrophage phagocytosis
	Macrophage bactericidal/tumorcidal activity
Host resistance assessment models	*Listeria monocytogenes*
	Plasmodium yoelli
	Trichinella spiralis
	Streptococcus pneumoniae
	Influenza virus
	PYB6 or B16F10 tumor cell challenge

by the model developed at the National Institute of Public Health and Environmental Protection (RIVM) in Bilthoven, The Netherlands (6,10).

Whereas the first-tier screening at RIVM consists of tests for general parameters of specific and nonspecific immunity, Tier I of the NIEHS-NTP panel includes functional tests in which an immune response is measured following in vivo antigenic challenge. These are generally considered the most sensitive indicators of immune integrity but are not routinely conducted as part of subchronic toxicology studies because of the potential for immunization and immunogenicity to compromise interpretation of other toxicity test results. If sufficient reason exists to pursue any tiered panel, the use of dedicated groups of animals will avoid this confounding variable.

Histopathology of lymphoid organs is a pivotal component in the RIVM screening battery (10). Routine histopathology of lymphoid organs has been shown to be useful in assessing the potential immunotoxicity of a chemical, particularly when these results are combined with the effects observed on lymphoid organs weights and under conditions where sufficiently high doses of the chemical are tested (10). In the RIVM panel, if the results in Tier I suggest immunotoxicity, then Tier II functional studies can be performed to confirm and further investigate the nature of the immunotoxic effect. Information on structure-activity relationships of immunotoxic chemicals can also lead to the decision to initiate functional evaluation. The choice for further studies depends on the type of immune abnormality observed. The second tier consists of a panel of in vivo and ex vivo/in vitro assays, including cell-mediated immunity, humoral immunity, macrophage and NK cell function, as well as host resistance assays (Table 2).

Recently, a database consisting of more than 50 compounds, which were evaluated in one or more tiers of the NIEHS/NTP panel, has been analyzed in an attempt to improve the accuracy and efficiency of screening chemicals for immunosuppression (11,12). The types of compounds in this database span a broad spectrum of agents, including environmental, industrial, and pharmacologic agents. Although these reports describe limitations existing in the datasets used in the analyses, a number of important conclusions were drawn from these data (11,12):

1. Assessment of as few as two or three immune parameters may successfully predict immunotoxicants in mice. In particular, enumeration of lymphocyte subpopulations by flow cytometry and quantitation of T-dependent antibody responses appear to be particularly predictive. Furthermore, commonly employed gross measures, such as lymphoid organ weights, appear somewhat insensitive as measures of immunotoxicity.

2. A good correlation existed between changes in the immune tests and altered host resistance. However, in many instances immune changes were observed in the absence of detectable changes in host resistance, suggesting that immune tests are, in general, more sensitive than the host resistance assays.

3. No single immune test was identified that could be considered highly predictive for altered host resistance in mice. However, combining several immune tests increased the ability to predict host resistance deficits, in some cases to about 80%.

4. Most immune function–host resistance relationships follow a linear rather than threshold model, suggesting that even small changes in immune function may theoretically manifest into some deficit in host resistance. However, because of the variability in the responses, it was not possible to establish linear or threshold models for most of the chemicals studied when the datasets were evaluated.

DOSING AND SPECIES CONSIDERATIONS

A variety of factors need to be considered when evaluating the potential of an environmental agent or pharmaceutical to adversely influence the immune system of experimental animals. As in most toxicological investigations, the selection of the exposure route should parallel the most probable route of human exposure. Treatment conditions should take into account the biophysical properties of the agent, including pharmacokinetics, metabolism, and mechanism of action, if available. Dose levels should be chosen that would likely establish distinct dose-response curves as well as a no-observable-effect level (NOEL). Although in some instances it may be necessary to include a dose level that induces some other manifestation of overt toxicity, immune changes observed at such dose levels should be interpreted cautiously because severe stress and malnutrition (and resultant cachexia) are known to impair immune responsiveness (13–15). Lastly, inclusion of a positive control group is also important to validate the robustness of the assay.

It is not surprising that the selection of the most appropriate animal model for immunotoxicology studies has been the subject of much deliberation. Assuming the species of primary interest is the human, toxicity testing should be performed in a species that will respond to the test chemical in a pharmacologic and toxicological manner similar to that anticipated in humans. For example, best efforts should be made to ensure that test animals and humans metabolize the chemical similarly and have comparable target organ responses and toxicity. Toxicological studies are often conducted in several animal species, most often employing a rodent and nonrodent species. Although some exceptions exist, for many immunosuppressive therapeutics rodent data on target organ toxicities and the comparability of immunosuppressive doses have generally been good predictors of subsequent clinical observations. Taking into account the toxicokinetic and pharmaco-kinetic differences that exist between experimental animals and humans (16), rodents continue to be very useful models for examining the immunotoxicity of non-species-specific compounds, based on established similarities of toxicological profiles as well as the relative ease of generating host resistance and immune function data. As novel xenobiotics continue to be produced, particularly recombinant biologics and gene therapy agents, comparative toxicological assessment should be seriously considered, because their safety assessment will likely present species-specific host interactions and toxicological profiles.

APPROACHES TO EVALUATING HUMORAL IMMUNITY

In risk assessment studies designed to evaluate the most sensitive and predictive tests for immunotoxicology, assessment of humoral immunity, via examination of antigen-specific antibody responses, has been shown to be the best single indicator to determine the potential for a compound to induce alterations in immune function (11). This is likely a reflection of the fact that measurement of the antibody response assesses more than B cell function, as both T cells and macrophage activity are generally required in mounting an effective antibody response. Macrophages have a significant role in antigen processing and presentation and may also modulate the antibody response via cytokine release. Antigen-specific T cells serve as a source of cytokines that ultimately stimulate (T_H) or down-regulate (T_S) the production of antibody. T helper cells produce a variety of cytokines, in particular, interleukin (IL)-4, IL-5, IL-6, and IL10, that regulate the proliferation, differen-tiation and class of antibody produced by B cells. Additional mechanistic information can also be obtained using T-independent antigens, such as lipopolysaccharide and dinitrophenol-ficoll. Because T cell help is not required, responses to T-independent antigens provide evidence of B cell, rather than T cell defects. It is worth noting that there are few naturally occurring T-independent antigens and that these antigens stimulate the production of only a single class (IgM) of antibody. There is a growing consensus that measurement of total IgM and IgG are of limited predictive value, particularly in the absence of the antigen-specific tests described below.

In laboratory rodents, primary antibody responses are commonly evaluated after in vivo immunization with a T-dependent antigen, such as sheep red blood cells (SRBC) or keyhole limpet hemocyanin (KLH). Cells producing antibody to SRBC can be quantified using a modification of the method first described by Jerne and Nordin (17), where they appear as a clear area or "plaque" in a mixture of antigen, lymphocytes and agar. Isolated splenic lymphocytes are the most common cell type employed in these types of studies, and data are typically expressed as the number of cells producing antibody per million viable cells and per spleen. Data for spleen cellularity and weight are also included in the evaluation, to correct for chemical-induced alterations in spleen cell number or as an indicator of overt toxicity to the whole animal. The enzyme-linked immunospot (ELISPOT) assay is another ex vivo method that can be used to quantify antibody production using antigen bound to a solid substrate. Although chemical-induced alterations in numbers of antibody forming cells or serum antibody levels are suggestive of defects in one or more of the cellular pathways contributing to the antibody response, techniques such as these are limited in that they do not identify the specific cellular target. Thus, in vitro methods to assess antibody production, which can be useful in determining the specific mechanism of immunosuppression, have been developed. In general, these studies use purified macrophages, B and T lymphocytes isolated from control animals, or animals treated in vivo with the chemical of interest in elegant separation-reconstitution experiments to identify the target cell type. This type of methodology has been used successfully to elucidate cell-specific toxicity for immunomodulatory compounds such as dideoxyinosine, carbon tetrachloride and 2,3,7,8-tetrachlorodibenzodioxin (TCDD) (18–20).

Enzyme linked immunosorbant assay (ELISA) assays, which evaluate antigen-specific antibodies in serum, are an excellent measure of in vivo antibody production and, depending on the kinetics of serum collection, can provide information on effects in specific antibody isotypes. Primary and anamnestic (memory-inducing) humoral immune responses in nonhuman primates are frequently evaluated using ELISA techniques. In rodents there is a high degree of correlation between the plaque assay and the SRBC ELISA (21); however, the kinetics may be slightly different across rodent species, and it is critical to ensure that quantitation occurs at the peak of the response for the species and isotype of interest. Use of ELISA techniques to evaluate antigen-specific antibody responses has become increasingly popular, as the potential for robotic automation and the availability of inexpensive microplate dilutors, pipetors, and ELISA readers has allowed for the generation of highly reproducible results for large numbers of samples in an ever decreasing time period.

Studies in humans have generally been limited to quantitating serum antibody titers to common vaccine antigens (e.g., tetanus) or evaluating in vitro production of antibody in response to similar antigens. Alternatively, *total* antibody secretion to nonspecific stimuli (e.g., pokeweed mitogen) can also be measured in vitro. These studies generally involve obtaining peripheral blood lymphocytes from human volunteers and culturing them in defined media for optimized time periods in the presence of either the specific antigens or mitogen. However, the latter assays are difficult to perform, due to the difficulty in obtaining enough responsive lymphocytes (22). Recent studies have made use of "humanizing" immunodeficient mouse strains, such as the CB-17 scid/scid (severe combined immunodeficient: SCID) mouse by engrafting with human immune cells, but the utility of these methods to examine chemical-induced alterations in humoral immunity may be limited by the high degree of variability in the reconstituted responses (23).

Vaccination represents the best opportunity for monitoring alterations in humoral immunity in humans. Secondary (recall and booster) responses appear to be less sensitive to chemical-induced perturbations than do primary responses (24); however, in cases of severe immunosuppression, response to recall antigens can be informative (25). In adults, postvaccination antibody responses to Epstein Barr virus, and influenza neoantigens may be useful to assess primary reactions (26,27). Changes in virus-specific immune responses or activation of latent viruses may provide an indication of mild to moderate immunosuppression in human populations (2). There is a growing realization that, as the developing immune system may be particularly vulnerable to immunotoxic agents, studies of primary immune responses in newborns and young children in conjunction with established vaccination programs (such as against measles, diphtheria, tetanus, and poliomyelitis) may offer a significant opportunity to assess chemical-induced alterations in immune status and improve public health.

APPROACHES TO EVALUATING CELLULAR IMMUNITY

A number of factors determine whether a specific antigen will induce a T cell-mediated response, a humoral immune response, or both. These factors include the route of exposure, the physicochemical attributes of the antigen, the nature of antigen processing and presentation, as well as the initial and ultimate distribution of the antigen within the host tissue. In light of this inherent complexity, some patterns do exist which may assist in identifying those antigens that generally elicit CMI. These include chemical agents and drugs that covalently bind to self-proteins, tissue-associated antigens, and certain antigenic determinants on persistent microorganisms, such as *Mycobacterium tuberculosis*.

At the heart of the initial T-cell interaction with antigen is the ability to recognize the foreign agent and become activated along a specific pathway, which results in functions dependent on cell contact (i.e., cytotoxicity) or functions resulting in amplification or suppression of the capacity of other cells through the release of soluble mediators, such as IL-1 2,4,5, and 6, and interferon (IFN)-γ. Work by Bottomly et al. (28) demonstrated that CD4 + Th cells can be further subdivided into two distinct populations, referred to as Th1 and Th2 cells. Th1 cells produce IL-2 and IFN-γ, whereas Th2 cells produce IL-4, IL-5, and IL-6. Changes in the normal homeostatic control of these cells, and their respective soluble mediators, may be the basis for a number of hypersensitivity diseases including allergy (29,30).

Assessment of T cell integrity is performed using a number of test methods, such as quantification of lymphocyte subsets or lymphoproliferation assays (31), that measure the blastogenic and proliferative capacity of splenic or circulating lymphocytes to selected plant lectins or mitogens (i.e., phytohemmagluttinin or concanavalin A). In light of the immune system's dependence on clonal expansion following antigen exposure, a decrease in lymphoproliferation is clearly an immunotoxic event. However, the predictive value of these nonspecific proliferative assays has been shown to be limited as compared with a number of other immune function tests (10). Other frequently employed methods used to detect T cell dysfunction are the mixed lymphocyte response (MLR) and the CTL assay (31,32). The MLR tests the proliferative response of T lymphocytes to surface major histocompatibility complex (MHC) antigens on allogeneic cells and provides a sensitive indicator for CMI. Clinically, the MLR measures those cellular events involved in graft rejection and graft versus host reactions and have been shown to be predictive of host response to organ transplants. T lymphocytes with cytotoxic effector function are generated in response to a variety of stimuli, including allogeneic cell surface MHC determinants, certain mitogenic lectins, chemically or virally modified autologous or syngeneic cells, as well as unique tumor associated antigens. The differentiation of CTL from their precursors involves a highly complex series of cellular interactions and production of soluble mediators, ultimately resulting in the production of effector cells capable of recognizing and lysing the target. Assessment of CTL function is measured by the MHC restricted lysis of sensitive target cells and has been recently reviewed by House and Thomas (32).

APPROACHES TO EVALUATING NONSPECIFIC IMMUNITY: MACROPHAGES, NK CELLS, AND NEUTROPHILS

A comprehensive assessment of macrophage function requires multiple tests that take into consideration their heterogeneous function, origin, and activation state. The concept of macrophage activation, developed in the 1960s on the basis of work of Mackaness and colleagues (33), is central to any analysis of isolated macrophages. Although many mechanistic studies have been performed with activated macrophages stimulated to accumulate in the peritoneal cavity, an applied approach warrants evaluation of macrophages derived from the organ(s) most closely associated with chemical exposure because macrophages derived from different sites of the body may be functionally and phenotypically distinct. The unique environment each tissue macrophage operates within probably drives such heterogeneity. For instance, whereas many macrophages operate in a relatively anaerobic state, the alveolar macrophage resides in an environment with comparatively high oxygen levels, which may be related to its relative robust reactive oxygen production compared to the peritoneal macrophage. Techniques are available to obtain highly enriched macrophage populations from many organs (34). Furthermore, the cells are well suited to short-term culture and activation by such mediators as IFN-γ and lipopolysaccharide (35).

The methods employed to evaluate the functional status of macrophages following exposure to suspected immunotoxicants vary considerably, ranging from phagocytic indices, release of a growing list of soluble mediators, or complex bactericidal or tumoricidal activities, including the release of reactive oxygen or nitrogen (36–38). Table 3 lists a number of the biological capacities and functions of macrophages commonly evaluated in immunotoxicological investigations.

Considering the established role of NK cells in neoplastic immunosurveillance, an adequate understanding of chemical-induced suppression of NK cell activity may provide insight into the mechanism(s) by which certain chemicals exert their carcinogenic effects. Immunotoxicologic investigations frequently include the evaluation of NK cell integrity in a functional manner, using cytotoxicity assays, as well as quantitatively through lymphocyte subset analysis of circulating blood. The NK cell cytotoxicity assay is one of the more easily conducted functional tests performed in an immunotoxicological assessment and can be performed using human peripheral cells and readily available target cells, such as the K562 cell line, or using rodent spleen cells with the YAC-1 tumor cell line (39).

A variety of methods are available to assess the function of neutrophils, including chemotaxis, phagocytosis, and the respiratory burst (40–42).

Table 3 Immunobiological Functions and Capacities Associated with Macrophages

Function/capacity	Examples
Interaction with lymphocytes	Antigen processing in conjuction with MHC complex
Production of soluble mediators	Interleukins
	TNF
	Fibronectin
	Arachondonic acid metabolites
	Platelet activating factor
Scavenger	Antigen uptake incorporation and catabolism within phagolysosomes
Host defense	Phagocytosis
	Tumor cytostasis or cytocidal activity
	Bactericidal activity
	Reactive oxygen and reactive nitrogen production

Abbreviations: MHC, major histocompatibility complex; TNF, tumor necrosis factor.

APPROACHES TO EVALUATING HYPERSENSITIVITY RESPONSES

Xenobiotics that induce hypersensitivity responses can be either low molecular weight, highly reactive molecules (haptens), or proteins that produce a unique and antigen-specific immune response. The clinical/diagnostic characteristic that sets these responses apart from immune mechanisms involved in host defense is that the reaction is characteristically inappropriate and often leads to tissue damage. Clinical differentiation of allergic responses from nonimmune irritant responses is based on the requirement for a prior, sensitizing exposure or increasing severity of the lesion on subsequent exposure to small quantities of the antigen. Chemical-induced hypersensitivities can be considered to fall into two general categories distinguished both mechanistically and temporally; (1) delayed-type hypersensitivity (DTH), which is a CMI-based response that occurs within 24–48 hours after reexposure to the eliciting agent; and (2) immediate hypersensitivity, which is mediated by Ig (most commonly IgE) and manifests within minutes following exposure to an allergen. The type of immediate hypersensitivity response elicited depends upon the interaction of the sensitizing antigen or structurally related compound with antibody. In contrast, DTH responses are characterized by T lymphocytes bearing antigen-specific receptors that, on contact with cell-associated antigen, respond by secreting cytokines. Hypersensitivity responses usually occur at potential xenobiotic portals of entry, which explains why the skin and respiratory tract are very common disease targets. Mononuclear phagocytes have a major role in mediating local responses, initially via antigen processing and later via the release of reactive oxygen species and cytokines that modulate the recruitment and activation of additional cell types, including neutrophils and lymphocytes. In addition to leukocytes, local cell types are often involved in the response including keratinocytes, epithelial cells and fibroblasts.

Historically, the guinea pig has been used to test for potential sensitizers. In the induction phase (primary exposure period), the guinea pigs are treated with the test agent, followed by reexposure(s) (challenge phase) to the same test compound, normally after a period of 10–14 days. Erythema and edema are measured at the site of the challenge exposure with a nonirritating concentration of the test compound. Many variations in procedures for guinea pig hypersensitivity assays have been studied (e.g., Buehler occluded, guinea pig maximization, split adjuvant), details of which can be found elsewhere (43). These guinea pig models are very sensitive, and it has been suggested that in light of this, they may produce more false positives than is desirable. This argument may not be completely convincing when one considers the notable heterogeneity of immune responses in the human population.

Many efforts have been made to substitute the guinea pig assays with mouse models. Gad et al. (44) proposed a mouse ear swelling test (MEST). This procedure is similar technically to the guinea pig assay in that both induction and challenge phases are required, but measuring an increase in ear thickness when the material for challenge is applied quantitates the response. One of the more intensively studied methods is the local lymph node assay (LLNA) (45). In this procedure, the test material is applied topically in three successive daily applications to both ears of the test species, usually the mouse. Control mice are treated with the vehicle alone. After five days of exposure, mice are injected with radioisotopically labeled DNA precursors (e.g., ^{3}H-thymidine), and single-cell suspensions are prepared from the lymph nodes draining the ears. At least one concentration of the test chemical must produce a threefold increase or greater in lymphocyte proliferation in the draining lymph nodes of test animals, compared with vehicle-treated control mice, to be considered a positive. The primary advantage of this assay is that it minimizes the manipulation of animals.

DEVELOPMENTAL IMMUNOTOXICITY

It is well established that diseases associated with abnormal immune function, including common infectious diseases and induction of asthma, are considerably more prevalent at younger ages. Several factors are thought to account for this increased susceptibility, including functional immaturity of the immune system and age-related differences in the integrity of the host's anatomical and functional barriers. Although not established absolutely, it is generally believed that the immature immune system is also more susceptible to xenobiotics than the fully mature system and that sequelae of developmental immunotoxicant exposure may be particularly persistent, in contrast to effects observed following adult exposure that generally occur at higher doses and are expected to resolve soon after exposure ends. Based on experimental animal studies, perturbations of the developing immune system may be manifested as a qualitative difference (i.e., affecting the developing immune system without affecting the adult immune system) or a quantitative difference (i.e., affecting the developing immune system at lower doses than in adults) (46–48). Immune maturation may simply be delayed by xenobiotic exposure and recover to normal adult levels over time or, if exposure interferes with a critical step in the maturational process, life-long defects in immune function may follow. These defects may be expressed as immunosuppression or as dysregulation of the immune system, resulting in decreased resistance to infection or failure to switch from the functional phenotype that is normally associated with allergy and asthma to the adult phenotype that efficiently combats infections. Immunosuppression is clearly an adverse event, given the known link between even moderate suppression of immune function and the incidence of infections (49).

Adult levels of antigen-driven immune function are the result of a process that begins with the appearance of hematopoietic stem cells, first detectable late in the first trimester. Early in the second trimester of rodents these cells migrate to the fetal spleen and liver and begin to differentiate and mature, although most hematopoietic activity is dedicated to the production of red blood cells at this stage of development. Progenitor cells from the bone marrow (prothymocytes) migrate to the thymus, the central lymphoid organ where the process of T lymphocyte maturation takes place. B lymphocyte progenitors are also produced at this time and migrate to the spleen and lymph nodes, peripheral lymphoid organs that are the main sites for antigen trapping and presentation to cells that will eventually mature into antibody secreting cells. During the last trimester, immature lymphocytes expressing antibody on the cell surface (B cells) and T cells are present in the spleen but in very small numbers. Although certain immune responses can be elicited in newborn rodents, maturation of the immune response continues after birth, attaining adult levels at about the time of sexual maturation in humans and rodents (although humans are more immunologically mature at birth than are rodents). An excellent review of immune system ontogeny in various species is available (50).

To date, the majority of developmental immunotoxicity studies have been designed to detect immunosuppression in offspring of exposed dams, or, occasionally, in directly exposed newborns, once the animals reach immunologic maturity. Fewer studies have addressed the effects of developmental exposure on allergy or autoimmunity, in part because there are fewer assays available and in part because suppression has long been assumed to be the most likely outcome of developmental exposure.

Although not studied in as much detail as adaptive immunity, innate immune function is believed to be less developed in newborns compared to adults (50). For example, granulocytes that provide protection against extracellular bacteria are less efficient at migrating to sites of bacterial colonization and at engulfing and killing bacteria than the same cells in adults. Fewer circulating NK cells are present in cord blood than in adults, and these cells are likewise less efficient than their adult counterparts.

It has yet to be established whether conducting screening tests only in adults is sufficient to detect chemicals that may be developmental immunotoxicants. Although most of the compounds that cause immunosuppression following developmental exposure also affect function in adults at some dose, effective doses and persistence of effects can vary significantly, depending on when exposure occurs (50). Acknowledging the potential shortcomings of adults only testing, the U.S. Food and Drug Administration testing guidelines for new drugs includes a provision for developmental testing of drugs with demonstrated effects on adult immune function, particularly if the drug is likely to be used during pregnancy (51).

IMMUNOMODULATION IN HUMAN POPULATIONS

Evaluation of immunotoxicity in the general population is notably more complex than in animals, given the limited number of noninvasive tests and wide "normal" range of biological responses in the general population. In addition, with the exception of controlled clinical studies, exposure levels of the agent (i.e., dose) are typically difficult to verify. As such, the most reliable data will be obtained if immune function studies are performed in recently exposed populations or when body burdens of contaminants can be assessed. Because many immune tests performed in humans have a certain degree of overlap (redundancy), it is also important that a positive diagnosis of immune dysfunction be based not on a single change but on a profile of changes, similar to those used clinically to define immunodeficiency (e.g., low CD4:CD8 ratios accompanied by changes in skin tests to recall antigens). The World Health Organization (WHO) has prepared a monograph providing testing schemes and their respective merits and pitfalls for examining immune system changes in humans (52). It should be noted that the selection of many of these assessments were derived from observations in patients with primary immunodeficiency disease, individuals who suffer from a degree of immunosuppression considerably more severe than that induced by chemicals (immunomodulatory drugs excluded) and that are the result of metabolic or genetic defects that are unlikely to be present in individuals exposed to xenobiotics. In light of the difficulties that exist in identifying chemical-induced immunosuppression in humans, establishment of exposure levels (e.g., blood or tissue levels) of the suspected chemical(s) is essential in determining a cause-effect relationship between exposure to xenobiotics and altered immune function.

In human immunological studies it should not be necessary to observe clinical diseases before considering detected defects in immune function to be biologically meaningful. Uncertainties exist regarding whether the relationship between immune function and clinical disease follow linear or threshold models. If the relationship were linear, then even minor changes in immune function would relate to increased risk of disease and may be detected if the population examined is large enough. Although the relationship at the low end of the dose-response curve is unclear, at the high end of the curve (i.e., severe immunosuppression), clinical disease is readily apparent, best exemplified by increased incidence of infections and neoplasia in therapeutically immunosuppressed transplant patients. Nevertheless, suppressed immune function has been detected in a population living near a Superfund site contaminated with pesticides, volatile organics, and metals (53). Reduced resistance to herpes virus infection was also linked to blood levels of DDE (a long-lived metabolite of DDT) in a subpopulation of individuals living close to the site (54). Reduced resistance to infection has also been documented in chronically stressed populations experiencing mild to moderate levels of immunosuppression (55).

The Agency for Toxic Substances and Disease Registry with the CDC (ATSDR/CDC) and National Research Councils subcommittee on Biologic Markers in Immunotoxicology have proposed testing batteries that attempt to address many of the above described problems and pitfalls by implementing a comprehensive state-of-the-art immunological evaluation in conjunction with more traditional tests (56,57). Many of these tests are similar to those used to identify chemical-induced immunosuppression in laboratory animals and should help to predict the probability of developing suppressed host resistance or clinical disease in humans, and, comparable to animal investigation, these tests are also recommended in a tiered approach.

REGULATORY ISSUES IN IMMUNOTOXICOLOGY

Environmental Chemicals

The earliest codified immunotoxicology test guidelines were developed to augment toxicological assessment of chemicals with the potential for large-scale human exposure. In 1996 the Office of Prevention, Pesticides and Toxic Substances (OPPTS) of the U.S. Environmental Protection Agency (EPA) published guidelines titled *Biochemicals Test Guidelines: OPPTS 880.3550 Immunotoxicity* (58), which described the preferred study design for evaluating potential immunotoxicity in biochemical pest control agents. The panel of tests included in this guideline includes standard toxicology tests as well as functional tests that evaluate both humoral and CMI function (the exceptions being primarily cytokine quantification and flow cytometry). A second document was published concurrently entitled *Biochemicals Test Guidelines: OPPTS 880.3800 Immune Response* (59). This companion document provided the rationale for why pesticides must be tested for immunotoxicity, more detailed explanations for testing strategies, and additional details on advanced (mechanistic) tests including host resistance and bone marrow function. In 1998, EPA followed up with *Health Effects Test Guidelines: OPPTS 870.7800*

Immunotoxicity (60), which described immunotoxicology testing for nonbiochemical agents that would be regulated by EPA. This document provided descriptions of both why and how, with a much more abbreviated panel of testing to be performed. The testing approach mandated by 870.7800 has stood up well in intervening years and reflects the more limited, case-by-case approach currently favored. Most notably, the functional assessment is pared down to T-dependent antibody formation (plaque assay), NK cell function, and quantitation of T and B cells; this combination is derived from the early work of Luster et al. (11), demonstrating the greatest predictivity of known immunotoxicants using these three assays. The study design described in this document is amenable for testing a wide range of industrial and environmental chemicals.

In Europe, the Organization for European Cooperation and Development (OECD) regulates testing of chemicals for toxicity. OECD Guideline 407 entitled *Repeated Dose 28-day Oral Toxicity Study in Rodents* (61), although not specific for immunotoxicology, includes a variety of toxicological endpoints that can provide early evidence of immune system alterations. These guidelines do not include functional assays to directly measure any immune deficit.

Food Additives

After industrial and environmental chemicals, food additives might possibly have the greatest potential for human exposure. In the United States, these chemicals are regulated by the FDA's Center for Food Safety and Applied Nutrition. In March 1993 the FDA published the *Draft Redbook II*, which recommended safety-testing practices for food additives. This document contained an extensive description of immunotoxicology testing; although Redbook II was never finalized, the approach was described in some detail in a number of publications (62,63). In general, these guidelines resembled the "tier" approach used by the National Toxicology Program. However, Redbook emphasized a stepwise approach, beginning with Retrospective Level I (Expanded) studies utilizing data obtained in standard toxicology testing as an initial indicator of potential immunomodulation. Subsequent stages included Enhanced (Expanded) Level I, Level II, and Enhanced (Expanded) Level II testing designs. This approach was very much case-by-case, with each level predicated on findings in its predecessor. In 2001, FDA began offering an electronic version of Redbook, titled *Toxicological Principles for the Safety of Food Ingredients (Redbook 2000)* (64). As of the writing of this review, the guidelines for immunotoxicity studies exist only in outline form in Redbook 2000.

Pharmaceuticals

In the United States, safety testing of small molecule pharmaceuticals is the purview of the United States Food and Drug Administration Center for Drug Evaluation and Research (FDA/CDER). In October of 2002, CDER released a document entitled *Guidance for Industry: Immunotoxicology Evaluation of Investigational New Drugs* (51). This document describes a number of adverse events, including immunosuppression, immunogenicity, hypersensitivity, autoimmunity, and adverse immunostimulation in detail, and provides not only approaches but also suggested methodology for evaluating each type. The FDA/CDER guidance advocates the use of information derived from standard repeat-dose toxicity studies to provide early evidence of immunotoxicity, with subsequent evaluations to be rationally designed to use a minimum number of animals and resources while deriving the maximum amount of information. The implications of the guidance were discussed subsequent to their publication by their primary author (65).

In Europe, the Committee for Proprietary Medicinal Products (CPMP) regulates safety testing for pharmaceuticals. In October of 2000, CPMP published *Note for Guidance on Repeated Dose Toxicity (CPMP/SWP/1042/99)* (66); although the primary purpose of this particular document was to describe an overall approach to safety testing of pharmaceuticals, it was important as the first guidance document mandating specific immunotoxicology screening for pharmaceuticals. An appendix in this document describes a staged evaluation, emphasizing that information gained in standard toxicology evaluation can be useful as a primary indicator for immunotoxicity. Functional tests could be incorporated to gain additional information, first as an initial screen and then progressing to extended studies as indicated. A second CPMP document that includes reference to immunotoxicity assessment is *Note for Guidance on the Quality, Preclinical and Clinical Aspects of Gene Transfer Medicinal Products (CPMP/BWP/3088/99)* (67), is currently in draft form. This document recognizes the possibility of adverse immunological events as a consequence of gene transfer therapy, although it makes no specific recommendations for testing.

In 1999, the Japanese Pharmaceutical Manufacturers Association (JPMA) published two documents, International Trends in Immunotoxicity Studies of Medicinal Products (68) and Survey on Antigenicity and Immunotoxicity Studies of Medicinal Products (69). These comprehensive documents provided a survey of immunotoxicology methods and study designs in use in Japan and elsewhere, without advocating or requiring any studies per se. An Interim Draft Guidance for Immunotoxicity Testing, which describes the current thinking on such testing has been prepared; however, at this time the draft guidance document has not been published and is not readily available for review. Thus, as of 2004, there are no published Japanese guidance documents specifically regulating immunotoxicology evaluation.

Biologics/Biotherapeutics

Biologicals, biologics, or biotherapeutics (for the purposes of this review defined as therapeutics derived by biotechnology-based methodology) often present a unique challenge for immunotoxicity assessment for two primary reasons. First, many of these agents (e.g., cytokines and other immunomodulatory molecules) are intended to therapeutically modulate the immune response; therefore, it can be difficult to differentiate between the agent's efficacy and a truly adverse reaction. Second, because many of these agents are proteins or peptides, their introduction into a host often triggers an immune response directed against the molecule itself; this can lead to alterations in pharmacodynamics or to other adverse reactions (70,71). Thus, development of appropriate guidance on testing these agents has been challenging. The International Conference on Harmonization addressed this issue with the document *Preclinical Safety Evaluation of Biotechnology-Derived Pharmaceuticals S6* (72). This document includes sections on immunogenicity (as described above) as well as a brief mention of immunotoxicity studies. This document recognizes the challenges of using a structured tier approach, opting instead for thoughtful design of screening studies, followed by mechanistic studies to clarify any potential evidence of immunotoxicity. Table 4 lists additional regulatory resources which may be helpful in drug development efforts.

Alongside immunopharmacology, preclinical analysis of the immunotoxic potential of biotherapeutics can be a key component in drug development. Although regulatory guidance has been recently promulgated for drugs, the decision to commence nonclinical immunotoxicology studies during the course of biotherapeutic development is generally made on a case-by-case basis, depending on the targeted indication, compound class, and

Table 4 Useful Regulatory Documents in Biotherapeutic Drug Development

ICH S6 Document: Preclinical safety evaluation of biotechnology-derived pharmaceuticals
ICH S5a Document: detection of toxicity to reproduction for medicinal products
ICH S7A Document: safety pharmacology studies for human pharmaceuticals (section 2.8.2.4)
Guidance for industry: content and format of investigational new drug applications (INDs) for phase
    1 studies of drugs, including well-characterized, therapeutic, biotechnology-derived products
    (11/1995)
Guidance for industry: immunotoxicology evaluation of investigational new drugs (10/2002)
    (specifically for drugs, not biotherapeutics, but useful foundation for a case-by-case approach to
    biotherapeutics)
Guidance for industry: drugs, biologics, and medical devices derived from bioengineered plants for
    use in humans and animals (draft)
Draft guidance for industry—medical imaging drug and biological products part 1: conducting
    safety assessments (5/2003)
EMEA/CPMP—note for guidance on comparability of medicinal products containing biotechnology
    derived proteins as a drug substance (7/2002)

results of nonclinical studies (73). When the decision is made to assess immunotoxicologic potential, a wide range of methods and approaches are available (Table 2) (5,65,74,75). Although predictive methodology exists in assessing unintended immunosuppression, challenges still remain in assessing wayward immune stimulation, such as immunogenicity, allergic/anaphylactic reactions or autoimmunity. Recent work has suggested some improvements to traditional approaches (76). Evidence of immunotoxicity often results in supplementary mechanistic investigation, depending on the intended use of the therapeutic. Additional factors to consider include whether the effect is an exaggerated pharmacologic response or whether the disease state is likely to be uniquely influenced by the immunomodulation (e.g., HIV).

Biotechnology-derived therapeutics can be as simple as a 3-amino acid peptide or as complex as a humanized monoclonal antibody with remarkable specificity (Table 5). The complexity of biotherapeutic polypeptides is often amplified with secondary and tertiary structural features that can be intimately associated with pharmacologic activity. The coming age of generic biologics (perhaps properly termed "follow-on biologics") will

Table 5 Examples of Therapeutic Antibodies, Targets, Indications, and Immunogenicity

Therapeutic	Target	Indication	% of patients with immune response
ReoPro® (abciximab)	GPIIb/IIIa	Blood clots	6
Zenapax® (daclizumab)	IL-2R (CD25)	Transplantion	8.4
Remicade® (infliximab)	TNF-α	Crohn's disease, rheumatoid arthritis	10–60
Simulect® (basiliximab)	IL-2R (CD25)	Transplant rejection	1.5
Humira® (adalimumab)	TNF-α	Rheumatoid arthritis	12
Rituxan® (rituximab)	CD20	Non-Hodgkin's lymphoma	1.1
Herceptin® (trastuzumab)	HER-2/neu	Breast cancer	0.1
Campath-1H® (alemtuzumab)	CD52	Chronic lymphocytic leukemia	50

usher in new ways of looking at old problems, particularly the important roles of manufacturing methods and formulation influences on safety. Regardless of the approach taken to produce the biotherapeutic, it is fundamental that the identity, purity or impurities, potency, and excipient influences can be measured and controlled in a reproducible fashion.

Vaccines

As with a number of other biological agents, vaccines present a challenge for immunotoxicological evaluation because they are specifically designed to induce an immune response, a situation deemed undesirable (or potentially so) for most other agents. Because methodology is well established to evaluate the desirable immunomodulation produced by vaccines, the concern of regulatory agencies is the propensity of these therapeutics to produce undesired or deleterious effects on the immune system.

European regulation of vaccines is described in *Note for Guidance on Preclinical Pharmacological and Toxicological Testing of Vaccines* published by the CPMP (77). In this document, immunotoxicology is to be considered during toxicology testing. In particular, vaccines should be considered for immune-mediated effects on toxicity, such as antibody complex formation, release of cytokines, induction of hypersensitivity reactions, and association with autoimmunity.

FDA/CBER is tasked with regulating vaccines in the United States. One of the primary documents describing vaccine studies is Guidance for Industry for the Evaluation of Combination Vaccines for Preventable Diseases: Production, Testing and Clinical Studies (78). Immunogenicity in animals is covered in detail in the document, although immunotoxicity is not specified as an area of concern. On the other hand, Center for Biologics Evaluation and Research (CBER's) Considerations for Reproductive Toxicity Studies for Preventive Vaccines for Infectious Disease Indications (79), although intended primarily to assess effects of vaccination on reproductive function (including generalized toxicity, such as fetal malformations, etc.), acknowledges the potential immunological reactions resulting from the vaccination process to exert unintended consequences. No specific guidance is provided on methods or approaches to be used in this evaluation.

Devices and Radiological Agents

It has been recognized by the FDA that immunotoxicity may result not only from chemical or biological agents but also from medical devices that contact the body externally (via skin or mucosa), internally (implantable devices), or by external communication to the blood or tissue. In 1999, the FDA Center for Devices and Radiological Health (CDRH) published the guidance entitled *Guidance for Industry and FDA Reviewers: Immunotoxicology Testing Guidance* that addressed testing for medical devices (80). This guidance is based on General Program Memorandum G95-1, an FDA-modified version of International Standard ISO-10993, *Biological Evaluation of Medical Devices-Part 1: Evaluation and Testing* (81). The Immunotoxicology Testing Guidance provides detailed guidance for determining when immunotoxicity testing should be performed (including a flowchart and numerous tables) but does not provide details on which methods should be employed.

American Society for Testing and Materials

The American Society for Testing and Materials (ASTM) is a not-for-profit organization promoting the development of voluntary standards for materials, products, systems, and services. ASTM develops documents that serve as a basis for manufacturing, procurement, and regulatory activities. Because the ASTM standards are voluntary, they are included in this review only for the sake of completeness. The two relevant documents are F1905-98 (*Standard Practice for Selecting Tests for Determining the Propensity of Materials to Cause Immunotoxicity*) and F1906-98 (*Standard Practice for Evaluation of Immune Responses in Biocompatibility Testing Using ELISA Tests, Lymphocyte Proliferation, and Cell Migration*) (82,83).

Hypersensitivity

Although much attention is paid to immunosuppression (low immune response) in the majority of guidance documents, it is hypersensitivity (hyperactive immune response) that is the most common type of immunomodulation resulting from exposure to xenobiotics. The murine LLNA has taken priority in the assessment of contact hypersensitivity. Detailed explanations of this assay and its use are covered in the OECD 429 guideline, *Skin Sensitisation: LLNA* (84); the U.S. EPA document *OPPTS 870.2600 Skin Sensitization* (85), and the ASTM document *Standard Practice for Evaluation of Delayed Contact Hypersensitivity Using the Murine LLNA* (86). Systemic and respiratory hypersensitivity reactions also constitute a significant risk. However, at present, standardized methods are not available to screen for these effects.

CONCLUSIONS/FURTHER DIRECTIONS

Adverse effects on the immune system occurring from exposure to xenobiotics are manifest in a wide range of biological responses that share one common element, namely an alteration the normal homeostatic balance of immune system components. The diverse pathogenesis of these diseases necessitates that different testing strategies be employed for their assessment. Although sensitive and predictive diagnostic tools for the assessment of some alterations in immune function are well developed (i.e., contact hypersensitivity), measures to quantify immunosuppression in humans are still relatively insensitive. Gender, age, genetics, nutritional status, and other nonimmune factors influence immunologic health at the level of the individual and the population; these factors must all be taken into account when attempting to extrapolate data generated in young healthy laboratory animals exposed to a single chemical under laboratory conditions to the possible consequences for an individual exposed to one or more environmental agents or therapeutic drugs. In all likelihood it will be more difficult to detect low to moderate levels of immunosuppression, the scenario most likely following exposure to immunotoxic drugs or chemicals, and the ensuing health consequences, than the severe immunosuppression and related diseases resulting from severe congenital or acquired immune deficiencies. However, even small changes in the frequency or persistence of diseases caused by adverse immunomodulation could be significant at the population level in terms of the cost in health-care dollars and lost productivity.

With increasing public awareness of the potential for increased disease due to alterations in immune function, regulatory agencies have begun to require immune assessment as part of the registration process for chemicals, drugs, and devices. This must be balanced with the increasing pressure to reduce the use of animals, costs of testing, and so forth. New methodologies which will provide useful and predictive information as adjuncts to current tests (e.g., activation markers in phenotyping studies), in vitro models (i.e., use of primary cell cultures to assess immune function in the skin and lung), transgenic and knockout mice, and the use of molecular techniques (i.e., the use of cytokine profiles to assess potential hypersensitivity) need to be refined and subsequently validated to better assess the effects of low-level exposures to environmental agents.

REFERENCES

1. Seki Y, Kawanishi S, Sano S. Mechanism of PCB-induced porphyria and yusho disease. Ann NY Acad Sci 1987; 514:222–234.
2. Yang EV, Glaser R. Stress-induced immunomodulation and the implications for health. Int Immunpharmacol 2002; 2:315–324.
3. Burns LA, Meade BJ, Munson AE. Toxic responses of the immune system. In: Klassen C, ed. Casarett and Doull's Toxicology. The Basic Science of Poisons. 6th ed. New York: McGraw Hill, 2001:419–470.
4. Descotes J. Drug induced immune diseases. In: Dukes MGN, ed. Drug-Induced Disorders, Vol. 4. Amsterdam: Elsevier, 1990:1–222.
5. Dean JH. A brief history of immunotoxicology and a review of the pharmaceutical guidelines. Int J Toxicol 2004; 23:83–90.
6. Luster MI, Munson AE, Thomas PT, et al. Development of a testing battery to assess chemical-induced immunotoxicity: National Toxicology Programs guidelines for immunotoxicity evaluation in mice. Fundam Appl Toxicol 1988; 10:2–19.
7. Hinton DM. Testing guidelines for evaluation of the immunotoxic potential of direct food additives. Crit Rev Food Sci Nutr 1992; 32:173–190.
8. Sjoblad RD. Potential future requirements for immunotoxicology testing of pesticides. Toxicol Ind Health 1989; 4:391–395.
9. Straight JM, Kipen HM, Vogt RF, et al. Immune function test batteries for use in environmental health field studies, Public Health Service Publication Number: PB94-204328. U.S. Department of Health and Human Services: Washington, DC, 1994.
10. Van Loveren H, Vos JG. Evaluation of OECD Guideline #407 for Assessment of Toxicity of Chemicals with Respect to Potential Adverse effects to the immune system; National Institute of Public Health and Environmental Protection: Bilthoven, The Netherlands, 1992.
11. Luster MI, Portier C, Pait DG, et al. Risk assessment in immunotoxicology: sensitivity and predictability of immune tests. Fundam Appl Toxicol 1992; 18:200–210.
12. Luster MI, Portier C, Pait DG, et al. Risk assessment in immunotoxicology: relationships between immune and host resistance tests. Fundam Appl Toxicol 1993; 21:71–82.
13. Pruett SB, Collier S, Wu WJ, et al. Quantitative relationships between the suppression of selected immunological parameters and the area under the corticosterone concentration vs. time curve in B6C3F1 mice subjected to exogenous corticosterone or to restraint stress. Toxicol Sci 1999; 49:272–280.
14. Pruett SB, Ensley DK, Crittenden PL. The role of chemical-induced stress responses in immunosuppression: a review of quantitative associations and cause-effect relationships between chemical-induced stress responses and immunosuppression. J Toxicol Environ Health 1993; 39:163–192.
15. Pruett SB, Fan R, Myers LP, et al. Quantitative analysis of the neuroendocrine-immune axis: linear modeling of the effects of exogenous corticosterone and restraint stress on lymphocyte subpopulations in the spleen and thymus in female B6C3F1 mice. Brain Behav Immun 2000; 14:270–287.
16. Mordenti J, Chappell W. The use of interspecies scaling in toxicokinetics. In: Yacobi A, Skelly J, Batra VK, eds. Toxicokinetics and New Drug Development. New York: Pergamon Press, 1989:42–96.
17. Jerne NK, Nordin AA. Plaque formation in agar by single antibody producing cells. Science 1963; 140:405.

18. Phillips KE, Munson AE. 2'3'-Dideoxyinsine inhibits the humoral immune response in female B6C3F1 mice by targeting the B lymphocyte. Toxicol Appl Pharmacol 1997; 145:260–267.

19. Delaney B, Kaminski NE. Induction of serum-borne immunomodulatory factors in B6C3F1 mice by carbon tetrachloride. I. Carbon-tetrachloride-induced suppression of helper T-lymphocyte function is mediated by a serum-borne factor. Toxicology 1993; 85:67–84.

20. Dooley RK, Morris DL, Holsapple MP. Elucidation of cellular targets responsible for tetrachlorodibenzo-p-dioxin (TCDD)-induced suppression of the antibody response: II. Role of the T-lymphocyte. Immunopharmacology 1990; 19:47–58.

21. Temple L, Kawabata TT, Munson AE, et al. Comparison of ELISA and plaque-forming cell assays for measuring the humoral immune response to SRBC in rats and mice treated with benzo[a]pyrene or cyclophosphamide. Fundam Appl Toxicol 1993; 21:412–419.

22. Wood SC, Karras JG, Holsapple MP. Integration of the human lymphocyte into immunotoxicological investigations. Fundam Appl Toxicol 1992; 18:450–459.

23. Pollock PL, Germolec DR, Comment CE, et al. Development of human lymphocyte-engrafted SCID mice as a model for immunotoxicity assessment. Fundam Appl Toxicol 1994; 22:130–138.

24. Van der Heyden AA, Bloemena E, Out TA, et al. The influence of immunosuppressive treatment on immune responsiveness in vivo in kidney transplant recipients. Transplantation 1989; 48:44–47.

25. Raszka WV, Moriarty RA, Ottolini MG, et al. Delayed-type hypersensitivity skin testing in human immunodeficiency virus-infected pediatric patients. J Pediatrics 1996; 129:245–250.

26. Glaser R, Pearson GR, Bonneau RH, et al. Stress and the memory T-cell response to the Epstein-Barr virus in healthy medical students. Health Psychol 1993; 12:432–435.

27. Kiecolt-Glaser JK, Glaser R, Gravenstein S, et al. Chronic stress alters the immune response to influenza virus vaccine in older adults. Proc Natl Acad Sci 1996; 93:3043–3047.

28. Bottomly KA. A functional dichotomy of CD4+T lymphocytes. Immunol Today 1988; 9:268–274.

29. Finkelman FD, Katona IM, Mossman TR, et al. IFN-γ regulates the isotopes of Ig secreted during in vivo humoral immune responses. J Immunol 1988; 140:1022–1027.

30. Dearman RJ, Hegarty JM, Kimber I. Inhalation exposure of mice to trimellitic anhydride induces both IgG and IgE antihapten antibody. Int Arch Allergy Appl Immunol 1991; 95:70–76.

31. Dean JH, Cornacoff JB, Rosenthal GJ, et al. Immune system, evaluation of injury. In: Hayes AW et al., ed. Principles and Methods in Toxicology. 3rd ed. New York: Raven Press, 1994:1074–1075.

32. House R, Thomas P. In vitro induction of cytotoxic T-lymphocytes. In: Burleson, Dean, Munson, eds. In: Methods in Immunotoxicology, Vol. 1. New York: Wiley-Liss, 1995:159–172.

33. Mackaness GB. The monocyte in cellular immunity. Semin Hematol 1979; 7:172–184.

34. Lewis JG. Isolation of alveolar macrophages, peritoneal macrophages, and Kupffer cells. In: Burleson, Dean, Munson, eds. In: Methods in Immunotoxicology, Vol. 2. New York: Wiley-Liss, 1995:15–26.

35. Rosenthal GJ, Blaylock BB, Luster MI. Isolation and in vitro culture of mononuclear phagocytes. In: Tyson CA, Frazier JM, eds. In: Methods in Toxicology: In vitro Biological Systems, Vol. 1A. San Diego California: Academic Press, 1993:455–466.

36. Nelson DL, Lange RW, Rosenthal GJ. Macrophage nonspecific phagocytosis assays. In: Burleson, Dean, Munson, eds. In: Methods in Immunotoxicology, Vol. 2. New York: Wiley-Liss, 1995:39–57.

37. Rodgers KE. Measurement of the respiratory burst of leukocytes for immunotoxicologic analysis. In: Burleson, Dean, Munson, eds. In: Methods in Immunotoxicology, Vol. 2. New York: Wiley-Liss, 1995:67–78.

38. Dietert RR, Hotchkiss JH, Austic RE. Production of reactive nitrogen intermediates by macrophages. In: Burleson, Dean, Munson, eds. In: Methods in Immunotoxicology, Vol. 2. New York: Wiley-Liss, 1995:99–118.

39. Djeu JY. Natural killer activity. In: Burleson, Dean, Munson, eds. In: Methods in Immunotoxicology. Vol. 1. New York: Wiley-Liss, 1995:437–450.

40. Wilkinson PC. Assays of leukocyte locomotion and chemotaxis. J Immunological Methods 1998; 216:139–153.

41. Bassoe CF, Smith I, Sornes S, et al. Concurrent measurement of antigen- and antibody-dependent oxidative burst and phagocytosis in monocytes and neutrophils. Methods 2000; 21:203–220.

42. Van Eeden S, Klut ME, Walker BAM, et al. The use of flow cytometry to measure neutrophil function. J Immunol Methods 1999; 232:23–43.

43. Andersen KE, Maibach HI. Guinea Pig Sensitization Assays. Curr Probl Dermatol 1985; 14:263–290.

44. Gad SC, Dunn BJ, Dobbs DW, et al. Development and Validation of an Alternative Dermal Sensitization Test: Mouse Ear Swelling Test (MEST). Toxicol Appl Pharmacol 1986; 84:93–114.

45. Basketter DA, Scholes EW, Kimber I, et al. Interlaboratory evaluation of the local lymph node assay with 25 chemicals and comparison with guinea pig test data. Toxicol Methods 1991; 1:30–43.

46. Holladay SD, Luster MI. Alterations in fetal thymic and liver hematopoietic cells as indicators of exposure to developmental immunotoxicants. Environ Health Perspect 1996; 104:809–813.

47. Holladay SD, Smialowicz RJ. Development of the murine and human immune system: differential effects of immunotoxicants depend on time of exposure. Environ Health Perspect 2000; 108:463–473.

48. Luebke RW, Parks C, Luster MI. Suppression of immune function and susceptibility to infections in humans: association of immune function with clinical disease. J Immunotoxicol 2004; 1:15–24.

49. Luster MI, Germolec DR, Parks CG, et al. Are Changes in the Immune System Predictive of Clinical Disease? In: Tryphonas H, Fournier M, Blakley B et al., eds. Investigative Immunotoxicology. Boca Raton, FL: CRC Press, 2005:165–182.

50. Holsapple MP, West LJ, Landreth KS. Species comparison of anatomical and functional immune system development. Birth Defects Res B Dev Reprod Toxicol 2003; 68:321–334.

51. Guidance for Industry: Immunotoxicology Evaluation of Investigational New Drugs. U.S. Department of Health and Human Services, Food and Drug Administration Center for Drug Evaluation and Research (CDER). October 2002. (Accessed January, 2005, at http://www.fda.gov/cder/guidance/4945fnl.PDF.)

52. IUIS/WHO Working Group. Laboratory Investigations, Clinical Immunology. Methods, Pitfalls, and Clinical Indications, 1988; 49: 478–497.

53. Vine MF, Stein L, Weigel K. Plasma 1,1-dichloro-2,2-bis (p-chlorophenyl) ethylene (DDE) levels and immune response. Am J Epidemiol 2001; 153:53–63.

54. Arndt V, Vine MF, Weigle K. Environmental chemical exposures and risk of herpes zoster. Environ Health Perspect 1999; 107:835–841.

55. Yang EV, Glaser R. Stress-induced immunomodulation: impact on immune defenses against infectious disease. Biomed Pharmacother 2000; 54:245–250.

56. National Research Council. Biologic Markers in Immunotoxicology. Washington, DC: National Academy Press, 1992.

57. U.S Congress, Office of Technology Assessment, Identifying and Controlling Immunotoxic Substance, OTA-BP-BA-75 (Washington, DC: U.S. Government Printing Office), 1991.

58. Biochemicals Test Guidelines: OPPTS 880.3550 Immunotoxicity. United States Environmental Protection Agency, February 1996. (Accessed January, 2005, at http://www.epa.gov/opptsfrs/OPPTS_Harmonized/880_Biochemicals_Test_Guidelines/Series/880-3550.pdf.)

59. Biochemicals Test Guidelines: OPPTS 880.3800 Immune Response. United States Environmental Protection Agency, February 1996. (Accessed January, 2005 at http://www.epa.gov/oppts/oppts_harmonized/880_biochemicals_test_guidelines/series/880-3800.pdf.)

60. Health Effects Test Guidelines: OPPTS 870.7800 Immunotoxicity. United States Environmental Protection Agency, August 1998. (Accessed January, 2005, at http://www.epa.gov/docs/OPPTS_Harmonized/870_Health_Effects_Test_Guidelines/Drafts/870-7800.pdf.)

61. OECD Guideline for the Testing of Chemicals 407:Repeated Dose 28-day Oral Toxicity Study in Rodents. Adopted July 27th, 1995.

62. Hinton DM. Immunotoxicity Testing Applied to Direct Food and Colour Additives: US FDA 'Redbook II' Guidelines. Hum Exp Toxicol 1995; 4:43–45.

63. Hinton DM. U.S FDA "Redbook II" immunotoxicity testing guidelines and research in immunotoxicity Evaluations of Food Chemicals and New Food Proteins. Toxicol Pathol 2000; 28:467–478.

64. Toxicological Principles for the Safety of Food Ingredients: Redbook 2000. Draft. (Accessed January, 2005, at http://www.cfsan.fda.gov/~redbook/red-toca.html.)

65. Hastings KL. Implications of the new FDA/CDER Immunotoxicology guidance for drugs. Int Immunopharmacol 2002; 2:613–1618.

66. Committee for Proprietary Medicinal Products (CPMP). Note for Guidance on Repeated Dose Toxicity (CPMP/SWP/1042/99). October 2000.

67. Committee for Proprietary Medicinal Products (CPMP). Note for Guidance on the Quality, Preclinical and Clinical Aspects of Gene Transfer Medicinal Products (CPMP/BWP/3088/99). Draft.

68. International Trends in Immunotoxicity Studies of Medicinal Products. JPMA Drug Evaluation Committee Fundamental Research Group, Data 92. April 1999.

69. Survey on Antigenicity and Immunotoxicity Studies of Medicinal Products. JPMA Drug Evaluation Committee Fundamental Research Group, Data 93. April 1999.

70. Chamberlain P, Mire-Sluis AR. Understanding the implications of the immunogenicity of therapeutic proteins: a dialogue with the FDA. Global Outsourcing Rev, 2004; 6:16–24.

71. Bugelski PJ, Treacy G. Predictive power of preclinical studies in animals for the immunogenicity of recombinant therapeutic proteins in humans. Curr Opin Mol Ther 2004; 6:10–16.

72. ICH Topic S 6: Preclinical Safety Evaluation of Biotechnology-Derived Pharmaceuticals (CPMP/ICH/302/95). March 1998.

73. Dean J, Hincks J, Remandet B. Immunotoxicology assessment in the pharmaceutical industry. Toxicol Lett 1998 Dec. 28th; 102–103:247–255.

74. Talmadge JE. Pharmacodynamic aspects of peptide administration biological response modifiers. Adv Drug Deliv Rev 1998; 33:241–252.

75. Thomas PT. Nonclinical evaluation of therapeutic cytokines: immunotoxicologic issues. Toxicology 2002; 174:27–35.

76. Mire-Sluis AR. Recommendations for the design and opimization of immunoassays used in the detection of host antibodies against biotechnology products. J Immunol Methods 2004; 289:1–16.

77. Committee for Proprietary Medicinal Products (CPMP). Note for Guidance on Preclinical Pharmacological and Toxicological Testing of Vaccines (CPMP/SWP/4654/95). June 1998.

78. Guidance for Industry for the Evaluation of Combination Vaccines for Preventable Diseases: Production, Testing and Clinical Studies. U.S. Department of Health and Human Services, Food and Drug Administration Center for Biologics Evaluation and Research (CDER). April 1977. (Accessed January, 2005, at http://www.fda.gov/cber/gdlns/combvacc.pdf.)

79. Guidance for Industry: Considerations for Reproductive Toxicity Studies for Preventive Vaccines for Infectious Disease Indications. U.S. Department of Health and Human Services, Food and Drug Administration Center for Biologics Evaluation and Research. Draft version, August 2000. (Accessed January, 2005, at http://www.fda.gov/ohrms/dockets/98fr/001400gd.pdf.)

80. Guidance for Industry and FDA Reviewers: Immunotoxicology Testing Guidance. U.S. Department of Health and Human Services, Food and Drug Administration Center for Devices and Radiological Health. May 6, 1999. (Accessed January, 2005, at http://www.fda.gov/cdrh/ost/ostggp/immunotox.html.)

81. Required Biocompatibility Training and Toxicology Profiles for Evaluation of Medical Devices. May 1, 1995 (G95-1). (Accessed January, 2005, at http://www.fda.gov/cdrh/g951.html.)

82. American Society for Testing and Materials: Standard Practice for Selecting Tests for Determining the Propensity of Materials to Cause Immunotoxicity. F1905-98.

83. American Society for Testing and Materials: Standard Practice for Evaluation of Immune Responses in Biocompatibility Testing Using ELISA Tests, Lymphocyte Proliferation, and Cell Migration. F1906-98.

84. OECD Guideline for the Testing of Chemicals 429: Skin Sensitisation: Local Lymph Node Assay. Adopted April 24th, 2002.

85. Health Effects Test Guidelines: OPPTS 870.2600 Skin Sensitization. United States Environmental Protection Agency, March 2003. (Accessed January, 2005, at http://www.epa.gov/docs/OPPTS_Harmonized/870_Health_Effects_Test_Guidelines/Drafts/870-2600.pdf.)

86. American Society for Testing and Materials: Standard Practice for Evaluation of Delayed Contact Hypersensitivity Using the Murine Local Lymph Node Assay (LLNA). F 2148-01.

14

Inhalation and Pulmonary Toxicity Studies

Raymond M. David
*Health and Environment Laboratories, Eastman Kodak Company, Rochester,
New York, U.S.A.*

INTRODUCTION

Inhalation as a Route of Exposure Versus Pulmonary Toxicity

Inhalation as a route of exposure is used extensively in animal studies when it mimics the likely route of human exposure. In many cases, the effect to be evaluated is on an organ system other than the respiratory tract. For example, developmental toxicity, reproductive toxicity, and neurotoxicity have been evaluated in animals following inhalation exposure because the primary route of exposure for humans to the test substances is by inhalation (solvents, for example). On the other hand, the effect of interest may be on the lungs and respiratory tract (irritating gases or particulates, for example). Although the mechanics of the exposures are the same in both cases, the approach to the study design and the end points selected for evaluation will be quite different. The following provides some understanding of the principles that guide study design. The emphasis will be on pulmonary toxicity, but issues relevant for other end points, such as reproductive or developmental toxicity, will also be discussed.

In addition, the nature of the test substance can influence the study design and what end points should be evaluated. For example, gases or vapors typically enter the respiratory tract and are easily able to reach the alveoli for absorption into the blood; therefore, the likelihood that vapors can affect other organ systems is high. Frequently, animals are exposed to gases and vapors specifically to evaluate systemic end points. On the other hand, it is also true that very water-soluble gases will mix with the mucous in the upper respiratory tract where they can cause local irritation. Thus, even when the primary emphasis of the study is on nonrespiratory end points, the respiratory tract should be evaluated for possible effects. Exposure to aerosols (liquid or solid particles) often result in localized effects in the lungs and upper respiratory tract because the physics of aerosol particle movement dictates where the particle will be deposited. Typically, small particles (<5 μm diameter) can travel into the deep lung, whereas large particles (>5 μm) become deposited in the nose or pharynx because they cannot maneuver the bends and turns of the airways. Frequently, aerosol studies focus on respiratory tract effects. Regardless of where the particles deposit, however, the respiratory tract has mechanisms for removal that result in many particles being ingested or entering the lymphatic system leading to systemic effects. Consequently, even studies of particles should include evaluation of nonrespiratory tissues for possible effects. This is even more important for studies of very small particles than can be translocated to other parts of the body. Until recently, very small particles (nanoparticles, <0.1 μm diameter) were considered to move so easily in the air stream that there would be little or no deposition in the lungs. Investigators studying atmospheric, ultrafine particles (<0.1 μm diameter, now called nanoparticles) have shown that as size decreases, the particles behave more like gases, resulting in greater deposition in the nasopharynx and translocation to other organs, such as the brain or testes. Thus, studying the effects of nanoparticles suggests that all organs should be evaluated.

For a review of the basics of inhalation toxicity, effects on the respiratory tract, and factors that influence deposition and absorption of test substances, the reader is directed to one of several texts (1–3).

Decisions, Decisions!

There are many options for conducting any toxicity study and what end points to evaluate. For many test substances and study types, these options are limited either by the prevailing guidelines or by generally accepted methods. Inhalation toxicity studies conducted in fulfillment of regulations, such as for registration of test substances with competent authorities, should follow the appropriate guidelines (*vide infra*). On the other hand, the number of options for evaluating inhaled pulmonary toxicity of substances, such as fibers, consumer products, or nanoparticles, is greater than for other routes of exposure (at least until there are regulations requiring testing). As a result, it may be necessary to be creative and/or pragmatic in designing a study. Information and guidance are provided in this chapter for the variables to consider and what options are available based on the purpose of the study and the characteristics of the test substance. There may be options other than those listed here, and it is important to discuss the study design with the study director. In any case, it is recommended that the study design be reviewed carefully to make sure that it addresses all the issues of concern before proceeding.

One important issue to address in the final study design is whether the logistics of exposure, the number of animals needed, or the manpower needed to assess the desired end points requires conducting more than one study. Trying to assess too many end points when one is limited by the number of animals that can be exposed simultaneously may result in too few animals per end point, especially if the end points are mutually exclusive. For example, if one is using a nose-only exposure system that has a limited number of animal ports, it is unwise to try to capture too many end points and thus reducing the number of animals for each end point. Other end points may not be able to be added to the same study for technical reasons. For example, performing a bronchoalveolar lavage procedure (*vide infra*) and lung morphometrics procedures together is not possible because the lavage procedure may distort the architecture of the lung. In the case of a particle that poses technical problems to generating a test atmosphere, it may be easier to administer the particle directly into the lungs via intratracheal instillation to determine the intrinsic toxicity, followed by an inhalation study to focus on the end point of concern or long-term effect rather than attempting an inhalation study in which the generation of the particle is not well characterized.

CONTRACTING AN INHALATION STUDY

Just How Complicated Can This Be?

Why should studies conducted by inhalation exposure be any more complex than those conducted by other routes? One reason is that there are several factors that influence the amount of the test substance that gets to the target organ (i.e., bioavailability). First, inhalation exposures extend over several hours, much like slow infusion administration. As a result, there is a prolonged absorption phase that is limited by the availability of the test substance in the chamber. Bioavailability is therefore dependent on absorption and the amount of the test substance available in the chamber to enter the body. The test atmosphere (i.e., the mixture of test substance and air) is constantly being prepared or generated, which means that minor changes in the supply of air or test substance can alter the momentary or instantaneous concentration of the test atmosphere; thus, the bioavailability varies because the amount of test substance to which the animal is exposed can vary from moment to moment. In addition, the test substance is not instantly delivered to the animal the moment the generator is turned on (except perhaps for some nose-only exposure designs). This delay in delivery is particularly true for whole-body exposure systems that use large chambers, i.e., it takes time for the chamber to fill with the test substance. This equilibrium time (and the same time for termination of exposure) may pose logistical problems that are not associated with other routes of administration. For example, one cannot conduct detailed neurobehavioral evaluations or collect blood samples for pharmacokinetics immediately after exposure in a whole-body chamber because of the time it takes for the chamber to exhaust before the door can be opened. Because it takes time for the chamber to be depleted of the test atmosphere, one should not schedule complex end points requiring a lot of animal handling immediately after exposure. Typically, the earliest that the animals should be handled is 30 minutes after the end of the exposure (except for nose-only, which has a shorter exhaust period).

Inhalation exposures also require more analytical support than other routes of exposure. Constant checks and balances are necessary for the control of inhalation studies because of the variation in the quantity and characteristics of a test substance in the air. In general, everything that can be is measured or controlled. Nothing, not even measurements from sophisticated instruments, are taken at face value. Each piece of equipment, flow meter, and thermometer should be calibrated, and each chamber should be tested for distribution of test atmosphere. As a result of this checking and double checking, inhalation studies are time consuming, tedious, and generate volumes of data that ensure to whoever reviews the report that the biological responses observed could be reproduced because all of the variables were quantified or controlled.

How to Select a Contract Laboratory for Testing

The basic considerations for Good Laboratory Practices in selecting a contract laboratory have been reviewed in Chapter 1. Selecting an appropriate laboratory for an inhalation study is even more complex than for other types of studies because of all the variables involved in conducting the exposures. Questions such as "How can laboratories with inhalation capability be identified?" or "Do all laboratories that conduct inhalation studies have the same capability or experience?" are frequently asked. These are not easy questions to answer, and a number of approaches, such as questionnaires, have been used to aid the selection process. However, it is difficult to pose all the correct questions in a questionnaire because subsequent questions may depend on the initial answers. Telephone calls, followed by personal visits to potential contractors, are also recommended. It is advisable to make a list of questions that need to be answered before calling. It is also advisable to have information about the test substance to help the potential study director understand what obstacles he or she will face if generating a test atmosphere. Some basic questions are provided in Tables 1 and 2. When asking about experience with a specific type of test substance or test atmosphere, a negative response should not exclude

Table 1 Questions to Ask in Evaluating Laboratories

Objective	Questions
Does the lab have inhalation capability?	Do you have inhalation chambers? What type?
Is the capability adequate to conduct the intended study?	Could you conduct a study in which _____ number of animals are exposed simultaneously? If whole-body What size? How many chambers of each size? What is the maximum number of animals that can be exposed per chamber? If nose-only Flow-past or other type? Number of animals per unit? What type of restraint tubes and what sizes are they?
What is the generation capability/ experience?	What type of generation systems do you have? How much experience do you have with generating vapors or aerosols? What kind of aerosols: liquids or dusts? How many studies have you conducted of each? Do you have technical staff who can administer by intratracheal instillation or oropharyngeal administration?
Do they have adequate analytical capability for the intended study?	Can you monitor the concentration in each chamber/nose-only unit simultaneously? What kind of monitoring/analytical capability do you have? (Miran IR, online GC, RAM, microlaser particle counter, condensation-particle counter for small particles are all appropriate but not mandatory)
Do they have experience with this particular type of test substance?	Have you ever tested a test substance with these particular physical or chemical properties before?

Abbreviations: IR, infrared; GC, gas chromatography; RAM, real-time aerosol monitor.

a laboratory. A study director gains experience by working with a test substance (one does not obtain that knowledge otherwise), and there is no reason why the test substance in question cannot be the first. On the other hand, it may take longer for the study to start if a laboratory does not have experience with a specific type of test substance. Bear in mind that the preliminary test period allows the study director to become completely familiar with the characteristics of the test substance. This period will be longer than normal if the laboratory has never worked with this type of test substance. Such a delay may need to be factored into the selection process.

Much of the process of selecting a laboratory depends on working with the study director. The creativity of the study director working with the technical staff will be the key to a good study. Generally, the more input a study director has in the preliminary

Table 2 Issues to Review at a Site Visit

Question	Issue
Is room air or outside air used for the chamber?	Outside air is preferred rather than room air unless adequately conditioned. On the other hand, outside air needs to be adequately filtered.
Is the air (HEPA) and charcoal filtered? How close are the filters to the chamber inlets?	HEPA and charcoal filtering is desirable as close to the chamber as reasonable. Charcoal needs to be replenished occasionally depending on the chemical load. Are there charcoal filters on the exhaust to prevent test substance from entering the air intakes to the chamber?
Where are the animals housed relative to the exposure room?	Typically, animals are housed in a room separate from location where the exposures occur to avoid any incidental exposure from residual test substance in the chamber.
Do the chambers look clean?	They should. How often are they cleaned? Between each exposure (not necessary but good practice)? Between each test substance (mandatory)?
Are the chambers constructed or a nonreactive material?	Stainless steel is common, but any nonreactive material is okay as long as it can be cleaned.
Can all or most of the animals be easily observed during exposure?	Observations of individual animals can be important especially when conducting a neurotoxicity or acute toxicity study.

Abbreviation: HEPA, high efficiency particle air.

testing, especially if the test substance is unusual, the better the results of study. The study director needs to understand the problems surrounding generation of the test atmosphere. In addition, the sponsor needs to feel that the study director has a good grasp of the technical difficulties involved with generating the test atmosphere and that the study director has considered methods to circumvent those difficulties.

Once the laboratory is selected, the timeline for getting the study conducted should be discussed with the study director. One should have realistic expectations. Frequently, inexperienced sponsors underestimate the problems that can arise in trying to generate a test atmosphere, and in how long it may take to resolve those problems. It is not uncommon for preliminary work to require 2–4 weeks, taking into account determining analytical procedures, test atmosphere generation, distribution of test substance in the chamber, etc. All of these considerations will need to be addressed even for a single-exposure study. How much time it takes to complete the study (i.e., receive a study report) will vary, but several weeks for an acute study is not uncommon. More time is required for an acute study in which subsequent exposure concentrations are determined by the results of previous exposures. These studies generally take longer because the study director does not set the next exposure level until he/she sees the results of the previous exposure level.

STUDY DESIGN

What Study Design Should Be Used?

To design a good study, the first step is to clearly identify the purpose of the study, i.e., is the study conducted for regulatory submission (agricultural chemical, industrial chemical, or pharmaceutical), for consumer protection, or for occupational hazard assessment (respiratory or systemic toxicity). One of the primary reasons to identify the purpose is to determine under which regulatory guideline (if any) the study must be conducted. There remain subtle differences between study designs that vary with the regulatory agency and the country. Consult a recent copy of whichever regulatory guideline is appropriate. The U.S. Environmental Protection Agency (EPA) guidelines are online at: (4) FDA guidance documents for nonpharmaceuticals can be found online at: (5,6).

For pharmaceuticals, the guidance document is at: (7). Guidance documents for Organization for Economic Cooperation and Development (OECD) protocols are available for purchase at: (8). If the study report is to be submitted to several regulatory bodies or to regulatory bodies in different countries, the OECD guideline should be acceptable worldwide.

Regulatory guidance documents specify the numbers of animals per group, length of exposure, and some of the parameters that the competent authorities find necessary to evaluate the quality of the study. In this regard, they are useful. On the other hand, the documents do not always provide enough guidance on end points for evaluation, so it is important to incorporate the correct end points for the issues of concern. It is best to discuss this with the study director. Some ideas for end points, depending on the questions or issues of concern, are provided in a later section of this chapter.

For some test substances, such as pharmaceuticals that are administered via specialized devices (e.g., pulse inhalers), there are no specific testing guidelines. It may be advisable, therefore, to utilize a study design that resembles a standard guideline. The only variation from that guideline might be in the means of administration (and characterization) of the test atmosphere. Because each delivery device might pose unique problems for the investigator, it is difficult to provide general guidance concerning these types of studies. Regulatory guidance/guidelines are listed on Table 3, which are based on the nature of the test substance and end points of interest.

In the event that a consumer product is being tested, the protocol design may require some creativity. For example, the purpose of the study may be to compare the effects of different products, or it may be to compare the effects of a specific product to a reference material. In these cases, the study design need not be more elaborate than a published guideline study, with the substitution of the reference and test products for the different exposure concentration levels. Thus, one might design the study to use available systemic and pulmonary end points (depending on the end points of interest) with a control group(s) (air and/or vehicle control), one test group exposed to the test product, and one test group exposed to the reference material. The key to interpreting this type of study is to adjust the exposure levels of the reference and test products to ensure that the concentrations are equivalent. Many times, equivalent exposures are difficult to accomplish, especially if the test and reference products are mixtures of varying components. In such cases, multiple concentrations of each material should be used—a practice that should be used for all such studies.

Studies of particles of unusual sizes, such as fibers or very small particles (ultrafine or engineered nanoparticles), pose other problems primarily because these materials can be difficult to generate in an atmosphere. Other approaches have been taken to evaluate the toxicity of these materials. For fibers, the EPA published the consensus findings of a workshop of experts (9), which suggested using acellular in vitro tests as a screen for persistence, the key to long-term effects, followed by direct instillation into the lungs and bronchoalveolar lavage. Some have suggested that this approach is also appropriate for ultrafine or nanoparticles. Unfortunately, there is no consensus of how the results of in vitro studies correlate with in vivo effects for small particles. So the best study design for nanoparticles may be direct instillation into the respiratory tract followed by

Table 3 Study Guidance Depending on the Nature of the Test Substance and End Point

End point of interest	Gas (vapor), liquid, nonfibrous solid	Nanoparticle[a]	Fiber[a]
Pulmonary toxicity	Acute inhalation toxicity: OPPTS 870.1300, OECD 403 28-day or 14-day repeated dose inhalation toxicity: OECD 412 90-day inhalation toxicity: OPPTS 870.3465, OECD 413	Intratracheal instillation followed by bronchoalveolar lavage and histopathology (similar to OPPTS 870.1350)	Acellular dissolution in vitro Intratracheal instillation followed by bronchoalveolar lavage and histopathology Combined chronic toxicity/carcinogenicity testing of respirable fibrous particles: OPPTS 870.8355
Pulmonary sensitization	Dermal exposure to liquid or solid and measurement of serum IgE, IL-4, IL-13 levels according to Dearman et al. (1992, 2003) and Guo et al. (2002) followed by measurement of serum IgE, IL-4, IL-13 levels Inhalation exposure to gas/vapor followed by measurement of serum IgE, IL-4, IL-13 levels	Not applicable	Not applicable
Systemic toxicity	28-day or 14-day repeated dose inhalation toxicity: OECD 412 90-day inhalation toxicity: OPPTS 870.3465, OECD 413	28-day or 14-day repeated dose inhalation toxicity: OECD 412	Combined chronic toxicity/carcinogenicity testing of respirable fibrous particles: OPPTS 870.8355
Reproductive/ developmental toxicity	Reproductive/developmental toxicity screening test: OPPTS 870.3550, OECD 421	Questionable applicability unless distribution studies determine that nanoparticles can reach reproductive tissues or affect pituitary-gonadal hormone axis	Questionable applicability

(Continued)

Table 3 Study Guidance Depending on the Nature of the Test Substance and End Point (*Continued*)

End point of interest	Gas (vapor), liquid, nonfibrous solid	Nanoparticle[a]	Fiber[a]
	Combined repeated dose toxicity with the reproduction/developmental toxicity screening test: OPPTS 870.3650, OECD 422		Questionable applicability
	Prenatal developmental toxicity study: OPPTS 870.3700, OECD 414		
	Reproduction and fertility effects: OPPTS 870.3800, OECD 416		
Neurotoxicity	Acute and 28-day delayed neurotoxicity of organophosphates substances: OPPTS 870.6100, OECD 418, 419	Neurotoxicity screening battery: OPPTS 870.6300, OECD 424	
	Neurotoxicity screening battery: OPPTS 870.6300, OECD 424		
	Schedule-controlled operant behavior: OPPTS 870.6500		

[a] Use of intratracheal or other direct administration into the pulmonary tract may be appropriate.

bronchoalveolar lavage, such as what is suggested by the EPA testing guideline Office of Prevention, Pesticides and Toxic Substances (OPPTS) 870.1350.

How Long to Expose the Animals?

All regulatory guidelines require a 4-hour/day exposure for acute studies and a 6-hour/day exposure for repeated exposures. When evaluating exposure time for whole-body chambers, one must bear in mind the time required for the concentration in the chamber to reach steady state (this is not a consideration for nose-only exposure systems). Usually, four air changes are allotted to achieve steady state, which often translates to ~30 minutes. The actual time of exposure is usually from the time the generator is turned on until the time the generator is turned off.

If the purpose of the study is not for submission to a competent authority, but rather to evaluate worker and consumer safety, one has more flexibility to expose the animals for longer or shorter periods of time per day. Of course, using a guideline can always be defended. On the other hand, using a guideline for a pesticide may not answer the question regarding consumer safety. A 4-hour or 6-hour exposure might either overestimate or underestimate the hazard, depending on the population at risk. The exposure period and design of the study should take into account the population. Workers may be exposed to relatively low concentrations for at least 6 hours per day with occasional bursts of high concentrations for short periods of time (1 hour). In contrast, consumers are rarely exposed to the neat chemical and generally not for long periods of time (e.g., hairspray). Thus, depending on the population to safeguard, it may be wise to conduct two studies: one in which animals are exposed to high concentrations for only 1 hour (a Department of Transportation type of study design) that is designed to provide information to establish short-term exposure limits or acute exposure guidance limits, and another in which animals are exposed for 6-hours per day for several weeks to provide information on cumulative toxicity.

Consumer safety studies are even trickier because it is best to generate the test substance in a way that most closely mimics consumer exposure conditions. For example, if a product is sold in an aerosol spray can, it may be wise to expose animals to the test atmosphere generated from aerosol spray cans rather than one generated with a laboratory nebulizer that is designed to produce aerosol particle of a particles size range. The reason for this is that mass-produced nebulizers on spray cans may not produce particles in the same size range as a laboratory nebulizer. Thus, the laboratory nebulizer might not truly reflect the particles to which the consumer is exposed. In addition, most self-pressurized containers cannot generate a consistent size distribution of particles for long periods of time because the propellant tends to decrease the temperature of the can as it escapes, thus decreasing pressure and output. These containers are meant to be used for short bursts. Thus, the study design may need to mimic this intermittent exposure (i.e., short bursts of aerosol over short periods of time).

An Acute Study

The complexity and cost of an acute inhalation toxicity study surprises most first-time sponsors. What first-time sponsors forget is that all the characterization of the test atmosphere, problems with generation of the test atmosphere, and questions about how well the animals will tolerate exposure must be resolved prior to conducting this brief exposure. Furthermore, minor variations in generator output are more troublesome because the staff only has the brief 4-hour exposure period to make adjustments so that the average hits the desired level. During repeated exposures, a slight variation in 1 hour has little impact when the exposure concentration is averaged over several days. In an acute study, the concentration has to reach the target and hold steady. Achieving and maintaining the target concentration is an important task in conducting an inhalation study because the concentration is the closest one has to a "dose." The actual concentration in the chamber should be within 10% of the target concentration.

In addition, acute studies are confounded by the fact that the biological responses are unknown. After all, the acute study is the first time animals have been exposed to the test substance, and the purpose is to evaluate lethal and other short-term effects. If the initial concentration is too toxic, subsequent exposures at lower concentrations will be needed, each requiring time for the staff to make adjustments in the generation procedures to achieve the desired concentration. Range-finding studies are not common prior to lethal concentration (LC_{50}) studies because the same effort is required for a full study. However, if a test substance is very toxic via oral ingestion, or is very irritating in a dermal test, exposing 1–2 animals may help establish the correct concentration range for a definitive LC_{50}. The recent OECD test guideline for inhalation toxicity studies (433) has proposed an alternative approach for conducting a series of exposures at prescribed levels and exposing a minimal number of animals. Fixed concentration of 100, 500, 2500, and 5000 ppm for gases; 0.5, 2, 10, and 20 mg/L for vapors; or 0.05, 0.5, 1, and 5 mg/L for aerosols is recommended. One animal per concentration can be used, but the main study might require a complete five animals per sex per group. It is not clear if this approach will reduce the effort needed to determine acute inhalation toxicity.

As mentioned above, the duration of exposure is fixed by the testing guideline. The Toxic Substances Control Act (TSCA) and Federal Insecticide, Fungicide, and Rodenticide Act (FIFRA) testing guidelines (now combined into an OPPTS guideline), as well as the OECD guideline, require a 4-hour exposure for acute studies—even though repeated exposure studies require 6-hour exposures. On the other hand, the DOT testing requirement is for only a 1-hour exposure. Exposure to pharmaceuticals can be for as long as 12 hours, depending on the manner of the test substance administration to humans.

One aspect of acute toxicity studies that may need to be considered is the effect of stress. This issue is particularly relevant for nose-only exposures that are generally more stressful than whole-body exposures because of the restraint (10). Animals tend to become stressed when first put into the restraint tubes. Stress can increase respiration that can lead to higher bioavailability, a higher internal dose, and potentially greater toxicity. One way to overcome the problem of stress-related increase in toxicity is to acclimate the animals to the restraint tubes. This can be done by placing the animals in the tubes and sham-exposing them to air for several hours on several days prior to the actual exposure to the test atmosphere. In this way, the stress of restraint is diminished.

A Repeated-Exposure Study

As mentioned previously, the regulatory guidelines require that repeated exposure studies be conducted for six continuous hours per day. Repeated-exposure studies (1-, 2-, 4-, 13-weeks, or longer) can be easier to conduct than single-exposure studies because the purpose is not to determine the acute life-threatening concentrations but, rather, to evaluate cumulative toxicity from repeated exposure to sublethal concentrations. In repeated-exposure studies, there is more time to characterize the test atmosphere and to make adjustments to keep within 10% of the target concentration. Furthermore, repeated-exposure inhalation studies are typically conducted over 5 days per week, not 7 days, as with oral toxicity studies. It's not clear why that is the practice, but it is common for laboratories to only expose animals Monday through Friday—unless the end point is developmental or reproductive toxicity, in which case animals need to be exposed daily for 7 days. As a result of the 5-day per week schedule, termination of the animals, relative to the last exposure is critical because it would not be appropriate to terminate animals on the Monday following two days of nonexposure. Animals can recover substantially over that time period, and it is best to terminate animals following at least 2 days of exposure.

Another aspect of repeated exposure studies is that, over the course of the study, the animals' placements in the chamber should be changed so that they are not in the same part of the chamber throughout the study. This concept of "rotation" in the chamber comes from the understanding that the concentration of the test atmosphere inside a whole-body chamber (or probably nose-only chamber) is not uniform. Occasionally, corners of the chamber have different concentrations than the middle (see below for further discussion of determining uniformity of concentration in the chamber). Therefore, it is advisable, over the course of a long-term study, to move animals around to different locations so that one animal is not exposed to slightly different concentration than another animal. Rotation is typically done on a weekly basis, even for a 28-day study.

THE TEST SUBSTANCE

Know the Test Substance

An inhalation study cannot be conducted without the sponsor and study director having a good grasp of the physical and chemical properties of the test substance. The test substance is going to be mixed or suspended in the air for long periods of time, so the study director needs to know the answer to several questions in order to generate a test atmosphere: Is it a gas, liquid, or solid at room temperature? Does it react with air, even in the presence of high humidity? Is it reactive with any of the components of the exposure system? If a liquid, will the test substance vaporize at a reasonable temperature? Does it react with air to form peroxides or a different chemical species? What is the lower explosive limit? If the liquid cannot be vaporized, is its viscosity low enough that it can be aerosolized (nebulized). Is it water soluble? If solid, is it already a particulate, and what is the size distribution of the particles? Can the test substance be compacted? Is it hygroscopic? The answers to these questions will determine if the study will be of a gas, liquid aerosol, or dust. This determination will, in turn, influence the study director's decision on the exposure system to use or if inhalation is even practical. Therefore, knowing the characteristics of the test substance ahead of time may make the whole process of planning for a study (and getting it started) go more smoothly. Some of the important questions about the test substance and how answers influence the study and selection of the exposure system are outlined in Figure 1.

To make matters more complex, the test substance may be any of the above (gas, liquid, solid) packaged in a unique delivery system, such as an inhaler or canister. For these types of products, the device is the generator of the test atmosphere (usually an aerosol). Some of the issues surrounding the use of such a device have been raised above. To reiterate, canisters or inhalers are designed to deliver bursts of aerosol for short periods of time (seconds), not continuous delivery over hours. In addition, as the propellant is released, the canister cools, reducing the pressure and output, and likely the particle size. Therefore, the two questions to be answered are: should the device be attached to a continuous supply of test substance under constant pressure so it can generate the test atmosphere continuously over the exposure period, or should the device be triggered to deliver bursts of test substance for the exposure period? There are no correct answers

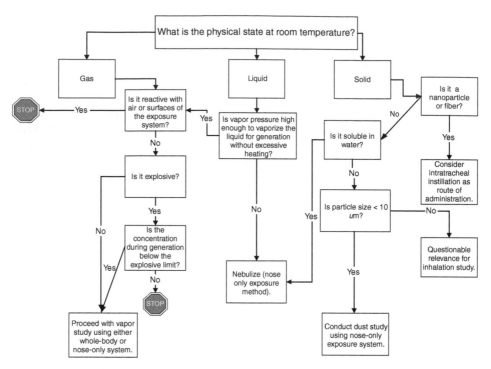

Figure 1 Decision tree for selecting the exposure system and nature of the generation system based on the physical and chemical properties of the test substance.

to these questions, and the answer may depend on the aerosol characteristics from each generation method.

Nanomaterials (particles with a diameter of <100 nm) and fibers present different problems for inhalation toxicity studies because both are difficult to generate as airborne atmospheres. Nanomaterials tend to agglomerate (coalesce into larger particles) when aerosolized using traditional aerosol generators (perhaps more so than typical dusts). These larger particles may be in the low micrometer diameter range and may not produce the same biological response as the nanosized particles. Electrospray atomizers can be used to generate an aerosol of nanomaterials without agglomeration, but there are few testing laboratories with this capability. Generating atmospheres for fibers may also be difficult, but there are methods and equipment available (9). An alternative method of administration for these materials is intratracheal instillation, which can be used in a preliminary test to understand intrinsic hazards. This technique involves anesthetizing the animal and delivering into the trachea a small volume (5 μL) of test substance suspended in saline. This tool has been used for many years to deliver known amounts of a test substance to the lungs. Because saline is the carrier, the lungs will respond to the presence of a foreign substance even in the absence of the test substance, so it is always important to have a vehicle control group (in addition to an untreated control group) to use for comparison.

How Much Test Material Will Be Needed for the Study?

Naturally, the characteristics of the test substance and the exposure system selected will determine how much test substance will be needed for the study. For example, for a 13-week or chronic vapor study in large chambers, more than one 55-gallon drum may be

Table 4 Quantities of Test Substance Needed for Inhalation Studies

Exposure system/ chamber size	Maximum number of rodents exposed	Likely air flow rate (Lpm)	Minimum amount of test substance per day[a] (g)
12 port nose only	12	10	6
0.5 m^3	20	100	40
1 m^3	30	200	80
4 m^3	100	800	300
8 m^3	300	1600	600

[a]Assumes a concentration of 1 mg/L for 6 hours.

needed. Large-scale nose-only (25–75 animal ports) will not be much different. Small-scale nose-only systems (12–24 animal ports) will use 25% or less of the amount of a whole-body chamber. If a liquid test substance is to be aerosolized, the amount need for an aerosol study could be less than 100 kg for a 13-week study. A guide for deciding the amount of test substance required is given in Table 4. For each exposure concentration, the amount of test substance required can be estimated by multiplying column four by the concentration in mg/L and adding 25% for technical development.

Dusts are a different story. Aerosolizing (or suspending, as the case might be) a dust presents an entirely different situation for the inhalation toxicologist. Typically, dust particles are not generated in the same sense that a liquid aerosol is generated. The dust generator does not produce a particle that has a diameter that is much different from the diameter of the original test substance (it at least it shouldn't), whereas the size of a liquid aerosol particle is determined primarily by the generator (nebulizer) used. In addition, dusts are very electrostatic, and the charge needs to be neutralized (or at least reduced) to prevent the dust from electrostatically adhering to every surface with which it comes into contact. Because of losses on surfaces, the maximal concentration of an atmosphere of dust tends to be much lower than that which can be achieved with a liquid. Therefore, in addition to the exposure system dictating the amount of test substance needed for a study, the amount will depend on whether the test atmosphere is a vapor, liquid aerosol, or dust and how it is generated.

Chemical Analysis

Good Laboratory Practice regulations require that the performing laboratory analyze all test substances for purity, identity, stability, concentration, and homogeneity in the vehicle. The same is true for inhalation studies, especially concerning concentration and homogeneity. The concentration of the test substance in air should be determined during the exposure using appropriate methods. The method used will need to be specific enough to clearly identify the test substance. How one analyzes the test atmosphere depends on the physical and chemical properties of the test substance. For vapors and gases, the method should be able to distinguish between potential materials in the chamber. Absorption in the infrared or ultraviolet ranges may not be adequate for this because the EPA does not consider the method to be specific enough for identification. Instead, wet chemical analysis or chromatography might be necessary. These methods (and the instruments that utilize them) can be used to monitor the instantaneous concentration, but they are not adequate to determine the "true" concentration. In these cases, gas chromatographs that draw directly from the chamber can be used to quantitate the amount of test substance in the air. The alternative is to capture or "grab" a sample into another container, such as a tedlar bag, and analyze it by gas chromatography or wet chemistry process. "Grab" samples don't provide instantaneous concentration so the frequency of sampling becomes important. Sampling once an hour is suggested for acute studies, although the EPA suggests only twice during the 4 hours, and sampling once a day is more common for repeated exposures.

For solid and liquid aerosols, real-time monitors can be used for monitoring the concentration, and frequently they are acceptable for concentration determination. It is also advisable to collect "grab" samples for gravimetric determination of the concentration. This provides validation of the real-time monitor. Chemical analysis of what is collected during gravimetric "grab" sampling is not frequently done but may be important. An additional parameter to measure for aerosols is the particle size distribution. Some real-time monitors provide this information. There has been debate about whether the particle size distribution is sufficiently accurate from these devices. It may be advisable to use the standard method of cascade impaction to determine the particle size. This methodology involves collecting the test atmosphere in a cascade impactor that can distinguish size based on mass. It is the "gold" standard for particle size determination. The frequency of particle size determinations is probably preferred less than that for concentration determinations. It is advisable to measure particle size at least twice during an acute 4-hour study, and at least once weekly for a repeated-exposure study or, better, once per day.

The EPA is particular about the particle size and how it relates to validity of the study. Particle sizes that are too large (median diameter of $> 3 \, \mu m$) are considered to be too large for inhalation studies because the particles may not reach the lower airways. Should preliminary testing of the particles indicate that the test atmosphere is made up of such large particles (usually solids because liquid aerosols are generally generated in the $2 \, \mu m$ range by most nebulizers), alternative methods of administration (such as intratracheal instillation) are advisable.

The homogeneity of the test substance concentration in air (or uniformity of the test concentration in the chamber) should be determined prior to initiating exposures of animals; this is typically part of the preexposure trials. The intent is to evaluate how well the test atmosphere is distributed in the chamber so that each animal is exposed to the same concentration. This evaluation should be conducted for large whole-body chamber studies; it is unlikely that the concentrations in each corner of the chamber where the animals are placed will be exactly the same. Fluctuations of 10%, relative to a reference point, are not uncommon. The extent of the fluctuation may depend on the type of chamber used. For nose-only chambers, homogeneity is less of an issue and harder to test because the apparent homogeneity may change as one samples the test atmosphere from one port. Sampling several ports simultaneously, or at very low flow rates may overcome this problem.

One last comment about analysis: the testing guidelines require that samples of the test atmosphere be taken from the "breathing zone" of the animal. This request is important for whole-body exposure systems but has little relevance for nose-only systems. The study director will likely have guidance on the location of sampling lines based on his/her own experience.

THE TEST SYSTEM

Rats or Mice?

Selecting the test species is a relatively straightforward decision. Rats and mice are perhaps the most commonly used animals for inhalation studies. Other species, such as guinea pigs or rabbits, can be used if there is a good reason, such as the end point to be evaluated requires a species other than rats and mice. However, for most testing guidelines, the rat is the species of choice. Mice may be unacceptable for some inhalation studies especially those in which the test substance is irritating to the mucus membranes because mice have a greater capacity to reduce their breathing rate when exposed to irritants. Reduced breathing rate means less material inhaled, which means lower absorbed dose. Thus, mice may not show as dramatic responses to irritants than rats.

In some cases, nonrodent species are required. Developmental and reproductive toxicity studies, and some studies for FDA, require the use of nonrodents. Large species, such as rabbits, dogs, and primates, pose problems to the inhalation toxicologist by virtue of their size. Exposure of rabbits to vapors as part of a developmental of reproductive toxicity study can be conducted in whole-body chambers. Special caging is needed, and the chamber size will need to exceed 3 m^3 if body burden is not to exceed 10%. Many facilities built in the 1970s and early 1980s contained chambers of that size. Nose-only chambers for rabbits are rare. Exposure of other species, such as dogs or primates, can be accomplished using masks (essentially nose-only). As with rodents, the animals need to be acclimated to wearing the mask (*vide supra*). Primates can also be trained to accept treatment via pulse inhalers, and exposure of dogs can be performed via implanted tracheal tubes. Intratracheal tubes for exposure, such as those described by Halpern and Schlesinger for exposure of rabbits might also be available (11). These novel exposure systems might be valuable for unique types of test substances that have characteristics that make standard exposure systems impractical. However, it is best to let the study director suggest using them rather than trying to find a laboratory that specializes in these types of systems. As mentioned previously, if the standard inhalation exposure systems are not practical, intratracheal instillation is an option. This technique has been used for many years to deliver known quantities of test substance to the lungs of animals.

Regardless of the species is selected, it is important to make sure that the animals are sufficiently old at the start of exposures as required by the testing guidelines. In fact, most testing guidelines require the animals to be 4–6 weeks of age, but 6–8 week-old animals tend to tolerate exposures better. This is especially true for nose-only exposures; if animals are too young (and too small), they will turn around in the restraining tube and face away from the test atmosphere. Older animals have more difficulty maneuvering in the restraint tube; so older animals might be better.

Once the species and age have been selected, the next question is how many animals to use in a study. To some extent, this is dictated by the testing guideline. So for acute toxicity studies in rodents, the requirement can range from 2–5 animals per sex, depending on the regulatory agency and guideline selected. For repeated-exposure studies (<13 weeks) 5 rodents per sex per group are required. For 13-week studies, 10 rodents per sex per group are required, and for lifetime exposures, usually 50 rodents per sex per group are necessary. If larger species are used, the number of animals required decreases (e.g., 12 rabbits for Segment II studies, and 5–7 dogs for short-term studies).

The exposure system, too, and the end points for evaluation also are factors. For whole-body exposure systems, the number of animals in a chamber should not exceed 5% of the total volume of the chamber, assuming the animal's volume is directly proportional to its weight. Thus, for a 1 m^3 chamber (1000 L) the total number of 250 g rats that can be exposed is 200. In practical terms, 200 animals in a 1 m^3 chamber is too many because each cage takes up more volume than each animal, so it is unlikely that one might overload the chamber except perhaps for large animals. For nose-only systems, the 5% rule doesn't apply. Instead, the number of animal ports dictates the number of animals to be used. Most nose-only systems have a minimum of 12 ports, which are often used to expose 10 animals leaving two sampling ports. The number of end points and type of end points also impacts the number of animals needed. Again, regulatory testing guidelines often specify the number of animals for each end point, but not always. Having sufficient numbers of animals for meaningful statistical evaluations is important. If the variability in a particular end point is high ($>20\%$) large numbers of animals may be needed to discern significant differences between the groups. It is important to remember that, as long as there is space available in the chamber, the effort to expose 20 animals is the same as the effort to expose one animal.

EXPOSURE SYSTEMS

Big Chambers or Nose Only?

Whole-body chambers are the most common system used and can vary in size from 0.5 to 18 m^3. The size of the chamber selected for the study depends on the number of animals per concentration group to be exposed. The type of system selected and finding a laboratory with that capability depends on the properties of the test substance. Whole-body chambers are most appropriate for vapors and gases. If the test substance is an aerosol or fiber, however, a nose-only system may be more appropriate than whole-body chambers because substantial amounts of material can be deposited on the fur of the animal in whole-body chambers. Test substance deposited on the fur can be ingested through grooming. Although ingested test substance may not greatly influence the results of the study, there are cases where the effect of the test substance has been substantially altered (10), depending on the route of administration. Some laboratories have devised ingenious methods to overcome the problem of ingestion, including wrapping the animal so that only the head is exposed or washing the pelt following exposure. It seems easier to use a nose-only exposure system.

There is only one other factor that influences the selection of the exposure system; that is, the amount of test substance needed for nose-only versus whole-body exposure systems. As shown in Table 4, nose-only systems use far less material than whole-body systems. The use of less material may be important if testing a biochemical pesticide or a bioengineered pharmaceutical that is only available in small quantities.

Using a nose-only system usually causes great anxiety for the novice sponsor because the first question to ask is whether the regulatory agency will accept the data (this was probably more true in years past than today). It is true that most regulators are accustomed to inhalation studies using whole-body chambers, but the testing guidelines do provide for the use of nose-only when appropriate, and most regulators now accept the advantages of nose-only exposure. Using a nose-only exposure system does bring with it unique issues and problems that may need to be considered. The first issue is that animals have to be restrained during exposure, as mentioned earlier. Restraints vary from immobilizing the neck to placing the animal into a tube. Any form of restraint brings with it stress, which can result in an increased respiratory rate that could lead to greater amounts of test substances being inhaled. Acclimation to the restraint can reduce the severity of the stress response and can virtually eliminate it. So, if nose-only exposure systems are selected, make sure that the animals are acclimated for several days prior to exposure, even for an acute study.

Another factor to contend with is heat stress from tube restraints. Most tube restraints are made from plastic (PVC) or polycarbonate and can retain the animal's body heat. Although personal experience has demonstrated that the temperature inside the tube increased only 1–2°C, this may be unacceptable for some types of studies. Although, keeping the tail out of the tube or even keeping it in cool water can easily dissipate body heat.

CHARACTERIZING THE EFFECTS OF EXPOSURE

Systemic Toxicity

Once the purpose of the study has been defined, select the biological end points to evaluate the questions and concerns about the test substance. For regulated studies, most biological end points are specified by the guideline that is most appropriate. Systemic end points, such as clinical observations, body weight measurements, feed consumption determination, clinical pathology (clinical chemistry and hematology), and anatomical pathology (histopathology) are commonly included and, unless there are good reasons to exclude them, should be included in all study designs. Clinical observations can be tricky for whole-body inhalation studies, at least during exposure, because all of the animals might not be visible. In those cases, the appearance and reactions of most of the animals should be applicable for the entire group. Some laboratories have means of evaluating sedation during exposure by scratching lightly on the chamber wall and judging how quickly the animals respond to the stimulus. Observation of animals during nose-only exposures is restricted by the animal's ability to maneuver within the restraint, but experienced technicians can judge the animal's alertness. When interpreting in-life data, one needs to bear in mind that feed and water are withdrawn during exposure. Thus, body weight and feed consumption often remain steady or decrease slightly Monday to Friday (exposure days) but rebound on the weekend when animals are not exposed and have *ad libitum* access to feed and water. Likewise, organ weights (especially adrenal weight), clinical chemistry, and even histopathology may reflect the stress of exposure, particularly when nose-only exposure systems are used.

As mentioned earlier, when to terminate animals relative to the last exposure can be an important factor in observing changes in clinical chemistry or histopathology. Exposures for repeated-exposure studies are typically carried out 5 days per week (except for reproductive and developmental studies that require 7 days per week). Terminating animals on a Monday after 2 days of rest during studies of short-term exposures of less than 4 weeks can allow some parameters to recover. It may be better to expose the animals an extra 2 days the following week, prior to termination, to see the full impact of exposure.

There are cases where the health concern is not related to the lung, and inhalation exposure simply reflects the route of human exposure. For example, inhalation exposure can be used as a route of administration for neurotoxicity, reproduction, and developmental toxicity studies. When designing these studies, one must take into account the logistics of exposure, and how the exposure system may influence the study design. For example, labor- or time-intensive neurotoxicity end points, such as functional observational battery, cannot be conducted on a large number of animals 6 hours after a 6-hour exposure without interfering with the light/dark cycle. So, it is best to be creative in addressing the end points selected and to work within the logistics of exposure. One approach that has been used is to skip exposure days during procedures that require more than 1 hour (12,13). It may also be necessary to deviate from timetables that are spelled out in the guidelines if they do not make sense for the exposure regimen that you have established. Likewise, when conducting a reproductive or developmental toxicity study of an aerosolized material, the use of nose-only inhalation may introduce some potential artifact caused by the stress of restraining the animals.

Pulmonary Toxicity

Other end points specifically designed to evaluate pulmonary toxicity can be added without changing the scope of the study because the lungs might not be a simple portal of entry. For histopathology, one important caveat is to make sure that the histopathology is appropriate for the respiratory tract (i.e., include the nasal cavity, larynx, trachea, and various planes of the lungs along the airways). The lungs and nasal cavity should be sectioned to provide the best possible evaluation of the tissue (14). Traditional methods for evaluating pulmonary toxicity include weighing the lungs prior to fixation and routine histopathology. Although weighing the lungs appears to be straightforward, there are occasional difficulties dissecting away extraneous tissue (the esophagus, for example), which leave the lungs or trachea perforated and makes inflation with formalin fixative more difficult. Usually, experienced laboratories have learned to overcome such difficulties without sacrificing accuracy in the organ weight. Preserving the lungs for histologic evaluation might also present some difficulties. The generally accepted method to fix the lungs is to inflate them with fixative. How much fixative to add might vary from laboratory to laboratory, but 1.5 to 2 times the collapsed size is not uncommon. Inflating the lungs with too much fixative may damage the architecture of the alveoli and make the pathologist's evaluation difficult. Conversely, insufficient fixative might be so destructive that the tissue cannot be adequately evaluated because it is not properly fixed.

An additional pulmonary end point is bronchoalveolar lavage, a procedure that washes out free lung cells, proteins, and debris from the lungs (15,16). The procedure is used postmortem in rodents but must be done immediately after euthanasia before the cells die. Usually the lungs and trachea are excised from the thorax, and a blunt-end needle is inserted into the trachea and tied off. A small amount of saline (physiological, usually Dulbecco's) is infused into the excised lungs, and the lungs massaged to distribute the fluid. The amount of saline infused is important. Typically, a volume of no more than 5 mL is used for rats and $\sim$1.5 mL is used for mice. Care must be taken to reduce leakage. Loss of fluid can be corrected by measuring the volume retrieved. The washings are analyzed for total and differential cell counts, total protein and albumin concentrations, and the activities of lactate dehydrogenase (LDH), alkaline phosphatase, and N-acetylglucose aminidase, among others. Typically, the first wash (or first and second) contains the highest concentration of analytes for biochemical analysis, so this wash is separated from the remaining washes. Cells from the first wash are combined with the subsequent washes for counts. Bronchoalveolar lavage has been used to evaluate the pulmonary toxicity of a variety of inhaled materials in animals and humans (16). In most cases, increases in enzyme activity can be related directly to damage of specific cell types in the lung. Changes in free lung cell numbers can indicate inflammation. The EPA has recently incorporated this procedure into an acute inhalation exposure guideline (OPPTS 870.1350), which can be used to help understand the effects of environmental air pollutants. The end points that are recommended in the guideline are minimal, so adding others will provide a better understanding of the pulmonary response to exposure. Some suggested end points and how to interpret changes are shown in Table 5.

For solid particles such as fibers and nanoparticles, additional tests can be performed in vitro which shed light on potential for pulmonary toxicity. For fibers, dissolution time in aqueous media has been suggested as a parameter that influences pulmonary toxicity (9). The concept is that if fibers persist, they have greater potential for long-term effects. Other tests using macrophages have also been suggested to evaluate if fibers can be engulfed and relocated out of the lungs or if macrophages release inflammatory elements as they try to engulf fibers. The fact that these tests can be performed outside of the animal makes them

Table 5 End Points for Bronchoalveolar Lavage

Parameter	Reflective change	Indicative of
Total free cell number (macrophages and neutrophils)	Increase	Inflammation
Number of neutrophils	Increase	Inflammation
Lactate dehydrogenase activity	Increase	General cell damage, usually of bronchial epithelium
Total protein concentration	Increase	General cell damage, usually of bronchial epithelium
Albumin concentration	Increase	Increased capillary permeability
N-acetyl glucosaminidase activity	Increase	Increased phagocytic activity by macrophages
Alkaline phosphatase activity	Increase	Type II cell damage
Fibronectin, collagenase, histamine	Increase	Fibrosis

attractive as screening tools. Some have suggested that similar tests can be used to screen nanoparticles for potential pulmonary toxicity. Although the effects of nanomaterials on cells in culture have been studied and reported by various investigators, there is no consensus on how predictive of effects in vivo such in vitro tests will be for nanomaterials.

Pulmonary Sensitization

Another end point that is useful is the measurement of immunoglobulin E (IgE) levels in the blood as an indicator of pulmonary sensitization. Pulmonary sensitization can be a serious workplace issue, and a method for evaluating the potential for pulmonary sensitization might help complete a workplace safety study (17). Several methodologies have been developed to evaluate pulmonary sensitization (18–20), but care should be used in adapting any method to the test substance in question because the methods might be most appropriate only to specific classes of chemicals. However, serum IgE measurement is, by no means, the only method that has been used for detection of pulmonary sensitization. Recent studies have demonstrated that cytokine levels (IL-4, IL-6) are also sensitive indicators of respiratory sensitization. Interestingly, Ig. and IL increases occur following dermal exposure, so detecting pulmonary sensitizers does not always require inhalation exposure of the animals.

Respiratory/Pulmonary Irritation

Evaluating the irritation potential of a test substance is often accomplished using standard dermal irritation studies. However, these studies do not adequately predict the respiratory tract response when exposed to irritating chemicals. Alarie (21) described the physiological responses following exposure to irritating chemicals. These responses can be characterized by measuring changes in respiration (22), and such changes have been proposed as a means of categorizing the toxicity of chemicals (23). Although using changes in respiration as a tool might be valuable, it is not easy to incorporate measurement of respiration into the standard inhalation toxicity study. Such evaluations are better performed within a specific study designed only for that purpose.

THE REPORT AND DATA INTERPRETATION

Any report sums up the study design and results. In general, reports for inhalation studies contain more detailed explanation of materials and methods than do most other studies because the methods vary significantly from laboratory to laboratory and from test substance to test substance. Make sure the report contains adequate details on the characterization of the test substance, test atmosphere generation, chamber design and sampling ports, analytical methods, etc. Table 6 provides some suggestions as to what information should be contained in the report. There is probably no such thing as too much information. It may also be helpful to have some description of validation/calibration procedures, especially if the results are going to be viewed as controversial (positively or negatively). There is a Standard Evaluation Procedure (SEP) for inhalation toxicity studies written by the EPA that can be very helpful in making sure that the report will meet standards (24). If the EPA or other government agency will review the study, it is recommended to read the SEP because it contains examples showing what might make a study invalid in the minds of the regulators, which are therefore issues to avoid or address. Appropriate information to include in the report is identified in Table 5. In addition, inadequate analytical information (test substance characterization) or inadequate sampling from the breathing zone of the animal may invalidate a study. For aerosols, if the median particle diameter is greater that 3 μm, or is not determined by cascade impaction, the study might be deemed invalid.

Interpreting the data with respect to effects on the respiratory tract can be complex because of the variables that need to be taken into account with regard to the test

Table 6 Important Information for Materials and Methods Section of Report

Section of the materials and methods	Information to include
Chamber	Size and configuration
	Construction material
	Placement of inlet and outlet relative to the animals
	Location and number of animals in the chamber
	Rotation scheme over the course of the study
Air supply	Type of filtration and proximity to chamber inlet
	Source of air supply; airflow per unit time and how was it determined (how often is the instrument calibrated or checked?)
	Measurements of chamber air temperature and relative humidity
Generation	Type of generator used; if vapor study, are particles present; if particle study, what is size distribution and how was it measured
	Diagram of system
	Physical parameters of generation: total air flow, air pressure (or pressure differential), rate of feed flow for test substance
Analytical	Instrumentation and detection limits; can the test substance be identified analytically?
	Frequency of sampling; frequency of calibration check
	How calibration curve was established
	Obtain sample procedures (if applicable)
	Type of monitoring device and location of sample lines: how close to the breathing zone; homogeneity (uniformity) of concentrations inside the chamber relative to a reference point (no more than 10%)

substance deposition or absorption. Recently, the International Programme on Chemical Safety developed a document containing the "Scientific Principles And Methods For Assessing Respiratory Tract Injury Caused By Inhaled Substances" that provides an excellent overview for evaluating study data. In general, responses of the respiratory tract range from irritation to inflammation to severe edema. Very water-soluble reactive gases may produce irritation in the nasopharyngeal region, as evidenced by nasal discharge to hyperplasia of the squamous epithelium or respiratory epithelium of the nasal cavity. As the reactivity increases, one may observe hyperplasia of the olfactory epithelium. Squamous metaplasia of the epithelium has been observed following prolonged low-level exposure to irritating substances. The location of the metaplasia might reflect deposition of the substance, which might be affected by the physical state of the substance [i.e., a vapor (gas) or particle]. Mucus discharge might reflect severely irritating substances that cause severe inflammation in the epithelium, whereas edema might be the result of increased permeability of the capillaries in the alveoli. Fibrosis is a long-term response that requires a significant time period to be observed histologically. One can get an early indication of fibrotic changes using bronchoalveolar lavage, a technique that is easily extrapolated from animals to humans because the effects and changes in the end points are similar. Sustained elevations in all parameters (LDH activity, protein level, N-acetylglucosaminidase activity, B-glucuronidase activity) and release of fibronectin have been associated with the development of fibrosis (25,26). Table 6 lists the end points that can be measured in lavage fluid. Interpreting the changes in parameters from lavage fluid is relatively straightforward.

REFERENCES

1. Kennedy GL, Jr., Valentine R. Inhalation toxicology. In: Hayes AW, ed. Principles and Methods in Toxicology. 3rd ed. New York: Raven Press, 1994.
2. Gad SC, Chengalis CP. Acute inhalation testing. In: Gad SC, Chengalis CP, eds. Acute Toxicology Testing Perspectives and Horizons. Caldwell, New Jersey: The Telford Press, 1989.
3. McClellan RO, Henderson RF. In: McClellan RO, Henderson RF, eds. Concepts in Inhalation Toxicology. New York: Hemisphere Publishing Corp., 1989.
4. http://www.epa.gov/docs/OPPTS_Harmonized/870_Health_Effects_Test_Guidelines/html.
5. http://www.cfsan.fda.gov/~dms/guidance.html.
6. http://vm.cfsan.fda.gov/~redbook/red-toca.html.
7. http://www.fda.gov/cder/guidance/index.htm.
8. http://www.oecd.org/findDocument/0,2350,en_2649_34377_1_1_1_1_1,00.html.
9. U.S. EPA Workshop Report on Chronic Inhalation Toxicity and Carcinogenicity Testing of Respirable Fibrous Particles, 1996; EPA-748-R-96-001.
10. Tyl RW, Ballantyne B, Fisher LC, et al. Evaluation of the developmental toxicity of ethylene glycol aerosol in CD-1 mice by nose-only exposure. Fundam Appl Toxicol 1995; 27:49–62.
11. Halpern M, Schlesinger RB. Simple oral delivery device for inhalation exposure of rabbits to aerosols. J Toxicol Environ Health 1980; 6:751–755.
12. David RM, Tyler TR, Ouellette R, et al. Evaluation of subchronic neurotoxicity of N-Butyl acetate vapor. NeuroToxicology 1998; 19:809–822.
13. David RM, Bernard LG, Banton MI, et al. The effect of repeated methyl iso-butyl ketone vapor exposure on schedule-controlled operant behavior in rats. NeuroToxicology 1999; 20:583–594.
14. Haschek WM, Witschi HP. Respiratory system. In: Haschek WM, Rousseaux CG, eds. Handbook of Toxicologic Pathology. New York: Academic Press, 1991.
15. Bond JA, Wallace LA, Osterman-Golker S, et al. Assessment of exposure to pulmonary toxicants: use of biological markers. Fundam Appl Toxicol 1992; 18:161–174.

16. Reynolds HY. Bronchoalveolar lavage. Am Rev Respir Dis 1987; 135:250–263.
17. Kimber I, Wilks MF. Chemical respiratory allergy. Toxicological and occupational health issues. Hum Exp Toxicol 1995; 14:735–736.
18. Sarlo K, Clark ED. A tier approach for evaluating the respiratory allergenicity of low molecular weight chemicals. Fundam Appl Toxicol 1992; 18:107–114.
19. Dearman RJ, Spence LM, Kimber I. Characterization of murine immune responses to allergenic diisocyanates. Toxicol Appl Pharmacol 1992; 112:190–197.
20. Ritz HL, Evans BLB, Bruce RD, et al. Respiratory and immunological responses of guinea pigs to enzyme-containing detergents: a comparison of intratracheal and inhalation methods of exposure. Fundam Appl Toxicol 1993; 21:31–37.
21. Alarie Y. Sensory irritation by airborne chemicals. Crit Rev Toxicol 1973; 2:299–363.
22. Kane LE, Barrow CS, Alarie Y. A short-term test to predict acceptable levels of exposure to airborne sensory irritant. Am Ind Hyg Assoc J 1979; 40:207–229.
23. Schaper M. Development of a database for sensory irritation and its use in establishing occupational limits. Am Ind Hyg Assoc J 1993; 54:488–544.
24. Gross SB, Vocci FJ. Standard evaluation procedure. Inhal Toxicol Test 1988. EPA-540/09-101.
25. Lindenschmidt RC, Driscoll KE, Perkins MA, et al. The comparison of a fibrogenic and two nonfibrogenic dusts by bronchoalveolar lavage. Toxicol Appl Pharmacol 1990; 102:268–281.
26. Driscoll KE, Maurer JK, Lindenschmidt RC, et al. Respiratory tract response to dust: relationahsips between dust burden, lung injury, alveolar macrophage fibronectin release, and the development of pulmonary fibrosis. Toxicol Appl Pharmacol 1990.

15

Cancer Risk Assessment of Environmental Agents: Approaches to the Incorporation and Analysis of New Scientific Information

William H. Farland and William P. Wood
Office of Research and Development, U.S. Environmental Protection Agency, Washington, D.C., U.S.A.

Kerry L. Dearfield
Office of the Science Advisor, U.S. Environmental Protection Agency, Washington, D.C., U.S.A.

INTRODUCTION

The objective of the U.S. Environmental Protection Agency's (EPA's) risk assessments was to support environmental decision making. Assessments of risks to environmental agents serve not only the regulatory programs of EPA but also state and local agencies, as well as international communities that are addressing environmental issues. The components of health risk assessments include information on whether a chemical produces adverse health effects and who might be susceptible, how the frequency of adverse effects changes with dose, and to what degree and under what conditions people may be exposed as pollutants travel in the environment. The primary sources of information for judging human hazard and/or risk are human epidemiological and animal toxicological studies and other empirical information, such as genotoxicity, structure-activity relationship, and exposure data. Risk assessments often rely on studies in animals because human data are not available. The health-related information available on environmental agents is typically incomplete. Moreover, health risk assessments on environmental agents must usually address the potential for harm from exposure levels found in the environment that are usually considerably lower than concentrations at which toxicity is found in laboratory animal or epidemiological studies. Thus, the extrapolations that are required to characterize human risk (i.e., from high to low doses, from nonhuman

Disclaimer: Although this chapter has been subjected to review and approved for publication, it does not necessarily reflect the views and policies of the U.S. Environmental Protection Agency. The opinions expressed within this article reflect the views of the authors. The U.S. government has the right to retain a nonexclusive royalty free license in and to any copyright covering this chapter.

species to human beings, from one route to another route of exposure) inherently introduce uncertainty.

Given that extrapolations must be performed, risk assessment is complex and often controversial. EPA develops risk assessment guidelines to provide staff and decision makers with guidance and perspectives necessary to develop and use effective health risk assessments. Guidelines encourage consistency in procedures to support decision making across the many EPA programs. They also encourage approaches to the incorporation of new, emerging forms of scientific information, such as genomics and other potential biomarkers of exposure or effects. The following lists the risk assessment guidelines that EPA published:

Carcinogenicity (1,2)
Mutagenicity (3)
Developmental toxicity (4)
Reproductive toxicity (5)
Neurotoxicity (6)
Exposure (7)
Complex mixtures (8)

EPA recently issued new cancer risk assessment guidelines to bring current and relevant science into future assessments and to promote research that applies new knowledge to specific pollutants (2). There have been significant gains in our understanding of the cellular and subcellular processes that result in cancer, and these advances have enabled research on the ways environmental contaminants act on cells to cause cancer or stimulate its growth. These new guidelines are discussed here as an illustration of how new scientific evidence and analysis approaches are impacting and improving the characterization of potential human risk and, in particular, cancer risk from environmental agents.

Human health risk assessment approaches are evolving in a number of ways (Table 1). Risk analyses historically relied to a large degree on observations of frank toxic effects (e.g., tumors, malformations). Risk assessments are moving from this phenomenological approach by identifying the ways environmental agents are changed through metabolic processes, the dose at the affected organ system or even at the cellular or subcellular (molecular) level, and how an agent produces its adverse effects at high doses and at low ones. This understanding of how an agent produces its toxic effect is beginning to break down the dichotomy that has existed between assessments of cancer and noncancer risks. Of equal importance, the "one-size-fits-all" approach is being replaced by emphasizing the ascertainment of risk to susceptible populations or life-stages.

Table 1 Current Trends in Health Risk Assessment

Historical approach	Emerging emphasis
Phenomenological studies	Mechanism studies
Separate assessments and approaches for cancer and noncancer risks	Integrative health assessments and harmonization of approaches for cancer and noncancer risks
Risk to general populations	Risk to susceptible populations
Single chemical exposure and single pathway	Multiple chemical exposures via multiple pathways
Risk characterization	More expanded characterizations of human risk

In 1996, EPA published a national agenda to protect children from toxic agents in the environment (9). Supplemental guidance for assessing susceptibility from early life exposures to carcinogens was recently published along with the new EPA Cancer Guidelines (10). In addition, EPA continued to research the implications of age, pre-existing disease, and life-stage on susceptibility to environmental agents.

Risk Assessment Paradigm

Since the early 1980s, EPA has followed the basic human health risk assessment paradigm put forth by the National Academy of Sciences' National Research Council (NRC) (11). The paradigm describes a four-step process to analyze the data and then summarize the implications from the data in a risk characterization that others, such as risk managers, other discipline-related technical experts, and the public, can easily follow and understand. For each step, the relevant and scientifically reliable information is evaluated. In addition, the related uncertainties and science policy choices are described. The four steps, paraphrased for cancer risk assessment, are:

1. Hazard Identification—the determination of whether a particular chemical may or may not be causally linked to cancer under some situations.
2. Dose-Response Assessment—the determination of the relation between the magnitude and nature of exposure and the probability of occurrence of cancer.
3. Exposure Assessment—the determination of the extent of human exposure before or after application of regulatory controls.
4. Risk Characterization—the description of the nature and often the magnitude of human risk to cancer, including attendant uncertainty.

This chapter discusses the incorporation of newer scientific information and analysis approaches in the context of the risk paradigm—hazard identification, dose-response assessment, and exposure assessment and subsequent risk characterization (Fig. 1). Examples are provided to illustrate these approaches in cancer risk assessment.

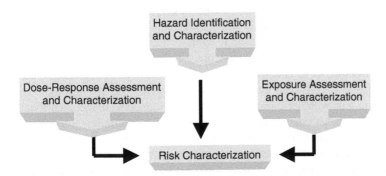

Figure 1 The elements of the risk paradigm. Health risk assessment is organized by the paradigm put forward by the National Academy of Sciences' National Research Council (11,12), which defines four types of analysis: hazard identification, dose-response assessment, exposure assessment, and risk characterization.

HAZARD IDENTIFICATION/HAZARD CHARACTERIZATION

In its 1994 report about the use of science and judgment in risk assessment, the NRC recommended that EPA incorporate technical characterizations of risk that are both qualitative and quantitative in its assessments (12). Thus, hazard identification, as well as dose-response and exposure analyses, is changing by the increased emphasis on providing characterization discussions. These technical characterizations essentially reveal the thought process that leads to the scientific judgments of potential human risk. The technical hazard characterization explains the extent and weight of evidence, major points of interpretation and rationale, strengths, and weaknesses of the evidence and discusses alternative conclusions and uncertainties that deserve serious consideration. It moves away from the simple "yes/no" presentations of the past when identifying potential cancer hazard. The technical hazard characterization, along with those for the dose-response and exposure assessments, are the starting materials for the risk characterization process (see section Risk Characterization of this chapter) that completes the risk assessment. As shown in Figure 2, this concept of technical hazard characterizations is incorporated into EPA's newly revised *Guidelines for Carcinogen Risk Assessment* (2).

Expanding Role of Mechanistic Data

Hazard identification is moving beyond relying on traditional toxicology by using a weight-of-evidence (WOE) approach that considers all relevant data and the mode of action (MOA) of the given agent. It is the sum of the biology of the organism and the chemical properties of an agent that leads to an adverse effect such as cancer. Thus, it is an evaluation of the entire range of data (e.g., physical, chemical, biological, toxicological, clinical, and epidemiological information) that allows one to arrive at a reasoned judgment of an agent's potential to cause human harm. For example, EPA made a major change in the way hazard evidence is weighed in reaching conclusions about the human carcinogenic potential of environmental agents (2,11). Rather than relying almost exclusively on tumor findings, the full use of all relevant information is promoted and an understanding of how the agent induces tumors is emphasized. In the new EPA *Guidelines for Carcinogen Risk Assessment* (2), a short WOE narrative is derived from the longer technical hazard characterization. The WOE narrative is intended for risk managers and other users, and it replaces the previous six alphanumeric classifications found in earlier EPA cancer guidelines: A, human carcinogen; B1/B2, probable human carcinogen; C, possible human carcinogen; D, not classifiable, and E, evidence of noncarcinogenicity (1). This narrative explains in nontechnical language the key data and conclusions, as well as the conditions for hazard expression. Conclusions about potential human carcinogenicity are presented by route of exposure. Contained within this narrative are simple likelihood descriptors that essentially distinguish whether there is enough evidence concerning human hazard (i.e., "Carcinogenic to Humans," "Likely to Be Carcinogenic to Humans," or "Not Likely to Be Carcinogenic to Humans") or whether there is insufficient evidence to make such a call (i.e., the descriptor makes a statement about the database, for example, "Inadequate Information to Assess Carcinogenic Potential," or a database that provides "Suggestive Evidence of Carcinogenic Potential"). Because one encounters a variety of data sets on agents, these descriptors are not meant to stand alone; rather, the context of the WOE narrative is intended to provide a transparent explanation of the biological evidence and how the conclusions were derived. Moreover, these descriptors should not be viewed as classifications (like the alphanumeric system), which often obscure key scientific differences among chemicals. The new WOE narrative also presents conclusions about

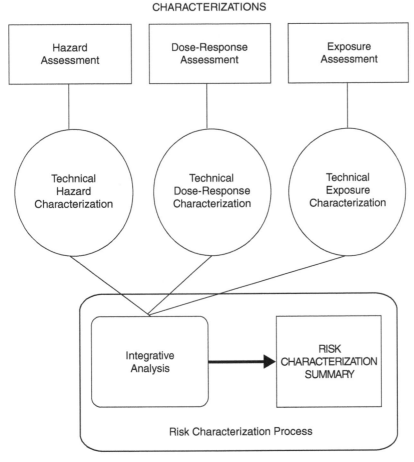

CHARACTERIZATIONS

Figure 2 The risk characterization process: the framework of the Environmental Protection Agency *Guidelines for Carcinogen Risk Assessment* (2) is based on the paradigm put forth by the National Research Council (11). This framework puts an emphasis on characterizations of hazard, dose-response, and exposure assessment. These technical characterizations integrate the analyses of hazard, dose-response, and exposure, explain the weight of evidence and strengths and weaknesses of the data, as well as discuss the issues and uncertainties surrounding the conclusions. The technical characterizations themselves are integrated into the overall conclusions of risk that are presented in an integrative, overall risk characterization (13).

how the agent induces tumors and the relevance of the MOA to humans and recommends a dose-response approach based on the MOA analysis (discussed below).

Mode of Action Analysis

The use of MOA in the assessment of potential carcinogens is now the main approach for analyzing the relevance of a chemical's ability to induce cancer. This emphasis arose because of the significant scientific breakthroughs that have developed concerning the causes of cancer induction. Without MOA information, EPA generally takes conservative (public health–protective) default positions regarding the interpretation of toxicologic and epidemiologic data: animal tumor findings are judged to be relevant to humans, and cancer risks are assumed to conform with low-dose linearity. Elucidation of a MOA for a particular cancer response in animals or humans is a data-rich determination. Usually, significant information will need to be developed to support the position that a MOA underlies a particular process leading to cancer at a given site.

From the EPA Cancer Guidelines (2), the term *"MOA"* is defined as a sequence of key events and processes, starting with interaction of an agent with a cell, proceeding through operational and anatomical changes, and resulting in cancer formation. A "key event" is an empirically observable precursor step that is itself a necessary element of the MOA or is a marker for such an element. MOA is contrasted with "mechanism of action," which implies a more detailed understanding and description of events, often at the molecular level, than is meant by MOA. The toxicokinetic processes that lead to formation or distribution of the active agent to the target tissue are considered in estimating dose but are not part of the MOA, as the term is used here. There are many examples of possible modes of carcinogenic action, such as mutagenicity, mitogenesis, inhibition of cell death, cytotoxicity with reparative cell proliferation, and immune suppression. It should be noted these MOAs are not necessarily mutually exclusive.

The EPA Cancer Guidelines provide a general framework (Table 2) in which toxicology and other relevant information can be analyzed to assess whether a plausible MOA is supported for a chemical induction of cancer (2). This framework also should be used to determine if there are sufficient data to establish a MOA for that chemical. The framework provides a transparent, consistent, and practical approach for analyzing the scientific information needed to assess a chemical's carcinogenic MOA. The derivation of the framework is based upon earlier international efforts to develop a systematic approach to evaluate MOA relevant information (14,15). It should be noted that this general framework can be used to evaluate MOA(s) for a number of adverse health effects in addition to cancer. Both national and international efforts are underway to enhance the MOA framework; for example, to refine the approach to understanding the relevance of the MOA in animals to human cancer hazard and risk (16). This framework helps elucidate the thought process necessary to establish the causality of an effect. In addition, it can be used to identify data gaps and to suggest research that will be useful in filling the gaps.

Once the analysis for carcinogenic MOA is performed and the MOA for cancer is found relevant to humans, quantitative estimates for human risk are usually calculated and extrapolated from the higher doses usually seen in the test systems to the usually lower

Table 2 Elements of the Mode of Action Framework

Description of the hypothesized mode of action
  Summary description of the hypothesized mode of action
  Identification of key events
Discussion of the experimental support for the hypothesized mode of action
  Strength, consistency, and specificity of association
  Dose-response concordance
  Temporal relationship
  Biological plausibility and coherence
Consideration of the possibility of other modes of action
Conclusions about the hypothesized mode of action
  Is the hypothesized mode of action sufficiently supported in the test animals?
  Is the hypothesized mode of action relevant to humans?
  Which populations or life stages can be particularly susceptible to the hypothesized mode of action?

Source: From Ref. 2.

doses seen in human exposure scenarios (discussed in more detail in section Dose-Response Assessment/Dose-Response Characterization). Generally, for cancer induction with a mutagenic-based MOA, the underlying assumption is that the low-dose extrapolation will be characterized by a linear extrapolation of the dose response relationship (2,17). However, there will be instances where the MOA might indicate a nonlinear dose-response relationship to lower doses for tumor induction. If more than one MOA is found plausible, both linear and nonlinear extrapolations may need to be considered. Finally, the MOA may not completely inform the extrapolation and the low-dose response relationship may remain unknown. In the absence of nonconclusive MOA information, therefore, the general default is to assume a linear extrapolation for regulatory purposes (2,17).

Understanding of MOA can be a key to identifying processes that may cause chemical exposures to differentially affect a particular population segment or life stage. For example, some MOAs are anticipated to be mutagenic and are assessed with a linear approach for most, if not all, parts of the population. This is the MOA for radiation and several other agents that are known carcinogens. Other MOAs can support differential susceptibilities and low-dose extrapolations for different segments of the population or human life stages. The low-dose extrapolation may then be characterized with either linear or nonlinear approaches for those particular susceptible populations or life stages after a rigorous analysis of the available data.

When a particular MOA is being assessed for the first time, the analysis will generally require a data-rich set of information to establish the validity and acceptability of that MOA. This is to ensure that the support underlying that particular carcinogenic MOA is understood as much as possible and there is indeed scientific consensus for the MOA for that tumor induction. This is considered by many as "setting the bar relatively high" for regulatory acceptance of a MOA to inform potential human risk. This is a necessary approach to make sure such regulatory agencies as EPA do not promulgate rules and regulations on less than solid, sound supporting science. Subsequent analyses focusing on the same MOA for other chemicals may not need such a data-rich set of information to support the MOA for that chemical. It may be only necessary to demonstrate that several key events and other elements found in the MOA framework are operative to satisfy the scientific community that that MOA is the main, plausible MOA for tumor induction. The following subsections provide several examples of a MOA analysis for particular tumor types.

α_{2u} Nephropathy and Kidney Cancer

The development of male rat kidney tumors mediated by α_{2u}-globulin is one of the more thoroughly studied MOA processes in cancer toxicology. Exposure to several agents, such as 2,2,4-trimethylpentane, unleaded gasoline, and d-limonene, have been reported to result in an accumulation of protein droplets containing α_{2u}-globulin in the epithelial cells of the proximal convoluted tubules of male rat kidneys (18–21). This protein accumulation is thought to result in renal cell injury and proliferation and eventually renal tubule tumors. Female rats and other laboratory animals do not accumulate this protein in the kidney and, when exposed to α_{2u}-globulin inducers, do not develop an increased incidence of renal tubule tumors. The manner in which the human male responds to such agents is uncertain. This MOA appears to be specific to the rat, given the results from studies of other laboratory species and given the high doses that are needed to produce an effect in the male rat.

In 1991, EPA concluded that the sequence of events proposed to link α_{2u}-globulin accumulation to nephropathy and renal tubule tumors in the male rat was plausible, although not totally proven; that the α_{2u}-globulin response following chemical administration appears to be unique to the male rat; and that the male rat kidney response to chemicals that induce α_{2u}-globulin is probably not relevant to humans for purposes of risk assessment (21). However, when chemically induced α_{2u}-globulin kidney tumors are present, other tumors in the male rat and any tumor in other exposed laboratory animals may be important in evaluating the carcinogenic potential of a given chemical. Some investigators think that the issue of α_{2u} nephropathy and kidney cancer is not resolved and have proposed alternative hypotheses (22). Should significant new information on α_{2u}-globulin kidney tumors become available, EPA will update its policy position accordingly.

Perturbation of Pituitary-Thyroid Homeostasis and Thyroid Cancer

The MOA in which antithyroid compounds induce thyroid tumors is also reasonably well understood, even though the precise molecular events leading to thyroid follicular cell tumors are not totally described. Experimental findings in rodents have shown that perturbation of hypothalamus-pituitary-thyroid homeostasis leads to elevated thyroid-stimulating hormone (TSH) levels, which in turn results in increased DNA synthesis and cell proliferation, and eventually to thyroid gland tumors (23–26). Thus, thyroid tumors are secondary to a hormone imbalance. Agents with antithyroid activity include sulfamethazine and other thionamides. There is uncertainty whether prolonged stimulation of the human thyroid by TSH may lead to cancer. Because this possibility cannot be dismissed, it is presumed that chemicals that produce thyroid tumors in rodents may pose a carcinogenic risk to humans. Humans (including other primates) are thought to be substantially less sensitive than rats to this mechanism.

One factor that may account for the interspecific difference in sensitivity concerns the influence of protein carriers of thyroid hormones in the blood. Rodent thyroid hormones are more susceptible to removal from the body because of the lack of a high-affinity binding protein, which humans possess (27). In the rat, there is chronic stimulation of the thyroid gland by TSH to compensate for the increased turnover of thyroid hormones. This may render the rat more sensitive to disturbances in TSH levels. EPA issued science policy guidance on the consideration of thyroid carcinogenesis in risk assessment (26). Briefly, chemicals that produce rodent thyroid tumors should be presumed to pose a hazard to humans; evaluations of human thyroid cancer risk from long-term perturbations of pituitary-thyroid function in rodents should incorporate considerations about potential interspecific differences in sensitivity and evaluate the applicability of potential human exposure patterns in relation to the findings in animal models. Dose-response approaches should be based on MOA information; application of nonlinear approaches is appropriate for those nonmutagenic chemicals shown to cause a hormonal imbalance. However, those antithyroid compounds with mutagenic activity need to be carefully evaluated on a case-by-case basis.

Bladder Calculi and Tumors

Another situation for which the rat appears to be quantitatively more sensitive than humans is the induction of bladder tumors secondary to bladder calculi-induced hyperplasia. Cohen and Ellwein (28) reported that if the administered dose of a chemical (e.g., melamine, uracil, calcium oxalate, orotic acid, glycine) is below the level that causes calculus formulation, there is no increase in irritation or cell proliferation; consequently, there is no increase in bladder tumors. Thus, calculus-forming compounds would have a biological threshold of response. EPA considered this in its assessment of melamine (29).

Formaldehyde and Nasal Tumors

The understanding of formaldehyde carcinogenicity developed over a number of years since Kerns et al. (30) demonstrated that inhalation exposure to formaldehyde caused nasal squamous cell carcinomas in mice and rats. In 1991, the carcinogenicity of formaldehyde was reassessed using data from rats and monkeys: levels of DNA-protein cross-links (DPXs) were evaluated with a linearized multistage model (31). Using DPXs as a more precise measure of dose resulted in risk estimates that were significantly lower than those derived by using external exposure only. Although the mechanisms of formaldehyde carcinogenesis are not completely understood, data have continued to provide additional insight into the cancer risk associated with low-dose exposure to inhaled formaldehyde by defining more precisely the location of the nasal tumors in the rat, determining rates of cell proliferation in the nose, and establishing the delivered dose (i.e., levels of DPXs) to the target tissue as well as rates of repair of DPXs after repeated exposures (32–36). Precursor response data also may have implications in the estimation of risk to humans (36). In the rat, the dose-response relationships of induction of nasal tumors and of cell proliferation correspond and are both highly nonlinear (34,36). The DPXs do not accumulate, and although the dose-response relationship is linear in the range of tumor induction and increased cell replication, the slope is greater than at lower dose ranges due to saturation of detoxification (34,35). Although formaldehyde is a mutagenic carcinogen, the data on tumors, cellular kinetics, and molecular dosimetry indicate that the dose-response relationship in rats is not linear throughout the entire range but is subject to an upward curvature due to increased cell proliferation (36).

With the structure of the model used in this analysis, it was noted that the prediction of the tumor dose-response was extremely sensitive to cell kinetics. In recent work, Conolly et al. (37) extended their modeling work to humans. Positive maximum likelihood estimates (MLE) were obtained with this model. These MLE estimates were lower, for some comparisons by as much as 1,000-fold, than MLE estimates from previous cancer-dose response assessments for formaldehyde. Additional research and assessment work will be needed to put these modeling results in perspective and to address recent reports of an association between formaldehyde exposure and increased human risk for leukemia as well as for respiratory cancer (38,39).

Conditions of Hazard Expression

As mentioned earlier, hazard identification has expanded from simply identifying adverse effects to fuller technical characterizations of a particular hazard. One dimension critical to characterizing hazard potential is the concept of hazard expression (i.e., What are the circumstances under which a particular hazard is expressed?). For example, an agent may not carry the same hazard potential for different routes of exposure. Inhalation exposure to vinyl acetate (600 parts per million) produces statistically significant increases in nasal tumors in rats, whereas no statistically significant increases in tumors are observed when the compound is ingested orally via drinking water (40,41). Likewise, a compound's carcinogenicity may be dose limited. Although methylmercury has been shown to produce tumors in mice at high doses (42), it is unlikely to pose a hazard to humans at low doses. Conditions of hazard expression may not only involve exposure conditions (e.g., route, magnitude, or duration) but also may depend on biological and physiological processes.

Studies on metabolism may provide pertinent data about the circumstances that affect hazard expression. The biotransformation of many chemicals to reactive compounds is dependent on the presence of certain metabolic pathways (e.g., oxidative pathways involving P450 cytochromes or conjugation pathways involving glutathione S-transferases). For example, 1, 3-butadiene is carcinogenic in rats and mice, with mice being more sensitive to tumor induction than rats (43,44). It is thought that the carcinogenic potential of 1, 3-butadiene is dependent on metabolic activation to reactive metabolites, which interact with DNA. For example, metabolism of 1, 3-butadiene to reactive epoxides is substantially greater in mice than in rats (45–47). Thus, metabolizing enzymes can account for different susceptibilities among species. Other biological factors that can result in differences in sensitivity include age, sex, or preexisting diseases. These factors that may contribute to special sensitivity to a given agent are discussed further in the following section.

Variation in Human Susceptibility

Humans vary in their susceptibility to toxicity because of differences in age, gender, metabolism, genetic makeup, and/or preexisting disease conditions. Certain individuals may be at an increased risk because their activity patterns increase their exposure or because their proximity to a source means higher exposures to environmental contaminants. For example, a number of studies have shown the role of carcinogen-metabolizing enzyme polymorphisms in cancer susceptibility (48), of which the most convincing is for the association of the GSTMl homozygous genotype and the CYPlAl rare alleles with lung cancer in Japanese (49,50). Gene-environmental interactions have also been shown to be important to an elevated risk for developmental defects. For example, genetic variation of transforming growth factor alpha and maternal smoking have been associated with increased risk for delivering infants with cleft lip or palate (51,52). Human responses may vary due to environmental exposures during different periods of the life cycle. Exposures of the fetus or neonate may disrupt developing systems, thereby resulting in increased sensitivity later in life.

The causes of cancer encompass a variety of possible risk factors, including genetic predisposition, diet, lifestyle, associations with congenital malformations, and exposure to biological and physical agents and chemicals in the environment. Historically, the focus on cancer has been as a disease associated with aging, resulting from extended exposure duration with prolonged latency periods before the cancers appear. Because much of cancer epidemiology addresses occupational exposures and because rodent cancer studies are designed to last approximately a lifetime (two years) beginning after sexual maturity, the cancer database used by regulatory agencies and others for risk assessment focuses on adults.

Unequivocal evidence of childhood cancer in humans occurring from chemical exposures is limited (53). The relative rarity in the incidence of childhood cancers and a lack of animal testing guidelines with perinatal exposure impede a full assessment of children's cancer risks from exposure to chemicals in the environment. Established risk factors for the development of childhood cancer include radiation and certain pharmaceutical agents used in chemotherapy and some evidence in humans for adult tumors resulting from perinatal exposure, i.e., pharmacological use of diethylstilbesterol during pregnancy to prevent miscarriages. In addition to the limited human data, there are examples of transplacental carcinogens in animal studies, as well as studies suggesting that altered development can affect later susceptibility to cancer induced by exposure to other chemicals.

The methodology that has been generally used to estimate cancer risk associated with oral exposures relies on estimation of the lifetime average daily dose, which can account for differences between adults and children with respect to such exposure factors as eating habits and body weight. However, susceptibility differences with respect to early life stages historically have not been taken into consideration because cancer slope factors are based upon effects observed following exposures to adult humans or sexually mature animals. One element in extending analyses to children is to evaluate the extent to which exposures early in life would alter the incidence of cancers observed later in life, compared with the incidence observed with adult-only exposures (53,54).

Cancer risk to children in the context of EPA's Cancer Guidelines (2) includes both early-life exposures that may result in the occurrence of cancer during childhood and early-life exposures that may contribute to cancers later in life. Because a much larger database exists for chemicals inducing cancer in adult humans or sexually mature animals, it was necessary to determine whether adjustment of such adult-based cancer slope factors would be appropriate when assessing cancer risks associated with exposures early in life. The analysis undertaken by EPA has been described in detail (10,55).

Beyond the analysis of early life exposure studies in animals, there are conceptual biological rationales that would suggest DNA-damaging agents would have greater impacts on early life stages. Growth involves substantial levels of cell replication, even in organs that in adults are only very slowly replicating, thus increasing the likelihood that a cell will undergo division before the DNA damage caused by the mutagen has been repaired. Increased replication also can lead to a greater division of initiated cells, leading to a larger number of initiated cells per specified dose. These periods of cell replication can vary for different tissues. Tumor promotion processes can be very dependent upon the duration of promotion, initiation processes can occur in relatively brief periods (e.g., the single-dose studies in animals or radiation exposure in humans). Most tumors take extended periods to develop, making damage that occurs earlier in life more likely to result in tumors prior to death than would exposures that occur later in life. Although some of these observations may also pertain to other modes, all of them (with some differences among tumor sites) appear to be potentially relevant to a greater susceptibility to mutagenic MOAs during early-life stages (vs. later-life stages).

EPA's analysis of early-life animal exposure studies demonstrated a greater susceptibility to chemicals with a mutagenic MOA. Based on this analysis, EPA developed a set of age dependent adjustment factors that are applied to the cancer slope factors from adult animal studies to account for exposure during childhood to chemicals with a mutagenic MOA. The information on life-stage susceptibility for chemicals inducing cancers through MOAs other than direct DNA interaction is more varied, showing an increase in tumor incidence during perinatal exposure versus exposures of mature animals in some cases, no tumors from perinatal exposure, no enhanced effect, and different tumors from perinatal exposure versus adult exposure. These variations are likely a result of the differences in the MOAs of these chemicals and the pharmacokinetic differences in doses during different periods of life. At the present time, the available studies covering chemicals acting through nonmutagenic MOAs are not sufficient to develop age dependent adjustment factors for these other MOAs. The available data suggest, however, that other MOAs warrant further research and analysis as well as new toxicity testing protocols that consider early life-stage dosing.

Integrative Analysis of Cancer and Noncancer Health Effects

In evaluating health risks posed by environmental agents, EPA considers both cancer and noncancer effects. Some of the noncancer effects specifically considered are developmental and reproductive toxicity, neurotoxicity, immunotoxicity, and respiratory toxicity, as well as systemic organ toxicities. Historically, assessments have been done separately and very differently for cancer and noncancer health effects. An important new direction is to harmonize approaches to cancer and non-cancer assessments. The National Academy of Sciences (12) noted the importance of an approach that is less fragmented, more consistent in application of similar concepts, and more holistic than separate end point–specific approaches.

EPA's revised cancer guidelines emphasize the importance of understanding a chemical's MOA in characterizing risk. In recent years, research efforts have identified many toxicological responses that are not unique to a particular end point but are common across various noncancer effects as well as carcinogenicity. For example, chemically induced toxicity can cause cell death. Surviving cells may then compensate for that injury by increasing cell proliferation (hyperplasia), which may underlie many types of toxic responses. If this proliferative activity continues unchecked, it may result in tumors. Chemicals may modulate or alter gene expression via receptor interactions. Thus, receptor-mediated pathways may play a role in both carcinogenesis and other organ system toxicities. For example, 2,3,7,8-tetrachlorodibenzo-p-dioxin and dioxin-like compounds bind to the *Ah* receptor, which may represent the first step in a series of events leading to cellular and tissue changes in normal biological processes. Thus, dioxin (and dioxin-like compounds) may exert its carcinogenic, immunological, and reproductive effects via *Ah* receptor-dependent events (56–58).

It is generally felt that through a better understanding of various MOAs and the extension of the MOA framework for cancer to noncancer end points that assessors will be better positioned to apply an integrative set of principles to all risk assessments. This advance will help not only in hazard characterization through identification of common precursors and key events in the causal chain leading to toxicity but also in the quantification of risk through selection of an appropriate point of departure (POD) [e.g., benchmark dose (BMD)] for low-dose extrapolation that reflects not only the full range of toxicities but also a dose-response relationship that is driven by an understanding of the underlying MOA rather than whether the effect is merely carcinogenicity or some noncancer end point.

DOSE-RESPONSE ASSESSMENT/DOSE-RESPONSE CHARACTERIZATION

Historically, dose-response assessment has been done very differently for cancer and non-cancer health effects. For nearly two decades, EPA modeled tumor risk by a default approach based on the assumption of low-dose linearity. To estimate human cancer risk, the linearized multistage model was applied, which extrapolates risk as the 95% upper-bound confidence interval (1,59,60). The standard practice for noncancer health assessment assumed the existence of a nonlinear dose-response curve for adverse effects. Acceptable exposures for chemicals causing noncancer effects have been estimated by applying uncertainty factors (UFs) to a determined *no-observed-adverse-effect level* (NOAEL), which is the highest dose at which no adverse effects have been detected. If a NOAEL cannot be established, then a *lowest-observed-adverse-effect level* (LOAEL) is determined for the critical effect. The UFs may be as much as 10 each and are intended to account for limitations in the available data, such as human variation, interspecific differences, lack of chronic data, or lack of certain other critical data. In the reference concentration (RfC) method, the composite UF for interspecific differences is three because of dosimetric adjustments (61,62). The NOAEL (or LOAEL) is divided by UFs to establish a reference dose (RfD) for oral exposures or a RfC for inhalation exposures, which is an estimate (with uncertainty spanning perhaps an order of magnitude) of daily exposure (RfD) and continuous exposure (RfC) that is likely to be without an appreciable risk of deleterious effects during a lifetime (61–65). The RfDs and RfCs are not derived using composite UFs greater than 3000. Alternatively, the NOAEL can be compared with the human exposure estimate to derive a margin of exposure (MOE).

Modeling in the Range of Observation for Both Cancer and Noncancer Risk

EPA human health risk assessment practices are beginning to come together. The modeling of observed response data to identify points of departure in a standard way, will help to harmonize cancer and noncancer dose-response approaches and permit comparisons of cancer and noncancer risk estimates.

Benchmark Dose Approach

The traditional NOAEL approach for noncancer risk assessment has often been a source of controversy and has been criticized in several ways. For example, experiments involving fewer animals tend to produce larger NOAELs and, as a consequence, may produce larger RfDs or RfCs. The reverse would seem more appropriate in a regulatory context because larger experiments should provide greater evidence of safety. The focus of the NOAEL approach is only on the dose that is the NOAEL, and the NOAEL must be one of the experimental doses. Moreover, it also ignores the shape of the dose-response curve. Thus, the slope of the dose-response curve plays little role in determining acceptable exposures for human beings. These and other limitations prompted development of the alternative approach of applying UFs to a BMD rather than to a NOAEL (66). Essentially, the BMD approach fully uses all of the experimental data to fit one or more dose-response curves for critical effects that are, in turn, used to estimate a BMD that is typically not far below the range of the observed data. The BMD approach allows for a more objective approach in developing allowable human exposures across different study designs encountered in non-cancer risk assessment.

The BMD is defined as a statistical lower confidence limit (CL) on the dose producing a predetermined level of change in adverse response (BMR) compared with the response in untreated animals (66). The choice of the BMR is critical. For quantal end points, a particular level of response is chosen (1%, 5%, or 10%). For continuous end points, the BMR is the degree of change from controls and is based on what is considered a biologically significant change. The methods of CL calculation and choice of CL (90%, 95%) are also critical. The choice of extra risk vs. additional risk is based to some extent on assumptions about whether an agent is adding to the background risk. Extra risk is viewed as the default because it is more conservative. Several RfCs and a RfD based on the BMD approach are included in EPA's Integrated Risk Information System database[a]. These include methylmercury based on delayed postnatal development in humans, carbon disulfide based on neurotoxicity, 1, 1, 1, 2-tetrafluoroethane based on testicular effects in rats, and antimony trioxide based on chronic pulmonary interstitital inflammation in female rats. It should be noted that the BMD approach is still under discussion and development, including for modeling cancer dose-response curves for cancer assessments supported by a nonlinear MOA (66–69).

---

[a] IRIS can be accessed via the Internet at http://www.epa.gov/iris.

Two-Step Process for Cancer Dose-Response Assessment

The principle underlying EPA's current approach to dose-response assessment is to use approaches that include as much information as possible. The preferred approach is to use a biologically based dose-response model. Biologically based modeling is potentially the most comprehensive way to account for the biological processes involved in a response. Such models seek to reflect the sequence of key precursor events that lead to cancer. These models can contribute to dose-response assessment by revealing and describing relationships between internal dose and cancer response. Because the parameters of these models require extensive data, it is anticipated that the necessary data to support these models will not be available for most chemicals and that modeling in the observed range will probably be done most often with an empirical curve-fitting approach. EPA applies a two-step process that distinguishes between what is known (i.e., the observed range of data) and what is not known (i.e., the range of extrapolation) (2,13).

The first step involves modeling response data in the empirical range of observation (Fig. 3) to establish a POD near the lower end of the observed range. The POD is used as the starting point for subsequent extrapolations and analyses. For linear extrapolation, the POD is used to calculate a *slope factor*, and for nonlinear extrapolation the POD is used in the calculation of a RfD or RfC. In a risk characterization, the POD is part of the determination of a MOE. The lowest POD is used that is adequately supported by the data. If the POD is above some data points, it can fail to reflect the shape of the dose-response curve at the lowest doses and can introduce bias into subsequent extrapolations. On the other hand, if the POD is far below all observed data points, it can introduce model uncertainty and

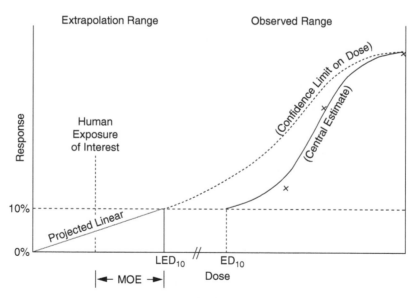

Figure 3 Dose-response assessment: the dose-response assessment of cancer and noncancer end points is to begin with modeling response data in the observable range (2,66). The dose-response assessment is a two-step process; in the first step, response data are modeled in the range observation, and in the second step, the POD below the range observation is determined. The LED_{10} (effective dose corresponding to the lower 95% limit on a dose associated with 10% increase in response) is suggested as the POD for extrapolation to the origin as the linear default or for a reference dose and/or margin of exposure analyses as the nonlinear default. *Abbreviations*: POD, point of departure; MOE, margin of exposure. *Source*: From Ref. 2.

parameter uncertainty that increase with the distance between the data and the POD. Use of a POD at the lowest level supported by the data seeks to balance these considerations. It uses information from the model(s) a small distance below the observed range rather than discarding this information and using extrapolation procedures in a range where the model(s) can provide some useful information. The POD for extrapolating the relationship to environmental exposure levels of interest, when the latter are outside the range of observed data, is generally the lower 95% CL on the lowest dose level that can be supported for modeling by the data. When tumor data are used, a POD is obtained from the modeled tumor incidences. Conventional cancer bioassays, with approximately 50 animals per group, generally can support modeling down to an increased incidence of 1–10%; epidemiologic studies, with larger sample sizes, below 1%. Various models commonly used for carcinogens yield similar estimates of the POD at response levels as low as 1%. Consequently, response levels at or below 10% can often be used as the POD. As a modeling convention, the lower bound on the doses associated with standard response levels of 1%, 5%, and 10% can be analyzed, presented, and considered. For making comparisons at doses within the observed range, a standard POD is suggested as the lower 95% CL on a dose associated with 10% extra risk (LED_{10}).

The Range of Extrapolation for Cancer Risk

The second step involves extrapolation below the range of observation (Fig. 4). The purpose of low-dose extrapolation is to provide as much information as possible about risk in the range of doses below the observed data. As mentioned earlier, a biologically based or case-specific model is preferred for extrapolating low-dose risk. If the available data do not permit such approaches, the cancer guidelines provide for several default extrapolation

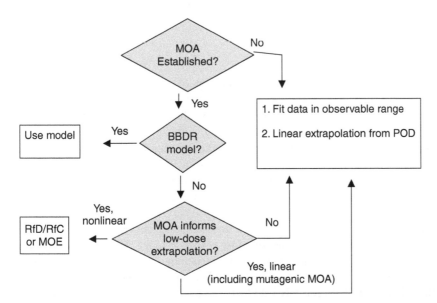

Figure 4 Extrapolation below the range of observation. There are several possible ways to extrapolate from the observed data to the lower doses humans will presumably experience: use of a biologically based dose-response model (if data are available), a linear approach (if the data indicate a linear response, or as a default if no data are available), a nonlinear approach (if the data indicate this), or both linear and nonlinear approaches (if both are plausible).

approaches (linear, nonlinear, or both), which begin with the POD. The approach for extrapolation below the observed data considers the understanding of the agent's MOA at each tumor site. MOA information can suggest the likely shape of the dose-response curve at lower doses. *Linear extrapolation* should be used when there are MOA data to indicate that the dose-response curve is expected to have a linear component below the POD. When the weight of evidence evaluation of all available data are insufficient to establish the MOA for a tumor site and when scientifically plausible based on the available data, linear extrapolation is used as a default approach, because linear extrapolation generally is considered to be a health-protective approach.

A *nonlinear approach* should be selected when there are sufficient data to ascertain the MOA and conclude that it is not linear at low doses *and* the agent does not demonstrate mutagenic or other activity consistent with linearity at low doses. For cases where the tumors arise through a nonlinear MOA, an oral RfD or an inhalation RfC, or both, are developed in accordance with EPA's established practice for developing such values. This approach expands the past focus of such reference values (previously reserved for effects other than cancer) to include carcinogenic effects determined to have a nonlinear MOA. As with other health effects of concern, it is important to put cancer in perspective with the overall health impact of an exposure by comparing reference value calculations for cancer with those for other health effects.

Both linear and nonlinear approaches may be used when there are multiple MOAs. If there are multiple tumor sites, one with a linear and another with a nonlinear MOA, then the corresponding approach is used at each site. If there are multiple MOAs at a single tumor site, one linear and another nonlinear, then both approaches are used to decouple and consider the respective contributions of each MOA in different dose ranges. For example, an agent can act predominantly through cytotoxicity at high doses and through mutagenicity at lower doses where cytotoxicity does not occur. Modeling to a low response level can be useful for estimating the response at doses where the high-dose MOA would be less important.

Modeling of Precursor Response Data

The EPA Cancer Guidelines (2) encourage modeling of not only tumor data in the observable range but also other responses thought to be important precursor events in the carcinogenic process (e.g., DNA adducts, gene or chromosomal mutation, cellular proliferation, hyperplasia, hormonal or physiological disturbances, receptor binding). The modeling of important precursor response data makes extrapolation based on default procedures, discussed earlier, more meaningful by providing insights into the relationships of exposure and tumor response below the observable range. In addition, modeling of nontumor data may provide support for selecting a certain extrapolation procedure (linear vs. nonlinear). If the nontumor end point is believed to be part of a continuum that leads to tumors, such data could then be used to extend the dose-response curve below the observed tumor response to provide insight into the low-dose response range. For example, studies using DNA adducts can be conducted with doses overlapping with the observed tumors down to environmental exposure levels. Several studies have demonstrated the merit of examining the relationship between DNA adduct concentration and tumor incidence for more accurate low-dose extrapolations (70). However, when using DNA adducts (as a dosimeter) to extend the observable range, it is important to have a reasonable understanding of the target cell and the adduct involved in the carcinogenic process. In addition, changes in cell proliferation rates can cause a steep upward curvature of the dose-response curve, and thus need to be factored into the evaluation of risk (71). The role of cell proliferation in changing the cancer dose-response curve has been shown for 2-acetylaminofluorene for bladder tumors (72) and for formaldehyde for nasal tumors (36).

Precursor response data may be modeled and used for extrapolation instead of the available tumor data. Currently, it is not anticipated that precursor response data will be used in lieu of tumor data for many compounds because of the more stringent conditions that must be demonstrated. To be acceptable for extrapolation, the MOA and the role the precursor event plays in the carcinogenic process must be understood. Furthermore, the precursor response should be considered to be more informative of the agent's carcinogenic risk. Precursor data should be from in vivo experiments and from repeat dosing experiments over an extended period of time: precursor data are most valuable if they are built into the design of the cancer bioassay. It is anticipated that the modeling of precursor response data will come into play predominantly for the nonlinear default approach, which must be based on a reasonable understanding of the agent's MOA in causing tumors. The most likely situations for which precursor response data are used to estimate risk involve those mechanisms for which tumor development is secondary to toxicity or disruption of a physiological process. For example, hyperplasia might be used in lieu of tumor data to extrapolate risk for a bladder carcinogen that causes calculi to form in the urine, or TSH levels might be used for a thyroid carcinogen that perturbs hypothalamus-pituitary-thyroid homeostasis. Alterations in TSH or thyroid hormone levels may result in other disease consequences. Early responses in the continuum of events that lead to organ pathology or resultant diseases, such as liver enzyme changes and liver histopathology, respiratory irritation, and respiratory tract damage, have been a consideration in noncancer risk assessment (64). Thus, the consideration of precursor response data in health risk assessment is not a new concept.

EMERGING DIRECTIONS IN EXPOSURE ASSESSMENT

Exposure is defined as the contact of a chemical, physical, or biological agent with the outer boundary of an organism (7). Application of exposure data to the field of risk assessment has grown in importance since the early 1970s because of greater public, academic, industrial, and government awareness of chemical pollution problems in the environment. In environmental health assessment one attempts to address the question of how many people are exposed to a pollutant and to how much. Information about the distribution of exposure to determine the causes of exposures for high-risk groups is a key element in the development of cost-effective mitigation strategies. In addition, information is needed on body burden and related factors in the general population to provide a baseline for interpreting the public health significance of measured exposures from site- or source-specific investigations. For example, body burden levels of environmental pollutants can put people near the linear part of the dose-response curve, even for a dose-response curve that is nonlinear.

In the past several years, aggregate exposure, the assessment of chemical mixtures, and cumulative risk have taken on increased importance, as evidenced by such reports as the NRC's *Pesticides in the Diets of Infants and Children* (54) and *Science and Judgment in Risk Assessment* (12), the National Academy of Public Administration's *Setting Priorities, Getting Results* (73), and the Presidential/Congressional Commission on Risk Assessment and Risk Management's *Risk Assessment and Risk Management in Regulatory Decision-Making* (74). In addition, recent U.S. legislation has mandated consideration of cumulative risk and variability factors in the risk characterization process. Specifically, the Food Quality Protection Act of 1996 (FQPA) (75) directs EPA in its assessments of pesticide safety to focus, in part, on the cumulative effects of pesticides that have a common mechanism of toxicity, considering aggregate dietary and non-occupational pathways of exposure.

Aggregate Exposure

Aggregate exposure refers to the combined exposures to a single chemical across multiple routes (oral, inhalation, and dermal) and across multiple pathways (food, drinking water, residential) (76). In the past, regulatory risk assessments have oftentimes focused on a single pathway or a single exposure route in setting environmental standards or approving product registrations. Increasingly, assessments are attempting to characterize risk across multiple exposure routes and pathways by not treating exposures from different pathways as independent events but rather as a series of sequential or concurrent events that may overlap or be linked in time and space.

The basic concept underlying aggregate exposure is that exposure occurs on an individual-by-individual basis. Estimates of an individual's exposure are developed to reflect consistent spatial, temporal, and behavioral and demographic characteristics and to move closer to describing the pattern of exposure actually encountered by individuals in the real world. The assessor builds the aggregate exposure assessment by focusing first on the individual and then a population of individuals. Generally, the aggregate exposure assessment begins with the identification of the toxicological end points of concern, proceeds toward the identification of possible exposure scenarios, assigns certain toxicological end points for each route of exposure, and, finally, defines a series of hypothetical, potentially exposed individuals by bringing together data sets or a series of professional judgments relating to the aggregate exposure assessment under consideration. Exposure scenarios are constructed to be internally consistent as to their temporal, spatial, and demographic characteristics. Each of the pathway analyses (e.g., food, drinking water, and residential) are linked to individual behavior patterns which are subsequently aggregated into a population-based approach.

Aggregate exposure techniques are in a state of transition and will require new ways to frame the data and to combine data from existing sources. Increasingly, assessors are turning to probabilistic techniques to replace deterministic estimates of exposure that should result in a better sense of the variability and uncertainty in such assessments.

Exposure to Mixtures

Mixtures risk assessments move beyond single chemical assessments (8,77). Mixtures are defined as any combination of two or more chemical substances, regardless of source or of spatial and temporal proximity, that can influence the risk of chemical toxicity in the target population. In some situations the mixtures are highly complex, consistently of scores of compounds that are generated simultaneously as by-products from a single source, e.g., coke oven emissions. In other cases, complex mixtures of related compounds are produced as a commercial product, e.g., PCBs. Another possibility consists of compounds, often unrelated chemically, that are present in the same geographical area that can result in combined exposures to humans.

Mixtures risk assessments usually involve substantial uncertainties, and although the problems have been recognized for a long time, advancement in the capability to assess mixtures has been slow. Studies of chemical mixtures have been carried out for decades, but most have been with simple binary mixtures of commercial chemicals rather than the complex mixtures typical of real world environmental conditions. Nevertheless, advances are being made in the area of research, toxicity testing, and guidance to risk assessors. When toxicity data on the mixture of concern are available, the preferred approach is to use these data directly. When toxicity data on the mixture of concern are not available, assessors will attempt to use data on a "sufficiently similar" mixture. Finally, when neither data set is available, the approach is generally to evaluate the mixture through an analysis of its individual components, assuming dose addition for similarly acting chemicals and response addition for independently acting chemicals.

Currently, chemical mixtures assessment is most focused on developing methodologies for chemicals that share a common MOA. Grouping of chemicals by a common MOA requires that each chemical produces a common toxic effect by the same, or essentially the same, sequence of biochemical events and that each chemical assigned to the group affects the same target site. A weight of evidence approach is generally utilized in establishing a common MOA where considerations are made concerning: common toxic effect (e.g., route specificity; species, sex, or strain differences; site and nature of effect), pharmacokinetics (e.g., metabolites), and pharmacodynamics (e.g., dose-response relationships).

Additivity, applied as dose addition to account for interactions, is the default assumption for estimating the toxicity of a mixture of chemicals acting through a common MOA. Under dose addition, the general procedure is to scale the doses of the components by their relative potency and add the scaled doses together. There are three approaches to dose addition that have commonly been used: relative potency factors (RPFs), toxicity equivalence factors (TEFs), and the hazard index (HI) (77). RPFs have been utilized in the case of organophosphates, TEFs have been used in the case of dioxins, furans, and some PCBs, and HIs have been used in a variety of other, less robust situations.

Cumulative Exposure

Ongoing development in the areas of aggregate exposure and chemical mixtures assessment is contributing to progress in formulating and conducting cumulative risk assessments. Cumulative risk assessment is defined as an analysis, characterization, and possible quantification of the combined risks from multiple agents or stressors (78). Although an assessment of a chemical mixture whose components operate through a common MOA is one form of a cumulative risk assessment, cumulative risk assessment recognizes that there is no limitation that chemicals of concern must act through a common MOA or that the "agents or stressors" be only chemicals. The possibility of combined effects from different types of stressors makes cumulative risk assessment different from many assessments commonly conducted today. Cumulative risk assessments may not always be quantitative because of the paucity of currently available techniques to combine disparate stressor types. Because cumulative risk assessments recognize that there can be a multitude of stressors acting on a population, there is increased emphasis on the specific populations potentially affected rather than on hypothetical individuals. Citizen concerns over a possible excess of cancers, birth defects, or other diseases in a particular community—as well as concerns over disparities of risk among various population subgroups, e.g., environmental justice cases focused on disparities in exposure of minority subgroups to pollutants—has emphasized the important role of cumulative risk assessment in answering the questions and issues being raised by the public.

Challenges posed by a multiple stressor, population based approach can be daunting, even if only a few of the stressors affecting a population are evaluated together. Cumulative risk issues are helping to focus research activities. Ongoing activities are being focused on improving understanding of the interactions among chemicals and are seeking to identify toxicologic principles of joint action that are applicable to mixtures involving many chemicals. Another focus is the development of biomarkers and biomonitoring techniques that are capable of addressing a diversity of stressors. Vulnerability of a population can be thought of as including susceptibility of individuals, differential exposures, differential preparedness to withstand the insult, and differential ability to recover. How these various factors interact to determine outcomes is poorly understood. Finally, research on how to combine disparate measures of risk and to create meaningful measures of cumulative risk is only in the early stages of development.

RISK CHARACTERIZATION

Risk assessment is an integrative process that culminates ultimately in a risk characterization, i.e., risk characterization is the final, integrative step of risk assessment. As defined in EPA's Risk Characterization Policy [see in USEPA (79)], *the risk characterization integrates information from the preceding components of the risk assessment and synthesizes an overall conclusion about risk that is complete, informative, and useful for decision makers.* In essence, a risk characterization conveys the risk assessor's judgment as to the nature and existence of (or lack of) human health risk(s). This component of the risk assessment process characterizes the data in nontechnical terms, explaining the key issues and conclusions of each component of the risk assessment and the rationale, strengths, and limitations of the data and the conclusions. Risk characterization is the product of risk assessment that is used in risk management decisions. The current emphasis on risk characterization is demonstrated in publications by EPA and the NRC (79,80).

For an integrative risk characterization, an *overall* risk characterization incorporates each individual characterization written for the other separate components of the risk assessment. For cancer risk, the individual characterizations accompany the hazard identification, dose-response assessment, and exposure assessment sections as described earlier. These separate, component characterizations carry forward the key findings, assumptions, strengths, and limitations, etc. (Table 3 for elements of a risk characterization to consider) for each section and provide a fundamental set of information used in an *integrative analysis* that must be conveyed in the final overall risk characterization.

Table 3   Elements of a Risk Characterization

Key information
Context
Sensitive subpopulations
Scientific assumptions
Policy choices
Variability
Uncertainty
Bias and perspective
Strengths and weaknesses
Key conclusions
Alternatives considered
Research needs

Source: From Ref. 79.

Table 4   Representative Default Assumptions for Cancer Risk Assessment

When cancer effects in exposed humans are attributed to exposure to an agent, the default option is that the resulting data are predictive of cancer in any other exposed human population

When cancer effects are not found in an exposed human population, this information by itself is not generally sufficient to conclude that the agent poses no carcinogenic hazard to this or other populations of potentially exposed humans, including susceptible subpopulations or lifestages

Positive effects in animal cancer studies indicate that the agent under study can have carcinogenic potential in humans

In general, although effects seen at the highest dose tested are assumed to be appropriate for assessment, it is necessary that the experimental conditions be scrutinized

When cancer effects are not found in well-conducted animal cancer studies in two or more appropriate species and other information does not support the carcinogenic potential of the agent, these data provide a basis for concluding that the agent is not likely to possess human carcinogenic potential, in the absence of human data to the contrary

The default is to include benign tumors observed in animal studies in the assessment of animal tumor incidence, if such tumors have the capacity to progress to the malignancies with which they are associated

The default option is that there is a similarity of the basic pathways of metabolism and the occurrence of metabolites in tissues in regard to the species-to-species extrapolation of cancer hazard and risk

An agent that causes internal tumors by one route of exposure will be carcinogenic by another route if it is absorbed by the second route to give an internal dose

A linear extrapolation approach is used when the mode of action information is supportive of linearity or mode of action is not understood

When adequate data on mode of action provide sufficient evidence to support a nonlinear mode of action for the general population and/or any subpopulations of concern, a different approach—a reference dose/reference concentration that assumes that nonlinearity—is used

Source: From Ref. 2.

In addition to the key findings and other points mentioned above, the risk characterization should also identify where science policy choices were made (e.g., use of default assumptions) and identify where uncertainties exist as well as the conclusions of the risk assessment. This includes the conclusions of the MOA analysis, how the data were considered based on the cancer assessment guidelines, and the uncertainty analyses. Because each risk assessment will be unique, professional judgment will be a necessary part of every assessment. However, the process of examining the data, utilizing the guidelines, presenting the analyses, and writing the risk characterization should be transparent, clear, consistent, and reasonable to anyone who wants to follow or examine the risk assessment.

While working through the various steps of the risk assessment paradigm, data gaps and research needs will become evident. To complete the risk characterization, a decision is usually made whether to pursue additional data because the data gap is deemed critical enough to complete the risk characterization or to invoke default assumptions to allow the risk characterization to be completed. If default assumptions are invoked, this needs to be made very clear in the risk characterization where they were invoked (17,79). Some of the major default assumptions used in cancer risk assessment are outlined in the EPA Cancer Guidelines (Table 4 for representative list of default assumptions).

SUMMARY

Compared with traditional approaches to health risk assessment, ongoing activities to assess the risk of environmental agents are including a more complete discussion of the issues and an evaluation of all relevant information, promoting the use of MOA information to reduce the uncertainties associated with using experimental data to characterize and project how human beings will respond to certain exposure conditions. This emphasis on mechanisms is to promote research and testing to improve the scientific basis of health risk assessment and stimulate thinking on how such information can be applied. As the science continues to evolve, the practice and policies of risk assessment will reflect these advances.

ACKNOWLEDGMENTS

The authors wish to acknowledge two of the authors of the previous version of this chapter, Drs. Vicki Dellarco and Jeanette Wiltse, for their initial insightful writing. We have used the previous version as the main basis for this updated explanation of EPA's incorporation of new scientific analysis approaches as issued in EPA's new *Guidelines for Carcinogen Risk Assessment*.

REFERENCES

1. USEPA (U.S. Environmental Protection Agency). Guidelines for carcinogen risk assessment. Fed Regist 1986; 51:33992–34003.
2. USEPA (U.S. Environmental Protection Agency), Guidelines for carcinogen risk assessment, U.S. Environmental Protection Agency, Risk Assessment Forum, Washington DC, EPA Publication No. EPA/630/P-03/001F (2005). Available online at http://www.epa.gov/cancerguidelines.
3. USEPA (U.S. Environmental Protection Agency). Guidelines for mutagenicity risk assessment. Fed Regist 1986; 51:34006–340012.
4. USEPA (U.S. Environmental Protection Agency). Guidelines for developmental toxicity risk assessment (notice). Fed Regist 1992; 56:63798–63826.
5. USEPA (U.S. Environmental Protection Agency). Reproductive toxicity risk assessment guidelines. Fed Reg 1996; 61:56274–56322.
6. USEPA (U.S. Environmental Protection Agency), Guidelines for neurotoxicity risk assessment. U.S. Environmental Protection Agency, Risk Assessment Forum, Washington, DC, EPA Publication No.630/R-95/001F (1998).
7. USEPA (U.S. Environmental Protection Agency). Guidelines for exposure assessment (notice). Fed Regist 1991; 57:22888–22896.
8. USEPA (U.S. Environmental Protection Agency). Guidelines for the health risk assessment of chemical mixtures. Fed Regist 1986; 51:34014–34025.
9. USEPA (U.S. Environmental Protection Agency), Environmental Health Threats to Children, EPA 175F-96-001, Office of the Administrator, U.S. Environmental Protection Agency, Washington, DC (1996).
10. USEPA (U.S. Environmental Protection Agency), Supplemental guidance for assessing susceptibility from early-life exposure to carcinogens, Risk Assessment Forum, National Center for Environmental Assessment, Washington, DC (2005) Available online at http://www.epa.gov/cancerguidelines.
11. NRC (National Research Council). Risk assessment in the federal government: managing the process. Committee on the Institutional Means for Assessment of Risks to Public Health, Commission on Life Sciences, NRC. Washington, DC: National Academy Press, 1983.
12. NRC (National Research Council). Science and judgment in risk assessment. Committee on Risk Assessment of Hazardous Air Pollutants. Commission on Life Sciences, National Research Council. Washington, DC: National Academy Press, 1994.

13. Wiltse J, Dellarco VL. The U.S. Environmental Protection Agency guidelines for carcinogen risk assessment: past and future. Mutat Res 1996; 365:3–16.

14. IPCS (International Programme on Chemical Safety), IPCS workshop on developing a conceptual framework for cancer risk assessment, February 16-18, 1999, Lyon, France. IPCS/99.6. World Health Organization, Geneva.

15. Sonich-Mullin C, Fielder R, Wiltse J, et al. International Programme on Chemical Safety IPCS conceptual framework for evaluating a mode of action for chemical carcinogenesis. Regul Toxicol Pharmacol 2001; 34:146–152.

16. IPCS (International Programme on Chemical Safety), Draft IPCS framework for analyzing the relevance of a cancer mode of action for humans (2005). http://www.who.int/ipcs/methods/harmonization/areas/cancer_framework/en/index.html.

17. USEPA (U.S. Environmental Protection Agency), An Examination of EPA Risk Assessment Principles and Practices, U.S. Environmental Protection Agency, Office of the Science Advisor, Publication No. EPA/100/B-04/001 (2004).

18. Swenberg JA, Short B, Borghoff S, Strasser J, Charbonneau M. The comparative pathobiology of α_{2u}-globulin nephropathy. Toxicol Appl Pharmacol 1989; 97:35–46.

19. Lehman-McKeeman LD, Rivera-Torres MI, Caudill D. Lysosomal degradation of α_{2u}-globulin and α_{2u}-globulin-xenobiotic conjugates. Toxicol Appl Pharmacol 1990; 103:539–548.

20. Dietrich DR, Swenberg JA. The presence of α_{2u}-globulin is necessary for d-limonene promotion of male rat kidney tumors. Cancer Res 1991; 51:3512–3521.

21. USEPA (U.S. Environmental Protection Agency), Alpha 2u-Globulin: association with chemically induced renal toxicity and neoplasia in the male rat, Risk Assessment Forum, Washington, DC, EPA Publication No. EPA/625/3-91/019f (1991).

22. Melnick RL, Kohn MC, Portier CJ. Implications for risk assessment of suggested nongenotoxic mechanisms of chemical carcinogenesis. Environ Health Perspect 1996; 104:123–134.

23. Hill RN, Erdreich LS, Paynter OE, et al. Review: thyroid follicular cell carcinogenesis. Fundam Appl Toxicol 1989; 12:629–697.

24. McClain RM. The significance of hepatic microsomal enzyme induction and altered thyroid function in rats: implications for thyroid gland neoplasia. Toxicol Pathol 1989; 17:294–306.

25. McClain RM. Thyroid gland neoplasia: non-genotoxic mechanisms. Toxicol Lett 1992; 64/65:397–408.

26. USEPA (U.S. Environmental Protection Agency), Assessment of thyroid follicular cell tumors, U.S. Environmental Protection Agency, Washington, DC, EPA Publication No. EPA/630/R-97/002 (1998).

27. McClain RM. The use of mechanistic data in cancer risk assessment: case example—sulfonamides. In: Olin S, Farland W, Park C, et al. eds. Low-Dose Extrapolation of Cancer Risks: Issues and Perspectives. Washington, DC: ILSl Press, 1995:163–173.

28. Cohen SM, Ellwein LB. Genetic errors, cell proliferation and carcinogenesis. Cancer Res 1991; 51:6493–6505.

29. USEPA (U.S. Environmental Protection Agency). Melamine: toxic chemical release reporting. Fed Regist 1988; 53:23128–23132.

30. Kerns WD, Pavkov KL, Donofrio DJ, Gralla EJ, Swenberg JA. Carcinogenicity of formaldehyde in rats and mice after long-term inhalation exposure. Cancer Res 1983; 43:4382–4392.

31. Hernandez O, Rhomberg L, Hogan K, et al. Risk assessment of formaldehyde. J Hazard Mater 1994; 39:161–172.

32. Casanova M, Morgan KT, Steinhagen WH, Everitt JI, Popp JA, Heck Hd'A. Covalent binding of inhaled formaldehyde to DNA in the respiratory tract of rhesus monkeys: pharmacokinetics, rat-to-monkey interspecies scaling, and extrapolation to man. Fundam Appl Toxicol 1991; 17:409–428.

33. Casanova M, Morgan KT, Gross EA, Moss OR, Heck Hd'A. DNA-protein cross-links and cell replication at specific sites in the nose of F344 rats exposed subchronically to formaldehyde. Fundam Appl Toxicol 1994; 23:525–536.

34. Heck Hd'A, Casanova M, Starr TB. Formaldehyde toxicity—new understanding. Crit Rev Toxicol 1990; 20:397–426.

35. Monticello TM, Swenberg JA, Gross EA, et al. Correlation of regional and nonlinear formaldehyde-induced nasal cancer with proliferating populations of cells. Cancer Res 1996; 56:1012–1022.

36. Conolly RB, Kimbell JS, Janszen D, et al. Biologically motivated computational modeling of formaldehyde carcinogenicity in the F344 rat. Toxicol Sci 2003; 75:432–447.

37. Conolly RB, Kimbell JS, Janszen D, et al. Human respiratory tract cancer risks of inhaled formaldehyde: dose-response predictions derived from biologically-motivated computational modeling of a combined rodent and human dataset. Toxicol Sci 2004; 82:279–296.

38. Hauptmann M, Lubin JH, Stewart PA, Hayes RB, Blair A. Mortality from lymphohemato-poietic malignancies among workers in formaldehyde industries. J Natl Cancer Inst 2003; 95:1615–1623.

39. Hauptmann M, Lubin JH, Stewart PA, Hayes RB, Blair A. Mortality from solid cancers among workers in formaldehyde industries. Am J Epidemiol 2004; 159:1117–1130.

40. Bogdanffy MS, Dreef-van der Meulen HC, Beems RB, et al. Chronic toxicity and oncogenicity inhalation study with vinyl acetate in the rat and mouse. Fundam Appl Toxicol 1994; 23:215–229.

41. Bogdanffy MS, Tyler TR, Vinegar MB, Capanini KW, Cascieri TC. Chronic toxicity and oncogenicity study with vinyl acetate in the rat: in utero exposure in drinking water. Fundam Appl Toxicol 1994; 23:206–214.

42. Blakley BR. Enhancement of urethane-induced adenoma formation in Swiss mice exposed to methyl mercury. Can J Comp Med 1984; 48:299–302.

43. IARC (International Agency for Research on Cancer). Occupational Exposure to Mists and Vapors from Strong Inorganic Acids and Other Industrial Chemicals. France: Lyon, 1992; 54:237–287.

44. NTP (National Toxicology Program), Toxicology and carcinogenesis studies of 1,3-butadiene in B6C3F1 mice (inhalation), U.S. Department of Health and Human Services, Public Health Service, National Institutes of Health, NTP TR434, NIH Publication No. 92-3165 (1991).

45. Dahl AR, Bechtold WE, Bond JA. Species difference in the metabolism and disposition of inhaled 1,3-butadiene and isoprene. Environ Health Perspect 1990; 86:65–69.

46. Dahl AR, Sun DJ, Birnbaum LS, et al. Toxicokinetics of inhaled 1,3-butadiene in monkeys: comparison to toxicokinetics in rats and mice. Toxicol Appl Pharmacol 1991; 110:9–19.

47. Csanady GA, Guerigerich FP, Bond JA. Comparison of the biotransformation of 1,3-butadiene and its metabolite, butadiene monoepoxide, by hepatic and pulmonary tissue from humans, rats, and mice. Carcinogenesis 1992; 13:1143–1153.

48. Gonzalez FJ. The role of carcinogen-metabolizing enzymes polymorphisms in cancer susceptibility. Reprod Toxicol 1997; 11:397–412.

49. Kihara M, Noda K. Risk of smoking for squamous and small cell carcinomas of the lung modulated by combinations of CYPIAl and GSTMl gene polymorphisms in a Japanese population. Carcinogenesis 1995; 16:2331–2336.

50. Nakachi K, Imai K, Hayashi S, Kawajiri K. Polymorphisms of the CYPIAl and glutathione S-transferase genes associated with susceptibility to lung cancer in relations to cigarette dose in a Japanese population. Cancer Res 1993; 53:2994–2999.

51. Khoury MJ, Gomez-Farias M, Mulinare J. Does maternal cigarette smoking during pregnancy cause cleft lip and palate in offspring? Am J Dis Child 1989; 143:333–337.

52. Ardinger HH, Buetow KH, Bell GI. Association of genetic variation of the transforming growth factor-alpha gene with cleft lip and palate. Am J Hum Genet 1989; 45:348–353.

53. Anderson LM, Diwan BA, Fear NT, et al. Critical windows of exposure for children's health: cancer in human epidemiological studies and neoplasms in experimental animal models. Environ Health Perspect 2000; 108:573–594 (Suppl 3).

54. NRC (National Research Council). Pesticides in the diets of infants and children. Committee on Pesticides in the Diets of Infants and Children. Commission on Life Sciences. Washington, DC: National Academy Press, 1993.

55. Barton HA, Cogliano VJ, Flowers L, Valcovic L, Setzer RW, Woodruff TJ. Assessing susceptibility from early-life exposure to carcinogens. Environ Health Perspect 2005; 113:1125–1133.
56. Kerkvliet NI. Immunotoxicology of dioxin and related chemicals. In: Schecter A, ed. Dioxin and Health. New York: Plenum Press, 1994:199–218.
57. Theobald HM, Person RE. Developmental and reproductive toxicity of dioxin and other Ah receptor agonists. In: Schecter A, ed. Dioxin and Health. New York: Plenum Press, 1994:309–335.
58. USEPA (U.S. Environmental Protection Agency), Exposure and Human Health Reassessment of 2,3,7,8-Tetrachlorodibenzo-p-Dioxin (TCDD) and Related Compounds, National Academy Sciences (NAS) Review Draft, Office of Research and Development, Washington, DC (2003).
59. Crump KS. An improved procedure for low-dose carcinogenic risk assessment from animal data. J Environ Pathol Toxicol 1981; 5:675.
60. Krewski D, Gaylor DW, Lutz WK. Additivity to background and linear extrapolation. In: Olin S, Farland W, Park C, et al. eds. Low-Dose Extrapolation of Cancer Risks: Issues and Perspectives. Washington, DC: ILSI Press, 1995:105–121.
61. Jarabek AM. Interspecies extrapolation based on mechanistic determinants of chemical disposition. J Hum Ecol Risk Assess 1995; 1:641–662.
62. USEPA (U.S. Environmental Protection Agency), Methods for Derivation of Inhalation Reference Concentrations and Application of Inhalation Dosimetry, EPA/600/8-90/066F, Office of Research and Development, Washington, DC (1994).
63. Barnes DG, Dourson ML. Reference dose (RfD): description and use in health risk assessments. Reg Toxicol Pharmacol 1988; 8:471–488.
64. Jarabek AM, Menache MG, Overton JH, Dourson ML, Miller FJ. The U.S. Environmental Protection Agency's inhalation RfD methodology: risk assessment for air toxics. Toxicol Ind Health 1990; 6:279–301.
65. Jarabek AM. The application of dosimetry models to identify key processes and parameters for default dose-response assessment approaches. Toxicol Lett 1995; 79:171–184.
66. USEPA (U.S. Environmental Protection Agency), The Use of the Benchmark Dose Approach in Health Risk Assessment, EPA/630/R-94/007, Office of Research and Development, Washington, DC (1995).
67. Allen BC, Strong PL, Price CJ, Hubbard SA, Daston GP. Benchmark dose analysis of developmental toxicity in rats exposed to boric acid. Fundam Appl Toxicol 1996; 32:194–204.
68. Barnes DG, Daston GP, Evans JS, et al. Benchmark dose workshop: criteria for use of a benchmark dose to estimate a reference dose. Reg Toxicol Pharmacol 1995; 21:296–306.
69. Kavlock RJ, Schmid JE, Setzer RW, Jr. A simulation study of the influences of study design on the estimation of benchmark doses for developmental toxicity. Risk Anal 1996; 16:391–403.
70. La DK, Swenberg JA. DNA adducts: biological markers of exposure and potential applications to risk assessment. Mutat Res 1996; 365:129–146.
71. Chen C, Farland W. Incorporating cell proliferation in quantitative cancer risk assessment: approaches, issues, and uncertainties. In: Butterworth B, Slaga T, Farland W, McClain M, eds. Chemical Induced Cell Proliferation: Implications for Risk Assessment. New York: Wiley Liss, 1991:481–499.
72. Cohen SM, Ellwein LB. Proliferative and genotoxic cellular effects in 2-acetylaminofluorene bladder and liver carcinogenesis: biological modeling of the ED01 study. Toxicol Appl Pharmacol 1990; 104:79–93.
73. NAPA (National Academy of Public Administration), Setting Priorities, Getting Results: A New Direction for EPA, Washington, DC, LCCN 95-68048 (1995).
74. PCCRARM (Presidential/Congressional Commission on Risk Assessment and Risk Management), Risk Assessment and Risk Management in Regulatory Decision-Making, Washington, DC (1997).
75. FQPA (Food Quality Protection Act), PL 104-170, August 3, 1996.

76. USEPA (U.S. Environmental Protection Agency). Guidance for performing aggregate exposure and risk assessments. Fed Regist 2001; 66:59428–59430.
77. USEPA (U.S. Environmental Protection Agency), Supplementary Guidance for Conducting Health Risk Assessment of Chemical Mixtures, Risk Assessment Forum, Office of Research and Development, Washington, DC, EPA/630/R-00-002 (2000).
78. USEPA (U.S. Environmental Protection Agency), Framework for Cumulative Risk Assessment, Risk Assessment Forum, Office of Research and Development, Washington, DC, EPA/630/P-02-001F (2003).
79. USEPA (U.S. Environmental Protection Agency), Risk Characterization Handbook, U.S. Environmental Protection Agency, Science Policy Council, Publication No. EPA 100-B-00-002 (2000).
80. NRC (National Research Council). Understanding risk: informing decisions in a democratic society. Committee on Risk Characterization, Commission on Behavioral and Social Sciences and Education. Washington, DC: National Academy Press, 1996.

16

Nonclinical Safety Testing of Pharmaceuticals

Amy L. Ellis and Kenneth L. Hastings
Office of New Drugs, Center for Drug Evaluation and Research, U.S. Food and Drug Administration, Silver Spring, Maryland, U.S.A.

INTRODUCTION

The principal goals of nonclinical safety testing of pharmaceuticals are to enable the intentional exposure of humans to test compounds and to demonstrate that a proposed drug product is reasonably safe for its intended use. These studies are conducted to determine whether a candidate pharmaceutical can be safely administered to humans and the conditions under which intentional exposure does not present unreasonable risk. Additional goals of toxicology studies with pharmaceuticals are hazard identification (determining the toxic potential of a test compound) and risk assessment (determining the conditions of exposure, including dose, duration, and route) that may produce adverse effects in humans.

Toxicology studies conducted for pharmaceutical development can be divided into three broad categories: (1) screening studies, (2) studies designed to support clinical trials, and (3) studies designed for product registration and labeling. Screening studies are used to choose compounds for further development. These can include pilot experiments not conducted under the Good Laboratory Practice regulations that may not be required to be submitted to regulatory authorities (e.g., in vitro or in vivo screens for specific pharmacologic or toxicologic activities, pilot experiments with such end points as unvalidated genomic biomarkers, etc.). Other studies (e.g., genetic toxicology assays) may function as screening tools but are also needed to support clinical studies with a drug and to write a label for the product. The nonclinical studies designed to support clinical use (both human trials and eventual product registration/labeling) of a proposed drug are of prime regulatory importance. Data from these studies are used to demonstrate that the drug appears reasonably safe for its intended use and to provide information useful in determining the risk/benefit ratio for the drug in the intended clinical population. Examples of studies needed to support clinical trials include acute toxicity and standard short-term repeat-dose toxicity studies, safety pharmacology studies, and genotoxicity tests. Some nonclinical studies conducted to support marketing applications and product labeling are not ethical to conduct in humans (e.g., reproductive toxicity, carcinogenicity), necessitating the use of animal models as surrogates.

This chapter will discuss the animal and in vitro toxicity studies commonly performed to support clinical trials and marketing of new human drug products in the United States. It will refer to a number of guidance documents available through the web site of the Food and Drug Administration's Center for Drug Evaluation and Research (CDER) (1). Many of the studies mentioned here will be necessary for the development of the majority of pharmaceuticals, but some drug products will require a different approach or some additional investigations (including so-called "special" studies that may include local tolerance, addiction liability, phototoxicity, immunotoxicity, and others), depending on individual circumstances. In general, most of the nonclinical study requirements for drug development in the U.S. will be similar to those in Europe and Japan, particularly in light of the ICH (International Conference on Harmonization of Technical Requirements for Registration of Pharmaceuticals for Human Use) guidelines negotiated by representatives from these three major pharmaceutical producing areas of the world. However, the reader should be aware that there are still a few differences between these regions in the exact types and timing of certain studies.

The nonclinical studies conducted to support the clinical testing and use of biologics (e.g., therapeutic proteins and monoclonal antibodies) will necessarily differ from those for the "small molecule" drugs (e.g., chemicals, small peptides, and oligonucleotides) that are the focus of this chapter. It can be challenging to identify animal models for toxicity studies with biologics that are pharmacologically and clinically relevant, and use of nonrelevant species is discouraged as the data can be misleading. For biologics, other testing strategies (e.g., use of surrogate proteins, transgenic animals, animal models of disease) may be used if no relevant animal species are identified. Some studies that are required to demonstrate the safety and toxicity of drugs are not generally necessary for biologics (e.g., standard assays for genotoxicity, biotransformation metabolism studies). The reader is referred to the references (2,3) for more detailed information on the nonclinical safety testing of biologics.

Other chapters in this book discuss the methodology of various toxicology studies in detail, and there are additional references that the reader may find helpful with regard to study conduct. These include a number CDER guidance documents that will be specifically cited below, draft Organization for Economic Cooperation and Development (OECD) guidelines for a variety of tests, and references (4,5), among many.

DIRECTION ON THE TIMING OF TOXICOLOGY STUDIES IN RELATION TO CLINICAL TRIALS

An important aspect of toxicology studies conducted for pharmaceutical development is the concept of timing with respect to clinical trials. A number of screening studies may be conducted to determine which drug candidates are likely to be successfully developed. These are generally referred to as discovery toxicology studies, and they are designed to help sponsors make very early decisions about drug candidate viability. Screening studies may include in vitro cellular toxicity studies, bacterial mutagenicity studies, and acute dose toxicity studies, usually conducted in rodents. The data from these studies rarely have impact on regulatory decisions. Rather, they may function as "gate-keeper" studies and are designed to discover compounds that have unacceptable properties (such as mutagenic potential). Once a candidate drug has been identified, nonclinical studies to support clinical trials are initiated.

Phase 1 clinical studies generally begin with a limited group of human subjects (often healthy volunteers) receiving a single dose of drug. A full package of nonclinical toxicology studies is not necessary to support this type of trial, although certain information is needed to choose a safe starting dose and to demonstrate that the exposure to drug does not present an unreasonable risk. The data that are usually required before the initial human exposure to a drug (Table 1) include information on safety pharmacology (effects of drug on the cardiovascular, nervous, and respiratory systems), some pharmacokinetic (PK) determinations [e.g., area under the curve—an expression of total drug exposure (AUC), and maximum concentration (C_{max})], acute toxicity data in two mammalian species, an assessment of local tolerance using the proposed clinical route of administration, and, at a minimum, in vitro genotoxicity tests for mutations and chromosome damage. Additional genotoxicity testing may be needed before Phase 1 if there are positive or equivocal results. Safety pharmacology testing may not be needed for products with very low systemic absorption or for cytotoxic oncology drugs given to end-stage cancer patients. Genotoxicity testing may not be necessary for oncology drugs from classes known to be mutagenic.

A very important issue in the design of first-in-man studies is the initial dose. CDER has developed guidance on this issue (6). This document provides a detailed, rational approach to using data obtained in nonclinical toxicology studies for setting a safe starting dose in healthy volunteers when a drug has never been administered to humans. There are several essential points to consider. The animal studies conducted to enable initial clinical trials should have included doses that were of a sufficient magnitude to produce toxicity or were a significant multiple ($\sim$100-fold) of any dose that would be considered for administration to humans (such as a maximum feasible dose). A no-observed-adverse-effect level (NOAEL, that is, a dose at which no significant toxicity was observed) should also have been identified in the nonclinical studies. This NOAEL should be converted to an equivalent human dose using an appropriate conversion factor. An appropriate method for dose extrapolation (animal to human) should be used for setting the initial clinical dose. The Guidance advocates the use of relative body surface area as the basis for dose comparisons. This human equivalent dose might be further modified using a safety factor depending on observations, such as the characteristics of toxicity (reversible, monitorable, etc.) and the steepness of the dose/response curve with respect to any dose-limiting toxicity. The animal studies can also be used to estimate a maximum tolerated dose for the test compound. When human PK data become available, clinical exposure can be compared with PK and toxicokinetic (TK) data obtained in animal studies.

As clinical studies proceed, they are often conducted at higher doses of drug and for longer durations; thus, additional nonclinical toxicological information is needed to support clinical testing. Repeated dose toxicity studies in at least two mammalian species (including one nonrodent, e.g., dog, rabbit, swine, primate) that are at least as long as the proposed clinical study (with a minimum of 2 weeks duration) will be necessary. In the case of a drug product that has demonstrated the potential for a significant therapeutic

Table 1 Minimum Nonclinical Data Needed for Most Drug Products Before Initial Human Exposure in the United States

Safety pharmacology	Cardiovascular, central nervous, and respiratory systems
Limited pharmacokinetics	C_{max}, AUC
Acute toxicity	2 mammalian species
Local tolerance	Using proposed route of clinical administration
In vitro genotoxicity	Mutations, chromosome damage

gain, clinical trials may be allowed to proceed for lengths of time beyond the duration of the available animal studies. Data on drug metabolism in animals should be submitted by the time human drug metabolism data are available so that they may be compared and suitability of the animal model can be determined. Prior to the initiation of Phase 2, the remaining studies in the genetic toxicology package must be submitted.

The need for, and timing of, carcinogenicity testing will depend on the properties of the drug, how it will be used in the clinic and for what length of time, and the level of concern regarding human exposure to the product. Results from carcinogenicity studies are not generally needed prior to the initiation of clinical trials. In some cases, the data may be submitted postapproval. Frequently, carcinogenicity data (if required), will be submitted at the time of NDA submission, although in some circumstances it will be needed prior to the initiation of Phase 3 clinical testing (depending on the length of the trial and information available about the drug).

In the United States, reproduction toxicity studies assessing potential drug effects on fertility and embryo-fetal development should be completed before women of childbearing potential are enrolled in Phase 3 studies. A study of pre- and postnatal development should be submitted with the marketing application, unless concerns about the drug product compel earlier submission.

The ICH M3 guidance (7), provides information regarding the timing of the nonclinical study submission to support clinical testing in the U.S., Japan, and Europe. The timing of these data submissions is not identical in the three regions.

STUDIES NEEDED FOR MOST NEW DRUG PRODUCTS

Table 2 provides a list of nonclinical studies that are needed for the majority of new drug products. Animal toxicity studies are usually conducted using the same route of administration that is planned for the clinical trials, as long as adequate systemic exposure of the animals can be achieved using that route. If a compound is to be administered orally or parenterally, it is not generally necessary to test the clinical formulation of the drug, but only the active component, assuming that all excipients have been used in approved products given by the same route of administration for at least an equal duration of therapy. For drug products given via inhalation, or administered directly to the eyes, skin, or ears, it is frequently necessary to use the clinical formulation for animal testing.

Safety pharmacology data are generally needed for all products with significant systemic exposure, with the exception of cytotoxic oncology drugs given to end-stage cancer patients. Such data may not be necessary for compounds that are applied topically (e.g., to skin, eyes, or ears) or, in some cases given orally, but not absorbed. Information regarding a drug's actions on the cardiovascular, respiratory, and central nervous systems

Table 2 Nonclinical Studies Needed for Most New Drug Products

Study	Common test systems[a]
Safety pharmacology core battery	Rats, dogs
Pharmacokinetic/metabolism	Rats
General toxicity (may include acute, subchronic, chronic)	Rats, dogs
Genetic toxicity studies (in vitro/in vivo)	In vitro assays, rodents
Reproduction toxicity studies	Rodents, rabbits

[a]Other species (e.g., primates, swine) may be the best choice under particular circumstances.

is most important. These systems comprise a so-called "core battery" for testing. For some products, data on effects on the renal and gastrointestinal systems is also desirable, especially if the drug will be given to patient populations with special sensitivities to pharmacologic effects on related organs. It is possible to obtain some information on safety pharmacology during the conduct of general toxicity studies, but studies devoted to specific end points may be needed if particular concerns arise. In general, initial monitoring of potential central nervous system (CNS) effects will be conducted in a rodent species using a standard functional observational battery. It is preferred that cardiac and respiratory parameters be measured in conscious animals. Dogs and swine are useful models for cardiovascular testing. Most safety pharmacology experiments that are conducted in vivo are single dose studies, but repeat-dose studies may occasionally be needed. If initial safety pharmacology studies demonstrate a cause for concern, more specialized follow-up studies with more intensive monitoring are necessary. Specific information regarding the timing and necessity of safety pharmacology studies may be found in the ICH S7A document (8).

Pharmacokinetic and metabolism studies are conducted in animal models to elucidate the absorption, distribution, metabolic, and excretion (ADME) profile in animals. When compared with human data, this information may aid in discerning which animal model is most clinically relevant. The majority of PK and metabolism studies are conducted following single doses of drug. Under special circumstances (e.g., compounds that have a long half life, are not completely eliminated from the body, or demonstrate unanticipated toxicity following accumulation), these studies should also be conducted after repeated dosing. Additional details regarding repeat dose PK studies may be found in the ICH S3B document (9).

An issue that occasionally arises in pharmacokinetic studies is *differential metabolism*. It is not unusual for animals to demonstrate quantitative differences in ADME parameters with respect to a given drug. As long as there are no substantial *qualitative* differences in drug metabolism and disposition, it is likely that at least one of the test species will be similar enough to humans that *quantitative* differences will be relatively unimportant. However, there are cases where a biotransformation product (usually assumed to be a metabolite) is observed in humans but has not been seen in any animals used in nonclinical toxicology studies. The type and extent of toxicity testing needed for *unique human metabolites* has been the source of much debate between CDER and sponsors. This has been discussed extensively in the literature (10–12), and CDER is in the process of developing guidance on this issue. The formation of unique human metabolites is a relatively unusual occurrence. When they are observed, sponsors are advised to meet with the appropriate CDER review division concerning the best approach to evaluating the potential toxicity of unique human metabolites. Under most circumstances it is likely that some nonclinical toxicity testing with the unique human metabolite will be needed.

General toxicity studies are conducted to identify and elucidate the undesired effects of drug substances. These may include acute (single dose or repeated doses given within 24 hours), subchronic (<6 months duration), and chronic studies (≥ 6 months duration). Some toxic effects may be an extension of the drug's pharmacologic properties, but others will be unrelated. In an adequate toxicity study, the doses chosen should allow the target organs to be identified and a no-observed-effect level (NOEL) or NOAEL determined. For at least some of the general toxicity studies conducted for a drug, it is useful to include recovery groups that are sacrificed a few weeks after the animals in the main study to provide information as to the reversibility of any toxic effect. Occasionally, some pharmaceuticals may demonstrate little or no toxicity under the conditions of the study. These should be dosed to a maximum feasible level or a level that exceeds clinical exposure (based on PK or TK analysis) by a substantial margin. The intended clinical use and route of administration of a product will influence the conduct of toxicity studies and can compel an expanded evaluation of certain end points. For example, studies of compounds given via inhalation will include an expanded histopathologic evaluation of the respiratory tract, and ophthalmic drug products will require additional evaluation of the eye, compared with most drugs administered via oral or IV routes.

During general toxicity studies, serum or plasma levels of a drug are frequently monitored and its C_{max} and AUC are determined. Metabolites that account for significant exposure and pharmacologic or toxicologic activity may also be monitored, as applicable. This TK assessment allows exposure to be compared to any toxic effects observed in the animals, permitting more precise calculations of NOEL or NOAEL than is possible when one relies only on nominal dose comparisons. For additional information see (13).

Acute toxicity studies may be used to support single dose clinical trials when expanded analyses, including histopathology are performed (14). Data from acute studies may be useful for setting doses for the initial clinical studies as well as multiple dose animal studies. Observations from acute animal toxicity studies may also provide information on toxic effects that may occur following an acute drug overdose.

The length of subchronic and chronic toxicity studies will usually be driven by the duration of clinical trials and the length of use being sought for the marketed product. Longer term animal studies may also be requested to elucidate toxic effects observed in a shorter study. In general, a 6-month chronic toxicity study is acceptable for rodents, and a 9-month study is usually an adequate length for nonrodents (15). Chronic toxicity testing may not be needed for drug products used only for short courses of therapy.

There are, however, several additional issues that should be considered in determining the length of chronic nonrodent toxicology studies. Although under ICH guidelines a 9-month repeat-dose toxicology study is generally considered sufficient to evaluate the safety of a drug that would be administered chronically to humans, under some circumstances this length may not be appropriate. For example, if the drug is the first in its pharmacologic or chemical class, the Agency may request a 12-month repeat-dose nonrodent toxicology study, especially if the size of the clinical safety database is small. This has occurred for drugs developed to treat serious indications that were evaluated under an accelerated approval process. In contrast, a 6-month nonrodent study might be acceptable for a drug belonging to a class that has been well-characterized, especially if dose-limiting toxicities indicate that a 9-month toxicology study would be unlikely to yield additional useful information (e.g., inadequate survival or high probability of early sacrifice).

Genotoxicity tests are used to detect a compound's capacity for inducing genetic damage. Compounds that are positive in these assays are believed to be more likely to cause cancer or heritable mutations than those that are negative. The standard battery of genetic toxicity tests that should be carried out for most drug products includes a bacterial reverse mutation test (e.g., Ames test in *S. typhimurium* and *E. coli*), a mammalian cell assay for chromosome damage (e.g., cytogenetic analysis of chromosome aberrations in cultured cells or mouse lymphoma tk $+/-$ assay), and an in vivo test for chromosome damage to rodent hematopoietic cells (e.g., detection of micronuclei in rodent bone marrow). At times, a test in the standard battery may not be appropriate for a particular drug; in such cases, a different test may be substituted. For example, bacterial mutation assays are not appropriate for some antimicrobial drugs that are robustly toxic to the bacterial species used in these studies, so a mutation assay using mammalian cells might be substituted. The mouse lymphoma tk $+/-$ assay may be a useful substitute in such cases, as it has the capacity to detect point mutations as well as chromosome damage.

As discussed previously, the in vitro assays for mutagenicity and chromosome damage must be submitted prior to the first human exposure to drug, and the remaining study(ies) must be submitted before Phase 2 clinical trials are initiated. Additional genotoxicity data may be requested depending on the results of the standard battery. This could include additional in vitro tests (possibly using a metabolic activation system other than the standard rodent S-9) or in vivo tests measuring genetic damage in target organs or changes in tumor-related genes. The ICH S2A and S2B guidance documents (16,17) may be consulted for further details. Genetic toxicity data are included in the labels of approved drug products.

Reproduction toxicity studies cover adult fertility and reproductive behavior as well as the continuum of development in drug-exposed offspring ranging from conception to sexual maturity (18). Traditionally, these studies have been designed to cover one of three periods: (1) fertility and early embryonic development (to implantation), (2) embryo-fetal development (implantation to closure of hard palate), and (3) pre- and postnatal development, including maternal function (implantation through weaning). However, these data requirements may be fulfilled using a variety of protocols; one study may cover a large number of end points, or a series of smaller studies may be designed to cover shorter windows of development. It is helpful to include the collection of TK data in the design of reproduction toxicity studies, allowing for more precise interspecies exposure comparisons.

Reproduction toxicity studies for drugs are conducted in mammals, with rats being used most frequently. A second species, often the rabbit, is usually needed to evaluate the teratogenic potential of a drug. It is important to set the high dose for reproduction toxicity studies to be large enough to allow for adequate exposure and induction of effects on parents or offspring, without inducing an excessive level of maternal toxicity that may confound study results. Small reductions in maternal body weight gain in the absence of any other drug effect will usually not be considered adequate to limit the high dose in most reproduction toxicity studies. Reproduction toxicity studies may not be needed, or may be limited in scope, for products with no or very low systemic exposure.

Information on adult male and female fertility may also be obtained from general repeat-dose toxicity studies of at least two week's duration. At necropsy, the testes and ovaries are collected, weighed, and examined microscopically, revealing any adverse drug effects following repeated exposure of the tissues. Additional details may be found in the ICH S5B guidance documents (19,20).

Data regarding a product's effects on fertility and the development of offspring exposed to a drug in utero are included in product labeling. Results of studies on embryo-fetal development are used to assign a pregnancy category for the drug label- especially in the absence of human data. When available, data comparing drug exposure in animals to that observed in humans are included in the label.

CARCINOGENICITY TESTING

Carcinogenicity bioassays are usually required for products that are used clinically for more than 6 months. This encompasses chronic intermittent as well as continuous exposures. Other information, including chemical structure/activity data, positive genetic toxicity study results, long-term tissue retention, or the observation of precancerous lesions in animal toxicity studies, may also drive the need for carcinogenicity testing, as will the intended clinical use of the drug and the patient population for which it is indicated.

For example, in some cases, unequivocally positive genotoxicants or members of certain chemical or pharmaceutical classes may be assumed to be carcinogenic and would not need to be tested for carcinogenic potential; approval would depend on risk/benefit analysis. Drug products administered to patients with life expectancies not exceeding 2–3 years will not require carcinogenicity testing. For products that will be given only to patients with serious diseases with limited therapeutic options, carcinogenicity data, if required, may be submitted postapproval.

Not all testing for carcinogenic potential need be conducted using the traditional 2-year rodent bioassay. Studies using genetically modified animals and other alternatives may be acceptable on a case-by-case basis. Results of carcinogenicity testing will be included in product labeling.

The specifics on carcinogenicity testing of pharmaceuticals can be found in another chapter of this book. Additional information may also be found in ICH and CDER guidance documents (21–25). Dose selection for carcinogenicity testing is extremely important, and sponsors developing products for the U.S. market are advised to submit protocols for carcinogenicity testing, including proposed doses and the rationale for choosing them, to the appropriate CDER division.

SPECIAL STUDIES

The need for most of these so called "special studies" is driven by data, including knowledge of class effects, how the product will be used clinically, and observations from general animal toxicity studies and early clinical trials. Some examples of special studies are listed in Table 3.

The local tolerance to a drug substance or product is usually investigated as part of a general toxicity study using the clinical route of administration. As discussed elsewhere in this chapter, expanded histopathologic evaluation of tissues at the site of administration is the usual practice. For compounds that are to be given intravenously, additional data demonstrating how surrounding tissues fare following extravasation is usually provided. Early in the development of products intended for intravenous, intramuscular or subcutaneous injection, it is not unusual for sponsors to conduct small pilot tests to evaluate the local effects of several different salts and/or formulations of a drug before choosing among them.

For drugs in structural or pharmacological classes known or suspected to be addictive to humans (i.e., those that would be scheduled under the Controlled Substances Act), nonclinical studies of abuse potential may be needed. These could include in vitro binding studies (to determine a compound's affinity for a specific receptor, transporter, or

Table 3 Special Studies

Study	Common test systems[a]
Local tolerance	Rodents, dogs
Abuse potential	Rodents, primates, in vitro binding
Ototoxicity	Guinea pigs
Immunotoxicity	Rodents
Juvenile animal toxicity	Rats, dogs
Phototoxicity	In vitro assays, rodents

[a]Other species (e.g., primates, swine) may be the best choice under particular circumstances.

ion channel), in vivo binding with imaging, and studies in animals. Animal studies encompass tests of self-administration (animals will perform a task for the reward of an IV dose of test compound), drug discrimination experiments (animals are trained to press one lever in response to exposure to drugs of a particular pharmacologic class and a different lever in response to placebo), tests of tolerance and physical dependence, and motor function testing. Results from test compounds are compared with those from drugs known to be abused by humans.

Drugs that will be administered into the ear to treat conditions where the tympanic membrane may not be intact often require a special evaluation for ototoxicity. This will generally include a functional test conducted in vivo such as auditory brainstem response, as well as postmortem gross and microscopic examination of the tissues of the middle and inner ears, including enumeration of cochlear hair cells. Intratympanic administration of test products to guinea pigs is a useful means to evaluate their direct ototoxic potential.

Immunotoxicology studies encompass tests to determine both immunogenicity and immunosuppression. Products that are applied topically undergo evaluation for dermal sensitization potential. Some tests that may be used to evaluate dermal sensitization include the guinea pig maximization test, Buehler assay, and the murine local lymph node assay. Drugs that are given via inhalation are analyzed for their respiratory sensitizing potential in vivo (often in the guinea pig), with the inhalational route of administration used for both induction and challenge. On occasion, adverse reactions that may be mediated by the immune system are observed in animals or humans, and certain tests may be useful investigative tools. These include the Coomb's test to see whether hemolytic anemia is immune-mediated, measures of drug-induced histamine release and complement activation, or looking for evidence of immune complex deposition in tissues affected by vasculitis. Observations from general toxicity studies (including evidence of myelosuppression, alterations in immune system organ weights and histology, decreased serum globulin levels, and increased incidences of infections or tumors) may suggest that a drug is suppressing the immune system. If the drug is suspected of being an immunosuppressant, immune function studies may be requested. One method for determining a drug's effect on immune function is to measure its effect on T-cell dependent antibody response using an anti–sheep red blood cell primary antibody response assay (plaque assay). Immunogens other than sheep red blood cells have been used successfully in immune function assays, often in concert with such techniques as enzyme-linked immunosorbent assay (ELISA) to measure antibody response. Immune cell phenotyping using flow cytometry or immunohistochemistry is useful when investigating drug-induced immunosuppression. Host resistance assays and other techniques may also be of value. If a product causes immunosuppression in adults and is likely to be used by pregnant women, immune function in F_1 offspring may also be evaluated; this can be done as part of a reproduction toxicology study. Additional information may be found in the CDER guidance document (26).

Studies in juvenile animals may be requested to support pediatric clinical trials or marketing if there is concern that a drug may be more toxic to juveniles than to adults or if there is information suggesting the target organs of toxicity could differ depending on age. Data from adult animals and humans can be very useful in helping to determine the need for juvenile animal studies, as can data from pre- and postnatal developmental toxicology studies when adequate exposure of the offspring can be demonstrated. For many drugs, juvenile animal testing is unlikely to be necessary. Products targeting organ systems that undergo significant postnatal development are of special concern, as are drugs that are used long-term during critical periods of development. One should bear in mind that what is considered long-term in a neonate or infant may be a considerably shorter period than would be considered long-term in an adult. Products that will be used primarily, if not exclusively in children, should be tested in juvenile animals. The age of the animals used for testing should be determined by the target organ(s) and developmental parameters of greatest concern and the age of the intended pediatric clinical population. Additional information may be found in the CDER guidance document (27).

Photoirritation testing should be considered for products that absorb light in the UVA, UVB, or visible ranges (290–700 nm) and are present at significant levels in the skin or eyes or are used for photodynamic therapy. It is important that any phototesting be conducted using appropriate wavelengths of light. Simulated sunlight is generally preferred; at a minimum, the absorption spectrum of the drug within the sunlight spectrum should be covered. A variety of approaches may be used to determine the phototoxic potential of a drug. In vitro screening assays, such as measuring neutral red uptake in cultured 3T3 cells, can be useful in cases where only a water soluble active ingredient in a drug product needs to be tested for photoirritation. A variety of animals (shaved, depilated, or bred to be hairless) have been used for short-term in vivo photoirritation testing, including mice, guinea pigs, rats, rabbits, and swine. For products applied topically to sun-exposed skin, the clinical formulation should be used for in vivo phototoxicity testing, as excipients can influence drug-induced photoirritation (e.g., by allowing greater penetration of drug into the skin) or be photoirritants themselves. The results of nonclinical photoirritation testing will frequently guide clinical testing of this nature. Nonclinical photoallergy testing is usually not performed due to a lack of reliable models. Photocarcinogenicity testing is generally needed for products that are intended to be used in sunlight (e.g., sunscreens), and it may also be needed for products whose clinical utility would be affected by a positive result. Additionally, sponsors may choose to test a drug that is known to be a photoirritant to demonstrate that it is not a photocarcinogen. Most nonclinical photocarcinogenicity testing has been conducted in hairless rodents, usually Skh1-*hr* mice. The use of skin biomarkers to evaluate the combined consequences of drug and UV exposure is a potential alternative to "classic" rodent photocarcinogenicity testing, and alternative bioassays, some using transgenic animals, are also being explored. On rare occasions, some nonphotoreactive drug products that are used chronically may need to be evaluated for their potential to enhance UV-induced skin carcinogenesis. These products might be members of structural or pharmacologic classes known to enhance UV-induced carcinogenicity (e.g., immunosuppressants), or they may be known to induce adverse changes in the protective properties of the skin (e.g., cause thinning of the epidermis or alter the optical properties of the skin). Additional information may be found in the CDER guidance document (28).

STUDIES FOR PREVIOUSLY APPROVED DRUGS

In cases where approved drug products are reformulated and/or given via new routes of administration, substantial nonclinical toxicity information is usually already available. If the previous nonclinical studies were adequate, it may not be necessary to conduct nonclinical studies other than "bridging studies" to test the local tolerance of the new formulation or dosing route and to determine whether these changes have altered the toxicologic profile of the drug. For example, when an approved systemic antimicrobial is reformulated for ophthalmic, otic, or pulmonary dosing, nonclinical studies are usually confined to irritation/sensitization testing and a repeat-dose toxicity study (or studies) using the new formula and route of administration. Additional end points may need to be examined in the new repeat-dose toxicity studies, as appropriate to the route of administration (e.g., ototoxicity testing for otic products, expanded examinations of the eyes or respiratory tract for ophthalmic or inhalation toxicity studies). Formulation and/or route switches for other classes of drugs would be handled similarly.

Sometimes approved products will be investigated for new clinical uses without undergoing any changes in formulation or route of administration. If the dose/exposure or duration of use of the product changes substantially, additional nonclinical toxicity testing may be needed if the nonclinical data on file are not adequate (e.g., doses or systemic exposure was too low or study duration was too short) to support the reasonable safety of the new clinical use.

If any of the previous nonclinical toxicity studies conducted to support the original clinical testing and approval of the product were deficient or are inadequate by current scientific standards, additional studies may be needed to address deficiencies.

THE VALUE OF NONCLINICAL TESTING?

There is some controversy regarding the usefulness of nonclinical toxicology studies in drug development. There has been some disagreement between regulators, the pharmaceutical industry, academicians, and consumer groups as to the minimum amount of information needed to safely initiate and extend clinical trials. In part, this may be due to different beliefs with regard to the amount of risk that clinical trial participants are willing to accept or the amount of risk that these participants should be permitted to assume. Another issue is the use of nonclinical data to perform risk assessment for potential toxicities when it is unethical to obtain the necessary data from clinical studies (e.g., reproductive toxicology and carcinogenicity). There is concern as to whether the data from these studies, and other nonclinical toxicology studies, are applicable to humans. For example, sometimes specialized animal studies (e.g., neurotoxicity or cardiotoxicity) have been conducted to explore adverse effects observed in clinical trials that were not detected in the initial standard animal toxicology studies. This is troubling because the implication is that the standard nonclinical studies were inadequate to demonstrate clinically important adverse effects.

In fact, the issue of how well data from nonclinical studies predicts clinical adverse effects is difficult to assess and few studies have sought to address this problem. A frequently cited review on this topic was conducted by a group of industry and academic scientists for the Health and Environmental Sciences Institute of the International Life Sciences Institute (29). Although this study has several methodological flaws (e.g., information on doses at which toxicities were observed was not obtained, so it is unclear if risk could be inferred based on relative exposures), it does provide insight as to the general usefulness of nonclinical studies. Twelve pharmaceutical companies provided complete nonclinical and clinical data sets on 150 compounds. Based on an extensive analysis, the authors concluded that human adverse effects were predicted by animal studies in 71% of cases. Hematologic, gastrointestinal, and cardiovascular toxicities were best predicted, whereas cutaneous, hepatic, and neurologic adverse effects were poorly predicted. In the latter cases, the issue of predictivity is complex. Most cutaneous reactions in this data set appeared to have an immunologic basis, and current animal models are not especially useful for predicting hypersensitivity reactions after oral or IV administration. In contrast, animal models are more successful at predicting hypersensitivity after application of topical drug products, but there were few of these products in the dataset examined by Olson et al. (29,30). The neurologic adverse effects not predicted by nonclinical testing included headache, nausea, dizziness, blurred vision, and similar clinical signs that animal models are not able to detect. The lack of concordance between some animal and human hepatotoxicity data is still a matter of extensive discussion and debate (31). In general, animal models appear to adequately detect most typical direct hepatotoxicants, but neither nonclinical studies nor clinical trials have been able to identify drugs that were later associated with rare or idiosyncratic hepatotoxicity (32,33).

SUMMARY AND FUTURE DIRECTIONS

Before pharmaceuticals can be tested in humans and marketed, their toxicity profiles must be evaluated. It is important to consider the needs of the clinical population that will receive the proposed drug product when weighing the potential risks and benefits of exposure. Minimal information is generally needed to initiate single-dose clinical studies, including acute toxicity data in two mammalian species (usually one rodent and one nonrodent), local tolerance assessment using the proposed clinical route of administration, basic safety pharmacology data (effects on cardiac, respiratory, and central nervous systems), some pharmacokinetics (e.g., AUC, and C_{max}), and in vitro genotoxicity tests for mutations and chromosome damage. Additional studies covering repeat dose general toxicity (preferably with exposure data), effects on reproduction, and in vivo genotoxicity are needed as clinical development proceeds. Carcinogenicity bioassays are necessary for products that will be used chronically or as directed based on results of genotoxicity testing for drugs that will be used short-term. Depending on the results of nonclinical and clinical testing, or based on other information regarding the drug's structural or pharmaceutical class, more specialized toxicity studies (e.g., addiction potential, immunotoxicity, phototoxicity, use of juvenile animals) may also be needed.

It is important for the regulatory toxicology community to keep abreast of improvements made in nonclinical testing and to remain open minded about using results from studies using new methodology to support pharmaceutical development. Researchers are working to identify and validate promising new serum biomarkers for a variety of organ specific toxicities. The fields of pharmacogenomics, proteomics, and metabonomics may also provide new markers for toxicity. Researchers hope that "-omic" data might provide the means for earlier detection of a toxic effect, may be more sensitive than conventional toxicology testing, and may provide information about the probable human relevance of an animal finding. Enhanced imaging techniques allowing visualization of organs without sacrificing animals may permit scientists to follow the development (and perhaps also the reversal) of drug-induced changes. In the future, some of these techniques could improve and advance nonclinical toxicity testing, transforming the state of the art.

REFERENCES

1. www.fda.gov/cder/guidance/.
2. Preclinical Safety Evaluation of Biotechnology-Derived Pharmaceuticals ICH S6 (Final, 7/97), available on the Internet from the FDA Center for Drug Evaluation and Research (www.fda. gov/cder/guidance/1859fnl.pdf).
3. Mathieu M, ed. Biologics Development: A Regulatory Overview 3rd ed. Waltham: Parexel International Corporation, 2004.
4. Redbook 2000, Toxicological Principles for the Safety Assessment of Food Ingredients, available on the Internet from the FDA Center for Food Safety and Applied Nutrition (www. cfsan.fda.gov/ ~ redbook/red-toca.html).

5. Hayes AW, ed. Principles and Methods of Toxicology. 4th ed. London: Taylor & Francis, 2001.

6. Guidance for Industry: Estimating the Maximum Safe Starting Dose in Initial Clinical Trials for Therapeutics in Adult Healthy Volunteers (Final, 7/05), available on the Internet from the FDA Center for Drug Evaluation and Research (www.fda.gov/cder/guidance/5541fnl.pdf).

7. Nonclinical Safety Studies for the Conduct of Human Clinical Trials for Pharmaceuticals ICH M3 (Final, 7/97), available on the Internet from the FDA Center for Drug Evaluation and Research (www.fda.gov/cder/guidance/1855fnl.pdf).

8. Safety Pharmacology Studies for Human Pharmaceuticals ICH S7A (Final, 7/01), available on the Internet from the FDA Center for Drug Evaluation and Research (www.fda.gov/cder/guidance/4461fnl.pdf).

9. Pharmacokinetics: Guidance for Repeated Dose Tissue Distribution Studies ICH S3B (Final, 3/95), available on the Internet from the FDA Center for Drug Evaluation and Research (www.fda.gov/cder/guidance/ichs3b.pdf).

10. Baillie TA, Cayen MN, Fouda H, et al. Drug metabolites in safety testing. Toxicol Appl Pharmacol 2002; 182:188–196.

11. Hastings KL, El-Hage J, Jacobs A, Leighton J, Morse D, Osterberg RE. Letter to the editor. Toxicol Appl Pharmacol 2003; 190:91–92.

12. Baillie TA, Cayen MN, Fouda H, et al. Letter to the editor. Toxicol Appl Pharmacol 2003; 190:93–94.

13. Toxicokinetics: The Assessment of Systemic Exposure in Toxicity Studies ICH S3A (Final, 3/95), available on the Internet from the FDA Center for Drug Evaluation and Research (www.fda.gov/cder/guidance/ichs3a.pdf).

14. Guidance for Industry: Single Dose Acute Toxicity Testing for Pharmaceuticals (Final, 8/96), available on the Internet from the FDA Center for Drug Evaluation and Research (www.fda.gov/cder/guidance/pt1.pdf).

15. Duration of Chronic Toxicity Testing in Animals (Rodent and Nonrodent Toxicity Testing) ICH S4A (Final, 6/99), available on the Internet from the FDA Center for Drug Evaluation and Research (www.fda.gov/cder/guidance/62599.pdf).

16. Genotoxicity Studies- Specific Aspects of Regulatory Genotoxicity Tests for Pharmaceuticals ICH S2A (Final, 4/96), available on the Internet from the FDA Center for Drug Evaluation and Research (www.fda.gov/cder/guidance/ichs2a.pdf).

17. A Standard Battery for Genotoxicity Testing of Pharmaceuticals ICH S2B (Final, 7/97), available on the Internet from the FDA Center for Drug Evaluation and Research (www.fda.gov/cder/guidance/1856fnl.pdf).

18. Detection of Toxicity to Reproduction for Medicinal Products ICH S5A (Final, 9/94), available on the Internet from the FDA Center for Drug Evaluation and Research (www.fda.gov/cder/guidance/s5a.pdf).

19. Detection of Toxicity to Reproduction for Medicinal Products: Addendum on Toxicity to Male Fertility ICH S5B (Final, 4/96), available on the Internet from the FDA Center for Drug Evaluation and Research (www.fda.gov/cder/guidance/ichs5b.pdf).

20. Maintenance of the ICH Guideline on Toxicity to Male Fertility: An Addendum to the ICH Tripartite Guideline on: Detection of Toxicity to Reproduction for Medicinal Products ICH S5B(M) (Amended, 11/00), available on the Internet from the ICH (www.ich.org/cache/compo/276-254-1.html).

21. The Need for Long-term Rodent Carcinogenicity Studies of Pharmaceuticals ICH S1A (Final, 3/96), available on the Internet from the FDA Center for Drug Evaluation and Research (www.fda.gov/cder/guidance/ichs1a.pdf).

22. Testing for Carcinogenicity of Pharmaceuticals ICH S1B (Final, 7/97), available on the Internet from the FDA Center for Drug Evaluation and Research (www.fda.gov/cder/guidance/1854fnl.pdf).

23. Dose Selection for Carcinogenicity Studies of Pharmaceuticals ICH S1C (Final, 3/95), available on the Internet from the FDA Center for Drug Evaluation and Research (www.fda.gov/cder/guidance/ichs1c.pdf).

24. Addendum to Dose Selection for Carcinogenicity Studies of Pharmaceuticals: Addition of a Limit Dose and Related Notes ICH S1C(R) (Amended, 7/97), available on the Internet from the FDA Center for Drug Evaluation and Research (www.fda.gov/cder/guidance/1858fnl.pdf).
25. Carcinogenicity Study Protocol Submissions (Final, 5/02), available on the Internet from the FDA Center for Drug Evaluation and Research (www.fda.gov/cder/guidance/4804fnl.pdf).
26. Immunotoxicology Evaluation of Investigational New Drugs (Final, 10/02), available on the Internet from the FDA Center for Drug Evaluation and Research (www.fda.gov/cder/guidance/4945fnl.PDF).
27. Nonclinical Safety Evaluation of Pediatric Drug Products (Final, 2/06), available on the Internet from the FDA Center for Drug Evaluation and Research (www.fda.gov/cder/guidance/5671fnl.pdf).
28. Photosafety Testing (Final, 5/03), available on the Internet from the FDA Center for Drug Evaluation and Research (www.fda.gov/cder/guidance/3640fnl.pdf).
29. Olson H, Betton G, Robinson D, et al. Concordance of the toxicity of pharmaceuticals in humans and in animals. Regul Toxicol Pharmacol 2000; 32:56–67.
30. Weaver JL, Staten D, Swann J, Armstrong G, Bates M, Hastings KL. Detection of systemic hypersensitivity to drugs using standard guinea pig assays. Toxicology 2003; 193:203–217.
31. Lee WM. Drug-induced hepatotoxicity. N Engl J Med 2003; 349:474–485.
32. Peters TS. Do preclinical testing strategies help predict human hepatotoxic potentials? Toxicol Pathol 2005; 33:146–154.
33. Lee WM, Senior JR. Recognizing drug-induced liver injury: current problems, possible solutions. Toxicol Pathol 2005; 33:155–164.

17

Health Risk Assessment Strategies in the Food and Cosmetic Industry

Steven M. Weisman and Linnea Steiger
Innovative Science Solutions, Morristown, New Jersey, U.S.A.

INTRODUCTION

The main purpose of the U.S. Food and Drug Administration (FDA) is to assure that consumers are protected from unsafe products, including drugs, cosmetics, foods, and dietary supplements. Drugs are subject to strict guidelines regarding both their efficacy and safety and are approved by the FDA prior to marketing. Cosmetics, dietary supplements, and foods (excluding food additives) on the other hand, although subject to regulations and guidelines regarding their safety, do not require premarket approval prior to release to the public. All of these products are regulated by The Center for Food Safety and Applied Nutrition (CFSAN), a Center of the FDA, which is responsible for regulating the safety of cosmetics, dietary supplements, and food products. This chapter reviews the history of the development of safety regulations and recommended safety testing procedures for cosmetics, dietary supplements, and foods. In addition, it details the various safety testing approaches, including those that are required, recommended, or most commonly utilized to establish the safety of these products.

HISTORY

Federal Food, Drug, and Cosmetic Act of 1938

President Franklin Roosevelt signed the Federal Food, Drug, and Cosmetic Act (FDAC) of 1938 as a response to the elixir sulfanilamide tragedy in 1937, where 105 deaths occurred due to the drug. The FDCA was essentially structured to strengthen the safety of the pharmaceutical industry by requiring pharmaceutical companies to submit safety information prior to any new drug approval (1). However, the FDCA affected all aspects of the FDA, creating a complex set of regulations for foods, drugs, cosmetics, and medical devices. The major change in the FDCA was that the FDA was no longer responsible for ensuring that a drug is either safe or unsafe; it was now the responsibility of the manufacturer; however, the FDA continued to be responsible for establishing that a conventional food product was unsafe. There was no specific provisions given on vitamins, minerals, or botanical products; although, it was stated that a food is misbranded if it claims to be "for special dietary uses" but its label does not reflect FDA-prescribed statements indicating its vitamin, mineral, and dietary properties (2). In addition, the FDCA clearly defines cosmetics by their intended use, as "articles intended to be rubbed, poured, sprinkled, or sprayed on, introduced into, or otherwise applied to the human body...for cleansing, beautifying, promoting attractiveness, or altering appearance" (3). The FDCA also identified and defined color additives, as any "dye, pigment, or other substance made by a process of synthesis or similar artifice, or extracted, isolated, or otherwise derived, with or without intermediate or final change in identity from a vegetable, animal, mineral, or other source, and ... when added or applied to a food, drug, or cosmetic, or to the human body or any part thereof, is capable of imparting color thereto ..." (3). In addition, the FDCA laid out the framework for safety analysis of color additives. Color additives are commonly found in both food and cosmetic products and are subject to premarket regulation.

Food Additives Amendment of 1958

As an amendment to the FDCA, the Food Additives Amendment of 1958 requires FDA approval for additives prior to their being utilized in a food product (1). In addition, this act also required the manufacturer to prove the additive's safety both in the method of utilization and in the desired dosage (4). However, there were two groups of exemptions to this amendment, which included all substances that either the FDA or the U.S. Department of Agriculture had determined were safe in a specific food prior to 1958 and all food additives that are "generally recognized as safe" (GRAS). GRAS substances are those whose use is considered safe by experts based on either an extensive history before 1958 or strong scientific evidence (5). In addition, this amendment included the Delaney Clause, which states that no residue from pesticides found to be carcinogenic in animals would be allowed in food additives (1).

The Dietary Supplement and Health Education Act of 1994

The Dietary Supplement and Health Education Act (DSHEA) of 1994 clearly defined a dietary supplement as a product other than tobacco that is intended to supplement the diet and contains one or more of the following ingredients: a vitamin, a mineral, an herb or other botanical, an amino acid, a dietary supplement for use by humans to supplement the diet by increasing the total dietary intake, or a concentrate, metabolite, constituent, extract or any combination of an ingredient previously mentioned (6). In addition, DSHEA established safety standards for dietary supplements. In general, a manufacturer is responsible for ensuring the premarket safety of their product, although the manufacturer is not required to reveal the basis of their safety determination. Under this act, the Secretary of the Department of Health and Human Services has the ability to declare that a product poses an imminent hazard, or the FDA can initiate an action in court alleging that a product is adulterated. In these cases, the basis of the safety profile information must be provided by the manufacturer. Additionally, DSHEA provides new requirements for dietary supplement constituents, which are considered "new dietary ingredients." "New dietary ingredients" are defined as ingredients that were not marketed on or before October 15, 1994. Under DSHEA these ingredients are considered to be adulterated unless one of two situations is present: the ingredient has been present in the conventional food supply where the food has not been chemically altered, or there is a "history of use or other evidence of safety establishing that the dietary ingredient when used under the conditions recommended or suggested in the labeling" (6). The manufacturer of new dietary ingredients must provide the FDA with the information that they relied on in concluding that the dietary supplement with this particular new ingredient is reasonably expected to be safe. The information must be submitted to the FDA 75 days prior to the marketing of the supplement; if no notification from the FDA is received during this time the manufacturer is free to market the supplement as submitted. It is important to note that this process is for new dietary supplement ingredients and not necessarily for new dietary supplement products. A new dietary supplement product may be marketed if all of its ingredients were marketed prior to October 15, 1994.

The Food and Drug Modernization Act of 1997

The only significant change in reference to food safety that this act changed was the elimination of the required premarket approval from the FDA for most packaging and any other substance that may come in to contact with food or has the possibility of migrating in to the food. Instead, this act established a process whereby the manufacturer is to notify the agency about its intent to use certain food contact substances (FCS), and unless the FDA objects within a 120-day period, the manufacturer may proceed in the marketing of the product (7).

Current Food and Drug Administration Structure

Currently the FDA has six product-oriented centers, with one being the CFSAN. CFSAN is responsible, along with the agency's field staff, to ensure that the nation's food supply is safe, sanitary, wholesome, and honestly labeled and additionally that cosmetic products are both safe and properly labeled. CFSAN is responsible for both food products and food additives, along with dietary supplements, cosmetics, and numerous other food related items. There are essentially two sets of regulations with respect to the safety of a cosmetic, dietary supplement, or food. First, there is a premarket phase, which includes the testing and risk-benefit analysis that is conducted prior to marketing. Secondly, there is postmarket phase, which includes safety surveillance of postmarketing. There are different safety regulations for different regulated product types, and each is subject to different laws, regulations, and policies, such as the "new dietary ingredient" regulations passed with DSHEA. Table 1 summarizes how the FDA approaches each of these product types.

Safety Testing

The topic of safety testing is extremely expansive and diverse and is further complicated by the diverse nature of the products regulated by CFSAN as discussed in this chapter. In general, there are two broad types of safety testing: hazard identification and risk assessment. Hazard identification is defined as the process of testing a substance to determine if it does or does not have adverse effects. It is essential that the hazard identification process be appropriately conducted and completed prior to marketing to determine whether a substance has various adverse properties prior to public marketing. These include carcinogenic and teratogenic properties, just to name two. The other type of safety evaluation is risk assessment, which demonstrates whether a substance is likely to be a problem in the "real world" given practical issues. These practical issues include how often people will come in contact with the substance and at what dose/concentration people will be exposed. For example, with food additives, specific safety testing has to address effects related to the amount of the additive that the consumer is generally exposed to (8). The results from these tests are then analyzed to determine whether this additive would be a

Table 1 Status of Food and Drug Administration Regulation for Cosmetics, Dietary Supplements, Foods, and Food Additives

Status	Cosmetics	Dietary supplements	Foods[a]	Food/color additives
Premarket approval required	No	No[b]	No[c]	Yes
Risk-benefit analysis conducted by Food and Drug Administration prior to marketing	No	No	No	No
Postmarket reporting or surveillance by industry required	Rarely	No	No	Rarely
Burden of proof for demonstration safety or lack thereof (postmarket)	Manufacturer	Food and Drug Administration	Food and Drug Administration	Manufacturer

Proposed framework for evaluating the safety of dietary supplements, Institute of Medicine 2002.
[a]Foods (including conventional foods and dietary supplements), unlike drugs, are considered to be safe (reasonable certainty of no harm), and thus risk-benefit analysis is not applicable.
[b]A 75-day premarket notification, but not premarket approval, is required for dietary supplements containing ingredients not marketed before 1994.
[c]In 2001 the Food and Drug Administration proposed a rule requiring marketers of food developed though biotechnology to notify the agency at least 120 days before commercial distribution and to provide information to demonstrate that the product is as safe as its conventional counterpart.

concern in the general population or not. It is necessary to realize that each substance is different and that the various methods of safety testing may or may not apply to it.

Cosmetics

Premarket Safety of Cosmetics

Cosmetics, excluding color additives, are not subject to any type of premarket approval, ingredient approval, regulation, or even risk-benefit evaluation. However, it remains the manufacturer's responsibility to ensure their safety. As such, cosmetics and cosmetic ingredients often have some level of safety testing. As briefly mentioned previously, color additives are often utilized in cosmetics and are subject to premarket approval, and therefore must be shown to be safe and listed in the Code of Federal Regulations prior to being utilized in any cosmetic product. The safety of color additives in cosmetics are generally evaluated by utilizing skin penetration studies, along with anticipated levels of use, and the concentration of any impurities.

Cosmetic manufacturers do have the ability to register their products in the Voluntary Cosmetic Regulation Program (VCRP), which is maintained by one of the FDA's offices. The underlying idea behind the VCRP is to protect the consumer while at the same time aid the cosmetic industry in making informed decisions with respect to the safety of their products (9). The benefit behind the VCRP is to help avoid problem ingredients, such as nonapproved color additives, or other restricted ingredients that the manufacturer may have been unaware of prior to marketing. In addition, VCRP aids both the consumer and retailer in the selection of safety-minded manufacturers. Unless the cosmetic manufacturer registers their product with VCRP, the FDA has no regulatory authority over the cosmetic during the premarketing stage (10). Regulations require that if a cosmetic product has not been subjected to any safety testing, its product label must read: "WARNING: The safety of this product has not been determined."

Standard Safety Tests Used for Cosmetics

Although, as stated previously, the safety of a cosmetic product does not need to be established in the premarketing phase, the majority of manufacturers do put their products through some safety testing before the product goes on the market. The most common safety tests conducted on cosmetics include eye and skin irritancy tests, phototoxicity tests, and acute toxicity testing. Each of these tests are reviewed below.

Eye Irritation Testing. The most common test for cosmetic products is the Draize Eye Irritancy Test, which is used most commonly for testing the irritancy of make-ups, shampoos, and deodorants (11). This test is preformed on albino rabbits, which are known to have very sensitive eyes, therefore yielding a low number of false negative results. The main objective of the Draize Eye Irritancy Test is to determine the level of irritation on a scale of 0–110, with 110 equaling complete destruction of the eye. The score is calculated from observation of damage to the cornea, conjunctiva, iris, or any associated discharge. This test aids the manufacturer in determining if a product that may potentially get into the eye is ultimately safe for the eye.

For humane reasons, the common practice in most laboratories is to conduct early in vitro screening of test materials before conducting the test on rabbits. A number of in vitro alterative assays have been validated and some are even "accepted" for regulatory purposes in Europe. Two of these in vitro tests include systems utilize excised animal tissues, the bovine corneal opacity and permeability test (BCOP) and the isolated rabbit eye test (IRE) (12–14). Another non-mammalian assay, the hen's egg test-chorioallantoic membrane (HET-CAM) has also gained general acceptance (15).

Skin Irritation Testing. The Draize Skin Irritancy test is very similar to its companion study, the Draize Eye Irritancy test (11). The skin irritancy test involves application of the substance in question to the shaved skin of an animal, usually a rabbit, mouse, or rat, and the researcher looks for signs of redness or blistering. This test is often performed for any substance or ingredient that would be exposed to the skin, including lotions, shampoos, make-up, and deodorant—essentially almost all cosmetic products.

Similar to method development used for in vitro eye irritation testing, much effort has been directed towards the development of an alternate test to the Draize Skin Irritancy Test, where all of the testing would be done with human tissue using an in vitro technique. This in vitro technique utilizes either a human skin model developed commercially or one that is constructed from epithelial cells. The researcher looks for irreversible damage to the skin through cell viability as well as optical density. In vitro irritancy testing is currently used by many manufacturers; however, there is ongoing discussion as to whether it truly provides comparable results. Two in vitro tests for skin corrosivity have been validated and are currently accepted by the European Commission (EC) for regulatory purposes (16–19). The first utilizes reconstructed human skin (EPISKIN™ or EpiDerm™). The second EC approved test utilizes excised rat skin and transcutaneous electrical resistance.

Phototoxicity Testing. Phototoxicity testing is very common in the cosmetic industry, due to the fact that most cosmetic products are applied to the skin, and therefore they often are exposed to direct sun. There are essentially two forms of phototoxicity testing: the traditional in vivo method and the newer in vitro method. A validated method in Europe includes an in vitro phototoxicity assay that uses the mouse fibroblast cell line (3T3) with neutral red uptake (NRU) as the end point for cytotoxicity (20,21).

Phototoxicity testing, also referred to as photosensitivity testing, is essential for all products that are utilized or come in contact with the skin, as evidenced by the fact that UV-associated skin injury can be caused by many substances. Mechanisms include inhibition of repair in skin cells, altering the protective function of the epidermis, and even suppressing the immune system. The methods associated with phototoxicity testing vary greatly based on the substance being tested, the potential use of the substance, and whether in vitro or in vivo testing is the desired method. An understanding of the risks associated with the product in combination with UV radiation is necessary to determine the safety profile of the cosmetic product ingredient in question.

Acute Toxicity Testing. Two acute toxicity tests are used to evaluate the lethal dose of a particular cosmetic product or ingredient. These include the LD_{50} test, and its newer derivative, the "limit" test (see Chapter 6 for more details) (22). These tests tend not to be conducted with cosmetic products as much as the previously mentioned tests; however, they are often performed by raw material producers on a regular basis. The goal of this test is to provide a "lethal dose" range of the particular substance following a single dose. This test is usually completed to address the risks of poisoning or accidental overexposure.

Postmarketing Surveillance of Cosmetics

Even though cosmetic products are not subject to premarket approval, the FDA still has responsibility of ensuring the safety of the pubic. The FDA does have the authority to request all safety data for a particular product in question, and the FDA may remove the cosmetic product from the market if there is evidence that it is unsafe. However, they must first prove in a court of law that the product may be injurious to users, improperly labeled, or violates the law.

As a supplement to the weak postmarket regulation provided by the FDA, in the U.S. there is a seven expert panel called the Cosmetic Ingredient Review (CIR), which was established in 1976 by the Cosmetic, Toiletry & Fragrance Association with support and oversight from the FDA and the Consumer Federation of America. The CIR conducts extensive literature searches and collects relevant safety data on particular ingredients of interest (23). Once the collection of material is complete, the CIR compiles a safety report, which they make available to the public, and publishes a copy in the *International Journal of Toxicology*. At the conclusion of their review, the CIR will give each ingredient it reviews one of four ratings; safe as used, safe with qualifications, insufficient data, or unsafe. The CIR usually only evaluates "high priority ingredients," because this process is extremely time consuming and it is not feasible for them to evaluate all the new products and ingredients which come out each year.

Dietary Supplements, Food, and Food Additives

Premarket Safety

The similarity of dietary supplements, foods, and food additives are largely due to the fact that they are consumed and, in general, are processed through the same mechanisms. These similarities can make their safety testing procedures analogous. Where these products differ is how they are handled in regulatory settings.

There are no provisions in the law for the FDA to "approve" a dietary supplement for safety or efficacy prior to the product reaching the consumer (2). Like cosmetics, the burden of proof is on the agency to determine that a product or ingredient is unsafe.

The dietary supplement manufacturer is responsible for ensuring that the dietary supplement is expected to be reasonably safe. The term "safe" in this context means that the ingredients in the supplement do not present a significant or unreasonable risk of illness or injury under the specified conditions of use that are recommended in the product labeling.

Food ingredients are also, for the most part, not subject to prior approval before being placed on the market. However, both FCS, and food additives, including color additives, may be subject to differing regulations. Food additives, unless they have been previously considered GRAS, must go through a premarket approval process. Much like food additives, color additives must also be approved in the premarketing stage. Generally, this is accomplished by establishing a safety profile through levels of exposure, presence of impurities, as well as long-term animal toxicity testing. Additionally, any substance intended for use as a component of materials used in manufacturing, packing, packaging, transporting, or holding food is considered a FCS. These are also subject to a premarket notification program, where the notification must contain sufficient information to show that the substance is safe with its intended use.

Safety Testing of Dietary Supplements, Food, and Food Additives

Although human testing is the most reliable, the available data can be minimal or nonexistent, especially for new ingredients. Thus testing in animals or in in vitro test systems is generally the approach taken. In terms of dietary supplements, the manufacturer is responsible for assessing the safety of the supplement, so they may conduct all of the tests listed below, several of them, or, in some instances may even conduct entirely different tests. Safety testing of food ingredients is generally done on an ingredient-by-ingredient basis. Food additives, including color additives, are subject to a premarket approval process, whereby a petition is submitted containing information on the additives safety, both from a toxicology and environmental perspective. The FDA suggests that prior to any toxicology testing involving food additives; the manufacturer should contact the Consumer Safety Officer assigned to that specific petition in CFSAN for guidance in determining what specific toxicology information is necessary to support the safety of the ingredient. For FCS there are minimum testing recommendations provided by the FDA that reflect the expected exposure levels of a person to the particular substance. For more information on the various studies associated with each range of exposure, one should consult the CFSAN Final Guidance for Industry Document (24).

Below are four broad categories of safety testing and procedures that are commonly utilized for dietary supplements and food ingredients, whether it be additives, FCS, or other various substances. The four categories of safety testing are; human, animal, bioavailability, and in vitro (2). Each category of testing is summarized below and followed by a synopsis of the most commonly utilized testing methods with respect to the relevant category. For more in-depth information on the study designs and protocol recommendations, please refer to the FDA's Redbook, 2000 (25) or other chapters in this book that cover these tests in more detail.

Human Testing. Human data can be derived from a number of sources. First, epidemiologic or clinical trials can be conducted to determine the potential for, and type of, adverse events associated with a particular product. Controlled clinical trials powered to identify expected rates of adverse events are generally required to obtain meaningful relevant data. Often these data are available in the published literature, or the trial investigators or manufacturers may be able to supply unpublished data, which may be useful in a study evaluation, even if the published material does not contain all of the information about the adverse events (26). Second, meaningful human data can be obtained from observational epidemiological research, which may be able to detect latent or delayed safety signals that could not be derived from clinical trials due to their relatively short length. Third, is the evaluation of the frequency of spontaneously reported adverse events received by the manufacturer or the FDA. These reports may be useful in determining if the supplement is associated with the event by examining case reports. Finally, there is historical information, primarily the experience from generations of use, that may guide safety conclusions for certain dietary supplements and foods.

Epidemiology testing is extremely important in assessing the safety of various dietary supplement and food ingredients. There are two main categories of epidemiology studies: descriptive and analytic (25). Descriptive studies generally utilize existing distribution of variables and do not test hypotheses; however, they are utilized to generate hypotheses and possibly provide evidence that may indicate whether further and lengthier tests are necessary. Generally, descriptive studies can be assessed in two ways: through correlational studies and through case reports. On the other hand, analytic studies are designed to examine associations and identify the effects of the risk factors, which ultimately contribute to the overall safety evaluation. There are three types of analytic studies: cross-sectional, perspective, and retrospective studies.

In Vivo and In Vitro Animal Testing.   There are wide array of in vivo and in vitro studies than can be utilized when evaluating the safety of dietary supplement ingredients, food, and food additives. These tests are usually classified as either toxicology or safety pharmacology studies. Animal model studies are often useful in predicting adverse events and/or toxicity of dietary supplements, food, or food additives. Animal studies serve as important signal generators, and in some cases may even stand alone as indicators of reasonable risk. In general, evidence of harm from the ingredient in animals is an important indicator of a possible safety risk for humans. Testing can include acute toxicity, subchronic toxicity, chronic toxicity, genetic toxicity, carcinogenicity, reproductive and developmental toxicity, neurotoxicity, and immunotoxicity. Details on specific testing requirements and protocol designs for these various studies can be found in other chapters in this book.

Acute toxicity tests (see Chapter 6) are usually conducted for all dietary supplement and food ingredients. There are numerous procedures that can be utilized for acute testing, including the up-and-down procedure, the acute toxic class method, and the fixed-dose procedure, which in general are the three most popular for dietary supplement and food ingredients. Acute toxicity testing is useful in developing a safe dosing plan for the ingredient and establishing its effect on human physiology if the ingredient were to be accidentally dosed above the recommended dosage (25). In addition, the results of such a study may be utilized to classify and label substances according to their toxicity, help design subsequent longer duration studies, and assess health risk to humans.

In most, if not all safety analyses, subacute/subchronic toxicity studies (see Chapter 7) are either required or recommended, depending on the ingredient. Required testing is usually between 14 to 28 days in duration and conducted in two species (25).

Chronic studies (see Chapter 7), if needed, are also usually 6 to 12 months in duration and conducted in two species. A majority of food ingredients, including additives, and contact substances, are subject to the long-term toxicity studies, due to the extreme importance of assessing long-term safety.

Genetic toxicity tests (see Chapter 8) are recommended for food ingredients in which the cumulative estimated dietary intake per person exceeds 1.5µg, which is equivalent to 0.5 parts per billion (ppb) in the total diet. These types of tests directly measure potential gene mutation and/or chromosomal effects.

Carcinogenicity studies (see Chapter 9) are often conducted on FCS; however, they may be done on other ingredients, in particular food additives, if results of genetic toxicity testing warrant it.

Both reproductive and developmental toxicity studies (see Chapter 11) are extremely important to assess any adverse effects of the ingredient on the reproductive system or fetal development. In general, some FCS with a higher exposure rate and potentially some food additives either require or recommend both of these studies.

Neurotoxicity testing (see Chapter 12) differs from all of the aforementioned testing methods and procedures. The approach to neurotoxicity testing generally follows a tiered approach, which allows for multiple decision points that can eliminate further testing (25). Due to the impact that nervous system toxicity can have on human health, assessing the neurotoxic potential of a chemical proposed for use as a food ingredient should be an essential element in that ingredient's toxicological profile (27).

The FDA suggests immunotoxicity testing (see Chapter 13) for some FCS and food additives, however not on a majority of them unless previous in vitro tests affirm the need for them (24).

In addition to the 'standard' toxicity testing described above, there is a wide range of in vitro assays that can be utilized to gain additional knowledge regarding the potential risk of adverse events of specific compounds. However, these assays are rarely used as stand-alone tests for regulatory purposes. In terms of dietary supplements, in vitro tests are helpful in predicting which dietary supplement ingredients may contribute to supplement-drug interactions. There are numerous assays that can be utilized to assess enzymes, receptors, tissues, or other biological end points that may provide useful information in the context of other data (Table 2) (2). The type of test often depends on the ingredient being tested, its potential use, and its proposed mechanism of action.

Table 2 Examples of Useful In Vitro Assays for Evaluating the Safety of Dietary Supplements

Useful in vitro assays	
Apoptosis induction	Histaminergic effects
ATP synthesis inhibition	Hormone receptor binding studies
Cell cycle effects	Immunosuppressant effects
Cell proliferation effects	Mitochondrial respiration inhibition
Cell transformation effects	Mitogenic effects
Cholinergic effects	Parasympatholytic and parasympatho-
Cholinesterase inhibition or induction	mimetic effects
Cytolytic effects	Pharmacokinetic alterations
Cytotoxic effects	Phototoxicity effects
Detoxification enzyme inhibition or induction	Prooxidation effects
DNA damage	Sympatholytic/sympathomimetic effects
Epstein–Barr virus activation	

Abbreviation: ATP, adenosine triphosphate.
Source: Proposed framework for evaluating the safety of dietary supplements, Institute of Medicine, 2002.

Postmarketing Surveillance

As previously noted, the manufacturers of dietary supplements and food products are responsible for ensuring the safety of their product and the ingredients that compose it. In addition, it is the responsibility of the FDA to demonstrate proof of safety or lack there of in reference to these products. Conversely, the manufacturer is responsible for demonstrating the safety or lack there of in the case of food additives. In addition to the FDA, food product safety is also controlled by many other organizations including; the U.S. Department of Agriculture, Centers for Disease Control, Cooperative State Research, Education, and Extension Service, and many more. In terms of FDA's postmarketing role in the dietary supplement industry, an issue arises when a dietary supplement is thought to be "unsafe" to the consumer. Under DSHEA, once the product is marketed the FDA has the responsibility of showing that a product is "unsafe" before it can take any action to restrict the product's use or even remove the product from the market.

INTERNATIONAL REGULATIONS

In Europe, the regulation of foods, dietary supplements, and cosmetics is similar to that of the United States With respect to dietary supplements, the European Union (EU) directive must be followed. This means that as of August 1, 2005, manufacturers, distributors, and retailers of food supplements must not sell or manufacturer supplements unless all of the ingredients have been listed in Annexes I and II of the directive (28). In terms of cosmetics, it is the responsibility of the manufacturer or the person placing the product on the market to be able to demonstrate that the product is safe for the consumer. This safety evaluation should be based on the safety of the individual ingredients and more specifically on their toxicological profile, chemical structure, and the anticipated level of exposure (29).

The Japanese regulations differ from both the EU and U.S. systems, particularly with regards to classification of cosmetics, and dietary supplements. In Japan, most dietary supplements fall into the herbal category, which is considered Kampo medicine. In general, Kampo drugs are formulas which on average contain about 5–10 different herbs (30). About 147 Kampo drugs are considered formulae and are registered by the Ministry of Health and Wellness (MHW) as ethical drugs. These Kampo drugs are regulated in the same manner as "Western drugs." This means that approval must be filed and depending on the length or treatment, and the various indications time-consuming expensive toxicology testing may have to be completed. In general, the tests required generally look for mutagenicity, carcinogenicity, and teratogenicity. Kampo drugs are also a part of a three system postmarketing system (30). The three parts of the postmarketing system are an adverse drug reaction monitoring system for hospitals, a pharmacy monitoring system, and an adverse reaction reporting from manufacturers. Similarly, cosmetics are also regulated by the MHW. Under the Pharmaceutical Affairs Law, the manufacturer or importer is required to submit complete formulations before a license to manufacturer or import the product can be granted (31). Postmarket monitoring of licensed cosmetic containing a new ingredient is regulated by the MHW on a case-by-case basis. It is important to note that there is a class of cosmetic that are called quasi-drugs. Included in quasi-drugs are medicated cosmetics, body deodorants, antiperspirants, mouthwashes, talcum powders, hair dyes, special bath preparations, and various hair products. The licensing process of this category is slightly different and takes a minimum of 6 months (31).

FUTURE TRENDS

The low level of "required" safety testing in this industry gives both the consumer and manufacturer tremendous responsibility and legal liability in determining the safety of their cosmetics, dietary supplements, and food products. Each year there are numerous reports of "unsafe" products or questions regarding products not subjected to as rigorous safety testing as other similar products on the market. In addition, the safety testing of some products can also lead to the identification of other safety hazards that may have previously gone unnoticed or newly arisen. For example, Bovine Spongiform Encephalopathy, more commonly referred to as mad cow disease, is not only a concern for food products but also more recently also for cosmetics and dietary supplements that contain bovine-derived ingredients. Another problem that safety testing usually fails to confirm is interactions between ingredients and/or products. A prime example of this is supplement–supplement interactions or supplement–drug interactions, which at times can be fatal. If such occurrences become common, the likelihood of new legislation or new testing regulations for these products increases.

REFERENCES

1. Schechtman LM. The safety assessment process- setting the scene: an FDA perspective. ILAR J 2002; 43:S5–S10.
2. Institute of Medicine National Research Council. Proposed Framework for Evaluating the Safety of Dietary Supplements, 2002.
3. Accessed September, 2004, at http://www.fda.gov/oc/history/historyoffda/section2.html.
4. Accessed September, 2004, at http://vm.cfsan.fda.gov/ ~ lrd/foodaddi.html.
5. Food and Drug Administration. Substances generally recognized as safe; proposed rule. Fed Regist 1997; 62:18937–189364.
6. Accessed September, 2004, at http://www.fda.gov/opacom/laws/dshea.html.
7. Accessed September, 2004, at http://www.fda.gov/cder/guidance/105–115.htm.
8. Accessed September, 2004, at http://www.cfsan.fda.gov/ ~ dms/opa-tg1.html.
9. Accessed September, 2004, at http://www.cfsan.fda.gov/ ~ dms/cos-regn.html.
10. Accessed September, 2004, at http://www.cfsan.fda.gov/ ~ dms/cos-206.html.
11. Accessed September, 2004, at http://www.cfsan.fda.gov/~dms/cos-205.html.
12. Liebsch M, Spielmann H. Currently available in vitro methods used in the regulatory toxicology. Toxicol Lett 2002; 127:127.
13. Spielmann H, Liebsch M, Kalweit S, et al. Results of a validation study in Germany on two in vitro alternatives to the Draize eye irritation test, the HET-CAM test and the 3T3 NRU cytotoxicity test. Altern Lab Anim 1996; 24:741.
14. Cooper KJ, Earl LK, Harbell J, Raabe H. Prediction of ocular irritancy of prototype shampoo formulations by the isolated rabbit eye (IRE) test and bovine corneal opacity and permeability (BCOP) assay. Toxicol In Vitro 2001; 15:95.
15. Djabari Z, Bauza E, Dal Farra C, Domloge N. The HET-CAM test combined with histological studies for better evaluation of active ingredient innocuity. Int J Tissue React 2002; 24:117.
16. European Commission. Test guideline B-40 skin corrosivity-in vitro method of annex V of the EU Directive 86/906/EEC for classification and labeling of hazardous chemicals. Off J Eur Comm 2002; L136:85.
17. ESAC-ECVAM Scientific Advisory Committee. Statement on the scientific validity of the rat skin transcutaneous resistance (TER) test and the EpiSkin™ test (in vitro tests for skin corrosivity. Altern Lab Anim 1998; 26:275.
18. ESAC-ECVAM Scientific Advisory Committee. Statement on the application of the EpiDerm™ human skin model for skin corrosivity testing. Altern Lab Anim 2000; 28:365.

19. Fentem JH, Archer GEB, Balls M. The ECVAM international validation study on in vitro test for skin corrosivity. 2. Results and evaluation by the management team. Toxicol In Vitro 1998; 12:483.
20. European Commission. Test guideline B-41 phototoxicity—in vitro 3T3 NRU phototoxicity test of annex V of the EU Directive 86/906/EEC for classification and labeling of hazardous chemicals. Off J Eur Comm 2000; L136:98.
21. Spielmann H, Balls M, Dupuis J, et al. A study on the UV filter chemicals from annex VII of European union directive 76/768/EEC, in the in vitro 3T3 NRU phototoxicity test. Altern Lab Anim 1998; 26:679.
22. Accessed September, 2004, at http://oacu.od.nih.gov/ARAC/iracld50.htm.
23. Accessed September, 2004, at http://www.cir-safety.org/info.shtml.
24. Accessed September, 2004, at http://www.cfsan.fda.gov/~dms/opa2pmnt.html.
25. Food and Drug Administration: Office of Food Additive Safety. Redbook 2000: Toxicological Principles for the Safety Assessment of Food Ingredients. Updated, 2004.
26. Ioannidis JP, Chew P, Lau J. Standardized retrieval of side effects data for meta-analysis of safety outcomes. A feasibility study in acute sinusitis. J Clin Epidemiol 2002; 55:619–626.
27. Leukroth RW. Predicting neurotoxicity and behavioral dysfunction from preclinical toxicologic data. Neurotoxicol Teratol 1987; 9:395–471.
28. Accessed January, 2005, at http://www.nnfa.org/services/government/pdf/Codex_EUdir.pdf.
29. Pauwels M, Rogiers V. Safety evaluation of cosmetics in the EU. Reality and challenges for the toxicologist. Toxicol Lett 2004; 151:7–17.
30. Accessed January, 2005, at http://www.who.int/medicines/library/trm/who-trm-98-1/who-trm-98-1.pdf.
31. Accessed January, 2005, at http://altweb.jhsph.edu/regulations/cosmetic-marketing.htm.

Index

Milton Keynes UK
Ingram Content Group UK Ltd.
UKHW052024071024
449327UK00027B/2420